TEXTBOOK OF PERINATAL EPIDEMIOLOGY

TEXTBOOK OF PERINATAL EPIDEMIOLOGY

EYAL SHEINER
EDITOR

Nova Science Publishers, Inc.

New York

Library of Congress Cataloging-in-Publication Data

Perinatal epidemiology / editor, Eyal Sheiner.
    p. ; cm.
  Includes bibliographical references.
  ISBN 978-1-60741-648-7 (hardcover)
  1. Fetus--Diseases--Epidemiology. 2. Pregnancy complications--Epidemiology. I. Sheiner, Eyal.
  [DNLM: 1. Pregnancy Complications--epidemiology. 2. Infant, Newborn, Diseases--epidemiology. WQ 240 P441 2009]
  RG627.P47 2009
  614.5'99232--dc22

                              2009042899

Published by Nova Science Publishers, Inc. ✦ New York

Contents

Preface

This unique book was conceived to satisfy the rising need for epidemiology oriented clinicians. While there are many books separately devoted to epidemiology, obstetrics, and perinatology, there are almost none bridging the gaps between these disciplines. This book synthesizes methodological issues in epidemiology along with the essential aspects of perinatal medicine in a straightforward accessible manner.

The first section mainly deals with epidemiological concepts: definitions of key terms, measures of disease frequency, study design and validity, measures of associations, types of statistical analyses (univariate, multivariate, decision analysis and meta-analysis) as well as practical SPSS approach to data. All these are presented by means of examples from the perinatal world.

The second section is of clinical orientation. It focuses on essential and controversial topics and includes preconceptional and early pregnancy concerns, maternal and fetal morbidities in addition to peripartum and neonatal complications. The book is concluded with timely and urging ethical issues in perinatal medicine.

Written by international experts, this sensible guide draws on methodological issues as well as evidence-based data in perinatal medicine. We aim to give a clear and comprehensive set of tools enabling a deeper understanding of perinatal epidemiology and practical research. The book is a valuable resource for a broad spectrum of clinicians and healthcare professionals dealing with perinatal medicine. Medical and nursing students as well as residents in obstetrics and pediatrics may largely benefit from it at various stages of their training.

Acknowledgment

The incentive for this book came from an invitation by Professor Ilana Shoham-Vardi, (Director, Epidemiology and Health Services Evaluation Department, Faculty of Health Sciences, Ben-Gurion University) to co-teach a course in Perinatal Epidemiology. While there are many books separately devoted to Epidemiology or Perinatology and Obstetrics, I realized, there are almost no available books that bridge these gaps, and bring together methodological aspects of Epidemiology with the essential aspects of perinatal medicine. Interestingly, while preparing this volume, I received notice from one of the authors regarding a book entitled "Perinatal Epidemiology" edited by Michael B. Bracken, that was published 25 years ago (1984) and is unfortunately out of print.

Through our strive to present a comprehensive and updated textbook, few topics were omitted. In these matters more information should be sought in specialized volumes or texts.

I thank all authors who contributed excellent chapters. It is hoped that this work does justice to their contribution.

To my family, with love
Eyal Sheiner, Be'er-Sheva, 2010

About the Editor

Eyal Sheiner, MD, PhD is a graduate of the Ben-Gurion University of the Negev, Be'er-Sheva, Israel. He is a professor of Obstetrics and Gynecology. Following his residency, he earned his doctorate in Epidemiology and Public Health. His PhD study at Rush University Medical Center (Chicago, Il) was supported by a grant from the Fulbright Visiting Scholar Program of the United States. Dr. Sheiner has published extensively in the area of perinatal epidemiology.

Section I: Concepts in Epidemiology

In: Textbook of Perinatal Epidemiology
Editor: Eyal Sheiner, pp. 7-14

ISBN: 978-1-60741-648-7
© 2010 Nova Science Publishers, Inc.

Chapter I

Introduction: Perinatal Epidemiology

*Eyal Sheiner**

What is Epidemiology?

Epidemiology, the science of epidemic, is basically the study of something that affects a population. Epidemiology deals with how disease, injury and clinical practice are distributed in populations and with the factors that influence or determine this distribution [1-3]. Many questions surround the epidemic of diseases: Who develops the disease? Where? When? How? Why did they develop the disease? [3]. Obviously, diseases are not randomly distributed in human populations, since there are several predisposing or protective characteristics (either genetic or acquired) for the disease [1]. Mostly, it seems that an interaction of genetic and environmental factors leads to the development of a disease [1]. Epidemiology also highlights the significance of disease control, i.e., measuring and identifying causes for diseases as well as interventions to improve health [3].

The specific objectives of epidemiology are to determine the following factors [1]:

1) *The cause of the disease:* e.g., human papillomavirus and cervical cancer. Infection with high-risk oncogenic HPV was found to be associated with precancerous lesions and cervical cancer [4].
2) *Prevalence*, the proportion of a population with a disease at a designated time, *and the incidence*, the rate of new cases during a period of time, *of the disease*. For example, cervical cancer is one of the most common types of cancer in women worldwide, with the highest rates observed in underdeveloped countries [4].
3) *Prognosis of the disease*

---

* For Correspondence: Eyal Sheiner, M.D, PhD, Department of Obstetrics and Gynecology, Soroka University Medical Center, P.O. Box 151, Beer-Sheva, Israel. Tel 972-8-6403551, Fax 972-8-6403294, E-mail sheiner@bgu.ac.il

4) *Effectiveness of preventive and/or therapeutic options:* e.g., advances in the understanding of the role of HPV in the etiology of high-grade cervical lesions [CIN 2/3] and cervical cancer have led to the development, evaluation and recommendation of two prophylactic HPV vaccines [4].
5) *Public policy related to disease prevention*

What is Perinatal Epidemiology?

Events during pregnancy have a direct influence on both the health of the mother and the health of the child. Indeed, during pregnancy the obstetricians are dealing with two patients: the mother and the unborn child (figure 1). Perinatal epidemiology deals with the epidemiology of the perinatal period, i.e., from 22 completed weeks of gestation to seven completed days after birth. Exposures of the mother, such as smoking and drug intake, which are carefully discussed in this book, might have direct and indirect influences on the fetus. Moreover, several types of maternal exposures might have influence late into the adolescent life of the child. Perinatal epidemiology integrates care of both mother and child and incorporates the obstetrician's concern for the parturients with the pediatrician's concern for the newborn.

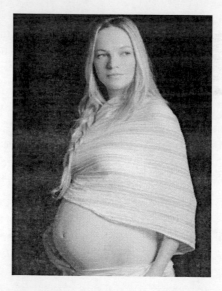

Figure 1. "…and she became pregnant and bore him a son." —Genesis 30:4–6 (by Ravit Veltman, with permission).

The improvement in perinatal health over the last decades is an impressive achievement of public health. Maternal and perinatal mortality rates have declined significantly over the years [5]. Nevertheless, statistics vary between countries. Awareness of the geographic gap in maternal mortality ratios led to the Safe Motherhood Initiative launched in 1987. The goal of this project was set at a 50–75% reduction in maternal mortality [5, 6]. Comparison of maternal mortality rates among populations must take into account different demopgraphic structures of the populations studied. Many parameters might bias this comparison, although age has the greatest influence upon mortality rates. For example, mortality rate in a low socioeconomic population may be surprisingly lower than in a high socioeconomic population only due to a much lower maternal age average in the low socioeconomic population.

Perinatal mortality (deaths) rate is regarded as one of the major health indicators that reflect achievement in health in the referring communities. Perinatal mortality is the sum of early neonatal mortalities and late fetal deaths and the denominator for perinatal mortality rate is the number of live births or live births plus fetal deaths. Most cases are attributed to prematurity (figure 2) and accordingly are associated with low birth weight (figure 3). For this reason, perinatal mortality rates reach 85% before 25 weeks of gestation, and are roughly 95% in newborns weighing less than 500 grams. On the other hand, mortality rises to 15% in fetuses with birth weights greater than 5500 grams.

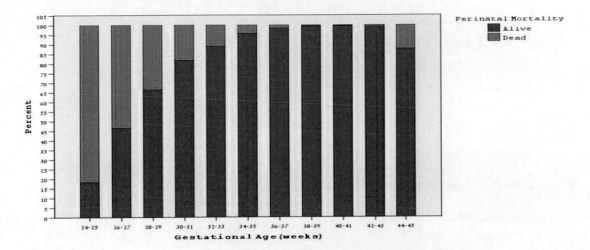

Figure 2. Perinatal mortality according to the gestational age; data from Soroka University Medical Center.

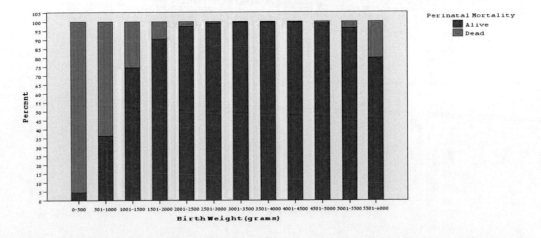

Figure 3. Perinatal mortality according to birthweight; data from Soroka University Medical Center

Medical litigation and concern regarding fetal well-being have, however, brought cesarean delivery to an epidemic (figure 4). Cesarean delivery (CD) rates have risen constantly in the last decade. Contributing factors are particular practice patterns and patient preferences, as well as the decrease in the rate of vaginal births after cesarean (VBAC) and decrease in vaginal births of breech pregnancies [7]. The steady increase in cesarean deliveries over the years is illustrated in figures 5 and 6. The rates of CD changed from an average of 10% between 1985 and 1989 to over 20% recently (figure 5). Figure 6 reflects trends for more births and more CDs over the years, and accordingly the percentage of CDs increase dramatically (total CDs in all years equals 100%).

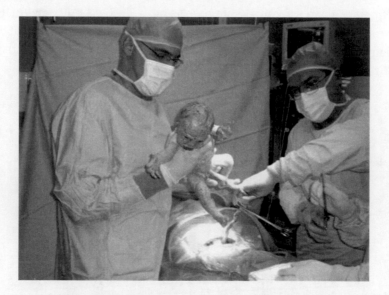

Figure 4. The final cut: The long and winding road towards parenthood sometimes ends in the operating room.

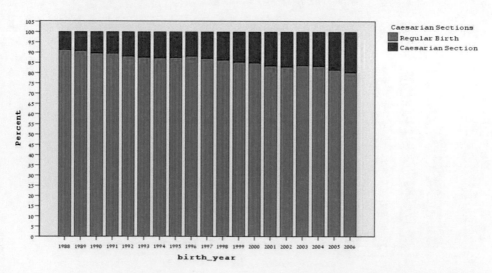

Figure 5. Cesarean section rates over the years (% for each year); data from Soroka University Medical Center.

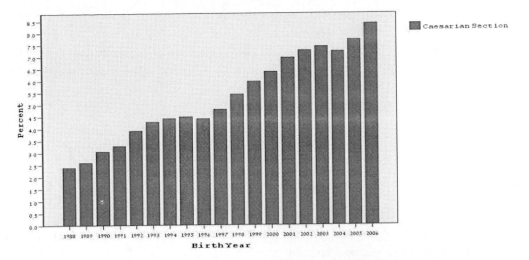

Figure 6. Distribution of all cesarean section cases over the years (% of total cesarean deliveries); data from Soroka University Medical Center.

Prevention Strategies

Epidemiologic analysis is a complex process. First, we have to determine if an association exists between exposure and disease (i.e., obesity and diabetes), and whether it is a causal association [1]. Descriptive statistics is the first step: once variables have been defined and measured, we need to draw conclusions from the data collected on these variables. Nevertheless, we must make sure that the data are valid and the differences are real. This is the time to examine potential biases, interactions and control for confounders using a multivariable analysis.

If we can identify high risk groups, we can move from observations to preventive actions and direct preventive efforts such as screening programs (i.e., Papanicolaou [Pap] smear: screening programs have significantly reduced the incidence and death rates in the Western world from cervical cancer) [8] or remove the risk factor if possible (i.e., smoking). Importantly, there are modifiable risk factors (such as obesity), but there are risk factors such as age (which can be associated with infertility, for example) that are not modifiable.

Two possible methods of prevention are a population-based approach vs. a high-risk approach [1]. It is difficult to reach a consensus regarding screening approaches since it is a matter of cost effectiveness as well. A measure that will be applied to the entire population must be inexpensive and minimally invasive [1].

Screening for gestational diabetes mellitus (GDM) is performed using the glucose challenge test (GCT). Screening recommendations range from the inclusion of all pregnant women (universal) to the exclusion of all women except those with highly specific risk factors (selective)—age: >25; obesity: BMI (body mass index) >30; ethnicity: Hispanic, Native American, Asian American, African-American; family history: first-degree relative; and previous GDM or large-for-gestational-age infant. Moreover, the cut-off value of the GCT matters as well: a value of 140 mg/dL will identify 80% of women with GDM, while a cut-off of 130 mg/dL will identify more than 80% of women with GDM (increased *sensitivity*, which measures the proportion of actual positives that are correctly identified as such, but decreased *specificity*, which measures the proportion of negatives that are correctly identified). In Israel, screening for GDM as well as the triple test (genetic screening for Down syndrome) are offered to all pregnant women.

Three types of preventions exist:

- Primary prevention: Action taken to prevent the occurrence of the disease,[1] such as folic acid for prevention of neural tube defects [9].
- Secondary prevention: Identification of a population in the pre-clinical phase of the disease, i.e., they do not yet have clinical symptoms [1]. In such cases, treatment is easier and more effective, and might prevent mortality. The effectiveness of anticoagulant therapy and thromboprophylaxis in patients with thrombophilia might serve as an example for secondary prevention.
- Tertiary prevention: Preventing complications in patients who have already developed signs and symptoms of the disease in order to prevent end-stage complications (such as renal failure in patients with type 2 diabetes with proper treatment) [1].

In this Book

Part 1: Epidemiology

The book starts with pure epidemiology and methodological issues. This part focuses on definitions, measures of disease frequency, prevalence and incidence of diseases, sensitivity and specificity of studies, and includes examples from the perinatal world. Perinatal events along the perinatal period are discussed in details. Multivariable analysis is essential to the study of perinatology. An important chapter explains what multivariable analysis is, why is it needed, what types of multivariable analyses are commonly used in perinatal research, how to understand and construct a multiple logistic regression model, how well the model predicts outcome, and whether the model is reliable.

SPSS examples provide the reader with the opportunity to repeat measurements and understand the statistical analysis. Other chapters discuss study design. While the randomized, double-blind placebo-controlled design has come to be regarded as the "gold standard" to which other designs of clinical research should be compared [10-12], it surely has limitations. A chapter dealing with RCT (randomized controlled trials) highlights the advantages, but also sounds a note of caution in the conduct and interpretation of the results of these trials. A chapter regarding decision analysis (i.e., a quantitative analysis that combines information, using a formal stepwise process, in an attempt to aid the process of decision making) follows. Decision analysis is an interesting type of study design that can provide useful insights, and is particularly helpful in circumstances in which an interventional or observational study design cannot provide the required information needed to differentiate between different tests or therapies.

Meta-analysis is a study that combines the results of several studies that address a set of related research hypotheses. Synthesis of available evidence remains essential for good clinical practice. A systematic review is a slightly different form of research that provides a summary of medical reports, using explicit methods to search, critically appraise and synthesize the published or unpublished evidence concerning a specific clinical question. Quantitative systematic review, or meta-analysis, combines different studies to produce an overall effect estimate of a specific treatment using explicit statistical techniques. The role of systematic reviews and meta-analyses has been increasingly endorsed in the practice of evidence-based decision making. The chapter provides an overview of basic and quantitative methods and issues needed to be considered for the conduct of a meta-analysis.

Part 2: Perinatal Epidemiology

The second part of the book focuses on clinical topics and includes essential chapters dealing with conditions directly affecting maternal well-being, fetal well-being and combined factors.

Critical maternal conditions and diseases that have direct effect on the fetus: These include hypertensive disorders, diabetes mellitus, thrombophilia, maternal obesity during pregnancy, preterm delivery, placental abruption and placenta previa.

Maternal exposures that might affect the fetus: These include drugs, smoking and even ultrasound.

- Maternal considerations: These include maternal mortality, fertility and abortions, ectopic pregnancies, post-partum hemorrhage and cesarean deliveries (specifically due to deliveries of breech gestations).
- Fetal issues: Perinatal mortality, twins gestation, shoulder dystocia, epidemiology of birth defects, intrauterine growth restrictions (IUGR), cerebral palsy (CP) and gender differences in perinatal medicine are discussed.

Obviously, most cases are interrelated, and categorizing them is artificial and incorrect. When the mother is jeopardized, the fetus is at risk. When the mother has uncontrolled disease, delivery even of a premature baby is sometimes the only option (as in severe preeclampsia). Maternal hypertensive disorders can result from thrombophilia and can cause IUGR. Likewise, fetal conditions such as birth defects can lead to the same entity. Even without labor induction, uncontrolled maternal disease can cause preterm delivery, which is a major risk factor for CP as well as perinatal mortality.

Studies regarding the health of the mother and fetus are well within the field of perinatal epidemiology, which has evolved into a major sub-specialty of epidemiology and an important component of perinatal medicine [13]. This book attempts to draw all relevant materials in epidemiology and perinatal medicine together to present a comprehensive appraisal of perinatal epidemiology.

Part 3: Ethics in perinatal research

At the end of the book, ethics in perinatal research is discussed: Less than optimal treatment of pregnant and fetal patients may lead to serious clinical sequelae. Clinical concerns lend urgency to the need to conduct well-designed clinical investigations of interventions with pregnant women and fetuses to improve the outcomes of perinatal medicine. Investigators in perinatal research must address and responsibly manage ethical challenges related to the protection of both the pregnant patient's and fetal patient's health-related interests. The chapter identifies the international consensus that has formed on ethics of perinatal research, focusing on research of fetal interventions and obstetric ultrasound.

References

[1] Gordis L. *Epidemiology*. Philadelphia: Saunders, Elsevier, 2009.
[2] Jekel F, James., Katz L, David., Elmore G, Joann., Wild M, Dorothea. *Epidemiology, Biostatistics, and Preventive Medicine*. Philadelphia: Saunders, Elsevier, 2007.
[3] Webb P, Bain C, Pirozzo S. *Essential Epidemiology*. Cambridge, UK: Cambridge University Press, 2005.
[4] Oaknin A, Barretina MP. Human papillomavirus vaccine and cervical cancer prevention. *Clin Transl Oncol* 2008;10:804-11.
[5] Schneid-Kofman N, Sheiner E. Frustration from not achieving the expected reduction in maternal mortality. *Arch Gynecol Obstet* 2008;277:283-4.
[6] Freedman LP, Graham WJ, Brazier E, et al. Practical lessons from global safe motherhood initiatives: time for a new focus on implementation. *Lancet* 2007;370:1383-91.
[7] Menacker F, Declercq E, Macdorman MF. Cesarean delivery: background, trends, and epidemiology. *Semin Perinatol* 2006;30:235-41.
[8] Lowy DR, Solomon D, Hildesheim A, Schiller JT, Schiffman M. Human papillomavirus infection and the primary and secondary prevention of cervical cancer. *Cancer* 2008;113:1980-93.
[9] Cordero JF, Do A, Berry RJ. Review of interventions for the prevention and control of folate and vitamin B12 deficiencies. *Food Nutr Bull* 2008;29:S188-95.
[10] Beswick AD, Rees K, West RR, et al. Improving uptake and adherence in cardiac rehabilitation: literature review. *J Adv Nurs* 2005;49:538-55.
[11] Cook NR, Cohen J, Hebert PR, Taylor JO, Hennekens CH. Implications of small reductions in diastolic blood pressure for primary prevention. *Arch Intern Med* 1995;155:701-9.
[12] Hennekens CH, Buring JE, Hebert PR. Implications of overviews of randomized trials. *Stat Med* 1987;6:397-409.
[13] Bracken B, Michael. *Perinatal Epidemiology*. Oxford: Oxford University Press, 1984.

In: Textbook of Perinatal Epidemiology
Editor: Eyal Sheiner, pp. 15-21

ISBN: 978-1-60741-648-7
© 2010 Nova Science Publishers, Inc.

Chapter II

Perinatal Events along the Perinatal Period: Measures and Definitions

Ilana Shoham-Vardi[*]

1. The Time Frames of the Perinatal and Neonatal Periods

According to latest version of the International Classification of Disease and Causes of Death (ICD-10) [1], the World Health Organization (WHO) defines the perinatal period as the time that "commences at 22 completed weeks (154 days) of gestation (the time when birth weight is normally 500 g), and ends seven completed days after birth". The last seven days of the perinatal period overlap the first week of the neonatal period, which ends at 28 completed days after birth. This overlapping period is known as the early neonatal period, while the last three weeks of the neonatal period are known as the late neonatal period.

Events occurring around conception and during the early stages of pregnancy are outside the perinatal period, which begins at the lowest threshold for fetal survival. As medical technology has progressed in the last 20 years, the threshold of fetal survival has been lowered, but current opinion holds that the threshold for survival is 23–24 weeks of gestation [2]. Differences exist between countries regarding the legal definition of the lowest limit of the perinatal period [3]. These differences affect medical practices regarding treatment of very premature infants, as well as international comparisons and assessment of time trends of perinatal statistics.

---

[*] For Correspondence: Ilana Shoham-Vardi, PhD; Associate Professor, Department of Epidemiology and Health Services Evaluation, Faculty of Health Sciences, Ben Gurion University of the Negev, Beer-Sheva, Israel; E-mail: vilana@bgu.ac.il

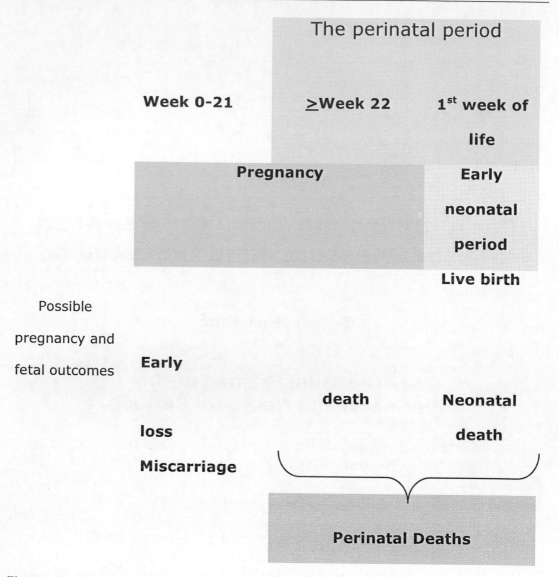

Figure 1. Gestational, perinatal and neonatal periods and outcomes of pregnancy.

The lowest limit of this time frame is set in terms of gestational age, while the upper limit is set by the newborn age, regardless of gestational age. The simultaneous use of these two time scales has recently been addressed as a methodological issue in perinatal epidemiology [4]. Thus, a live birth can, by definition (see below), occur at any time in pregnancy, while the outcome of pregnancy resulting in a non live birth is classified by WHO according to the length of gestation. Pregnancy outcomes in early pregnancy (<22 weeks of gestation) are defined as outside of the perinatal period, since such pregnancies very rarely end in a live birth. The most common outcome at that stage of pregnancy is "early pregnancy loss", which often goes unrecognized. In studies with careful monitoring by daily urine samples of women trying to conceive, it was shown that about one-third of conceptions are not carried to delivery and two-thirds of those losses occur before they are recognized [5].

2. Pregnancy Outcomes in the Perinatal Period

2.1 Definitions

- Live birth: The WHO defines a live birth as "the complete expulsion or extraction from its mother of a product of conception, irrespective of the duration of the pregnancy, which, after such separation, breathes or shows any other evidence of life, such as beating of the heart, pulsation of the umbilical cord, or definite movement of voluntary muscles, whether or not the umbilical cord has been cut or the placenta is attached; each product of such a birth is considered liveborn" [1]. In 1992, a revision to this definition was made in the United States. Two main changes were made: (1) Spontaneous fetal deaths were distinguished from induced terminations of pregnancy and excluded from fetal death statistics, and (2) a more restricted description was added to the term "signs of life": heartbeats are to be distinguished from transient cardiac contractions and respirations are to be distinguished from fleeting respiratory efforts or gasps [6].
- Fetal death: When a pregnancy over 22 weeks of gestation does not result in a live birth, the outcome of pregnancy is termed fetal death or stillbirth, defined by WHO as "death prior to the complete expulsion or extraction from its mother of a product of conception, irrespective of the duration of pregnancy; the death is indicated by the fact that after such separation the fetus does not breathe or show any other evidence of life, such as beating of the heart, pulsation of the umbilical cord, or definite movement of voluntary muscles" [1].
- Neonatal death: A death of a live-born during the first 28 completed days of life. The neonatal period is subdivided into early neonatal, the first seven days of life; and the late neonatal period, 7–28 completed days of life. Early neonatal deaths are counted as perinatal deaths.
- Perinatal death: Fetal deaths + early neonatal deaths
- Infant death: Death of a live-born infant during the first year of life, including neonatal deaths and post-neonatal deaths. Only deaths in the first week of life are counted as perinatal deaths.

2.2 Reporting Requirements

It is important to note that neither WHO definition of live birth nor those of fetal death are dependent on gestational age. The reporting requirements (and the vital statistics of these outcomes), however, are defined by gestational age and/or birth weight. WHO recommends that all fetuses and infants weighing at least 500 g at birth should be included in the statistics whether alive or dead. Fetal deaths occurring before 22 completed weeks of gestation or weighing less than 500 g are to be reported separately as *miscarriages or spontaneous abortions*. Moreover, for international comparisons, WHO sets the limit of reporting at 28 weeks gestation and/or 1000 g at birth.

2.3 International Comparison of Definitions of Perinatal Events

The US reporting requirements, which were revised in 1995, state that all spontaneous fetal deaths (to be distinguished from induced abortions) weighing 350 grams or more—or, if weight is unknown, having completed 20 weeks of gestation—should be reported as fetal deaths [6]. These requirements, however, vary among countries [3] and in the US between states [3,7]. In the National Vital Statistics Reports of the 2004 perinatal mortality data [7], two different definitions of perinatal mortality are used: Definition I (generally used for international comparisons): fetal deaths of 28 weeks of gestation or more and infant deaths under 7 days; Definition II: fetal deaths of 20 weeks of gestation or more and infant deaths under 28 days.

In Australia since 2006, the lowest limit for reporting fetal deaths was set at 20 weeks or 400 grams [8]. In the UK, the lowest limit for reporting fetal deaths is 24 completed weeks of gestation [9]. An effort has been made by members of the European Union through the Euro-Peristat project to create uniform European standards to report perinatal information. In a recent report summarizing the project [10], the lower limit for calculating perinatal mortality was set at 28 weeks of gestation.

2.4 Measures of Perinatal Mortality

There are several measures of perinatal mortality that are commonly used in vital statistics. Table 1 shows how the measures are calculated in terms of numerator and denominators. All measures are usually expressed per 1000 either live births or total births (including live births + fetal deaths), usually in a year, in a defined population.

Table 1. Commonly used measures of perinatal mortality.

Measure	Numerator	Denominator	10^x
Fetal death ratio	Fetal deaths	Live births	1000
Fetal death rate	Fetal deaths	Total births (live births+fetal deaths)	1000
Early neonatal mortality rate	Early neonatal deaths	Live births	1000
Perinatal mortality rate	Fetal deaths + Early neonatal deaths	Total births (live births + fetal deaths)	1000

3. Definitions of Gestational Periods

The period of gestation is traditionally divided into three periods: preterm, term and post-term. Table 2 shows the WHO definitions of these periods.

Table 2. Division of the gestational period according to WHO definition.

Pre-term	Before 37 completed weeks (less than 259 days) of gestation
Term	Completed 37 weeks –up to 41 weeks (259–293 days) of gestation
Post-term	42 completed weeks or more (294 days or more) of gestation

Crucial to these definitions is the timing of conception and estimating the length of time between conception and any event during pregnancy, i.e., determining gestational age. According to the WHO definition, the duration of gestation is measured from the first day of the last normal menstrual period, which is counted as day zero. Gestational age is expressed in completed days or completed weeks; thus, week 1 of gestation begins on day 7 (after completion of gestational week zero), and is completed on day 13. When information on last menstrual period is unavailable or unreliable, gestational age is determined by other means. The most widely-used method in developed countries is an ultrasound assessment during the first 20 weeks of pregnancy, when the inter-pregnancy variance in fetal size is negligible.

Several studies compared pregnancy dating in cohorts of pregnant women whose pregnancy was assessed by reliable information about last menstrual period (LMP) and by ultrasound during the first 20 weeks of gestation. Systematic differences were noted between the two most common methods of dating [11]. Ultrasound dating, which is based on comparing fetal measurements to standard fetal week-specific growth distributions, tends to slightly underestimate the gestational age of small fetuses, resulting in overestimate of preterm births, especially in population groups with smaller fetuses [12]. A recent study, however, has shown that rates of both preterm and post-term estimates were higher if dating was LMP-based in comparison to ultrasound-based dating [13]. LMP vs. ultrasound estimates were, respectively, 8.7% vs. 7.9% preterm (<37 weeks), 81.2% vs. 91.0% term (37–41 weeks), and 10.1% vs. 1.1% post-term (≥42 weeks). Studies based on artificial reproductive technologies-conceived pregnancies provide a unique opportunity to study the quality of dating methods, as the date of conception is not based on recall of LMP but rather on the actual date of fertilization. A study done on such a cohort revealed that inaccuracies in data entry are another source of error causing misclassification of gestational age [14]. Errors in gestational age estimates were also noted in a study done on a large cohort in Sweden [15]. Such errors, if likely to occur in specific populations more than in other populations, may bias our estimates of differences among population groups and trends in preterm births [16].

4. Definitions of Birth Weights

Birth weight is the first weight of the fetus or newborn obtained after birth. Table 3 presents the division of the gestational period according to WHO definitions. The definitions of "low", "very low" and "extremely low" birth weight overlap (i.e., "low" includes "very low" and "extremely low", while "very low" includes "extremely low").

Table 3. Classification of birth weight according to WHO definition.

Low birth weight	Less than 2500 grams (up to and including 2499 grams)
Very low birth weight	Less than 1500 grams (up to and including 1499 grams)
Extremely low birth weight	Less than 1000 grams (up to and including 999 grams)

References

[1]   http://www.icd10.ch/ebook/FRetENetGe_OMSetDIMDI_FR/ICD10_Volume_2_Par_ 5.7.1.asp

[2]   Pignotti MS, Donzelli G. Perinatal care at the threshold of viability: an international comparison of practical guidelines for the treatment of extremely preterm births. *Pediatrics.* 2008; 121(1):e193-8.

[3]   Nguyen RHN, Wilcox AJ Terms in reproductive and perinatal epidemiology: II, Perinatal terms. 2005; *J Epidemiology Community Health* 59:9196-921

[4]   Joseph KS. Incidence based measures of birth, growth restriction, and death can free perinatal epidemiology from erroneous concepts of risk. *J Clinical Epidemiol* 2004; 57:889-897

[5]   Wang X, Chen C, Wang L, Chen D, Guang W, French J. Conception, early pregnancy loss, and time to clinical pregnancy: a population-based prospective study. *Fertil Steril.* 2003;79:577-84.

[6]   *National Center for Health Statistics.* Model state vital statistics act and model state vital statistics regulations. Washington: Public Health Service. 1995

[7]   MacDorman MF, Munson ML, Kirmeyer S. Fetal and perinatal mortality, United States, 2004. *Natl Vital Stat Rep.* 2007;56:1-19.

[8]   http://www.health.nsw.gov.au/policies/pd/2006/PD2006_006.html

[9]   *Office for National Statistics. Mortality Statistics:* Childhood, infant and perinatal. Review of the national Statistician on death in England and Wales, 2006 (Series DH3. no 39)

[10] *European Perinatal Health Report. 2008.* http://www.europeristat.com/publications/ european-perinatal-health-report.shtml

[11] 11.Lynch CD, Zhang J.The research implications of the selection of a gestational age estimation method. *Paediatr Perinat Epidemiol.* 2007;21 Suppl 2:86-96.

[12] Yang H, Kramer MS, Platt RW, Blondel B, Bréart G, Morin I, Wilkins R, Usher R.How does early ultrasound scan estimation of gestational age lead to higher rates of preterm birth? *Am J Obstet Gynecol.* 2002 ;186:433-7.

[13] Dietz PM, England LJ, Callaghan WM, Pearl M, Wier ML, Kharrazi M. A comparison of LMP-based and ultrasound-based estimates of gestational age using linked California livebirth and prenatal screening records. *Paediatr Perinat Epidemiol.* 2007;21 Suppl 2:62-71.

[14] Callaghan WM, Schieve LA, Dietz PM.Gestational age estimates from singleton births conceived using assisted reproductive technology. *Paediatr Perinat Epidemiol.* 2007;21 Suppl 2:79-85.

[15] Haglund B:Birthweight distributions by gestational age: comparison of LMP-based and ultrasound-based estimates of gestational age using data from the Swedish Birth Registry. *Paediatr Perinat Epidemiol.* 2007 ;21 Suppl 2:72-8.

[16] Qin C, Dietz PM, England LJ, Martin JA, Callaghan WM.Effects of different data-editing methods on trends in race-specific preterm delivery rates, United States, 1990-2002. *Paediatr Perinat Epidemiol.* 2007;21 Suppl 2:41-9.

In: Textbook of Perinatal Epidemiology
Editor: Eyal Sheiner, pp. 23-32

ISBN: 978-1-60741-648-7
© 2010 Nova Science Publishers, Inc.

Chapter III

Observational Study Design in Perinatal Epidemiology

Ilana Shoham-Vardi[*]

Definitions

- Cohort: A group of people who share a common characteristic within a defined period.
- Cohort study: A comparison of incidence of a defined clinical outcome in exposed and unexposed persons.
- Case-control study: A comparison of prevalence of exposure in persons with a defined disease or clinical condition (cases) with prevalence of exposure in persons without the disease or condition (controls).

Introduction

Epidemiological studies are designed to test hypotheses regarding the etiology of disease by studying the patterns and strength of associations between exposures and defined health outcomes, and to provide the most valid estimate of this association. Perinatal epidemiology is mainly focused on the examination of exposures that are hypothesized to affect perinatal outcomes. There is, however, a growing body of research that focuses on perinatal events and fetal environment as exposures that affect health outcomes later in life [1,2]. This chapter will review the most common study designs used in observational perinatal epidemiology.

[*] For Correspondence: Ilana Shoham-Vardi, PhD; Associate Professor, Department of Epidemiology and Health Services Evaluation, Faculty of Health Sciences, Ben Gurion University of the Negev, Beer-Sheva, Israel; E-mail: vilana@bgu.ac.il

Cohort Studies

Cohort studies compare incidence of a defined clinical outcome in exposed and unexposed persons. Study participants are assessed at baseline to determine (1) their eligibility status according to predefined inclusion and exclusion criteria and (2) their exposure status to hypothesized risk factor(s). Disease occurrence is monitored and incidence rates are computed for the exposed and unexposed groups and compared. The most common measures of association in cohort studies are risk ratios or relative risks.

Relative risk

Incidence in exposed / Incidence in non-exposed

Cohort studies can be either prospective or retrospective (see below), but in all cohort studies the measure of disease occurrence is incidence: i.e., the new occurrence of disease in persons free of disease at the time exposure is assessed.

Table 1. Cohort Studies Design.

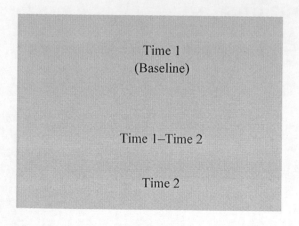

Time 1
(Baseline)

1. Determining participation eligibility (inclusion/exclusion criteria)

2. Measure of exposure to hypothesized risk factor/s (exposed/unexposed)

Time 1–Time 2

Follow-up period

Time 2

Measure of disease occurrence

Prospective cohort studies: In this type of study, the researcher defines a cohort in which incidence of disease is to be assessed. After the cohort has been defined by meeting eligibility criteria, exposure status of all cohort members is measured and participants are classified into exposed and unexposed. After the baseline assessment, the researcher actually follows in real time the disease experience of exposed and unexposed study participants and determines the incidence of disease at some defined point of time in the future.

One of the most problematic issues in conducting prospective cohort studies is the length of time between the assessment of exposure status and the occurrence of disease. The EPIC study [3], for example, is a large multi-center study designed to investigate the relation between diet, nutritional and metabolic characteristics, various lifestyle factors and the risk of cancer. It is expected to conduct lifetime follow-up on about 400,000 middle-aged participants. In perinatal epidemiology, where the variable of interest often is the outcome of pregnancy, the follow-up period is relatively short, allowing studies of the effects of prenatal exposures and pregnancy outcomes to be designed as prospective cohort studies. In a study conducted in Sweden, 866,188 women with singleton pregnancy were followed from the first antenatal visit to delivery. The study showed that mothers with chronic hypertension had an increased risk of perinatal mortality of their male, but not of their female, offspring [4]. Another example is a study showing an association between elevated free fatty acids measured at 30 weeks of pregnancy and the risk for preterm delivery [5], or a study conducted in Denmark on large cohort of pregnant women showing that level of high stress assessed at week 30 is associated with an increased risk for stillbirth [6]. In all of these studies, the length of follow-up needed was relatively short.

Studies of "time to pregnancy" aiming at detection of factors associated with the likelihood of conception and carrying a pregnancy to delivery are usually conducted as prospective cohort studies. A cohort of 443 women with pelvic inflammatory disease (PID) was followed up for 84 months to assess rates of pregnancy and recurrence of disease. Exposure was defined as the highest tertile level of antibody titers to chlamydia measured in the final follow-up year. The investigators concluded that the level of antibodies to *C. trachomatis* was associated with reduced likelihood of pregnancy and elevated risk of recurrent PID [7].

As the interest in the fetal origin of adult disease has been growing in recent years, several large-scale prospective cohort studies have been carried out to test hypotheses regarding the risks associated with various fetal environments and perinatal events. The Generation R Study is a study based on a cohort of 9,778 mothers in the Netherlands designed to assess characteristics and events in fetal life and early postnatal life that impact growth, development and health status in childhood and young adulthood [8]. The Jerusalem Perinatal Study has been following a population-based cohort of 80,936 offspring born in Jerusalem between 1964 and 1976. This study has demonstrated, among other findings, that birth weight is inversely associated with the risk of mortality in male adults age 15+ [9]. About 55,000 pregnancies resulting in live births comprised the cohort in the Collaborative Perinatal Project, which was originally designed to study the causes of neurological defects. Children were actively followed until age 7–8 years. A recent report has suggested an increased risk of childhood cancers in children with a documented birthmark, as compared with children with no birthmarks [10].

Retrospective cohort studies: Cohort studies can be conducted in a retrospective way when information about exposure had been collected for an entire cohort in the past. The researcher can use this information at a later point when all or some incident events had already occurred. These studies depend on valid documentation of the exposure of interest in the past; thus, they can be carried out in a relatively short time, as the period between exposure and disease occurrence had already elapsed at the time the study is carried out.

This study design is frequently used in perinatal epidemiology where prenatal information is routinely collected and documented in a uniform way for large cohorts of women. Availability of this kind of information allows testing new hypotheses about risk factors and incidence of disease without starting a new cohort study. It is especially useful when rare exposures are studied. A retrospective cohort study was conducted to examine the association between gestational weight gain and perinatal outcomes in women with gestational diabetes mellitus [11]. The cohort comprised all women (n=31,074) participating in a program for women with gestational diabetes in California between 2001 and 2004. Information about gestational weight gain was available for all program participants, and was retrieved from medical records after all study participants had already given birth. The study found that women who had gestational weight gain above the Institute of Medicine (IOM) guidelines had a higher risk of undesirable outcomes including preterm delivery, having macrosomic neonates, and cesarean delivery, while women who gained weight below IOM recommendations were more likely to have small-for-gestational-age neonates.

A large number of studies were conducted in Soroka University Medical Center (SUMC), Beer Sheva, Israel, which is the only tertiary hospital serving the entire population of Southern Israel (about 13,000 birth annually), and where prenatal information is available for population-based nonselective cohorts of births. Most women in the area attend maternal and child clinics for prenatal care. Thus, prenatal information is available to almost all women and is part of the computerized database of all birth records. Such a setting allows for the study of rather rare exposures, such as deep venous thrombosis [12] and Familial Mediterranean Fever during pregnancy [13], both of which were found to be associated with risk for preterm births.

Retrospective cohort studies can be conducted by linking databases such as the Swedish Conscript Study, where birth information from the Swedish Birth Register was individually linked to the Swedish Conscript Register, resulting in a cohort of 168,068 males. This study revealed that males born small for gestational age were at increased risk of subnormal intellectual performance compared to males born with adequate weight for gestational age [14].

Comparison of prospective and retrospective cohort studies: Cohort studies examine the effect of exposure on incidence of disease. The difference between these two types of studies is the way information becomes available to the researcher, but not in the way information had originally been collected. In both types of studies, exposure information is recorded before disease occurrence. Prospective cohort studies are also called concurrent cohort studies, as the follow-up is conducted in real time, while in retrospective cohort studies, also called historical cohort studies, the follow-up period had been completed at the time the study was initiated. Sometimes retrospective studies are the first stage in a multistage study and are continued with an active prospective follow-up for an additional period of time for studying participants who had not developed the disease at the time the retrospective study had been performed.

Case-Control Studies

When the disease of interest is rare, a cohort study might not be an efficient study design, as it requires following large number of people for long periods of time. In case-control studies, we compare persons with a defined disease or clinical condition (cases), and persons without the disease or condition (controls). We then measure retrospectively past exposures, which are hypothesized to be related to the disease. Our hypothesis is that exposures which are risk factors for the disease will be more prevalent among cases than among controls.

Since exposure information is collected retrospectively, after the disease status is known, the evidence of an association between exposure and disease is considered to be weaker than that obtained form cohort studies. Since in case-control studies we cannot measure incidence, relative risks or risk ratios cannot be computed. The most common measure of association used in case-control studies is Exposure Odds Ratio (the ratio of exposure odds in cases relative to odds of exposure in controls).

	DISEASE STUATUS	
EXPOSURE	CASES	CONTROLS
Present	a	c
Absent	b	d
Total	a+b	c+d

Odds of Exposure among cases: a / (a+b) : b/ (a+b) = a / b

Odds of Exposure among controls: c / (c+d) : d/ (c+d) = c / d

Exposure Odds Ratio

$$(a / b) : (c / d) = (a \times d) / (b \times c)$$

It can be shown that case-control studies that are properly conducted, i.e., the cases are representative of persons with the disease and controls of persons without the disease, and we study a rare disease, the exposure odds ratio (OR) is a good estimate of the relative risk, which would have been obtained from a cohort study.

The main advantages of case-control studies is that they are usually smaller and can be conducted in a relatively shorter time and consequently require less resources than cohort studies. However, case-control studies, more than cohort studies, are considered to be prone to selection and information biases (see Chapter 6). In perinatal epidemiology, case-control studies are usually conducted when a rare clinical condition is investigated. For example, a national case-control study was conducted in France to assess the role of ethnicity and nationality in maternal mortality, which is a very rare occurrence in France [15]. The study comprised a total of 267 cases of maternal deaths from 1996 to 2001 and a representative sample (n = 13,186) of women who gave birth in 1998 as controls. The study found that women from sub-Saharan Africa and women from Asia, North and South America were more likely to die postpartum than women born in France (odds ratios were 5.5 and 3.3, respectively).

The choice of appropriate controls is the major challenge in case-control studies. Controls should be chosen from the same population that gave rise to the cases. For example, if cases were identified through prenatal clinics, controls should be chosen from women attending the same clinics but without the condition ; if cases were identified at birth, controls should also be identified at birth at the same hospitals, etc. Case-control studies often choose more than one control per case. This is done to increase the statistical power of the study. There are case-control studies that use different control groups which allow controlling for different confounders, or to test a hypothesis under different conditions. A population-based case-control study is being conducted in Hungary to study risk factors for birth defects. In a recently published study, all cases (n=111) of isolated congenital cataract were compared to 111 matched controls without the defect to 37,837 population controls without any defects and to 22,744 malformed controls with other nonocular abnormalities [16].

Matched case-control studies: In order to make case-control studies more efficient, controls are sometimes not randomly chosen from the non-diseased population but are chosen to match cases in one or more characteristics. The matching factors are usually known risk factors that have already been shown to be associated with the disease. Matching such factor(s) reduces the variability in the study population, but creates a situation in which controls are not a representative sample of all non-diseased persons, and this needs to be accounted for when conclusions are drawn from a matched case-control study. The decision to use matching in choosing controls should be made after consideration of the advantages and disadvantages of matching in each particular study.

In a recently published case-control study of vascular dysfunction and cardiovascular risk factors in mothers of growth-restricted offspring, cases were 28 women with infants born at term below the 5th percentile of weight for gestational age and controls were 29 mothers of term infants born at the 25th–90th percentile of weight for gestational age [17]. Controls were matched to cases by age at index pregnancy, parity, body mass index and gestational age at booking prenatal care, and gestational age at delivery. Cases were found to have significantly higher proportions of perturbation of metabolic and vascular function than controls 3–4 years after the index birth. In the latter study, intensive and expensive testing was done that would not be feasible in a larger study. Matching helped to reduce the number of participants needed for the analysis, as many possible confounders were eliminated. While matching can make a study more efficient, it can introduce a selection bias if any of the matching factors is too closely associated with the exposure of interest; this is called "over-matching", and may cause an underestimation of a true difference between cases and controls. For example, if one of the cardiovascular risk factors studied were too closely associated with parity, which was one of the matching factors, the difference observed in the study between cases and controls might be smaller than that in the target population because the controls that were chosen through the matching process were too similar to the cases.

Controls can be individually matched to cases, i.e., each case will have its matched control/s (individual matching), or the control group can be chosen in such a way that the frequency distribution of the matching factors is similar in both study groups. When individual matching is employed, procedures appropriate for non-independent samples statistical analysis should be used.

Special designs of case-control studies in perinatal epidemiology: The most frequently special design case-controls studies used in perinatal epidemiology, are the "nested case-control" design and the "case cohort" designs [18].

Nested Case-Control studies: In these case-control studies, the two study groups are drawn from a large cohort study when a sufficient number of cases have occurred. Controls are drawn from the rest, non-diseased cohort members. A nested case-control study was conducted in Sweden to investigate prenatal, perinatal and neonatal risk factors for neuroblastoma [19]. Cases (n=245) were identified through the Swedish Cancer Register. The list was linked with the Swedish Medical Birth Register, and five living controls per case were randomly selected from the birth registry, matched by gender and age. The researchers concluded that neuroblastoma in infancy, but not with diagnoses at one year or older, are associated with some markers of prenatal, perinatal and neonatal distress. In this study, information about exposure was obtained from available medical records. In other nested case-control studies, this design is used when information regarding exposure is unavailable and needs to be collected for both cases and controls. Drawing the cases and controls from a large representative cohort may reduce the potential selection bias, which is often an issue in case-control studies.

Case Cohort Design : When cases are drawn from an ongoing cohort, controls can be drawn from the "risk set", i.e., all of the population at risk at the time a case is identified. The concept of "risk set" is illustrated in Figure 1.

Risk set 1

	W28	W29	Risk set 1 W30	W31	W32	Risk set 2 W33	W34	W35	Risk set 3 W36	W37	W38	W39	W40
A	0	0	0	0	0	X							
B	0	0	0	0	0	0	0	0	0	0	0	0	0
C	0	0	X										
D	0	0	0	0	0	0	0	0	0	0	0	0	0
E	0	0	0	0	0	0	0	0	X				
F	0	0	0	0	0	0	0	0	0	0	0	0	0
G	0	0	0	0	0	0	0	0	0	0	0	0	0
H	0	0	0	0	0	0	0	0	0	0	0	0	0

Stillbirth X	Ongoing Pregnancy 0

Figure 1. A Hypothetical Case Cohort Study of Stillbirth

In this cohort of eight pregnancies (A–H) that were followed from week 28 to week 40, three cases of stillbirth occurred. During week 30, when the first stillbirth (C) occurred, all other pregnancies were undelivered. The risk set at week 30 comprised all eight pregnancies, of which pregnancy C was the case and all the rest served as controls. Note that pregnancies A and E, which later became cases, served as controls for case C. The risk set for the second stillbirth included only seven pregnancies, of which A became a case, while C was not included in the risk set, as at that time it was no longer at risk. Pregnancy E, however, was included in the risk set. At the time stillbirth E occurred, the risk set included only six pregnancies, of which E was the case and the other five pregnancies (B, D, F, G and H) served as controls. In a regular case-control study, only the latter five pregnancies would have served as controls.

This methodology has been used in perinatal epidemiology, as it allows for optimal utilization of exposure information. In a study investigating risk factors for stillbirth, cases were identified through perinatal databases in Nova Scotia and Eastern Ontario, Canada

1991–2001 [20]. Exposure information was measured retrospectively from a sample of cases and controls. To account for differing lengths of gestation at the time of stillbirth, survival analysis approach was used, comparing cases to a comparison group (risk set) which included an original control group and a random sample of pregnancies which became cases in a later gestational week.

Cross-Sectional Studies

In cross-sectional studies, exposure and outcomes are assessed at the same time. This study design provides a low level of evidence because the temporal direction cannot be determined. The cross-sectional approach is used in population surveys, which provide important information on prevalence of risk factors in sub groups of the population. This information enables the identification of populations at risk. Information obtained from large monitoring of ongoing surveys such as the National Health Interview Survey (NHIS) [21], Behavioral Risk Factor Surveillance System (BRFSS) [22], Pregnancy Risk Assessment Monitoring System (PRAMS) [23] in the US and the Peristat survey in Europe [24] serve as the basis for initiation and evaluation of significant public health interventions.

Ecological Studies

Ecological studies are based on comparing disease occurrence or prevalence in units of populations (countries, neighborhoods, towns, geographic areas, etc.) that are characterized by some exposure that is hypothesized to affect the likelihood of disease. Unlike all other study designs discussed so far, in ecological studies we do not study individuals but units of population; thus, neither disease status nor exposure status are determined at the individual level. This type of study is used for generating hypotheses and to evaluate community interventions. An ecological study design was recently used to evaluate a national public health intervention in Brazil [25]. The findings from this study, which compared infant mortality rates in municipalities with varying degrees of exposure to the public health intervention, demonstrated an inverse association between infant mortality rates and level of coverage of the national intervention program.

Comparing the use and Strength of Evidence of Different Study Designs in Observational Perinatal Epidemiology

Four major categories of observational study designs were described: cohort, case-control, cross-sectional and ecological studies. Cohort studies provide the strongest type of evidence, as it follows the natural process from exposure to disease occurrence. Cohort studies are especially useful in perinatal epidemiology, as follow-up time in many studies is relatively short. The main difficulty with cohort studies is that they might lengthy, if conducted prospectively , and costly if large number of persons are to be followed. Cohort studies, relative to other observational study designs, are less prone to biases, as exposure status is determined before disease status is known. The main threat to validity in cohort studies is selection bias, which may be caused by selective participation in the study and/or selective drop from follow-up.

Case-control studies require fewer resources, as they are conducted on relatively small samples and for short periods of time. They are particularly efficient in the study of rare outcomes, but are more prone to both selection and information bias. If properly conducted, they can provide a valid estimate of association between exposure and disease. In contrast to cohort and case-control studies, cross-sectional and ecological studies cannot provide etiological evidence, but are very useful in providing population-based data on the prevalence of a variety of exposures and clinical conditions, and as a basis for evaluating interventions and changes at the population level.

References

[1] Gardiner HM.Early environmental influences on vascular development. *Early Hum Dev*. 2007 Dec;83(12):819-23.

[2] Kajantie E. Fetal origins of stress-related adult disease. *Ann N Y Acad Sci*. 2006 Nov;1083:11-27.

[3] Riboli E, Kaaks R. The EPIC Project: rationale and study design. European Prospective Investigation into Cancer and Nutrition. *Int J Epidemiol*. 1997;26 Suppl 1:S6-14.

[4] Zetterström K, Lindeberg SN, Haglund B, Hanson U. The association of maternal chronic hypertension with perinatal death in male and female offspring: a record linkage study of 866,188 women. *BJOG*. 2008 Oct;115(11):1436-42.

[5] Chen X, Scholl TO. Association of elevated free fatty acids during late pregnancy with preterm delivery. *Obstet Gynecol*. 2008 Aug;112(2 Pt 1):297-303.

[6] Wisborg K, Barklin A, Hedegaard M, Henriksen TB Psychological stress during pregnancy and stillbirth: prospective study. *BJOG*. 2008 Jun;115(7):882-5.

[7] Ness RB, Soper DE, Richter HE, Randall H, Peipert JF, Nelson DB, Schubeck D, McNeeley SG, Trout W, Bass DC, Hutchison K, Kip K, Brunham RC. Chlamydia antibodies, chlamydia heat shock protein, and adverse sequelae after pelvic inflammatory disease: the PID Evaluation and Clinical Health (PEACH). *Study. Sex Transm Dis*. 2008 Feb;35(2):129-35.

[8] Jaddoe VW, van Duijn CM, van der Heijden AJ, Mackenbach JP, Moll HA, Steegers EA, Tiemeier H, Uitterlinden AG, Verhulst FC, Hofman A. The Generation R Study: design and cohort update until the age of 4 years. *Eur J Epidemiol*. 2008 Dec 20.

[9] Friedlander Y, Paltiel O, Deutsch L, Knaanie A, Massalha S, Tiram E, Harlap S. Birthweight and relationship with infant, child and adult mortality in the Jerusalem perinatal study. *Paediatr Perinat Epidemiol*. 2003 Oct;17(4):398-406.

[10] Johnson KJ, Spector LG, Klebanoff MA, Ross JA. Childhood cancer and birthmarks in the Collaborative Perinatal Project. *Pediatrics*. 2007 May;119(5):e1088-93.

[11] Cheng YW, Chung JH, Kurbisch-Block I, Inturrisi M, Shafer S, Caughey AB. Gestational weight gain and gestational diabetes mellitus: perinatal outcomes. *Obstet Gynecol.* 2008 Nov;112(5):1015-22.

[12] Ben-Joseph R, Levy A, Wiznitzer A, Holcberg G, Mazor M, Sheiner E. Pregnancy outcome of patients following deep venous thrombosis. *Matern Fetal Neonatal Med.* 2008 Dec 16:1-5.

[13] Ofir D, Levy A, Wiznitzer A, Mazor M, Sheiner E. Familial Mediterranean fever during pregnancy: An independent risk factor for preterm delivery. *Eur J Obstet Gynecol Reprod Biol.* 2008 Dec;141(2):115-8.

[14] Lundgren EM, Cnattingius S, Jonsson B, Tuvemo T. Birth characteristics and different dimensions of intellectual performance in young males: a nationwide population-based study. *Acta Paediatr.* 2003 Oct;92(10):1138-43.

[15] Philibert M, Deneux-Tharaux C, Bouvier-Colle MH. Can excess maternal mortality among women of foreign nationality be explained by suboptimal obstetric care? *BJOG.* 2008 Oct;115(11):1411-8.

[16] Vogt G, Puhó E, Czeizel AE. Population-based case-control study of isolated congenital cataract. *Birth Defects Res A Clin Mol Teratol.* 2005 Dec;73(12):997-1005.

[17] Kanagalingam MG, Nelson SM, Freeman DJ, Ferrell WR, Cherry L, Lowe GD, Greer IA, Sattar N. Vascular dysfunction and alteration of novel and classic cardiovascular risk factors in mothers of growth restricted offspring. *Atherosclerosis.* 2008 Oct 14.

[18] Szklow M. & Nieto FJ. (2007) *Epidemiology Beyond the Basics*, 2nd Edition. Sudbury MA, Jones and Bartlett Publishers.

[19] Bluhm E, McNeil DE, Cnattingius S, Gridley G, El Ghormli L, Fraumeni JF Jr. Int J Cancer. 2008 Dec 15;123(12):2885-90. Prenatal and perinatal risk factors for neuroblastoma. *Int J Cancer.* 2008 Dec 15;123(12):2885-90.

[20] Dodds L, King WD, Fell DB, Armson BA, Allen A, Nimrod C. Stillbirth risk factors according to timing of exposure. *Ann Epidemiol.* 2006 Aug;16(8):607-13.

[21] www.cdc.gov/nchs/nhis

[22] *http://www.cdc.gov/BRFSS/*

[23] *http://www.cdc.gov/prams/*

[24] *http://www.europeristat.com/*

[25] Aquino R, de Oliveira NF, Barreto ML. Impact of the family health program on infant mortality in Brazilian municipalities. *Am J Public Health.* 2009 Jan;99(1):87-93

In: Textbook of Perinatal Epidemiology
Editor: Eyal Sheiner, pp. 33-40

ISBN: 978-1-60741-648-7
© 2010 Nova Science Publishers, Inc.

Chapter IV

Randomized, Double-Blind, Placebo Controlled Trials: Are they really the "Gold" Standard ?

Anthony Odibo[*]

Definitions

- Randomized controlled trials (RCT): Studies investigating efficacy or effectiveness of treatment, involving random allocation of different interventions (treatments or conditions) to patients, ensuring that known and unknown confounders are evenly distributed between treatment groups.
- Double-blind trial: The researcher and the patients do not know whether the treatment is a drug rather a placebo (or new vs. old drug). Double-blind trials tend to give accurate results since the researcher cannot possibly consult the patient, directly or otherwise, and cannot give in to patient pressure to give him the new treatment.

Introduction

Clinical research, including those in perinatology, attempt to mimic the laboratory model of research design by employing rigorous methods to reduce the introduction of bias and confounding into the final outcome. The randomized, double-blind placebo-controlled design has come to be regarded as the "gold-standard" to which other designs of clinical research

[*] For Correspondence: Anthony Odibo, MD, MSCE, Division of Maternal Fetal Medicine, Department of Obstetrics and Gynecology., Washington University in St Louis, 4990 Children's Place, St Louis MO, 63110, odiboa@wudosis.wustl.edu

should be compared.[1] This chapter highlights the advantages of the randomized controlled trial (RCT) compared with other study designs, but also sounds a note of caution in the conduct and interpretation of the results of these trials and begs the question that they may not always represent the "gold-standard".

An Overview of Randomized-Controlled Trials

When properly conducted, a RCT provide the most reliable basis for evaluating the efficacy and safety of new treatments. They provide the most convincing demonstration of causality. The main reason for randomization is to avoid bias due to imbalance of known and unknown confounders between the groups being studied.[2] Typical examples of study designs using the RCT approach include: comparing a new drug vs placebo; new combinations of drugs vs single drug; new surgical procedure or device.

A detailed discussion of RCT is beyond the scope of this chapter, however, a brief description of the process will be provided as a backdrop for the limitations to be highlighted later on.

In designing a RCT, the primary end point is crucial. The end-point must be well-defined, reproducible, clinically relevant and easily achievable.[2] The sample size consideration for the study is usually driven by the chosen end-point. Typical end-points can be continuous or ordinal data, may involve the use of rates of events or time-to event considerations. When the primary clinical outcome may involve a very long period to conduct or if very expensive, it is not uncommon to use surrogate markers that may provide quicker results.

When using surrogate markers certain principles must be considered. An ideal surrogate marker should be reproducible, easily measured, occur at a stage that is earlier than the main clinical outcome of interest, and of course related to the clinical outcome. The surrogate outcome should be amenable to treatment in trials involving therapy. Examples of surrogate markers or end-points include: the use of CD4 counts or viral load as indicators of response to HIV therapy, low density lipoproteins (LDL) as surrogates for cardiac events in studies involving heart disease or tumor size as a measure of response to chemotherapy.

There are other important practical issues that need to be addressed at the planning phase of a RCT. These include choosing the proper control groups; deciding on the method of randomization such as the use of coin flip, random table numbers or computer generated random numbers; the appropriateness of blinding and method of blinding including placebo or sham surgery; the number of study arms which is most commonly a two-arm study, but some may employ a cross-over design using an appropriate wash-out period. Finally, the study planning committee needs to decide what they actually want to accomplish with the study. Do they want to prove that a new therapy is superior or equally efficient compared with an established therapy? The sample size consideration can be influenced by such decisions of equivalence/non-inferiority versus superiority designs.[2]

The overall strengths of RCT is that they are the best design for evaluating a causal relationship in a study and for controlling bias and that they can be used to measure multiple outcomes. The RCT design however can be expensive, may encounter certain ethical hurdles that make their conduct difficult and there may be issues with compliance depending on the group to which subjects are randomized and whether their underlying medical condition is apparently improving or worsening. The strengths and weakness of RCT are depicted in Table 1. There are certain biases that can result from poor conduct of RCT including detection or classification bias, co-interventions and contaminations. This chapter will assume that the RCT is well conducted but highlight the possible systematic errors that could occur in an ideal RCT.

Table 1. The strengths and weaknesses of randomized controlled trials.

Strengths	Weaknesses
Best design for evaluating causal relationship	Ethical issues with randomization
Can control bias	Expensive to conduct
Can measure multiple outcomes	Issues with compliance

The Discrepancy Debate

The implied objectivity of a double-blind RCT is the differential outcomes that it can detect when compared with other research designs.[3] It had always been assumed that other study designs tend to overestimate treatment effects when compared with the RCT.[4] This discrepancy in treatment effects between RCTs and other research designs has been termed the "masking bias" and is generally accepted as evidence of the objectivity of blinded RCTs.[5]

In the report of the first study that introduced the term "double-blind" to clinicians, Gold and colleagues also introduced the "discrepancy debate" using the pilot study of the cardiac drug Khellin.[6,7] The pilot study of Khellin involved 19 patients and demonstrated dramatic improvement in cardiac indices compared with placebo. A larger double-blind study involving 39 patients showed no benefit in the use of the cardiac drug compared with placebo.[7] In short, most of the early studies establishing the objectivity of RCT proved that the more rigorous and stringent the methodology, the less efficacious the therapy and reinforced the belief that less rigorous methods produced higher estimates in favor of therapy.[8-13]

However, recently conducted systematic reviews of study designs have compounded the discrepancy debate in that they confirm that poor methodology in other study designs could bias results but in either direction of over-estimating or under-estimating the treatment effect when compared with RCT.[14-17] These systematic reviews resulted in a modified proposition of the discrepancy argument and Kuntz and Oxman now propose the RCT as the "best protection against the unpredictability of bias".[14]

Can the Process of RCT Result in Significant Bias?

In clinical research, we are dealing with conscious beings and some form of uncertainty could cloud even the most rigorous scientific process. The proponents of the discrepancy debate assume that deficiencies such as selection and measurement bias are responsible for the differences seen between RCT and other research designs. However, even the ideal experimental conditions can have unpredictable influence on clinical outcomes.

The set up for most RCTs are not the same as those in regular clinical settings and this can on its own result in biased results.[18,19] The participants in RCTs can also exhibit similar unconscious responses that distort the results as we see with other study designs. The knowledge that the subjects have a chance of receiving either a placebo or the actual therapy introduces uncertain perceptions in the patient enough to decrease the response of either the placebo or the medication.

The preferences of the patients are taken away by the RCT process and could result in confusion, demoralization and even poor compliance, all of which may influence the study results. These have been termed "resentful demoralization" and "voluntary submission" by certain authors.[20, 21] There is also the potential that post-randomization processes such as increased vigilance may result in increased drug effect or decreased placebo effect or vice versa.[22] Some of these factors may distort the underlying statistical assumption that the "placebo effect" in the treatment arm is similar to that in the placebo arm.[23]

The Possibility of a "Masking Bias" in Rcts

The ideal method of testing the "gold-standard" and verify the validity of the masked RCT study is to design a study where both the patients and the dispensing physicians are unaware that they are involved in a blind RCT. This has been termed the "platinum standard" by Kaptchuk.[3] Such a study may however, be impossible due to ethical barriers. As an alternative certain studies using some form of "deception" to evaluate the possibility of masking bias have been performed.[6, 24]

In one study, 30 matched hospitalized patients with insomnia were randomized to a double-blind RCT. One group of patients were informed they were in a RCT comparing place to a hypnotic drug ("benzodiazepine") while the other matched group were not informed of being in a study. Eventually, both groups received a single dose of a placebo. The control group that were unaware of being in a study reported a higher hypnotic effect compared with the first group.[24] In another study involving cancer patients receiving naproxen versus placebo, who were randomly chosen to be informed of being in a RCT or not, the "placebo" was significantly more effective in the informed group than naproxen in the uninformed group! [25] These two studies were performed in France before informed consent became mandatory.

Although the result of the insomnia and the pain studies above were opposite, the second study proved that awareness of being in a masked RCT compared with uninformed involvement in RCT produce disproportionate effects on the placebo and active drug. This would also suggest that a significant difference in the placebo response of the treatment arm versus the placebo arm unlike the traditional statistical assumption.

There are many other examples in the literature that confirm that for many active drugs that can be distinguished by the subject if they know what to expect, complete concealment can dramatically change the pharmacological effects.[26-29]

It must be emphasized that these effects of "deception" or concealments described above mainly concern short term effects and may not apply to RCTs evaluating long-term outcomes.[3]

Other Sources of Bias in Rcts

While patients are randomized in RCTs, in most cases, the investigators are not. It is a known fact that most researchers are different from the typical clinician and studies have shown that different researchers have different abilities to elicit placebo effect on subjects.[18] In one study, it was shown that with the same placebo, two different researchers either consistently increased or consistently decreased patient's gastric secretion! [30] The above has been described as "investigator self-selection" bias. Different styles of health care provision can result in measurable differences in outcomes and such effects have been confirmed in studies where the physician was made an independent variable.[31, 32] One suggestion for addressing this effect is to have a "physician run-in phase in RCTs to eliminate the influence of practitioners on the integrity of RCTs.[33]

The psychosocial literature have several examples that demonstrate that the process of negotiating therapy between patients and their physicians affects not only compliance but also hard outcomes such as survival.[34, 35] The process of randomization in RCTs removes such patients' preferences and could introduce a type of "preference bias". Such influences are more typical in studies involving un-blinded studies involving behavioral changes such as dieting and exercise.[36]

Other human influences can creep in and influence the outcomes of RCTs. It is common knowledge that the typical patient that consent to participate in a RCT, is usually different from the average patient. Many eligible subjects may decline participation and his can potentially bias the trial results. One study showed that the typical patients that consent to studies involving therapy are less affluent and less educated while the opposite is the case for typical consenters to prevention trials.[37] Such "consent" or "non-consent" bias may result in different outcomes in RCT when compared with typical clinical scenarios. The above examples of bias in RCTs are highlighted in Table 2.

Table 2. Potential factors resulting in bias in a well conducted randomized controlled trial.

Experimental conditions of RCT are not similar to typical clinical scenarios

Patients preference and "resentful demoralization"

Post-randomization influences on the "placebo effect"

Investigator "self-selection" bias

"Consent" versus "non-consenting" bias: subjects in RCT are atypical patients

Examples from Perinatal Literature

Due to practical and ethical difficulties with blinding during pregnancy, some of the examples above are not easily demonstrated in the perinatal literature. There are however, some indirect, but unproven evidence that can be examined.

The trial by Meis et al on behalf of the MFMU network, concluded that 17-hydroxy progesterone can prevent preterm birth in the treatment group. While it does not detract from the positive effect of therapy in the treatment group, the preterm delivery rate of 54.5% in the control group was much higher than would be expected.[38] The unanswered question is whether the placebo had additional detrimental effect in addition to the prior history of preterm birth in both groups.

Another consideration from the perinatal literature is in regard to studies comparing treatments for prevention of preterm birth such as cerclage to bed rest.[39,40] The assumption is that bed rest is not an intervention and therefore is comparable to a placebo. However, there are no trials out there comparing bed rest to routine activities for prevention of preterm birth that we are aware of. This may really be an example of poor choice of a control group rather than an inherent bias in RCT.

Conclusion

This chapter has highlighted the limitations of RCT, but it must be emphasized that RCTs are still the closest approximation to laboratory experiments. It has been demonstrated that blinded and un-blinded RCTs can introduce inherent sources of bias. The main aim of this chapter is to bring the attention of researchers to these potential sources of bias in the conduct and interpretation of RCTs. A secondary aim is to propose that when a well designed RCT is impossible, findings from properly conducted cohort studies should not be underestimated.

References

[1] Hennekens CH, Buring JE, Hebert PR. Implications of overviews of randomized trials. *Stat Med*. 1987;6(3):397-409.

[2] Rothman KJ, Greenland S: Matching. In Rothman KJ, Greenland S. Modern Epidemiology, 2nd edition. Philadelphia: *Lippincott Williams and Williams*; p147-161.

[3] Kaptchuk TJ. The double-blind, randomized, placebo-controlled trial: Gold standard or golden calf? *J Clin Epid* 2001; 54: 541-549.

[4] Sibbald B, Roland M. Why are randomized controlled trials important?. *Br Med J.* 1998; 316:201–202.

[5] Schulz KF, Chalmers I, Hayes RJ and D.G. Altman, Empirical evidence of bias. Dimensions of methodological quality associated with estimates of treatment effects in controlled trials. *J Am Med Assoc*. 1995; 273: 408–412

[6]   Kaptchuk TJ. Intentional ignorance: a history of blind assessment and placebo controls. *Bull Hist Med*. 1998; 72:389–433.

[7]   Greiner T, Gold H, Cattell M, Travell J, Bakst H, Rinzler SH, Benjamin ZH, Warshaw LJ, Bobb AL, Kwit NT, Modell W, Rothendler HH, Messeloff CR, Kramer ML. A method for the evaluation of the effects of drugs on cardiac pain in patients with angina on effort. A study of Khellin (Visammin). *Am J Med*. 1950; 9:143–155.

[8]   Foulds GA. Clinical research in psychiatry. *J Ment Sci*.1958; 104:259–265.

[9]   Glick BS, Margolis R. A study of the influence of experimental design on clinical outcome in drug research. *Am J Psychol*. 1962; 118:1087–1096.

[10] Astin A, Ross S, Glutamic acid and human intelligence. *Psychol Bull*. 1960; 57: 429–434

[11] Wechsler H, Grosser GH, Greenblatt M. Research evaluating antidepressant medications on hospitalized mental patients: a survey of published reports during a five-year period. *J Nerve Ment Dis*. 1965; 141:231–239.

[12] Grace ND, Muench H, Chalmer TC. The present status of shunts for portal hypertension in cirrhosis. *Gastroenterology*. 1996; 50: 684–691.

[13] O'Brien WM. Indomethacin: a survey of clinical trials. *Clin Pharm Ther*. 1967; 9: 94–107.

[14] Kunz R, Oxman AD. The unpredictability paradox: review of empirical comparisons of randomized and non-randomized clinical trials. *Br Med J*. 1998; 317:1185–1190.

[15] Recurrent Miscarriage Immunotherapy Trialists Group. Worldwide collaborative observational study and meta-analysis on allogenic leukocyte immunotherapy for recurrent spontaneous abortion. *Am J Reprod Immunol*. 1994; 32:55–72.

[16] Miller JN, Colditz GA, Mosteller F. How study design affects outcomes in comparisons of therapy. II: surgical. *Stat Med*. 1989; 8:455–466.

[17] Ottenbacher K. Impact of random assignment on study outcome: an empirical examination. *Control Clin Trials*. 1992;13:50–61

[18] Black N. Why we need observational studies to evaluate the effectiveness of health care. *Br Med J*. 1996; 312:1215–1218.

[19] McPherson K. The best and the enemy of the good: randomised controlled trials, uncertainty, and assessing the role of patient choice in medical decision making. *J Epidemiol Comm Health*. 1994; 48: 6–15

[20] Torgerson DJ, Sibbald B. What is a patient preference trial? *Br Med J*. 1998; 316: 360.

[21] Silverman WA, Altman DG. Patients' preferences and randomized trials. *Lancet*. 1996; 347:171–174.

[22] Kempthorne O. Why randomize? *J Stat Plan Inf*. 1977; 1:1–25.

[23] Kaptchuk TJ. Powerful placebo: the dark side of the randomized controlled trial. *Lancet*.1998; 351:1722–1725.

[24] Dahan R, Caulin C, Figea L, Kanis JA, Cauline R, Segrestaa JM. Does informed consent influence therapeutic outcome? A clinical trial of the hypnotic activity of placebo in patients admitted to hospital. *Br Med J*. 1986; 293:363–364.

[25] Bergmann JF, Chassany O, Gandiol J, Deblois P, Kanis JA, Segrestaa JM, Caulin C, Dahan R. A randomized clinical trial of the effect of informed consent on the analgesic

activity of placebo and naproxen in cancer pain. *Clin Trials Meta-Anal.* 1994; 29: 41–47.

[26] Kirsch I, Weixel LJ. Double-blind versus deceptive administration of a placebo. *Behav Neurosci.* 1988; 2:319–323.

[27] Hughes JR, Gulliver SB, Amori G, Mireault GC, Fenwsick JF. Effect of instructions and nicotine on smoking cessation, withdrawal symptoms and self-administration of nicotine gum. *Psychopharmacology.* 1989;99:486–491.

[28] Kirsch I, Rosadino MJ. Do double-blind studies with informed consent yield externally valid results?. *Psychopharmacology.* 1993;110:437–442

[29] Dinnerstein AJ, Lowenthal M, Blitz B. The interaction of drugs with placebos in the control of pain and anxiety. *Perspect Biol Med.* 1966;10:103–114.

[30] Wolf S. Part IV. Placebos: problems and pitfalls. *Clin Pharmacol Ther.* 1962; 3: 254–257.

[31] LeBaron S, Reyher J, Stack JM. Paternalistic vs. egalitarian physician styles: the treatment of patients in crisis. *J Fam Med.* 1985; 21:56–62.

[32] Sarles H, Camatte R, Sahel J. A study of the variations in the response regarding duodenal ulcer when treated with placebo by different investigators. *Digestion.* 1977;16:289–292.

[33] Shapiro AK, Shapiro E. The powerful placebo: from ancient priest to modern physician, *The Johns Hopkins University Press*, Baltimore (1997).

[34] Horwitz RI, Viscolli CM, Berkman L, Donaldson RM, Horwitz SM, Murray CJ, Ransohoff DF, Sindelar J. Treatment adherence and risk of death after a myocardial infarction. *Lancet.* 1991; 336:543–545.

[35] Horwitz RI, Horwitz SM. Adherence to treatment and health outcomes. *Arch Intern Med.* 1993; 153:1863–1868.

[36] Brewin CR, Bradley C. Patient preferences and randomised clinical trials. *Br Med J.* 1989; 299: 313–315

[37] McKee M, Gritton A, Black N, McPherson K, Sanderson C, Bain C. Interpreting the evidence: choosing between randomized and non-randomized studies. *Br Med J.*1999; 319:312–315.

[38] Meis PJ, Klebanoff M, Thom E, Dombrowski MP, Sibai B, Moawad AH, Spong CY, Hauth JC, Miodovnik M, Varner MW, Leveno KJ, Caritis SN, Iams JD, Wapner RJ, Conway D, O'Sullivan MJ, Carpenter M, Mercer B, Ramin SM, Thorp JM, Peaceman AM, Gabbe S; National Institute of Child Health and Human Development Maternal-Fetal Medicine Units Network. Prevention of recurrent preterm delivery by 17 alpha-hydroxyprogesterone caproate. *N Engl J Med.* 2003;349(13):1299.

[39] Berghella V, Odibo AO, Tolosa JE.. Cerclage for prevention of preterm birth in women with a short cervix found on transvaginal ultrasound examination: a randomized trial. *Am J Obstet Gynecol.* 2004;191(4):1311-7

[40] Berghella V, Odibo AO, To MS, Rust OA, Althuisius SM. Cerclage for short cervix on ultrasonography: meta-analysis of trials using individual patient-level data. *Obstet Gynecol.* 2005;106(1):181-9.

In: Textbook of Perinatal Epidemiology
Editor: Eyal Sheiner, pp. 41-54

ISBN: 978-1-60741-648-7
© 2010 Nova Science Publishers, Inc.

Chapter V

Data Analysis

*Julia Harris and Eyal Sheiner**

From the Department of Obstetrics and Gynecology, Soroka University Medical Center, and the Faculty of Health Sciences, Ben-Gurion University of the Negev, Beer-Sheva, Israel.

Introduction

The use of clear and appropriate statistics in medical research is crucial for the generation of applicable and useful outcomes that can benefit the medical community. In order to produce such statistics, it is necessary to master the basic principles of biostatistics. It is important to understand the appropriate application of these statistics so that presented results can be unambiguous and accessible to healthcare providers internationally. Firstly, one must be comfortable with the terminology and tools that make up basic biostatistics.[1]

Variables

Variables, or measurable characteristics of a sample population, are categorized based on how they can be quantified and compared. These categorizations help to determine what type of statistics can be garnered from data as well as to illustrate to an audience what type of data was gathered regarding a certain variable. A continuous variable has numerical values that exist on an uninterrupted ordinal scale. An example is birth weight (figure 1)[2], or cervical length (figure 2)[3]. It is important to note that continuous variables are measured on a scale

* For Correspondence: Eyal Sheiner, M.D, PhD, Department of Obstetrics and Gynecology, Soroka University Medical Center, P.O Box 151, Beer-Sheva, Israel., Tel 972-8-6403551 Fax 972-8-6403294, E-mail: sheiner@bgu.ac.il

with comparable intervals. For example, a baby of 3.0 kilograms is exactly one half the weight of a baby weighing 6.0 kilograms.

Variables that are not continuous are considered discrete; the values of discrete variables are often referred to as ordinal or categorical. A discrete variable has values that are non-numerical and are not quantifiably comparable as their intervals are not equivalent. Discrete variables can be further categorized by the number of outcomes they include. For example, sex is a dichotomous variable; there are two possible outcomes for this variable within a data set. Variables are also divided into quantitative and qualitative variables based on whether they measure a countable characteristic (i.e. number of births) or a characteristic with no ordering or numerical value attached to its outcome (i.e. religion).

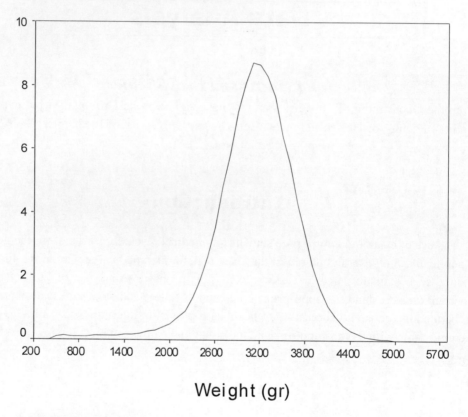

Weight (gr)

Figure 1: Birth weight distribution of 199,093 deliveries in the Soroka University Medical Center, Beer-Sheva, Israel during the years 1988-2007.[2]

The complex application of multiple characterizations of a variable can be found in a study titled *Gender Does Matter in Perinatal Medicine,*[4] where gender is used as a discrete, qualitative, dichotomous variable. This article found that the gender of a fetus (i.e. male vs. female) can be used as an indicator for increased risk of perinatal complications such as gestational diabetes mellitus, fetal macrosomia and failure to progress during the first and second stages of labor.

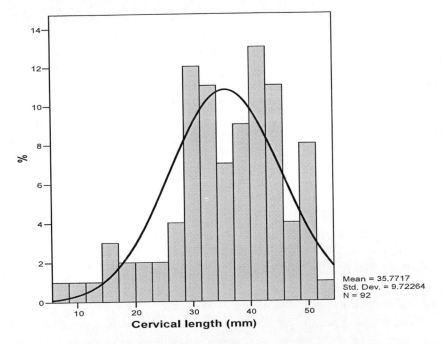

Figure 2: Cervical length in millimeters, measured by ultrasound, among 92 women with idiopathic polyhydramnios.[3]

Descriptive Statistics

Once variables have been defined and measured, the next step is to draw conclusions from the data collected. Firstly, one must describe the data using what is called descriptive statistics. These statistics serve to summarize the basic features of the sample population from which the data was obtained. The descriptive statistics that best portray the sample depend upon the types of variables collected. If the study involves continuous variables, the most important and most commonly used descriptive statistics are the mean, median and mode.

$$\bar{x} = \frac{1}{n} \sum_{i=1}^{n} x_i = \frac{1}{n}(x_1 + \cdots + x_n).$$

The mean is calculated as follows (see above): one divides the summation of the values of a given variable by n (the number of participants) for which said variable was collected. This statistic is used to express the "average," the most reflective value for a given population. Another statistic commonly employed as a representative value for a given sample population is the median. This statistic is the value which divides the data set into two; half of the values for the variable lie above the median and half lie below. If n is an even number, to obtain the median one must calculate the mean of the two values which saddle the centermost data point (the greatest value of the lower half of the data set and the least value of the upper half of the data set). Thirdly, there is a statistic called the mode. The mode is the most commonly found value for a given variable.

The best way to demonstrate the use of descriptive statistics is to observe their direct application in research. Figure 3 represents the thermal index for bones (TIB) measured during B-mode ultrasound studies.[5] TIB expresses the potential for rise in temperature at the ultrasound's focal point. In this TIB data set, the mean and mode were similar (i.e. 0.3). When a data set yields such results, called a "unimodal" distribution, the mode can be very useful. A unimodal distribution is a data set that contains a highly concentrated set of values for a single variable (figures 1,2 and 4).

Another useful descriptive statistic commonly used in medical studies is a proportion. The proportion refers to the number of observations with a certain characteristic divided by the total number of observations made; similar to a percentage. This can be a practical measure when dealing with a variable that has only integral values, such as the proportion of fatalities from uterine cancer in which metastases had occurred. In this case, the proportion would be equivalent to what is referred to as the case-fatality rate (of uterine cancer), or the number of fatalities per number of cases with the same pathology. A case fatality rate can be further qualified by non-integral, qualitative values such as the type of cancer, resulting in a complex statistic which states the proportion of a subpopulation of patients selected based on a qualitative parameter. Proportions also serve as another measure of variance; one can determine if a proportion of a specific population that contracts an illness is larger than average (by comparing to a national or international statistic) or larger than would be expected to occur by chance. These concepts will be elaborated below.

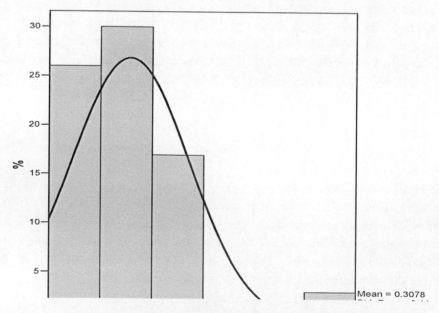

Figure 3: Distribution of TIB variations during B-mode ultrasound studies.[5]

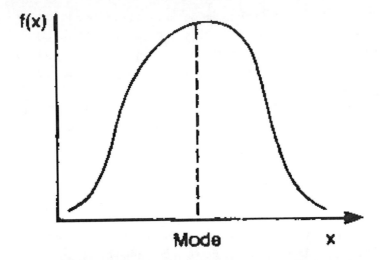

Figure 4: Normal distribution curve.

When using descriptive statistics to summarize a data set, the goal is either to show similarity within a data set or to show difference, which is referred to as variability. The mean, median and mode are measures of central tendency and thus are considered to represent similarity within a data set which can be contrasted by measures of statistical variability. The most common statistics that fall into the latter category are: standard deviation (SD), standard error (SE), interquartile range, range, variance and the coefficient of variation.

Measures of Statistical Variability

Standard deviation (SD) is the average distance that values fall from the mean. SD is calculated by summing the squared distances from the mean, dividing this sum by n or by n - 1 and taking the square root of the entire value. The value of n-1 is often used as the SD denominator because it accounts for a loss in the degrees of freedom, the number of observations that are free to vary. Every time that a calculation is done, a degree of freedom is lost in the manipulation of the data set and therefore needs to be taken into account by subtracting one from the value of n, yielding a more accurate statistic. Within samples that are normally distributed (figures 1 and 4), 68.0% of the sample will fall within one SD, 95.0% of the sample population will fall within 1.96 SDs, and 95.4% will fall within two SDs. These values can also be called confidence intervals (CIs) and are used to describe the population from which the sample is drawn.

Confidence intervals are used to make statements such as the following: with a 95% CI, it can be assumed that the mean birth weight of a population is between 3510 and 4490 grams. In this example, the mean birth weight of the sample (note: a sample is a slice taken from a larger population in the hopes of obtaining data reflective of the population which cannot be studied in its entirety) was 4000g, with an SD of 250g. Therefore, the body making this statement has 95% confidence that the stated range of values: 3510g - 4490g, should include the mean birth weight of the population based on the strength of statistical evidence. How is this conclusion made? The SD, 250g, is multiplied by 1.96 in order to give a 95% CI of 490g which is applied to either side of the mean, giving the range 3510g - 4490g. This range has a 95% chance of containing the mean birth weight of the population from which this sample was drawn.

Another value of interest, used in many statistical formulas is the variance (v). This value is obtained by squaring the SD. Variance therefore increases on an exponential scale whereas SD only increases incrementally, hence variance can be used to emphasis the variability within a data set. When the SD is divided by the square root of n, the resulting number is the standard error (SE) of the population. SE is used in many statistical tests, it can be viewed as the amount of variation contributed by each participant (see statistical tests section below for examples).

Interquartile range, another descriptive statistic of interest, is based on quartiles which are the subsections of the data set that result when it is divided into four equal sections called the first, second, third and fourth quartiles. The distance between the first and third quartiles is called the interquartile range, another measure of statistical dispersion. Range, which is incorporated into the interquartile range, is the distance between the smallest and largest values of a given data subset. The last descriptive statistic of interest is the coefficient of variation, which is the ratio of the SD to the mean.

It is important to remember that variation in a clinical study can reflect one of two concepts: errors in data/data collection, or true variation within the population. It is not easy to differentiate these two types of variation without collecting more data from the same sample population. Simply keep in mind that variation in data, just as any observation one draws from a data set, may or may not be reflective of true characteristics of the population. Repetition of results has always been heralded in all sectors of science due to the fact that results obtained can always be due to the unforeseen interference of associated factors.

Errors

Errors in data are important and can also serve as tools for the interpretation of data. Type I errors, also known as false-positives occur when a certain disease or condition is said to be found in a patient who does not have this malady. Type II errors, commonly referred to as false-negatives, occur when a patient is not diagnosed for an illness which he or she possesses (Table 1).

Table 1: Comparing the results of a test with the actual disease status.

	Disease	No Disease
Positive Test	True Positive (TP)	False Positive (FP)
Negative Test	False Negative (FN)	True Negative (TN)

Sensitivity= TP/(TP+FN); Specificity=TN/(TN+FP)

When the efficacy of a diagnostic test is evaluated it is useful to compare the sensitivity, the percent of patients who have the disease that are correctly identified, of an exam to the number of false-negative diagnoses. When a ratio is made between the false-negative error rate and sensitivity (sensitivity of a test/ false negative error rate) this value is called the likelihood ratio (LR). An LR involving the false-positive error rate also exists and is referred to as the LR+ or the positive likelihood ratio. When a diagnostic test yields an LR greater than 1, it is considered a valid exam.

When the LR- is graphed, the result is called a receiver operating characteristic curve (ROC; figure 5[6]). This curve can be used to identify an appropriate cut-off point for a diagnostic exam or to draw other conclusions that can be obtained from the relationship between sensitivity (true-positive rate) and the false-positive rate. For example, ROC analysis was employed to investigate the ability of birth weight to predict shoulder dystocia.[6,7] This study included the area under the curve (AUC) of the ROC due to its high predictive value of birth weight: AUC 0.92, 95% CI 0.90-0.93; p<0.001.[6,7]

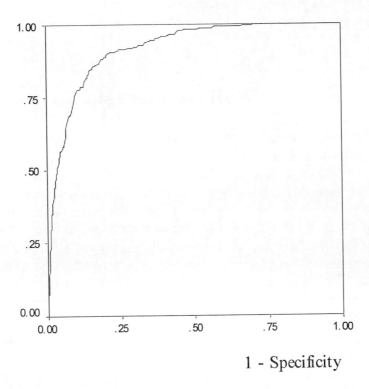

1 - Specificity

Figure 5: A receiver operating characteristic curve analysis of birth-weight in prediction of shoulder dystocia; based on analysis of 245 shoulder dystocia cases.[6]

In use of ROC to obtain cut-off points, one must graph a variety of false-positive error rates from numerous studies against the sensitivity of these exams. The point closest to the top left corner of the graph will be the most accurate cut-off point because it has the highest sensitivity and the lowest false-positive error rate of the data graphed (i.e. data coming from numerous previously conducted studies). By employing such a cut-off point, one is choosing a limited data range with a high probability of including accurately diagnosed subjects.

Distributions

The analyses thus far discussed regarding continuous quantitative variables operate on a very important assumption, that the data are normally distributed (figure 4). When a given characteristic is measured in a population it is expected that the values obtained will congregate around a given number (the mean and/or median). Additionally, it is assumed that when plotted on a continuous scale, the experimental data will have a characteristic bell shaped curve surrounding this central value. This bell-shaped curve (figures 1 and 4), called the normal distribution has been found repeatedly in many studies and its presence allows for the efficacy of the various statistical tests and measures (of continuous variable) thus far mentioned. All statistical tests which rely on a normal distribution (or more rarely on another assumption about the data) are called parametric statistical tests.

Non-parametric statistical tests do not make such assumptions. These tests are useful for ranked data or data lacking numerical indices. For the purposes of perinatal epidemiology, only four of the most common and most relevant non-parametric tests will be discussed: the Kruskal-Wallis, the Mann-Whitney U or Wilcoxon rank sum test, chi-squared tests and Mantel-Haenszel.

Null Hypothesis

After variables have been identified, but before data is collected, it is customary to present a hypothesis, an educated prediction of outcomes. For the purposes of statistics, one must present two hypotheses, a null hypothesis and an alternative hypothesis. Commonly, a null hypothesis states that a statistically significant difference will not be found between the experimental group and the control group. The alternative hypothesis is that a difference of statistical significance will be found. Once the data has been collected and statistical tests are run that evaluate the presence of a statistically significant difference between the two experimental groups, the null hypothesis is either rejected or accepted. If the null hypothesis is rejected, the alternative hypothesis is not yet proved to be true, but rather is accepted as likely due to the statistical evidence.

Statistical significance is based on the idea that an event occurred more often in a sample population than would have occurred due to chance alone. Empirically, statistical significance is based upon parameters specified prior to collection of data. Firstly, an α value must be selected. This value represents the highest rate of false-positive errors that would be acceptable in the study to be conducted. A value of 0.05 is almost always used, which means that a type I error (a false-positive) can occur less than 5% of the time. This value is more commonly referred to as the p value of the study. It is stated that when p is less than 0.05, the result obtained can be considered statistically significant. If a researcher decides to employ the use of an α value greater than 0.05, he or she should justify the decision to do so, as most statistics only acknowledge significance when p is less than 0.05.

Statistical Tests

Once a *p* value has been identified, and data has been obtained, it is possible to perform statistical tests. The most commonly used tests in medical research are t-tests and z-tests. The t-test, also known as the Student's t-test, is employed when comparing the means of two groups (most often, a control group and an experimental group). These groups are selected from a normally distributed population for which the SD is unknown and therefore must be estimated from the data which ideally should have a small sample size (relative to the population). To summarize, the t-test compares the means of two groups that come from a small sample size taken from a normally distributed population for which the SD is unknown. The z-test, on the other hand, is used when comparing proportions however; all of the conditions of the t-test apply.

Both the t-test and the z-test involve the calculation of a ratio called a critical ratio. This ratio should involve the comparison of a certain parameter within the study to the standard error (SE). In the case of z and t-tests, the parameter chosen is always the difference between two means one (as in t-tests) or two proportions (as in z-tests). One of the means or proportions is the control group, or a "standard population," that is compared to a mean or proportion from the experimental group. The following equation is used: Critical Ratio= difference between two means or proportions/SE of the difference between the two means or proportions.

Nonparametric Tests

There are many other statistical tests which can be used. However, for the purposes of perinatal epidemiology the most relevant tests outside of t-tests and z-tests are Mann-Whitney U, Kruskal-Wallis, Chi-squared tests and the Mantel-Haensze, all of which can employ the use of nonparametric data. The Mantel-Haenszel test is also known as the Cochran-Mantel-Haenszel (CMH) test, it is used to compare two groups on a binary response.

Mann-Whitney U also called Mann-Whitney-Wilcoxon is similar to the Student's t-test in that it tests whether there is significant difference between two groups of data, most commonly the control and test groups. A null hypothesis is employed that states these data are similar enough that they could have been drawn from the same group. If the data are categorical, they need to be ranked and the mean ranks of each data set are compared to determine "difference" among them. If there is a large different between the ranks of these two data sets, the null hypothesis is rejected. Additionally, a t-test using the assigned ranks as if they were numerical observations can be done to ensure the significance of the Mann-Whitney result. In a recent study, a Mann-Whitney test was used to determine if there was a significant difference in the Bishop scores of occiput posterior (OP) positioned births and non-OP positioned births.[8] The study found there was no difference; therefore, according to the definition above, the null hypothesis was accepted.

A Kruskal-Wallis test is used to compare three or more groups of ordinal data (the version of this test that employs continuous data is called ANOVA). This test, like Mann-Whitney requires that ranks are assigned to the data. In Kruskal-Wallis the ranks of each data set are summed, and the means are calculated and compared to determine if the groups differ more than could be expected by chance. In one-way ANOVA, the same procedure is carried out with numerical, continuous data; this test usually employs the use of a statistical analysis program to ensure accuracy.

Statistical Models

There are a variety of models created from mathematical equations that are used to explain data so that predictions can be made from the data and extended to the population at large. One such model incorporates the concept of null and alternative hypotheses, beginning with the statement that two variables are independent. If this statement can be sufficiently proven, the null hypothesis (no difference exists) is rejected and the alternative accepted. When utilizing this type of model, it is common to employ the use of a Chi-squared test ($\chi 2$). The Chi-square test is meant to prove the independence of two variables in a study. The model, in this case independence, provides an expected set of values. When one graphs the data values obtained in a study alongside those "expected" values based on a particular model, chi-square tests whether the data obtained fits sufficiently into the predicted model, it is a "goodness-of-fit" test. This test shows how far off the obtained values are from those values predicted using the chosen model. The outcomes measured in this case are referred to as "O" for obtained and "E" for expected values. Therefore the equation for chi-square is: $\chi 2 = \sum [\frac{(O-E)2}{E}]$. When a Chi-square value is small it means the outcomes are close to the expected, therefore the null hypothesis can be rejected and if $\chi 2$ is large, the null hypothesis will be accepted with a failure to prove independence.

An example of the use of chi square appear in an article by Eden et al. (2008) entitled: *Examining the value of electronic health records on labor and deliver*.[9] In this paper the use of an electronic health record (EHR) is tested in a labor and delivery unit. The chi square test was used to compare documentation quality before and after EHR implementation. Using the distance between O and E before and after, it was found that the chi square value was significantly reduced after the implementation of the EHR.

It has been shown that linear regression as a model of statistical analysis is also of great importance to perinatal epidemiology. Logistic regression involves the prediction of outcomes based on a set of numerous variables that may be of numerical or categorical origin. In the case of Peregrine et al.,[8] the measured outcome was mode of delivery which was predicted using the following 3 criteria variables: abdominal palpitation of spine position, ultrasonography of head position, and ultrasonography of spine position; all before labor induction. These measurements were all compiled and due to the known increase in cesarean delivery rate for each of these data, it was estimated that the 289 participants of this study would have an 80% probability of a clinically significant increase in observed cesarean delivery rate from 30% (the average rate at this time for the unit where the research was being carried out) to 45%. On an individual basis, one can calculate the probability of an outcome based on a known alteration in the probability of a measured characteristic using the formula: $\frac{1}{1+e^{-z}}$; where z, the increase in probability, is determined from prior studies. When one uses multiple variables in a logistic regression, such as the example above, it is more common to employ the use of a statistical analysis program.

An additional measure of risk, associated with statistical modeling is an odds ratio. This ratio compares of the odds (probability) of an event occurring in two different populations. If the ratio is equal to 1, the event has an equal likelihood of occurring in both populations. An odds ratio greater than one indicates an increase in the probability that the given event will occur in the first population; subsequently, when the ratio is less than one the event is more likely in the second population. The odds ratio can never be less than zero.

In a recent study, odds ratios were employed to demonstrate whether English proficiency and progesterone/estriol levels were found to be correlated with increased odds in preterm birth in acculturated Hispanic populations in the United States of America. An adjusted odds ratio of 4.03 was found for those patients proficient in English, while the lowest quartile of the progesterone/estriol ratio also yielded an increased adjusted odds ratio of 2.93. This means that those patients who spoke English well along with those with lower progesterone/estriol ratios were more likely to have preterm births than those with poorer English skills and higher hormonal ratios.

Presenting Results

Once the data have been collected and tested the next step is the presentation of results. There are a variety of ways to present results, however it is important to choose the form which represents the given data in a clear and accurate manner. For example, when one performs an ROC curve it is common to include a line graph which plots the false-positive error rate (x-axis) against sensitivity (y-axis).

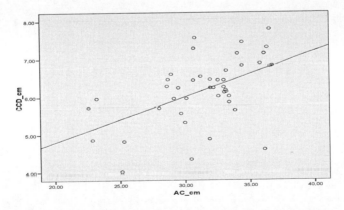

Figure 6: Correlation between the fetal cheek-to-cheek diameter (CCD) and abdominal circumference (AC).[11]

Another example of the use of a line graph that involves frequency can be found in figure 1, where the line graph shows birth weight on the x-axis and the percent (frequency) on the y-axis. This is a good way to show descriptive characteristics such as the mode and median birth weights. Figure 6 demonstrates a way to present linear correlation between two variables studied: fetal cheek-to-cheek diameter (CCD), an indicator of subcutaneous tissue mass in the fetus that can be evaluated by ultrasound, and abdominal circumference (AC). The correlation between CCD and the AC is graphically presented below in figure 6 (Pearson correlation coefficient of 0.47; P=0.01).[11]

A simple way of showing frequency of an event is a histogram (figures 2, 3, & 7). For example, one can graph the cases a disease such as idiopathic oligohydramnios, and its frequency of occurrence per month (see figure 7). [12] In this case, each month yields a bar whose height is reflective of the quantity of babies born with certain condition.[12] The most common way to display results in medical research is a chart which shows the various percentages, SDs, means or individual values obtained for various variables measured in various populations or sections of a population. This can be seen in nearly all scientific published articles.

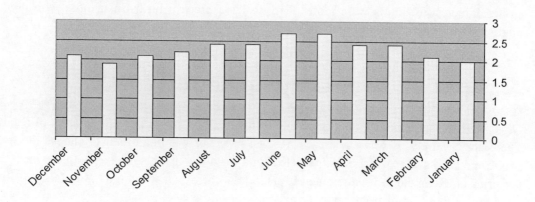

Figure 7: The distribution of cases of idiopathic oligohydramnios during the year.[12]

Sample Size Determination

The sample size, *n*, chosen in research is an essential but not sufficient characteristic to constitute a legitimate scientific study. When designing a study, there are numerous crucial components such as bias-limiting criteria and ethical protocols that contribute to the value and validity of the study. Furthermore, there are standards that must be adhered to in order to verify that the observations made were frequent enough to consider them reflective of a true scientific phenomenon. Fortunately, there are ways to ensure that one has included enough participants in a study to deem one's conclusions generalizable to the greater population.

Firstly, one must determine what it is that he or she would like to prove with a given study. In the article *Method of placental removal during cesarean delivery and postpartum complications*,[13] the authors wanted to determine if two methods of placental removal resulted in differential occurrences of postpartum complications such as wound infection and postpartum fever. In order to do so they needed to use two groups of women each exposed to a different type of placental removal. In order to determine how many women would be needed in each group, the following items needed to be considered: what difference (%) should be demonstrated in the outcomes of each groups' treatment, what type of power and what level of statistical significance (probability that results obtained are true) are desired by the researchers.

The first criteria, statistical significance is called "α" or the "p-value." This number comes from what is considered an acceptable type I error rate. Type I errors, ("error of the first kind," an α error, or a "false positive") are false conclusions of differences between two groups being compared, when none exists. This is the error of rejecting a null hypothesis when it is actually true. A type I error in the study above would have been to claim that both methods of placental removal resulted in different postpartum outcomes, when in actuality, no differences existed.

The next component that contributes to sample size is the power that one hopes to achieve in the study. This value comes from what is referred to as 1- β, or one minus the type II error rate. Type II error ("error of the second kind," a β error, or a "false negative") is the error of failing to reject a null hypothesis when it is false. This is the error of failing to observe a difference that exists between two groups. Using the study above as an example, a type II error would have resulted if there was a difference between the amount of postpartum fever and wound infection experienced by those women who received each type of placental removal, when no difference was reported in the study. If the β value (type II error rate), is the chance (probability) that a study makes a type II error, then the chance of not performing a type II error is 1-β. The third and final criteria noted above is the difference one wants to find between the two groups being compared. The sample size of a study is based on the power of the study (chance of not making a type II error), the statistical significance of the study (p-value) and difference in outcome observable between study groups.

In the study mentioned above, it was determined that a minimum of 150 women were needed in each group in order to show a difference in outcome of 15%, a probability of 95% and a power of 80%. The number referred to as "probability" here, is the chance that a type I error will not occur, therefore it is 1-α and not α, the p-value which in the case would be 0.05, the standard p-value used in most medical studies.

Once the α value, power and expected difference are known, the actual sample size number usually comes from a chart or most recently comes from an analytical computer program such as PS[14] which calculates power and sample size. One can refer to a sample size chart or a power-analysis program prior to determining the sample size, for instance in the article *Early maternal feeding following caesarean delivery: a prospective randomized study,*[15] an analytical program was used to determine how many patients would be necessary in each group in order to show a two-fold difference of patient satisfaction (a dichotomous yes/no variable) with a statistical significance of $\alpha = 0.05$ and a power of 80%. This is an example of working backwards from specific goals of power, p-value and ideal difference between groups to determine what sample size would satisfy these criteria. Alternatively, there are situations when only 80 patients are eligible for a specific study and one must use a chart or a power-analysis program in reverse to determine what maximum difference it is possible to demonstrate between groups if each group is comprised of 40 people.

References

- Jekel JF, Katz DL, Elmore JG, Wild DMG. *Epidemiology, biostatistics and preventive medicine. 3rd Edition*, Saunders Elsevier, Philadelphia, PA 2007.

- Sheiner E, Mazor-Drey E, Levy A. Asymptomatic bacteriuria during pregnancy. *J Matern Fetal Neonatal Med* 2009 May;22:423-7.

- Hershkovitz R, Sheiner E, Maymon E, Erez O, Mazor M. Cervical length assessment in women with idiopathic polyhydramnios. *Ultrasound Obstet Gynecol* 2006;4:1-4

- Sheiner E., Levy A., Katz M., Hershkovitz R., Leron E., Mazor M. Gender Does Matter in Perinatal Medicine. *Fetal Diagnosis and Therapy* 2004; 19:366-369.

- Sheiner E, Shoham-Vardi I, Pombar X, Hussy MJ, Strassner HT, Abramowicz JS. An increased thermal index can be achieved when performing Doppler studies in obstetrical ultrasound. *J Ultrasound Med* 2007;26:71-6.

- Sheiner E, Levy A, Hershokovitz R, Hallak M, Hammel R, Katz M, Mazor M. Determining factors associated with shoulder dystocia: a population-based study. *Eur J Obstet Gynecol Reprod Biol* 2006;126:11-5.

- Levy A, Sheiner E, Hammel RD, Hershkovitz H, Hallak M, Katz M, Mazor M. Shoulder dystocia: a comparison of pateints with and without diabetes. *Arch Gynecol Obstet* 2006; 273:203-6.

- Pererine E., O'Brien P., Jauniaux E. Impact on Delivery Outcome of Ultrasonographic Fetal Head Position Prior to Induction of Labor. *Obstet Gynecol* 2007; 109:618-25.

- Eden K, Messina R, Li H, Osterweil P, Henderson C, Guise J. Examining the value of electronic health records on labor and delivery. *Am J Obstet Gynecol.* 2008; 199:307.e1-9.

- Ruiz R. J., Saade G. R., Brown C. E., Nelson-Becker C., Tan A., Bishop S., Bukowski R. The effect of acculturation on progesterone/estriol ratios and preterm birth in Hispanics. *Obstet Gynecol.* 2008;111: 309-16.

- Kerrick H, Sheiner E, Mandell C, Strassner HT, Pombar X, Hussy MJ, Abramowicz JS. The fetal cheek-to-cheek diameter and abdominal circumference: are they correlated? *Arch Gynecol Obstet.* 2009;280:585-8.

- Feldman I, Friger M, Wiznitzer A, Mazor M, Holcberg G, Sheiner E. Is oligohydramnios more common during the summer season? *Arch Gynecol Obstet.* 2009;280:3-6.

- Merchavy S, Levy A, Holcberg G, Freedman EN, Sheiner E. Method of placental removal during cesarean delivery and postpartum complications. *Int J Gynaecol Obstet.* 2007;98:232-6.

- Dupont WD, Plummer WD: 'Power and Sample Size Calculations: A Review and Computer Program', Controlled Clinical Trials 1990; 11:116-28.

- Bar G, Sheiner E, Lezerovizt A, Lazer T, Hallak M. Early maternal feeding following caesarean delivery: a prospective randomised study. *Acta Obstet Gynecol Scand.* 2008;87:68-71.

In: Textbook of Perinatal Epidemiology
Editor: Eyal Sheiner, pp. 55-66

ISBN: 978-1-60741-648-7
© 2010 Nova Science Publishers, Inc.

Chapter VI

Interpretation of Research Findings

Ilana Shoham-Vardi[*]

Introduction

Epidemiological studies are designed to assess the association of an exposure and a disease or a clinical condition. Our aim in study design is to obtain the most valid and precise estimate of this association. In interpretation of the data, we are concerned about the extent to which the observed association in our study truly represents the association in the target population, as in most cases we study samples and not entire populations, and even when we do study entire populations we are concerned about whether the findings in this particular population can be generalized to other populations or even to the same population at a different point in time. Our first concern is the likelihood of having made a mistake when deciding to either reject (Type I error) or accept the null hypothesis (Type II error). We use a statistical test to address this concern. This chapter will address further issues of interpretation of research findings. These concerns cannot be left to the stage of data analysis, but should guide the study design at the initial planning stage. All studies have strengths and limitations and researchers should be aware of them when interpreting the study's results . This chapter addresses the issue of validity and the challenges facing the researcher in achieving validity. The readers should be reminded that this chapter is an overview of these rather complex issues as they relate to perinatal research. For a more in-depth discussion, readers are referred to comprehensive epidemiological methods texts such as Rothman [1], Szklow [2] and Kelsey [3].

[*] For Correspondence: Ilana Shoham-Vardi, PhD; Associate Professor, Department of Epidemiology and Health Services Evaluation, Faculty of Health Sciences, Ben Gurion University of the Negev, Beer-Sheva, Israel; E-mail: vilana@bgu.ac.il

Validity

- *Definition:* The extent to which our tool/instrument/method of measurement actually measures what we intend to measure.

In order to assess validity, we have to decide what is our "gold standard" – i.e the measure which gives us the result that is closest to the truth—in relation to which we will determine how good is the measurement we use in our study.

When our measurement is used to assess the presence or absence of a clinical condition or an exposure and we have a "gold standard", we use the terms *sensitivity* and *specificity* to assess the quality of our measurement:

- *Sensitivity:* The probability that a clinical condition is correctly assessed as "positive" by our measurement tool.
- *Specificity:* The probability that the absence of a clinical condition is correctly assessed as "negative" by our measurement tool.
- *Positive predictive value (PPV):* The probability that a case assessed as "positive" actually has the condition

The concepts of sensitivity, specificity and positive predictive value (PPV) are of particular importance in the context of screening tests, such as prenatal screening for birth defects. The most prevalent prenatal screening test is for Down syndrome. A definitive diagnosis can only be made on the basis of amniocentesis or chorionic villi sampling (CVS). Since these are costly and invasive procedures associated with a certain risk of procedure-related miscarriage, various screening protocols are used to screen and identify women at high risk for Down syndrome and to offer them a diagnostic test. Such screening programs are effective if false positive and false negative rates are low.

In a prospective cohort study of 4373 pregnancies of women who underwent an ultrasound screening for Down syndrome between 16 and 22 weeks of gestation, the validity of two markers of fetal aneuploidy were evaluated: absent or small nasal bone (NB) and increased nuchal fold (NF) (>5 mm and >6 mm). Absent NB was seen in 14/49 cases of Down syndrome for which the NB evaluation was available and NF of >6 mm was seen in 6 of 50 cases (12%) with Down syndrome [4].

Table 1.

Marker	Down Syndrome		
	Yes	No	
Positive (nuchal fold >5 mm)	6 (TP)	40 (FP)	46
Negative (nuchal fold ≤5 mm)	44 (FN)	4283 (TN)	4327
Total	50	4323	4373

Using NF > 5 mm as a cutoff point for a positive screen, six cases out of 50 pregnancies were true positives (TP), while 44 cases of Down syndrome were missed and therefore classified as false negatives (FN). A total of 46 cases had nuchal fold >5 mm, but 40 of those were seen in infants without Down syndrome, thus classified as false positives (FP). Most cases (n= 4283) were truly classified as negative (TN).

We can now calculate the probability that a case of Down syndrome will be detected by our test (Nuchal fold >5 mm), i.e., the sensitivity of the test, expressed as a percentage:

$$SENSITIVITY = \frac{6}{6+44}*100 = 12\%$$

We can calculate the probability that a case without Down syndrome will be correctly classified by our test as normal, i.e., the specificity of the test, expressed as a percentage:

$$SPECIFICITY = \frac{4283}{4283+40}*100 = 99\%$$

We can also ask the question what is the probability that a woman which screened positive (in our example: Nuchal fold >5 mm) actually carries a fetus with Down syndrome? This probability is a measure called positive predictive value:

$$Positive\ predictive\ value = \frac{TP}{TP+FP}*100$$

$$Positive\ predictive\ value = \frac{6}{6+40}*100 = 13\%$$

The probability that a positive test will actually be diagnosed as Down syndrome is rather low (13%).

Similarly, we can define the predictive value of a negative test:

$$Negative\ predictive\ value = \frac{TN}{TN+FN}*100$$

$$Negative\ predictive\ value = \frac{4283}{4283+44}*100 = 99\%$$

A growing number of epidemiological studies are based on information gathered from large computerized datasets and from national vital statistics computerized records such as birth certificates, notification of infant and fetal deaths, registries of birth defects, registries of very low birth weight infants, etc. The large number of cases, enabling the study of rare conditions and the non-selective population-based nature of such databases are their main advantages. As most of these databases were not originally meant for research purposes, much work has been done to validate the information derived from them [5-8].

Reliability

Often we are unable to truly validate information even when we have information from more than one source, because it is not possible to decide which is a measure that can be considered as the "gold standard". We tend to regard record-based information as superior to self-report, but this is not always justified. Which is a "better" source of information regarding having undergone a certain test in pregnancy: self-report of or data extracted from medical records? Information extracted from medical records will be a more valid source of information if we can be sure that the records contains all tests a patient may have had, as would be the situation if all tests are performed for a given population at a central lab or in a single clinic. Self report may be a more valid source of information in populations where some women may choose to undergo testing in several labs or clinics, not all of which made their records available to us. We need to have good understanding of our sources of information in order to decide which is more valid, but often we do not have enough information to make this decision. In this situation we can ask the question how reliable is the information obtained from these different sources of information, i.e., to what extent is there an agreement between the sources of information. This is also the case when we ask two physicians with the same levels of diagnostic skills to make a diagnosis of the same patient at the same time.

We define reliability as the extent to which information from different sources of information or from repeated measures of the same situation is identical.

The most common clinical situations where reliability is tested are the following:

- *Inter-rater reliability*: In studies based on diagnoses or clinical decisions made by different clinicians or in different study centers, we want to be sure that the same clinical information is interpreted in the same way by the different clinicians at the different sites.
- *Intra-rater, or test-retest reliability:* When a new diagnostic skill is introduced or a new research instrument, such as a questionnaire, is considered for use in a study, we want to make sure that the same test or questionnaire results obtained from the same person yield the same results if repeated, under the assumption that no change has occurred between the two measurements.

Statistical tools to assess reliability based on the comparability of two or more sources of information are available. For binary outcomes the most commonly used in the Kappa statistics, and for quantitative measures different types of correlation can be computed. The most commonly used are *Pearson correlation* for normally distributed variables and *Spearman correlation* for ordinal scale variables.

Kappa Statistics

A measure of agreement between two sources of information, adjusted for the proportion of agreement we would expect to occur by chance between those two sources of information.

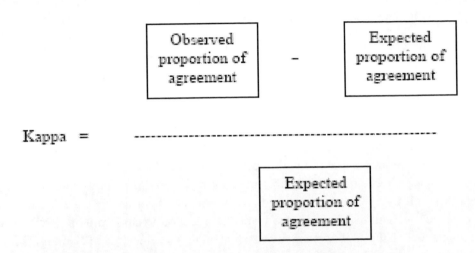

Two sources of information are considered in good agreement if the Kappa statistics are >0.75, fair agreement if Kappa is between 0.75–0.40, and if less than 0.40, poor agreement [9].

Nguyen and Baird [10] compared the reports of both men's and their partner's recall of time to pregnancy, and used the Kappa statistics to assess the reliability of report. The overall Kappa was 0.50 (95% CI 0.40–0.60), i.e., fair agreement.

It is important to note that valid sources of information are reliable; however, even excellent reliability does not necessarily indicate validity. Kelsey [3] gives an example of both man and wife interviewed about drinking habits of the husband. Their reports might be in perfect agreement, but both reports might be totally invalid.

Bias

The major threat to validity is a study design which leads to systematic wrong estimates of the parameters of interest. Bias in measurement is different from a random error. While random measurement error will on the average yield a correct estimate, bias would give us an estimate that is systemically different from the true value of the parameter.

Bias can result from two sources: a faulty study design where the study population is systematically different from the target population, or from measurement error where the information obtained is systematically different from the truth. The first kind of bias is called selection bias and the second is called information bias. Bias is more likely to occur in retrospective case-control studies than in large, population based studies, but it is possible even in prospective population-based cohort studies.

Selection Bias

Selection bias will occur when the study population is chosen in a way that distorts the true association between the exposure and outcome of interest. In perinatal epidemiology selection bias often occurs when we study populations for whom information is available, which are usually populations who seek medical care, for example women who seek prenatal care. Women can seek prenatal care for a variety of reasons. If one or more of these reasons are unknown to the researchers, and thus unmeasured, is associated with the outcome of interest, we will have a biased estimate of the association between exposure (prenatal care) and pregnancy outcomes. Frick and Lantz [11] present four scenarios leading to a biased estimate of the association between adequate prenatal care and adverse pregnancy outcomes. Favorable Selection: when women with favorable characteristics (for example: high level of education, high income) will be more likely than women with lower level of education or income to seek care and to comply with medical recommendation, and at the same time are more likely to have more favorable birth outcomes, regardless of prenatal care because they lead healthier lifestyles, are less exposed to risk factors such as violence, poor housing conditions, etc., we will overestimate the favorable effect of prenatal care on birth outcome. The opposite will happen if women who are at high risk due to social marginality and possible exposures which will place them at higher risk will not register for prenatal care (Estrangement Selection). Another way selection bias can affect our results is, according to Frick and Lantz [11], Adverse Selection, which will occur if factors that preselect women to prenatal care are risk factors for adverse pregnancy outcomes, such as bad obstetric history, chronic disease, etc. if such selection occurs we are likely to underestimate a favorable effect of prenatal care. If women with no risk factors tend to register late and choose to come for fewer visits (Confidence Selection), will result in underestimate of the effect of prenatal care on birth outcomes.

Selection bias affects cohort studies through selective participation and drop out from follow-up. Even population based data can lead to wrong inferences due to selection bias. Take, for example, epidemiological studies of congenital malformations. Often we use prevalence at birth data and tend to interpret them as if they were incidence data. It has been shown [12] that many pregnancies affected by birth defects tend to result in spontaneous abortions, sometimes in very early pregnancy losses. Moreover, a growing number of birth defects can now be prenatally diagnosed and couples may choose to terminate an affected pregnancy [13-14]. If we compare the prevalence at birth of a certain birth defect in two populations, which differ in the likelihood of prenatal diagnosis and termination of affected pregnancies, we can reach a conclusion that the population which is more likely to carry an affected pregnancy to birth is at higher risk, which is not necessarily true [15]. See, for example, the data in Table 2.

Another example of a selection bias was suggested in a recent study, based on the Texas birth defect registry, on the association between paternal age and birth defects in the offspring. The investigators found that some birth defects in offspring of younger fathers were more likely to be excluded from the database than those of older fathers, thus causing a biased estimate of the association of paternal age and birth defects [8].

Table 2. Percent of Neural Tube Defects (NTD) at birth from all diagnosed cases, by religion, national Israeli data [16].

	JEWS	NON JEWS
Anencephalus	20.3%	39.4%
Spina bifida	20.5%	56.5%

Information Bias

Information bias results from misclassification of disease and/or exposure status caused by faulty measurement tools. This type of bias can affect results of all types of research. Information bias can be either differential or non differential. *Non differential bias* occurs when the information regarding the study outcome variables (disease status in cohort studies, or exposure status in case control studies) is biased in the same direction and magnitude in the compared study groups (exposed and unexposed in cohort studies and in cases and controls in case control studies). Differential bias occurs in cohort studies, if disease status is assessed differently in exposed and unexposed subjects, and in case-control studies if exposure status is assessed differently in cases and controls.

In each situation, the bias will lead to misclassification. Misclassification can occur even when the same assessment method is used, but its validity differs among the study groups. One of the frequent examples of this problem is the use of pregnancy dating methods. It has been shown that using ultrasound for populations with either symmetrically large or small fetuses will be biased [17] For example, fetuses of smokers are known to be symmetrically small, thus the use of ultrasound to date pregnancies of smokers will tend to underestimate gestational age, consequently leading to a possible overestimate of prematurity in smokers [18]. Similarly, bias will occur while comparing rates of preterm birth among populations where different methods of dating are used, or comparing time trends in the rate of pre-term or post-term births when the most common methods of pregnancy dating have been changed [17].

Usually, when information bias affects the two study groups in the same direction and magnitude (non-differential bias), the result will be an underestimate of the true association between disease and exposure—i.e., in a cohort study, the relative risk (RR) and in case-control study, the odds ratio (OR) will be biased toward the null. This type of bias is considered a "conservative bias", if we can still uphold our hypothesis. But sometimes, especially when the association between the exposure and disease is weak and/or the sample size is too small a conservative bias may lead us to a wrong conclusion that there is no association when in fact there is.

When the bias affects each study group differently (differential bias) the effect on the RR or OR will vary according to the direction of the bias in the different study groups.

Recall Bias

Recall bias is a common problem in case-control studies which are based on obtaining information from study participants about past exposures. As at the time of interview the disease status is known, persons with the disease might tend to recall past events and report them more accurately than persons without the disease. Classic examples are case-control studies of birth defects. It has been repeatedly shown, by comparing self reported exposure information to medical records that women who had given birth to an infant with a birth defect tend to report differently than women who had a normal infant.[19]

Interviewer /Observer Bias

Interviewers may be more persistent in their effort to obtain information from cases than from controls. One way to avoid this kind of bias is to keep interviewers as much as possible "blind" to the disease status of the interviewee, or, if that is impossible, interviewers should at least be blind as to the main research hypothesis.[20] Similar problem can occur in cohort studies if different methods are used to assess disease status in exposed and unexposed study participants. For example, if in a prospective cohort study to assess the pregnancy outcomes of women with previous bad obstetric history in comparison with women with normal obstetric history, we follow a cohort of women who enrolled in prenatal care and collect information about pregnancy complications by way of self report in women with bad obstetric history (exposed) and from medical records for women without bad obstetric history (unexposed) an observer bias may occur.

Diagnosis /Detection/Referral Bias

This type of bias is caused when persons with known risks are more likely to be diagnosed, referred and thus diagnosed with the disease than persons without these risk factors, or when persons with a disease are more likely to be tested or questioned about their exposures than persons without the disease. Thus, this type of bias is both a selection and information bias. A recent systematic review examined the evidence of the possible teratogenic effect of paroxetine, a selective serotonin reuptake inhibitor (SSRI) commonly used as an antidepressant by women of childbearing age. The review concluded that the association shown by several studies of first-trimester exposure to paroxetine and an increased risk for cardiac malformations may result from a detection bias, since mothers using SSRIs in pregnancy were more likely to undergo ultrasound in pregnancy and their children were more likely to undergo echocardiograms in the first year of life than children of women who did not use SSRIs. Moreover, more women used the drug for anxiety or panic than women receiving other SSRIs [21].

How to Deal with Bias

Bias, unlike other problems that will be discussed later that may lead to wrong inferences, is caused by faulty study design either in the way the study population is chosen or in the way information is obtained, and therefore it cannot be corrected at the data analysis stage by statistical methods. Thus, careful consideration should be given at the stage of study design to avoid bias as much as possible. Randomized controlled trials (see Chapter 4) are designed to avoid bias, but almost all observational studies are prone to be affected by some sort of bias. It is therefore necessary to collect enough information which can help us to assess the possibility of bias, and to conduct, if necessary, sensitivity analyses, assuming various ways the study findings could have been affected by bias.

Confounding

The purpose of all epidemiological investigations is to get the best estimate of associations between risk factors (RF) and a disease (D). Confounding is a situation in which a wrong inference about the investigated association between a risk factor (RF) and the disease (D) is made because both RF and D are associated with a third variable that is a true risk factor for the disease. This third variable is called a confounder (C), and its presence can distort the true association between the risk factor and disease under investigation in different ways; it can cause a nonexisting association between RF and D to appear as if there is an association, and it can cause an existing association to disappear, but most frequently confounding causes over- or underestimation of a true association.

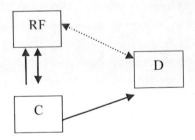

Unlike bias, which results from a faulty study design, confounding is caused by our inability, in observational studies, to take apart into simple components a complex reality. How can we test the effect of very young maternal age per se on birth outcomes in the US, where most teenage pregnancies are often characterized by unhealthy behaviors and limited access to health services characteristics that in and of themselves were shown to be associated with adverse pregnancy outcomes? Or, how can we test the effect of strenuous work in pregnancy on length of gestation if most pregnant women who hold physically strenuous jobs during pregnancy are exposed to other risk factors such as poverty, single motherhood and low level of education? One way is to study the relationship in populations where the exposure of interest is not associated with other known risk factors. An example is the study of Klebanoff, Shiono and Rhodas [22] on the association between strenuous work in pregnancy and preterm birth where the population exposed to physically strenuous work were pregnant female medical residents and the "unexposed" were pregnant wives of male residents. The researchers' conclusion that "working long hours in a stressful occupation has little effect on the outcome of pregnancy in an otherwise healthy population of high socioeconomic status" suggested that association between physical work and preterm birth reported in earlier studies might have been confounded by socioeconomic and other risk factors.

Another approach is to control for the confounding factors in appropriate statistical methods either by stratification (bivariate analysis) or by multivariable regression analyses. Stratified analysis allows the researcher to examine the pattern of association between the exposure of interest and the outcome in varying levels of the suspected confounder variable. If the same pattern of association is observed, it is possible to use the Mantel Haenszel technique to calculate an adjusted measure of association (relative risk or odds ratio). In a study comparing the risk of caesarian section (CS) in older primiparae (age>40) who conceived spontaneously and those who conceived by reproductive assisted technique, the authors conducted a stratified analysis to control for a variety of risk factors that may have been associated with both infertility and with indications for CS and found that, regardless of clinical conditions, nulliparous women who conceived after infertility treatment had an increased risk for CS delivery [23].

If different patterns of association are observed at different levels of the confounding variable, we conclude that an interaction, or effect modification, exists between the confounder variable and the exposure under study. A recent example was reported in a retrospective cohort study of twins of whom only one survived and the other died either intrapartum or neonatally [24]. The purpose of the study was to determine whether birth order is associated with mortality risk. While no association between birth order and the overall risk was found, birth order was found to significantly interact with gestational age. Among preterm deliveries, there was no association between birth order and risk of mortality, but in term deliveries the second twin was at a markedly increased risk of dying from intrapartum anoxia or trauma.

Multivariable regression analyses are used to control simultaneously for several potential confounders. Thus, the measures of association obtained from a multivariable regression represents the unique association of our exposure of interest and the outcome variable when all other confounder variables included in the model are held constant. Various multivariable regression models were developed to be applied for different research questions. (See chapter 7 for a detailed discussion of multivariable analysis.)

References

- Rothman K.J., Greenland S., & Lash T.L. (2008). *Modern Epidemiology,* 3rd Edition. Philadelphia, PA: Lippincott, Williams & Wilkins.

- Szklow M. & Nieto FJ. (2007) *Epidemiology Beyond the Basics*, 2nd Edition. Sudbury MA, Jones and Bartlett Publishers.
- Kelsey J. *Methods in Observational Epidemiology*, 2nd Edition 1996 Oxford University Press, Incorporated.
- Odibo AO, Sehdev HM, Gerkowicz S, Stamilio DM, Macones GA: Comparison of the efficiency of second-trimester nasal bone hypoplasia and increased nuchal fold in Down syndrome screening. *Am J Obstet Gynecol*. 2008;199(3):281.e1-5
- Melve KK, Lie RT, Skjaerven R, Van Der Hagen CB, Gradek GA, Jonsrud C, Braathen GJ, Irgens LM. Registration of Down syndrome in the Medical Birth Registry of Norway: validity and time trends. *Acta Obstet Gynecol Scand*. 2008;87(8):824-30.
- Ford JB, Roberts CL, Algert CS, Bowen JR, Bajuk B, Henderson-Smart DJ; NICUS group.Using hospital discharge data for determining neonatal morbidity and mortality: avalidation study. *BMC Health Serv Res*. 2007 Nov 20;7:188
- Lydon-Rochelle MT, Cárdenas V, Nelson JL, Tomashek KM, Mueller BA, Easterling TR. Validity of maternal and perinatal risk factors reported on fetal death certificates. *Am J Public Health*. 2005 Nov;95(11):1948-51. Epub 2005
- Archer NP, Langlois PH, Suarez L, Brender J, Shanmugam R. Association of paternal age with prevalence of selected birth defects. *Birth Defects Res A Clin Mol Teratol*. 2007 Jan;79(1):27-34.
- Fleiss JL. *Statistical methods for rates and proportions,* 2nd ed. New York, NY, John Wiley and Sons, 1981
- Nguyen RH, Baird DD.Accuracy of men's recall of their partner's time to pregnancy. *Epidemiology*. 2005 Sep;16(5):694-8.
- Frick KD. Lantz PM. Selection Bias in prenatal care utilization: An interdisciplinary framework and review of the literature. *Med Care Res Rev* 1996:53: 371-96.
- Rivas F, Dávalos IP, Olivares N, Dávalos NO, Pérez-Medina R, Gómez-Partida G,Chakraborty R.Reproductive history in mothers of children with neural tube defects. *Gynecol Obstet Invest*. 2000;49(4):255-60.
- Cragan JD, Roberts HE, Edmonds LD, Khoury MJ, Kirby RS, Shaw GM, Velie EM, Merz RD, Forrester MB, Williamson RA, Krishnamurti DS, Stevenson RE, Dean JH. Surveillance for anencephaly and spina bifida and the impact of prenatal diagnosis— United States, 1985-1994. *MMWR CDC Surveill Summ*. 1995;44(4):1-13.
- Van Allen MI, Boyle E, Thiessen P, McFadden D, Cochrane D, Chambers GK, Langlois S, Stathers P, Irwin B, Cairns E, MacLeod P, Delisle MF, Uh SH. The impact of prenatal diagnosis on neural tube defect (NTD) pregnancy versus birth incidence in British Columbia. *Appl Genet*. 2006;47(2):151-8.
- Zlotogora J, Amitai Y, Kaluski DN, Leventhal A. Surveillance of neural tube defects in Israel. *Isr Med Assoc J*. 2002;4(12):1111-4.
- Department for community genetics. Public Health Services, Ministry of Health. Israel. *Open Neural Birth Defects in Israel*. Jerusalem September 2002.
- Lynch CD, Zhang J The research implications of the selection of a gestational age estimation method. *Paediatr Perinat Epidemiol*. 2007 Sep;21 Suppl 2:86-96.

- Horta BL, Victora CG, Menezes AM, Halpern R, Barros FC: Low birthweight, preterm births and intrauterine growth retardation in relation to maternal smoking. *Paediatr Perinat Epidemiol.* 1997;11(2):140-51.

- Rockenbauer M, Olsen J, Czeizel AE, Pedersen L, Sørensen HT; EuroMAP Group. Recall bias in a case-control surveillance system on the use of medicine during pregnancy. *Epidemiology.* 2001 Jul;12(4):461-6.

- Watson LF, Lumley J, Rayner JA, Potter A.Research interviewers' experience in the Early Births study of very preterm birth: qualitative assessment of data collection processes in a case-control study. *Paediatr Perinat Epidemiol.* 2007 Jan;21(1):87-94.

- Bar-Oz B, Einarson T, Einarson A, Boskovic R, O'Brien L, Malm H, Bérard A, Koren G.Paroxetine and congenital malformations: meta-Analysis and consideration of potential confounding factors. *Clin Ther.* 2007 May;29(5):918-26.

- Klebanoff MA, Shiono PH, Rhoads GG. Outcomes of pregnancy in a national sample of resident physicians. *N Engl J Med.* 1990 Oct 11;323(15):1040-5.

- Sheiner E, Shoham-Vardi I, Hershkovitz R, Katz M, Mazor M. Infertility treatment is an independent risk factor for cesarean section among nulliparous women aged 40 and above. *Am J Obstet Gynecol.* 2001;185:888-92.

- Smith GC, Fleming KM, White IR. Birth order of twins and risk of perinatal death related to delivery in England, Northern Ireland, and Wales, 1994-2003: retrospective cohort study. *BMJ.* 2007;334(7593):576.

In: Textbook of Perinatal Epidemiology
Editor: Eyal Sheiner, pp. 67-82

ISBN: 978-1-60741-648-7
© 2010 Nova Science Publishers, Inc.

Chapter VII

The Importance of Multivariable Analysis for Conducting and Evaluating Research in Perinatology

Mitchell H. Katz[*]

Introduction

Multivariable analysis is essential to the study of perinatology. Why? Because many of the important outcomes in the field of perinatology for example, pre-eclampsia, prematurity, infants born small for gestational age, periventricular hemorrhage have multiple interrelated causes. Therefore, studies aimed at understanding and ultimately preventing negative outcomes and promoting successful ones must use multivariable analysis. Moreover, it is not just researchers who must be familiar with these models. As the number of articles using multivariable analysis increases in the literature, clinicians and other readers must be sufficiently familiar with the models to correctly interpret and apply the results.

Unfortunately, it is impossible to do justice to the topic of multivariable analysis in a single chapter. That's why I have written a book about it.[1] It is possible, however, to answer a number of key questions about multivariable analyses. In doing so, I have focused on examples from the perinatology literature in the hope that it will make the explanations more relevant for perinatologists.

What is Multivariable Analysis?

Multivariable analysis is a statistical tool for determining the unique contributions of a variety of factors to a single event or outcome. For example, a variety of factors are

[*] For Correspondence: Mitchell H. Katz, San Francisco Department of Public Health, San Francisco, CA 94102, USA. E-mail: mitch,katz@sfdph.org

associated with delivery of an infant small for gestational age, including maternal age, nulliparity, smoking, ethnicity, and administration of steroids. Depending on the context, these factors are referred to as risk factors, independent variables, explanatory variables, or treatment/intervention effects. Multivariable analysis enables us to determine the *independent* contribution of each of these risk factors to an outcome, such as the occurrence of an infant small for gestational age. (Outcome may also be referred to as the dependent variable or the response variable).

Why is Multivariable Analysis Needed?

There are four major reasons for performing multivariable analysis (Table 1).

Table 1. Why is multivariable analysis needed?

	Examples
Identify the unique contribution of a variety of risk factors to a single outcome.	Genital HSV infection, lack of antiretroviral prophylaxis, increased duration of membrane rupture, and increased gestational age are all independent risk factors for perinatal transmission of HIV. [2]
Identify and adjust for confounding	Pre-term delivery appeared to be associated with a higher rate of intraventricular hemorrhage because the association was confounded by gestational age. [3]
Develop a diagnostic/prognostic model	A logistic regression model using estimated fetal weight and the ductus venosus pulsatility correctly predicted a poor outcome in 66.7% of the cases of infants born to mothers with pre-eclampsia and a good outcome in 98.0% of the cases with an overall accuracy of 94.5%.[5]
Adjust models for variation in risk groups within treatment groups	Even in the absence of confounding, when using a non-linear model, adjust for baseline characteristics to avoid incorrect estimates of treatment effect.

First, to better understand and improve outcomes in perinatology, it is important to identify unique risk factors for positive and negative outcomes. For example, Chen and colleagues assessed risk factors for perinatal transmission of the human immunodeficiency virus.[2]

As you can see in Table 2, a bivariate analysis shows that there are four significant predictors of perinatal transmission: genital herpes simplex (HSV) infection during pregnancy, lack of zidovudine prophylaxis, a long delay in membrane rupture, and greater gestational age at delivery. But are these risk factors independent of one another? Does each contribute to an increase risk of HIV transmission or is it possible that some of the risk factors are redundant with one another (e.g., patients with HSV infection are also less likely to take zidovudine prophylaxis)?

Table 2. Bivariate Risk Factors for Perinatal transmission of HIV.

Maternal Variable	No. of Women*	No. of Infected Infants (%)	Odds Ratio	95% Confidence Interval	P
Diagnosis of genital HSV infection during pregnancy					
Yes	21	6 (28.6)	3.4	1.3-9.3	.02
No	381	40 (10.5)			
Lack of zidovudine prophylaxis during pregnancy / delivery					
Yes	124	21 (16.9)	2.0	1.1-3.7	.04
No	266	25 (9.4)			
Duration of membrane rupture (h)					
≥4	151	29 (19.2)	3.0	1.6-5.7	.001
<4	217	16 (7.4)			
Gestational age at delivery (wk)					
< 37	66	18 (27.3)	4.0	2.0-7.8	<.001
≥ 37	327	28 (8.6)			

*Numbers for some variables do not add up to total because of missing data
Data from Chen KT, Segúu M, Lumey LH, et al. Genital herpes simplex virus infection and perinatal transmission of human immunodeficiency virus. *Obstet Gynecol*. 2005;106:1341-8.

Table 3. Risk Factors for Perinatal Transmission of HIV.

Risk Factor	Adjusted OR	95% CI	P
Diagnosis of genital HSV infection during pregnancy	4.8	1.3-17.0	.02
Lack of zidovudine prophylaxis during pregnancy/ delivery	2.2	1.1-4.4	.02
Rupture of membranes ≥4 hours	2.5	1.3-5.0	.01
Delivery at < 37 weeks of gestation	3.4	1.6-7.0	.001

Data from Chen KT, Segúu M, Lumey LH, et al. Genital herpes simplex virus infection and perinatal transmission of human immunodeficiency virus. *Obstet Gynecol*. 2005;106:1341-8.

Answering this question requires multivariable analysis. Indeed, a multiple logistic regression (Table 3) indicates that each of these four variables contributes to HIV transmission. The analysis leads us to believe that to prevent perinatal transmission we should avoid or minimize all four of these risk factors.

In addition to identifying the unique contribution of different risk factors to a particular outcome, a second important function of multivariable analysis is to identify and adjust for *confounding*. Confounding occurs when the apparent association between a risk factor and an outcome is affected by the relationship of a third variable to the risk factor and to the outcome; the third variable is called a confounder. To be a confounder, a variable must be *associated with* the risk factor and *causally related to* the outcome (Figure 1).

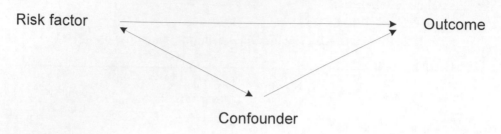

Figure 1. Relationship among risk factor, confounder, and outcome. [Reprinted with permission from Katz, MH. Multivariable Analysis: A Practical Guide for Clinicians (2nd edition). Cambridge: Cambridge University Press, 2006.].

To illustrate how multivariable analysis enables us to identify and adjust for confounding, let's examine the data from a study assessing whether outcomes are different for infants who have an indicated preterm delivery compared to those who had a spontaneous preterm delivery among neonates weighing < 1000 grams at birth.[3] The most common reasons for indicated preterm delivery were severe preeclampsia or eclampsia.

It would appear from the bivariate data shown in Table 4 that infants with indicated preterm delivery were less likely to have intraventricular hemorrhage than those with spontaneous preterm delivery. The 95% confidence interval for the bivariate odds ratio of 0.35 excludes 1, indicating that the association is statistically significant. However, infants who had an indicated preterm delivery were at a greater mean gestational age (28 weeks) than those with spontaneous preterm delivery (26 weeks).

Table 4. Does indicated pre-term delivery decrease neonatal morbidity in infants <1000 grams?

	Intraventricular hemorrhage (III/IV)		
	Yes	No	Total
Indicated pre-term delivery	9 (5.8 %)	147 (94.2 %)	156
Spontaneous pre-term delivery	38 (14.9%)	217 (85.1 %)	255
	47	364	411
	OR = 0.35 (0.16 – 0.76)		

Data from Kimberlin DF, et al. Indicated versus spontaneous preterm delivery: An evaluation of neonatal morbidity among infants weighing ≤1000 grams at birth. *Am J Obstet Gynecol* 1999;180:683-9.

When the investigators performed a multivariable logistic regression adjusting for gestational age they found that the difference in the frequency of intraventricular hemorrhage between those infants born following indicated preterm delivery and those born following spontaneous preterm delivery became smaller (odds ratio of 0.66) and the confidence intervals did not exclude one (0.34 − 1.31). In other words, the outcomes did not differ based on whether preterm delivery is indicated or spontaneous. What happened? Gestational age is confounding the association between indicated preterm delivery and intraventricular hemorrhage (Figure 2).

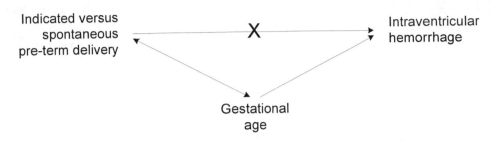

Figure 2. Gestational age confounds the relationship between indicated pre-term delivery and intraventricular hemorrhage.

Multivariable analysis is not the only statistical method for identifying and eliminating confounding. Stratified analysis also can be used to assess the effect of a risk factor on an outcome while holding other variables constant, thereby eliminating confounding. However, stratification works well only in situations where there are only one or two confounders. When there are many potential confounders, as is usually the case is perinatology, stratifying the sample for all possible confounders will create literally hundreds of groups in which the investigators would need to determine the relationship between the risk factor and the outcome. Because the sample sizes would be small, the estimates of risk would be unstable.

Given this discussion of the importance of multivariable analysis for minimizing confounding you may assume that you would not have to use multivariable analysis for a randomized controlled trial. After all, randomization produces unbiased groups; since group assignment is determined randomly it cannot be influenced by factors that favor one group over the other(s). Therefore differences between the groups, in response to an intervention, cannot be due to how the groups were assembled.

However, the reality is that the majority of randomized controlled trials perform multivariable analysis for one of a variety of reasons. First, it is possible that by chance (bad luck!) the randomized study groups differ on an important baseline characteristic. In this circumstance, you would use multivariable analysis to adjust for the difference. Second, even if the groups appear to be balanced, there may be small differences that together could bias your study. In some ways, adjusting for baseline differences using a multivariable model has become the standard of demonstrating that there is no confounding. If the unadjusted and the adjusted rates are the same, then you have evidence that there is no confounding due to these measured characteristics. Third, investigators may perform multivariable analysis in the context of a randomized controlled trial to identify additional independent predictors of outcome other than the randomized treatment. This is akin to using multivariable analysis to identify the unique contribution of a variety of risk factors to a single cause.

To illustrate the uses of multivariable analysis within a randomized study, let's look at a randomized controlled trial comparing the effect of preoperative vaginal preparation with povidone-iodine versus the standard abdomen only scrub on the rate of post-cesarean endometritis.[4] In a bivariate analysis women who received the vaginal scrub were significantly less likely to develop endometritis following cesarean section (odds ratio = 0.45; 95% confidence intervals 0.21-0.97). Since this was a randomized trial there should be no confounding. The authors checked to see if there were baseline differences between those subjects in the treatment group and those in the placebo group. None were statistically significant. However, there were some non-significant differences between the groups that could bias the estimate of the effect of a vaginal preparation on the rate of endometritis. Therefore the authors performed a multivariable analysis (shown in Table 5). As you can see, with adjustment for severe anemia, use of intrapartum internal monitors, and history of antenatal genitourinary infections, vaginal rub was protective for endometritis. The odds ratio (0.44) from the multivariate model was practically identical to that of the bivariate analysis, indicating that there was not confounding due to the other variables that were in the model. The fact that the other three variables in Table 5 were statistically significant indicates that these variables are also unique contributors to endometritis.

Table 5. Multivariate Analysis of Factors Affecting Risk for Postcesarean Endometritis (N=308).

Variable	Adjusted Odds Ratio	95% Confidence Interval
Vaginal scrub	0.44	0.193-0.997
Severe anemia (hematocrit <30%)	4.26	1.568-11.582
Use of intrapartum internal monitors	2.84	1.311-6.136
History of antenatal genitourinary infections	2.89	1.265-6.595

Data from Starr R, et al. Preoperative vaginal preparation with povidone-Iodine and the risk of postcesarean endometritis. *Obstet Gynecol*. 2005;105:1024-9.

A third reason to perform multivariable analysis is to develop a model containing multiple variables that can be used to diagnose conditions or to provide prognostic information about a particular condition. For example, Geerts and Odentaal used multiple logistic regression to predict a poor outcome in infants of women with pre-eclampsia.[5] A poor outcome was defined as perinatal mortality or evidence of neurologic compromise of the infant at discharge. The investigators found that the best model for predicting poor outcome was the combination of initial estimated fetal weight and final ductus venosus pulsatility index. It had a correct prediction of poor outcome in 66.7% of the cases, good outcome in 98.0% of the cases, and overall accuracy of 94.5%.

There are several differences between predictive/prognostic models and the explanatory models that we have been discussing so far. With predictive/prognostic models we are not as interested in the individual variables; in fact, it doesn't matter whether the variables are causally related to the outcome or not. Instead we are interested in how well the model predicts the outcome in a variety of settings; as is the case with the study by Geerts and Odentall,[5] some of the variables (e.g., pulsatility index) may be diagnostic tests rather than risk factors that are causally related to the outcome.

A fourth reason for conducting multivariable analysis is that variation in subjects' risk factors within study groups can result in incorrect estimates of the treatment effect in nonlinear models (e.g., logistic or proportional hazard regression) even when risk factors are balanced between the study groups.[6] In such cases, adjusting for risk factors in a multivariable model will yield more accurate estimates of the treatment effect.

What Types of Multivariable Analysis are Commonly Used in Perinatal Research?

Commonly used methods of multivariable analysis are shown in Table 6. As you can see the type of multivariable analysis to perform depends on the type of outcome variable you are using.

Table 6. Type of outcome variable determines choice of multivariable analysis.

Type of outcome	Example of outcome variable	Type of multivariable analysis
Interval	Gestational Weight	Multiple linear regression Analysis of variance
Dichotomous	Pre-eclampsia (Y/N)	Multiple logistic regression
Ordinal	Grade of intraventricular hemorrhage	Proportional odds regression
Nominal	Pre-term Pre-eclampsia, term Pre-eclampsia, small for gestational age neonate, normal pregnancy	Polytomous logistic regression
Time to occurrence of a dichotomous event	Establish prenatal care	Proportional hazards analysis
Rare outcomes and counts	Birth defects	Poisson regression

Linear regression and analysis of variance are used with interval (also called continuous) outcomes (e.g., gestational age). With interval variables, equal sized differences on all parts of the scale are equal. Gestational age is an interval variable because the difference between an age of 30 and 33 (3 weeks) is the same as the difference between an age of 33 and 36 (3 weeks).

Logistic regression is used with dichotomous outcomes (e.g., pre-eclampsia (yes/no)). Dichotomous variables, as implied by the name, are those variables that have only two values, such as yes/no, dead/alive.

Ordinal variables are analyzed using proportional odds regression. An ordinal variable has multiple values that can be "ordered" but unlike an interval variable there is not an equal size difference on each part of the scale. The difference between grade I and III intraventricular hemorrhage and II and IV ventricular hemorrhage is not the same amount of hemorrhage.

Nominal variables are analyzed using polytomous logistic regression. Nominal variables are categorical variables that cannot be ordered. They represent different states. For examples, Erez and colleagues used polytomous logistic regression to compare possible outcomes: delivery of a small for neonate gestational age, pre-term eclampsia, term eclampsia, and normal pregnancy.[7]

Proportional hazards regression is used when we are interested in the length of time to reach a discrete event (e.g., survival time). For example, Wy and colleagues used proportional hazards regression to identify neonatal and maternal predictors of death in infants born with a diagnosis of Hydrops Fetalis.[8] Poisson regression is used for rare outcomes such as birth defects or for analyzing the rates of outcomes (e.g., rates of pregnancies in a community over time).

What Independent Variables Should I Enter into a Multivariable Analysis?

For explanatory models each multivariable model should include the risk factor(s) and potential confounders. However, deciding which potential confounders to include is neither standard nor straightforward.

Ideally researchers should include in their models all those variables that have been hypothesized on theoretical grounds or shown in prior research to be confounders of the relationship being studied.

Although researchers should err on the side of including potentially important variables in the analysis, it is important to exclude extraneous ones. For example, seat belt usage should not be included in a model predicting early initiation of prenatal care, even though it may well be associated with this outcome. The reason is that seat belt use is not a potential cause of initiating prenatal care. It just happens that people who are more likely to comply with seat belts are also more likely to comply with recommendations about when to initiate prenatal care.

It is also important to exclude variables that are on the causal pathway of an outcome; these variables are referred to as intervening variables. For example, if you are testing the effectiveness of antiretroviral treatment on reducing the likelihood of transmission of the human immunodeficiency virus (HIV) from an infected mother to her fetus, it would be a mistake to include the change in the maternal viral load between initiation of treatment and delivery. Why? Because one of the mechanisms by which antiretroviral treatment prevents perinatal transmission is by reducing maternal viral load (Figure 3). If you adjust for the decrease in viral load, you will be adjusting away the effect you are trying to demonstrate. Of course, it would be okay to include maternal viral load prior to treatment as a risk factor in a model predicting treatment efficacy. It would also be okay to perform two models evaluating treatment efficacy with and without adjustment for change in maternal viral load. Comparison of the models would show how much of the effect of antiretroviral treatment is due to the effect of treatment on maternal viral load and how much is due to other ways that antiretroviral treatment prevents infection. For example, Sperling and colleagues, using a logistic regression model, estimated that decrease in viral load explained 17% of the treatment effect of zidovudine in preventing perinatal transmission.[9]

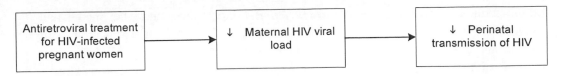

Figure 3. Maternal viral HIV viral load is an intervening variable between antiretroviral treatment and perinatal transmission.

When there are variables in the data set that are highly correlated to each other, you should include only one. The reason is that when two variables are highly correlated it is impossible for the model to identify the independent contribution of each a problem referred to as *multicollinearity*. For example, in a study of neonatal mortality, the investigators found that birth weight and gestational age were too closely related to one another to include both in the model.[10] They excluded gestational age because it had more missing data than birth weight.

After excluding extraneous variables, intervening variables, and redundant variables, you still may have too many variables in your model for your sample size. This can result in unreliable estimates and wide confidence intervals. As a rule of thumb, to have confidence in the results, there should be at least 20 subjects per independent variable eligible for inclusion into a linear regression model, and at least ten outcomes per independent variable eligible for inclusion into a logistic regression or proportional hazards model.[11-13] Sample size requirements for logistic regression and proportional hazards regression are expressed as outcomes per variable (rather than subjects per variable). The needed sample size is based on the less frequent state of the outcome. If only six babies suffer fetal demise, the model will have difficulty predicting how three variables independently predict demise even if there are 994 normal births.

Wide confidence intervals are a consequence of an insufficient sample size. Whenever you see confidence intervals that are clinically meaningless (risk between 0.8 and 22.0), it is likely that the sample size is insufficient for answering the question.

There are several techniques you can use to decrease the number of variables in your model. As discussed above, you should remove variables that are extraneous to your theory. Sometimes you can combine more than one variable into a scale. For example, education, income, ethnicity, and geographic location may be satisfactorily summarized by a variable measuring socioeconomic status. Another technique is to empirically test individual variables to determine whether they are confounders. Even if a variable is theoretically thought to be a confounder, if inclusion of the variable in the model makes no difference to the estimate of the risk between the independent variable(s) and the outcome of interest, it is not empirically functioning as a confounder and can potentially be excluded.[1]

It is also possible to reduce the number of variables in a model using automatic variable selection algorithms. These algorithms allow the computer to choose what variables to include in the model based on specific criteria. Variable selection methods include: *forward stepwise selection* (the variable with the strongest association with the outcome enters first, followed by the next strongest until all variables that are related to outcome, at an investigator specified significance level, have entered the model; if any of the variables that entered the model are no longer significant when the other variables are in the model, they will be sequentially deleted); ***backward deletion*** (all variables enter the model and are sequentially deleted starting with the variable having the weakest association with the outcome and continuing until the only variables left in the model are those related to outcome at an investigator specified level); and ***best subset*** (the subset of variables that maximizes the specifications chosen by the researcher).

Although, automatic variable selection techniques often produce models with a smaller number of independent variables, they have many serious limitations and should be avoided.[14-16] The variables that are retained in a model using automatic algorithms are not necessarily clinically more important than the variables that are excluded. If two variables are significantly associated with one another, the model will likely choose the one with the better statistical characteristics. It is much better for the investigator rather than the computer to determine which variables should be kept and which variables should be deleted.

In What Form Should Independent Variables be Entered into a Multivariable Model?

To enter an independent variable into a multivariable model it should be in the form of an interval or dichotomous variable. Nominal variables can never be entered in their original form. Instead, to enter a nominal variable into a multivariable model you must create multiple dichotomous variables (also referred to as "*dummy*" variables) to represent it. For example, the variable ethnicity, might be represented with four variables: Caucasian (yes/no), African-American (yes/no), Latino (yes/no), Asian (yes/no), with mixed ethnicity or other ethnicity as the reference group.

What Assumptions Underlie Multivariable Models?

Multivariable models are mathematical expressions. We choose particular models because we believe that the data will follow the form of that model. If the model does not fit the data, our understanding of the data will be distorted.

The underlying assumption of multiple linear regression is that as the independent variables increase (or decrease), the mean value of the outcome increases (or decreases) in a linear fashion. Although the relationship between the independent variable and the outcome must be linear, it is possible to model non-linear relationships by transforming the variables so that the independent variables have a linear relationship to the outcome. Readers will commonly see the use of logarithmic and spline transformations to model nonlinear relationships.

Logistic regression models the probability of an outcome, and how that probability changes with a change in the predictor variables. The basic assumption is that each one unit increase in a predictor multiplies the odds of the outcome by a certain factor (the odds ratio of the predictor), and that the effect of several variables is the multiplicative product of their individual effects. The logistic function produces a probability of outcome bounded by 0 and 1.

Proportional hazards models assume that the ratio of the hazard functions for persons with and without a given risk factor is the same over the entire study period. This is known as the *proportionality assumption*.[1, 17-19]

A major advantage of proportional hazards analysis is that it allows incorporation of subjects with varying lengths of follow-up. Varying lengths of follow-up occur commonly in longitudinal studies for several reasons including subjects being lost to follow-up, subjects developing a condition that makes it impossible to evaluate them for the study's outcome of interest, and subjects being enrolled in waves, resulting in some subjects having longer lengths of follow-up than other subjects.[20] Subjects who have not experienced the outcome of interest by the end of the study are referred to as censored observations.

In proportional hazards analyses censored subjects are assumed to have had the same course, if they hadn't been censored, as subjects who were not censored. In other words, the losses occur randomly, independent of outcome. It is this assumption that allows us to incorporate the follow-up time of censored subjects in the analysis. However, sometimes losses occur due to a systematic bias such as when persons who are lost to follow-up are more likely to have experienced the outcome of interest than those persons not lost to follow-up.

All of the multivariable statistics discussed thus far assume that observations are independent of one another; that is, the outcome for one subject is not influenced by the outcome of another subject. But in some perinatology studies the outcomes of some subjects may be correlated to each other (also referred to as clustered observations). For example, in a study of birth outcomes, some pregnancies will result in multiple births. It would not be correct to treat twins as two independent observations because they share the same mother and therefore the same physiology and depending on whether they are identical or fraternal twins, 50-100% of the genetics.

Although twinning may be the most obvious example of non-independent observations in the field of perinatology, there are a number of situations where observations may not be independent. For example, repeated observations of the same person (e.g., outcomes of different pregnancies) are not independent; we would expect that the second pregnancy of a woman would more closely resemble her first pregnancy than the pregnancy of a different woman. Also, women drawn from the same obstetrics practice are more likely to be similar to each other than women drawn from different practices.

When you have clustered observations, you need a multivariable technique that can incorporate clustered observations. Two such techniques are: *generalized estimating equations* and *mixed-effects models* (also known as mixed models, random effects regression models, random coefficient models, multilevel models and hierarchical models).[1, 21, 22]

How Should Interactions between Independent Variables be Interpreted?

An *interaction* occurs when the effect of a risk factor on an outcome is changed by the value of a third variable. As illustrated in Figure 4 the risk factor's effect on outcome (solid lines) differs depending on the value of the interaction variable. Note how the dotted line is the average of the two effects. Because the value of the third variable changes the effect of the risk on an outcome, interaction is often referred to as effect modification.

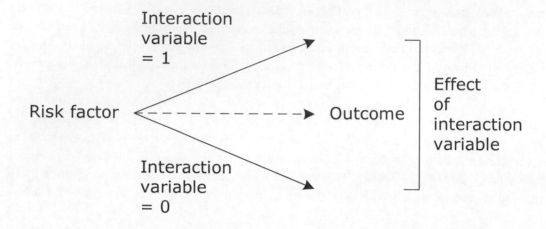

Figure 4. Illustration of an interaction effect. [Reprinted with permission from Katz, MH. Multivariable Analysis: A Practical Guide for Clinicians (2nd edition). Cambridge: Cambridge University Press, 2006.].

Interactions are different from confounding in that with interactions the relationship between the risk factor and the outcome is not due a third variable; rather the relationship varies depending on the value of the third variable. For example, Smith and colleagues assessed the ability of pregnancy-associated plasma protein A and alpha-fetoprotein in predicting preterm birth.[23] In a multivariate logistic model with the outcome of preterm delivery they entered two variables: pregnancy related plasma protein A and alpha-fetoprotein; the odds ratio associated with a low plasma protein A was 2.2 and the odds ratio associated with a high alfa-fetoprotein was 2.1. Because odds ratios in a logistic regression model have a multiplicative effect on outcome, the model containing these two variables would predict that a mother with an low plasma protein A level and a high alfa-fetoprotein level would have a risk of preterm delivery of 4.6 (2.2 x 2.1).

However, the reality was more complicated. The increase in risk was much higher in patients with both a low plasma protein A level and a high alfa-fetoprotein level than predicted by the product (4.6) of the odds ratios. The actual odds ratio for this group was 9.9. There was an interaction. The combination of a low plasma protein A level and a high alfa-fetoprotein level resulted in a higher risk of preterm delivery than you would think from the odds ratios of the individual variables. Interactions can be diagnosed by looking at the risk associated with different subgroups (e.g., the odds ratio associated with having only a low plasma protein A level, the odds ratio associated with having only a high alfa-fetoprotein level, and the odds ratio associated with having both risk factors). Interactions can also be diagnosed by entering into a multiple regression analysis the individual variables along with a product term. In the case of this example, you would enter plasma protein level (coded as 1 for low and 0 for high), alfa-fetoprotein level (coded as 0 for low and 1 for high) and the product term (plasma protein level x alfa-feto protein level).

Although the search for interactions can be clinically meaningful, as was the case in this study, readers should be skeptical of interaction terms that are not specified *a priori*. The reason is that when investigators search for interactions they are essentially performing subgroup analyses. The more interactions searched for, the more subgroups tested, and the greater the possibility that the relationship between the dependent variable and the outcome will differ, due to chance, in one or more of the different subgroups.

Does the Model Fit the Data?

The best way to assess whether the model fits the data is through residual analysis. *Residuals* are the difference between the observed and the estimated value.[1, 24] They can be thought of as the error in estimation. Large residuals suggest that the model does not fit the data. It may be that certain variables should be transformed (e.g., log transformation of an interval variable skewed to the right) or that the right variables are not in the model. Unfortunately, journals rarely print residual plots; the reader must rely on the investigators to have reviewed them.

How Well does the Model Predict Outcome?

To assess the power of a linear regression models model in predicting outcome, most investigators report the adjusted R^2. The value of R^2 ranges form 0 to 1; multiplied by 100, R^2 can be thought of as the percentage of the variance in the outcome accounted for by the independent variables. Because R^2 increases in value as additional variables are included in the model, adjusted R^2 charges a penalty for every additional variable included. In a model with a R^2 close to 1, the dependent variables taken together, accurately predict outcome.

For logistic regression models, investigators often report the **Hosmer-Lemeshow goodness-of-fit test**.[25] This statistic compares the estimated to observed likelihood of outcome for groups of subjects. In a well-fitting model, the estimated likelihood will be close to that observed. Readers should be aware that the Hosmer-Lemeshow goodness-of-fit test, along with other available goodness-of-fit statistics,[26] has significant limitations.

Although they exist, goodness-of-fit tests are rarely reported with proportional hazards regression. Instead, some investigators compare estimated to observed time to outcome in tabular form.[27] In a well fitting model, the estimated and observed times to outcome for different groups of subjects will be similar.

Although, goodness-of-fit statistics are an adequate measure of how well an explanatory model predicts outcome, predictive models require a more quantitative measure of their success in predicting outcome. This is commonly done with a logistic regression model by computing the sensitivity, specificity and accuracy of a model's predictions at a particular cut-point. The area under the receiver-operator characteristic (ROC) curves allow assessment of the predictive value of a logistic regression model over a variety of cut-offs of probability of outcome.[28, 29]

Is the Model Reliable?

Readers should see if the author has shown that a multivariable is reliable before accepting it at face value. The reliability of a model depends on its purpose. If it is an explanatory model, reliability means that a different set of data would likely yield the same terms in the model with similar coefficients. A reliable predictive model means that it predicts outcomes equally well in other settings or on data other than the ones in which it was developed.

Although, some decrement in performance is acceptable when a model is rerun with new data, a reliable model will perform well with new data. Unfortunately, it is not always possible for investigators to collect additional data. In these situations, investigators may report one of three alternative methods for assessing the reliability of a model: *split-group*, *jackknife*, and *bootstrap*.[1] With split-group validation the investigators divide the data set into two parts; the model is developed on the first dataset and then validated on the second dataset. With a jackknife procedure the investigator sequentially deletes subjects from a data set and repeatedly recomputes the model with each subject missing once. With a bootstrap procedure, the investigators take random samples of subjects from a data set with replacement (meaning that a subject may be chosen more than once). Although none of these methods can be considered definitive, if they closely approximate the original model, readers can have greater confidence in the results.

Conclusion

Multivariable analysis is critical to the field of perinatology. When performed and interpreted correctly, these models deepen our understanding of important perinatal outcomes. At the same time, it is important to remember the limitations of multivariable analysis. For example, although it is possible to adjust for known predictors of an outcome we can only adjust for those confounders that we know and have measured. Most importantly, models are only helpful to the extent that the data fit the assumptions of it.

References

[1] Katz MH. *Multivariable analysis: A practical guide for clinicians* (second edition). New York: Cambridge University Press, 2006.
[2] Chen KT, Segúu M, Lumey LH, et al. Genital herpes simplex virus infection and perinatal transmission of human immunodeficiency virus. *Obstet Gynecol.* 2005;106:1341-8.

[3] Kimberlin DF, Hauth JC, Owen J, et al. Indicated versus spontaneous preterm delivery: An evaluation of neonatal morbidity among infants weighing ≤1000 grams at birth. *Am J Obstet Gynecol* 1999;180:683-9.

[4] Starr R, Zurawski J, Mahmoud I. Preoperative vaginal preparation with povidone-iodine and the risk of postcesarean endometritis. *Obstet Gynecol*. 2005;105:1024-9.

[5] Geerts L, Odendaal HJ. Severe early onset pre-eclampsia: prognostic value of ultrasound and Doppler assessment. *J Perinatology*. 2007;27:335-342.

[6] Harrell FE., Jr. *Regression Modeling Strategies: With applications to linear models, logistic regression and survival analysis*. New York: Springer, 2001, p. 4.

[7] Erez O, Robero R, Espinoza J, et al. The change in concentrations of angiogenic and anti-angiogenic factors in maternal plasma between the first and second trimesters in risk assessment for the subsequent development of preeclampsia and small-for-gestational age. *J Matern Fetal Neonatal Med*. 2008;21(5):279-287.

[8] Wy CA, Sajous CH, Loberiza F, Weiss MG. Outcome of infants with a diagnosis of hydrops fetalis in the 1990s. *Am J Perinatol* 1999;16:561-7.

[9] Sperling RS, Shapiro DE, Coombs RW, et al. Maternal viral load, zidovudine treatment, and the risk of transmission of human immunodeficiency virus type 1 from mother to infant. *N Engl J Med*. 1996;335:1621-9.

[10] Phibbs CS, Bronstein JM, Buxton E, Phibbs RH. The effects of patient volume and level of care at the hospital of birth on neonatal mortality. *JAMA*. 1996;276:1054-49.

[11] Peduzzi P, Concato J, Kemper Ed, Holdord TR, Feinstein AR. A simulation study of the number of events per variable in logistic regression analysis. *J Clin Epidemiol*. 1996;49:1373-9.

[12] Peduzzi P, Concato J, Feinstein AR, Holford TR. Importance of events per independent variable in proportional hazards regression analysis II. Accuracy and precision of regression estimates. *J Clin Epidemiol*. 1995;48:1503-10.

[13] Harrell FE, Lee KL, Matchar DB, Reichert TA. Regression models for prognostic prediction: advantages, problems, and suggested solutions. *Cancer Treat Rep*. 1985;69:1071-7.

[14] Greenland S. Modeling and variable selection in epidemiologic analysis. *Am J Public Health*. 1989;79:340-9.

[15] Steyerberg EW, Eijkemans MJ, Habbema JD. Stepwise selection in small data sets: a simulation study of bias in logistic regression analysis. *J Clin Epidemiol*. 1999;52:935-42.

[16] Harrell F, Lee K, Mark D. Multivariable prognostic models: Issues in developing models, evaluating assumptions and adequacy, and measuring and reducing errors. *Statistics in Medicine*. 1996;15:361-87.

[17] Kahn HA, Sempos CT. *Statistical methods in epidemiology*. New York: Oxford University Press, 1989, pp. 193-8.

[18] Lawless JF. *Statistical models and methods for lifetime data*. New York: John Wiley and Sons, 1982, pp. 394-5.

[19] Kalbfleish JD, Prentice RL. *The statistical analysis of failure time data*. New York: John Wiley and Sons, 1980, pp. 89-98.

[20] Kelsey JL, Whittemore AS, Evans AS, Thompson WD. *Methods in observational epidemiology*. New York: Oxford University Press, 1996, pp. 130-4.

[21] Twisk JWR. Applied *Longitudinal Data Analysis for Epidemiology: A Practical Guide.* Cambridge University Press, 2003, pp. 62-92.

[22] Diggle PJ, Heagerty P, Liang K-Y, Zeger SL. *Analysis of Longitudinal Data* (second edn). Oxford: Oxford University Press, 2002, pp 141-189.

[23] Smith GCS, Shah I, Crossley JA, et al. Pregnancy-associated plasma protein A and alpha-fetoprotein and prediction of adverse perinatal outcome. *Obstet Gynecol.* 2006;107:161-6.

[24] Glantz SA, Slinker BK. *Primer of applied regression and analysis of variance.* New York: McGraw-Hill, 1990, pp. 110-80.

[25] Hosmer DW, Lemeshow S. *Applied Logistic Regression.* New York: Wiley, 1989, pp. 187-215.

[26] Hosmer DW, Hosmer T, Le Cessie S, Lemeshow S. A comparison of goodness-of-fit tests for the logistic regression model. *Statistics in Medicine.* 1997;16:965-80.

[27] Colford JM Jr, Tager IB, Hirozawa AM, Lemp GF, Aragon T, Petersen C. Cryptosporidiosis among patients infected with human immunodeficiency virus. Factors related to symptomatic infection and survival. *Am J Epidemiol.* 1996;144:807-16.

[28] Hanley JA, McNeil BJ. The meaning and use of the area under a receiver operating characteristic (ROC) curve. *Radiology.* 1982;143:29-36.

[29] Hsiao JK, Bartko JJ, Potter WZ. Diagnosing diagnoses. Receiver operating characteristic methods and psychiatry. *Arch Gen Psychiatry.* 1989;46:664-7.

In: Textbook of Perinatal Epidemiology
Editor: Eyal Sheiner, pp. 83-110

ISBN: 978-1-60741-648-7
© 2010 Nova Science Publishers, Inc.

Chapter VIII

Practical Guide for Data Analysis of Perinatal Epidemiology by SPSS®

Amalia Levy[*]

Introduction

As researchers, we usually start with scientific questions that lead us to our study hypotheses; we then plan and perform the study by collecting data from a subset of the population, our sample. Next, we analyze the collected data while using statistical tools to reach conclusions regarding the population.

This chapter gives a brief overview of the principles of data analysis within perinatal epidemiology studies; however, this will not include all of the important stages of a study. In addition, the examples shown in this chapter are the most common statistical tests in perinatal epidemiology only. In order to learn the most when reading this chapter, one needs a basic knowledge of statistics and SPSS®.

The Steps of Data Analysis

A typical data analysis includes three major steps:

1) Univariable analysis, which comprises mainly descriptive statistics and graphs describing the characteristics of the participants of a study. In this step, we begin by looking at the distribution of the variables as well as trying to discover and correct data errors that may occur. We also check whether our variable distributions are normal. Checking normality can be done by looking at the graphs, central tendency

[*] For Correspondence: Amalia Levy Ph.D, Department of Epidemiology and Health Services Evaluation, Faculty of Health Sciences, Ben Gurion University of the Negev, Beer-Sheva, Israel. E-mail: lamalia@bgu.ac.il

(mean, median, and mode), and the values of skewness and kurtosis, or by applying appropriate statistical tests.

2) Bivariable analysis tests the relationship between two variables or the differences between groups of people. For example, linear relationship is measured by a correlation, but the outcome can also be predicted by a single predictor using simple regression. Comparison of the means of two independent groups can be performed by student t-tests.

3) Multivariable analysis predicts an outcome from several predictor variables, or examines one variable in relation to the outcome variable while adjusting for all other variables (multiple regressions).

Choosing the Suitable Statistical Test

The principles of choosing the suitable statistical test for the three major steps mentioned above are provided in all statistics books.

Following are the principles, summarized very briefly:

1) The scientific study questions or the study hypothesis (relation between the variables, comparing groups or prediction).
2) The study type or outline (comparison between or within groups and the number of comparisons).
3) The variable type, such as continuous or categorical.
4) The variable distribution—whether a sample originates from a normally distributed population.
5) Sample size or number of observations in the compared groups, e.g., 30 or more observations per group.

Working with SPSS for Windows®

SPSS includes three types of files: the SPSS data editor, syntax, and the viewer (the output) [1–3].

The SPSS data editor is the file including all the study data that can be either imported from other types of files or entered directly to the SPSS file. The data editor has two views: the "data view" and the "variable view".

The data view is constructed of columns and rows: each column is a variable and each row is a participant in the study; as a result, each cell is a variable's value for a certain person in the study (Figure 1).

The second view is the variable view, which includes the variables' definitions, such as name, type, label, missing values, and measure (Figure 2).

We can shift from data view to variable view by clicking on the tabs shown in the bottom left side of the screen (see arrow in Figure 3).

	sno	gender	race	in_hosp_date	dis_date	i_b_date	m_b_date	ap1
1	1	2	1	02-JAN-2005	10-JAN-2005	04-JAN-2005	02-NOV-1972	8
2	2	1	2	09-JAN-2005	13-JAN-2005	09-JAN-2005	02-APR-1975	1
3	3	1	1	30-JAN-2005	01-FEB-2005	30-JAN-2005	16-MAY-1967	9
4	5	1	1	19-MAR-2005	24-MAR-2005	20-MAR-2005	24-FEB-1966	9
5	6	2	1	20-MAR-2005	25-MAR-2005	21-MAR-2005	01-JAN-1970	9
6	7	2	1	02-AUG-2005	07-AUG-2005	03-AUG-2005	21-OCT-1977	9
7	8	2	1	30-MAY-2005	04-JUN-2005	30-MAY-2005	26-JUN-1975	9
8	9	2	2	20-DEC-2005	24-DEC-2005	20-DEC-2005	02-JUN-1976	9
9	10	1	1	18-JUL-2005	25-JUL-2005	19-JUL-2005	08-DEC-1974	9
10	11	1	1	27-NOV-2005	28-NOV-2005	28-NOV-2005	15-AUG-1980	.
11	12	1	1	22-AUG-2005	28-AUG-2005	22-AUG-2005	07-FEB-1971	9
12	13	1	2	02-FEB-2005	06-FEB-2005	03-FEB-2005	12-APR-1976	9
13	14	1	1	07-FEB-2005	.	07-FEB-2005	22-JUL-1973	.
14	15	2	1	26-APR-2005	29-APR-2005	26-APR-2005	31-JAN-1969	9
15	16	1	1	04-NOV-2005	06-NOV-2005	04-NOV-2005	20-APR-1974	9
16	17	2	1	03-MAY-2005	06-MAY-2005	04-MAY-2005	26-JUN-1974	9
17	18	1	1	03-JAN-2005	05-JAN-2005	04-JAN-2005	20-MAY-1965	9
18	19	1	2	13-APR-2005	20-APR-2005	18-APR-2005	31-JUL-1974	9
19	20	2	1	25-JAN-2005	27-JAN-2005	25-JAN-2005	15-JUL-1978	9
20	21	1	1	16-JAN-2005	18-JAN-2005	16-JAN-2005	14-OCT-1975	9
21	22	1	2	09-MAR-2005	12-MAR-2005	10-MAR-2005	16-AUG-1983	9
22	23	2	1	14-NOV-2005	18-NOV-2005	15-NOV-2005	25-MAY-1971	9
23	24	1	1	20-NOV-2005	27-NOV-2005	23-NOV-2005	27-JAN-1972	.
24	25	1	1	20-NOV-2005	23-NOV-2005	21-NOV-2005	01-JUN-1971	9
25	26	1	1	30-JAN-2005	01-FEB-2005	30-JAN-2005	26-JAN-1973	9
26	27	1	1	03-JAN-2005	06-JAN-2005	04-JAN-2005	19-JUN-1972	9
27	28	1	2	22-NOV-2005	24-NOV-2005	22-NOV-2005	07-NOV-1981	9

Figure 1. The Data View of the SPSS Data Editor.

	Name	Type	Width	Decimals	Label	Values	Missing	Columns	Align	Measure
1	sno	Numeric	4	0	Serial number	None	None	8	Center	Nominal
2	gender	Numeric	1	0	Gender	{1, Male}...	None	8	Center	Nominal
3	race	Numeric	1	0	Race	{1, Caucasian }...	None	10	Center	Nominal
4	in_hosp_da	Date	11	0	Mother's hospitalization date	None	None	11	Center	Scale
5	dis_date	Date	11	0	Discharge date from hospitalization	None	None	11	Center	Scale
6	i_b_date	Date	11	0	Infant's birth date	None	None	11	Center	Scale
7	m_b_date	Date	11	0	Mother's birth date	None	None	11	Center	Scale
8	ap1	Numeric	8	0	Apgar at 1st minute	None	None	8	Center	Ordinal
9	ap5	Numeric	8	0	Apgar at 5th minute	None	None	8	Center	Ordinal
10	birth_weigh	Numeric	8	0	Birth-weight (in grams)	None	None	8	Center	Scale
11	ges_days	Numeric	8	0	Gestational age (in days)	None	None	8	Center	Scale
12	s_a_l_ges	Numeric	8	0	SGA/AGA/LGA	{1, SGA} ...	None	15	Right	Ordinal
13	APD	Numeric	8	0	Ante Partum Death	{0, No }...	None	8	Center	Nominal
14	IPD	Numeric	8	0	Intra Partum Death	{0, No }...	None	8	Center	Nominal
15	PPD	Numeric	8	0	Post Partum Death	{0, No }..	None	10	Center	Nominal
16	death_date	Date	11	0	Date of infant's death	None	None	10	Center	Scale
17	preg_num	Numeric	8	0	Number of pregnancies	None	None	8	Center	Scale
18	birth_num	Numeric	8	0	Number of births	None	None	8	Center	Scale
19	adver_obs	Numeric	8	0	Adverse obstetric history	{0, No }...	None	11	Center	Nominal
20	rec_abor	Numeric	8	0	Recurrent abortions	{0, No }...	None	8	Center	Nominal
21	pre_prema	Numeric	8	0	Previous premature labor	{0, No }...	None	13	Center	Nominal
22	infert_treat	Numeric	8	0	Infertility treatments	{0, No }...	None	8	Center	Nominal
23	poly	Numeric	8	0	Polyhydramnios	{0, No }...	None	8	Center	Nominal
24	oligo	Numeric	8	0	Oligohydramnios	{0, No }...	None	8	Center	Nominal
25	amniocynt	Numeric	8	0	Amniocyntesis	{0, No }...	None	12	Center	Nominal
26	PROM	Numeric	8	0	Premature rapture of membranes	{0, No }...	None	8	Center	Nominal

Figure 2. The Variable View of the SPSS Data Editor.

10	11	1	1	27-NOV-2005	28-NOV-2005
11	12	1	1	22-AUG-2005	28-AUG-2005
12	13	1	2	02-FEB-2005	06-FEB-2005
13	14	1	1	07-FEB-2005	.
14	15	2	1	26-APR-2005	29-APR-2005
15	16	1	1	04-NOV-2005	06-NOV-2005
16	17	2	1	03-MAY-2005	06-MAY-2005
17	18	1	1	03-JAN-2005	05-JAN-2005
18	19	1	2	13-APR-2005	20-APR-2005
19	20	2	1	25-JAN-2005	27-JAN-2005
20	21	1	1	16-JAN-2005	18-JAN-2005
21	22	1	2	09-MAR-2005	12-MAR-2005
22	23	2	1	14-NOV-2005	18-NOV-2005
23	24	1	1	20-NOV-2005	27-NOV-2005
24	25	1	1	20-NOV-2005	23-NOV-2005
25	26	1	1	30-JAN-2005	01-FEB-2005
26	27	1	1	03-JAN-2005	06-JAN-2005
27	28		2	22-NOV-2005	24-NOV-2005
28	29	2	2	23-FEB-2005	24-FEB-2005
29	30	2	1	21-MAR-2005	23-MAR-2005
30	31	2	2	25-AUG-2005	28-AUG-2005
31	32	2	2	14-MAY-2005	16-MAY-2005
32		2	2	14-AUG-2005	16-AUG-2005
33		2	2	19-NOV-2005	21-NOV-2005

Data View / Variable View

Figure 3. Shifting between Data View and Variable View.

The SPSS syntax is the file with the commands (as transformations) and procedures (the statistical analyses) [1–3]. We will create commands and procedures by using the SPSS dialog box. While using the dialog box, we can choose one of two options "OK" or "Paste". The recommended way of working is by clicking on the Paste tab rather than the OK tab because it creates documentation of written commands and procedures while OK does not. This is very important, especially when working on transformation variables. An example of syntax created automatically after choosing to work with the Paste option is shown in Figure 4.

The viewer is the SPSS output file [1–3]. In this file we will find the results after running the syntax file (see arrow in Figure 4). All commands and procedures will be performed on the data file, creating an output file. The next paragraphs will include examples of output files and further explanations.

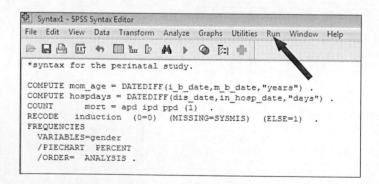

Figure 4. Example of a Syntax File.

Perinatal Data Analysis

Let us assume that we have a data file of a small obstetric department that includes information about 1200 mothers who gave birth during 2005. The data file includes variables such as demographic characteristics, chronic diseases, obstetric history, and information about the labor as well as the newborn (Addendum 1 includes the list of the study variables). In order to simplify the data analysis process, the data file consists of singleton births only.

Addendum 1. The Study Variables List.

Variable name	Variable label	Variable values
gender	Gender	1 Male, 2 Female
race	Race	1 Caucasian, 2 Afro-American
in_hosp_date	Mother's hospitalization date	
dis_date	Discharge date from hospitalization	
i_b_date	Infant's birth date	
m_b_date	Mother's birth date	
ap1	Apgar at 1st minute	
ap5	Apgar at 5th minute	
birth_weight	Birth-weight (in grams)	
ges_days	Gestational age (in days)	
s_a_l_ges_age	SGA/AGA/LGA	1 SGA, 2 AGA, 3 LGA
APD	Ante Partum Death	0 No, 1 Yes
IPD	Intra Partum Death	0 No, 1 Yes
PPD	Post Partum Death	0 No, 1 Yes
preg_num	Number of pregnancies	
birth_num	Number of births	
infert_treat	Infertility treatments	0 No, 1 Yes
poly	Polyhydramnios	0 No, 1 Yes
oligo	Oligohydramnios	0 No, 1 Yes
PROM	Premature rapture of membranes	0 No, 1 Yes
Cervical_incomp	Cervical incompetence	0 No, 1 Yes
placental_abru	Placental abruption	0 No, 1 Yes
placenta_previa	Placenta previa	0 No, 1 Yes
mal_presnt	Mal-presentation	0 No, 1 Yes
Malfor	Congenital malformations	0 No, 1 Yes
iugr	Intra uterine growth restriction	0 No, 1 Yes
fet_dist	Fetal distress	0 No, 1 Yes
miconium	Meconium stained amniotic fluid	0 No, 1 Yes
induction	Labor induction	0 No, 1 Yes
epidural	Epidural anesthesia	0 No, 1 Yes
general_anes	General anesthesia	0 No, 1 Yes
spontaneous_del	Spontaneous delivery	0 No, 1 Yes
cd	Caesarian delivery	0 No, 1 Yes
vacuum	Vacuum delivery	0 No, 1 Yes
post_pa_hemo	Post partum hemorrhage	0 No, 1 Yes
ret_placenta	Retained placenta	0 No, 1 Yes
Mild_pree	Mild preeclampsia	0 No, 1 Yes
severe_pree	Severe preeclampsia	0 No, 1 Yes
chr_htn	Chronic hypertension	0 No, 1 Yes
get_dm	Gestational diabetes mellitus	0 No, 1 Yes
dm	Diabetes Mellitus	0 No, 1 Yes
hemoglobin1	Maternal hemoglobin before delivery (g/dL)	0 No, 1 Yes
hemoglobin2	Maternal hemoglobin after delivery (g/dL)	0 No, 1 Yes

1. Descriptive Statistics

First of all, we would like to conduct a univariable analysis using mainly descriptive statistics [4]. The most common way is by using the "Frequencies" procedure. For example, we can present the gender distribution of the study's infants using a table and a chart [1–3].

After opening the data file we should click on *Analyze > Descriptive statistics>Frequencies* (Figure 5). Clicking on "Frequencies" will open the window shown in Figure 6. Now we choose the variables we would like to include in the procedure from the list on the left, simply by clicking on the variable name (Figure 6, 1) and then transferring it to the right window using the arrow button (Figure 6, 2). In all SPSS procedures the list on the left, presenting all the study variables, will appear in the same order as in the data file.

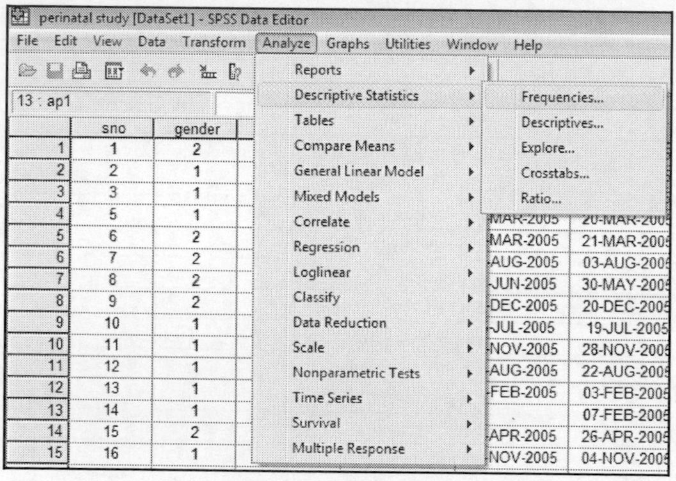

Figure 5. Descriptive Statistics of the Frequencies Procedure.

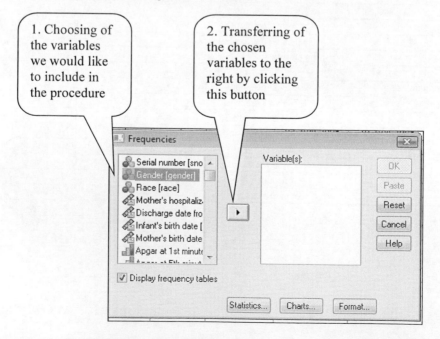

Figure 6. The Frequencies Procedure.

Now we can add the appropriate chart according to the descriptive statistics rules. In the Frequencies window we have to click on *Frequencies>Charts>Pie charts* (Figure 7). Now we can click on "Continue" and return to the main window. Clicking on Paste will automatically open a syntax file with the following text:

- FREQUENCIES
- VARIABLES=gender
- /PIECHART PERCENT
- /ORDER=ANALYSIS.

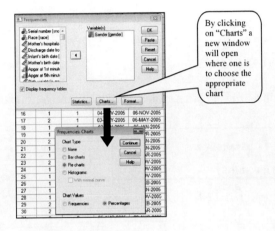

Figure 7. Adding a Chart to the Frequencies Procedure.

After running the Frequencies procedure, we will receive an output file that will look as shown in Figure 8.

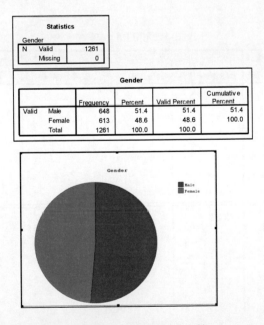

Statistics

Gender		
N	Valid	1261
	Missing	0

Gender

		Frequency	Percent	Valid Percent	Cumulative Percent
Valid	Male	648	51.4	51.4	51.4
	Female	613	48.6	48.6	100.0
	Total	1261	100.0	100.0	

Figure 8. The Output File Including the Frequencies Table and the Chart.

Frequencies

In the case of a continuous variable, such as birth weight, we can add statistics such as mean, median, mode, and standard deviation:

- Analyze> Descriptive statistics>**Frequencies>Statistics>mean, median**…

And the syntax will be:

- FREQUENCIES
- VARIABLES=birth_weight
- /STATISTICS=STDDEV MEAN MEDIAN MODE
- /ORDER=ANALYSIS.

The output will include the statistics table followed by the frequencies table (Figure 9).

Statistics

Birth-weight (in grams)

N	Valid	1261
	Missing	0
Mean		3157.27
Median		3215.00
Mode		3095
Std. Deviation		571.249

Birth-weight (in grams)

		Frequency	Percent	Valid Percent	Cumulative Percent
Valid	350	1	.1	.1	.1
	476	1	.1	.1	.2
	532	1	.1	.1	.2
	550	1	.1	.1	.3
	675	1	.1	.1	.4
	780	1	.1	.1	.5
	793	1	.1	.1	.6
	836	1	.1	.1	.6
	886	1	.1	.1	.7
	978	1	.1	.1	.8
	988	1	.1	.1	.9
	1008	1	.1	.1	1.0
	1158	1	.1	.1	1.0
	1160	1	1	1	1.1

Figure 9. The Output File Including the Statistics and the Frequencies Tables.

2. Transformations

Transformation is the creation of new variables according to the study hypothesis [1-3. For example, we calculate the mother's age (in years) at time of delivery, or the hospitalization duration (in days). In addition, we can create new variables by recoding the original variables, for instance, the variable of low Apgar scores (<7) at 1 minute and 5 minutes is created through the recoding of the original Apgar scores.

Another example of such transformation can be done when recoding the original birth weight variable to a low birth weight variable (<2500 g). Furthermore, we can construct a new variable, such as infant mortality, according to the APD, IPD, and PPD values, which had all been originally included in the data file.

Calculating the Mother's Age

The mother's age variable can be calculated by clicking the following [1-3].

- Transform> Compute…

The window shown in Figure 10 will then open. First, we type the "Target Variable" (Figure 10, 1)—for example, "mom_age"; next we choose the "Function group" needed (Figure 10, 2), which in this case of calculating the mother's age it is "Date Arithmetic"; afterwards we choose the function "Datediff" (Figure 10, 3) that calculates the time difference between any two dates, using any time units (years, months, or days…).

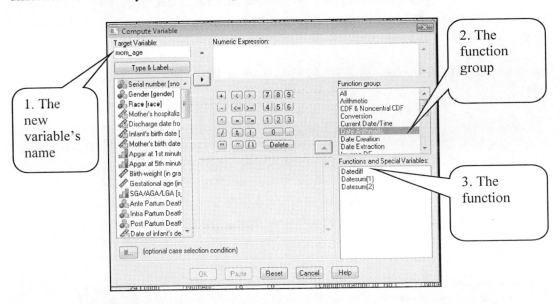

Figure 10. Computing Time Interval from two Date Variables.

After choosing "Datediff", we insert the "Numeric Expression" (Figure 11, 1). The pattern of the Numeric Expression should be as follows: datetime2, datetime1, "unit" (see arrow in Figure 11). For example, when calculating the mother's age (in years) at the time of giving birth, the pattern of the Numeric Expression is: infant's birth date, mother's birth date, "years" (Figure 11, 1).

Finally, we click the Paste button, which will result the following syntax:

- COMPUTE mom_age = DATEDIFF(i_b_date,m_b_date,"years").

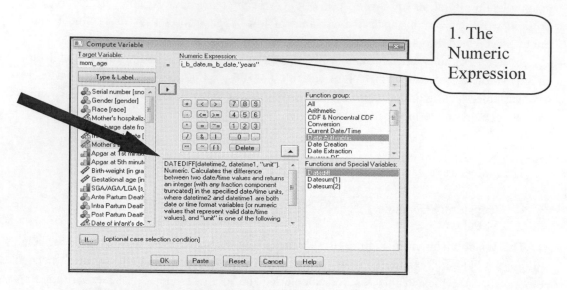

Figure 11. The Numeric Expression of the New Variable.

In the same way we can create a new variable of hospitalization duration (in days) by calculating the time difference between the mother's discharge date from the hospital and the mother's hospitalization date. In this case, the syntax is:

- COMPUTE hospdays=DATEDIFF(dis_date,in_hosp_date,"days".

Creating a New Variable – Infant Mortality

Sometime we create a new variable by summarizing other variables. For example, our data include three variables of infant mortality: APD, IPD, and PPD (Ante-Partum Death, Intra-Partum Death, and Post-Partum Death, respectively). After examining each of the original variables separately, we can create a new variable of infant mortality. Logically, if the answer to one of the original variables is "yes", the result of the new infant mortality variable would also be "yes". If our data have no errors, then only one variable can be "yes". We can count the number of positive answers and the total will represent the value of infant mortality.

In "Transform" click the following [1-3]:

- Transform> Count…

As shown in the window in Figure 12, we type the name of the target variable – for instance, "infant_mortality" (Figure 12, 1); then we define the variables that constitute the new variable (APD, IPD, and PPD) as depicted in Figure 12, number 2.

Next, we click on "Define Values" (see arrow in Figure 12) in order to define the values that are going to be counted, for instance in the example shown below, it is "1" (see arrow in Figure 13).

We can also define ranges of values if needed, as shown in Figure 13. After clicking on the "Continue" button, you then click on Paste, which will result the following syntax:

- COUNT infant_mortality=APD IPD PPD (1)

When running this syntax, the new variable will be created in the data file.

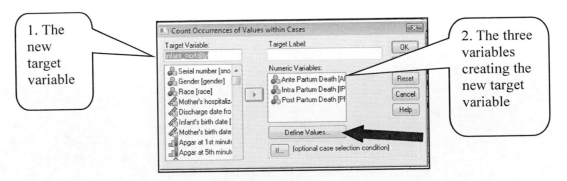

Figure 12. Creating New Variable by Counting Values

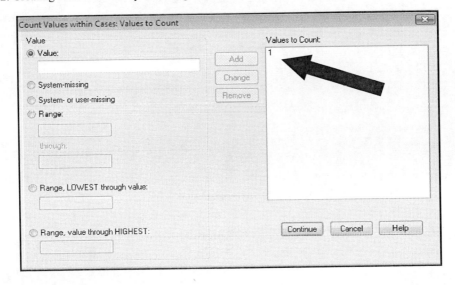

Figure 13. Defining the Values to be counted.

3. Bivariable Analysis

Bivariable analysis is the testing of the relationship between two variables or the differences between groups of the study participants.[4, 5] Two or more groups can be compared, for example, by the comparison of the variables' means. The decision to perform comparison of means should be done according to the statistical rules mentioned in the beginning of this chapter. For example, we can compare the birth weight of infants born with or without congenital malformations. When comparing between just two groups, the t-test is preferred. In the case of three or more groups, the One-Way ANOVA test is to be performed.

In order to compare the variables' means we do the following:[1–3]

•   Analyze> Compare Means>Independent-Samples T-Test…

As shown in Figure 14, you can choose from all the procedures for comparing means, including the Independent-Samples T-Test, the paired-samples T-Test, as well as the One-Way ANOVA.

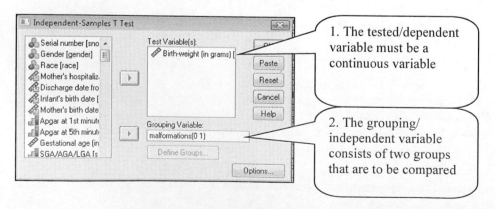

Figure 14. Comparison of Means Procedures.

When clicking on "Independent-Samples T-Test…" the window shown in Figure 15 will open. There, we will define the tested or the dependent variable (Figure 15, 1), in addition to the grouping variable or the independent variable (Figure 15, 2).

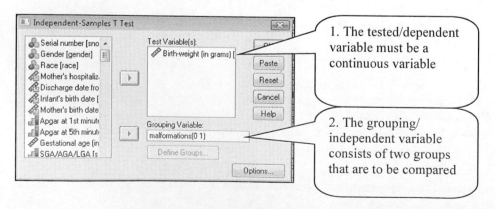

Figure 15. Defining the Test Variable and the Grouping Variable of the Independent Sample t-test Procedure.

Again, click on Paste, which will result the following syntax:

- T-TEST
- GROUPS=malformations(0 1)
- /MISSING=ANALYSIS
- /VARIABLES=birth_weight
- /CRITERIA=CI(.95).

Once the syntax is running, an output file will be created. An output file looks as depicted in Figure 16; it includes the descriptive statistics table and the t-test table.

From the descriptive statistics table we can see that newborns with congenital malformations have a lower mean birth weight (2903.68 g ± 849.47 g) compared to newborns without congenital malformations (3183.21 g ± 528.43 g) (Figure 16, 1). Examining the second table detects that "Leven's Test for Equality of Variances" is statistically significant (p < 0.001) (Figure 16, 2), meaning that we cannot assume equal variances (we reject the null hypothesis of equality of variances). As a result, we look at the second row of the t-test values. The result of the birth weight comparison according to the t-test procedure is statistically significant (p = 0.001) (Figure 16, 3).

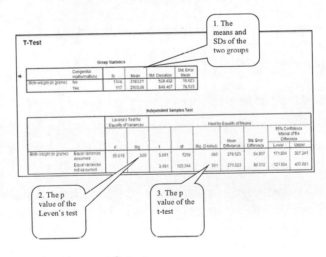

Figure 16. The Independent-Samples t-test Output.

The reported results should be written as follows: the mean birth weight of newborns with congenital malformations was found to be lower than newborns without congenital malformations (2903.68 ± 849.47 g and 3183.21 ± 528.43 g, respectively) (p = 0.001).

Occasionally, during the course of a study, certain observations are measured several times. The simplest situation is when we have a set of two repeated measurements; for example, in our study there are two hemoglobin test results, before and after delivery; therefore, we can examine the hypothesis of a decrease in hemoglobin level at the time of labor. In such a situation, the suitable statistical test is paired-samples t-test. Unlike in the previous example, we have two continuous variables that are measured at two different times during the study, instead of the comparison of the means of two groups.

In order to perform a comparison of two paired means, we will do the following:[1-3]

- Analyze> Compare Means> paired-samples T-Test

The screen shown in Figure 17 will appear. Only when choosing both of the variables (Variable 1, Variable 2) (Figure 17, 1), can we transfer the two to the "Paired Variables" on the right (Figure 17, 2).

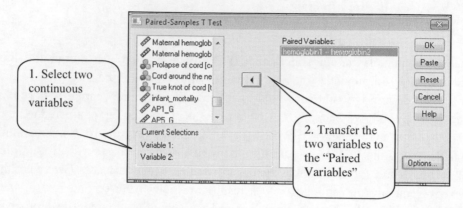

Figure 17. The Paired-samples t-test Procedure.

- T-TEST
- PAIRS=hemoglobin1 WITH hemoglobin2 (PAIRED)
- /CRITERIA=CI(.95)
- /MISSING=ANALYSIS.

Once the syntax above has been run, the output shown in Figure 18 will be created.

T-Test

The output of the paired-samples t-test (Figure 18) consists of 3 tables: the first table is the descriptive statistics of the two variables – the mean and the standard deviation of the hemoglobin levels, before and after delivery. Note how the mean of the hemoglobin after delivery is lower than the hemoglobin mean before delivery. The middle table presents the correlation between the variables, which were found to be statistically significant. The last table is the result of the paired t-test, which shows that the difference between the hemoglobin means, before and after delivery, is statistically significant ($p < 0.001$).

Bivariable analysis can also compare the proportions/rates of two categorical variables.[4, 5] For example, we would like to compare the proportions of cesarean deliveries in newborns with congenital malformations to newborns without congenital malformations. In this example, the two variables are referred to as "dichotomous variables", where these variables have only two groups; therefore, the suitable statistical tests are the chi-square test, or the Fisher's exact test, both of which examine the differences in qualitative variables.

Paired Samples Statistics

		Mean	N	Std. Deviation	Std. Error Mean
Pair 1	Maternal hemoglobin before delivery (gr/dl)	12.704	766	1.9757	.0714
	Maternal hemoglobin after delivery (gr/dl)	10.991	766	1.4630	.0529

Paired Samples Correlations

		N	Correlation	Sig.
Pair 1	Maternal hemoglobin before delivery (gr/dl) & Maternal hemoglobin after delivery (gr/dl)	766	.101	.005

Paired Samples Test

		Paired Differences					t	df	Sig. (2-tailed)
		Mean	Std. Deviation	Std. Error Mean	95% Confidence Interval of the Difference Lower	Upper			
Pair 1	Maternal hemoglobin before delivery (gr/dl) - Maternal hemoglobin after delivery (gr/dl)	1.7128	2.3372	.0844	1.5470	1.8785	20.283	765	.000

Figure 18. The Paired-samples t-test Output.

In order to perform the comparison above, do the following:[1-3]

- Analyze>Descriptive Statistics >Crosstabs…

The screen shown in Figure 19 will appear.

First choose the variables for the "Crosstabs" procedure (congenital malformations and cesarean delivery), then transfer them to the "Row" and "Column" (Figure 19, 1). After clicking on the "cells" button, check the relevant percentages, such as the percentage of the rows or of the columns (Figure 19, 2). The statistical tests can be added after clicking on "statistics" and checking "Chi-square" and "Risk" (Figure 19, 3).

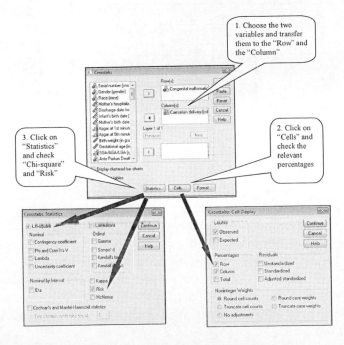

Figure 19. Crosstabulation, Chi-Square Test, and Risk Estimate Procedure.

Once the syntax below is running, an output file is created (Figure 20):

- CROSSTABS
- /TABLES=malformations BY cd
- /FORMAT=AVALUE TABLES
- /STATISTIC=CHISQ RISK
- /CELLS=COUNT ROW COLUMN
- /COUNT ROUND CELL

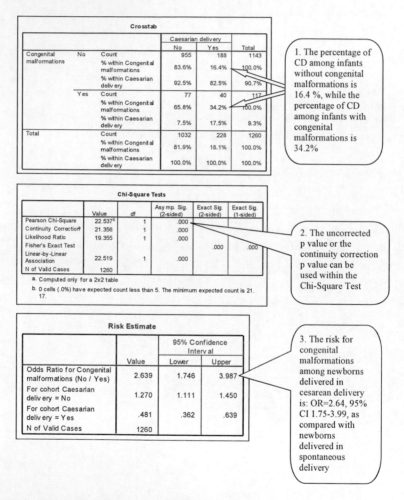

Figure 20. Crosstabulation, Chi Square Test, and Risk Estimate Output.

*Congenital Malformations * Caesarian Delivery*

In some studies the sample size is not big enough; therefore, the table will have over 20% of expected count with values less than 5. In such a case, the Fisher's exact test is the most suitable test. For example, if we compare the proportions of perinatal mortality by congenital malformations, we will obtain the tables shown in Figure 21. We can see that the rate of mortality is 1.0% among infants without malformations, while the rate is 11.1% among infants with malformations.

Congenital malformations * infant_mortality Crosstabulation

			infant mortality		
			.00	1.00	Total
Congenital malformations	No	Count	1133	11	1144
		% within Congenital malformations	99.0%	1.0%	100.0%
		% within infant_mortality	91.6%	45.8%	90.7%
	Yes	Count	104	13	117
		% within Congenital malformations	88.9%	11.1%	100.0%
		% within infant_mortality	8.4%	54.2%	9.3%
Total		Count	1237	24	1261
		% within Congenital malformations	98.1%	1.9%	100.0%
		% within infant_mortality	100.0%	100.0%	100.0%

Chi-Square Tests

	Value	df	Asymp. Sig. (2-sided)	Exact Sig. (2-sided)	Exact Sig. (1-sided)
Pearson Chi-Square	58.565[b]	1	.000		
Continuity Correction [a]	53.255	1	.000		
Likelihood Ratio	32.000	1	.000		
Fisher's Exact Test				.000	.000
Linear-by-Linear Association	58.519	1	.000		
N of Valid Cases	1261				

a. Computed only for a 2x2 table

b. 1 cells (25.0%) have expected count less than 5. The minimum expected count is 2.23.

Risk Estimate

		95% Confidence Interval	
	Value	Lower	Upper
Odds Ratio for Congenital malformations (No / Yes)	12.875	5.627	29.458
For cohort infant_mortality = .00	1.114	1.045	1.188
For cohort infant_mortality = 1.00	.087	.040	.189
N of Valid Cases	1261		

Figure 21. Crosstabulation, Fisher's Exact Test, and Risk Estimate Output.

In the second table (Figure 21) we notice that the Fisher's exact test p value should be used, and not the p value of Pearson's chi-square test.

The last table (Figure 21) presents the risk of mortality, which is OR=12.87, 95% CI 5.63–29.46, and is a measurement of the strength of the association between the presence of a factor and the occurrence of an event. If the confidence interval for the statistic includes a value of 1, one cannot assume that the factor is associated with the event. The odds ratio (OR) can be used as an estimate of relative risk when the occurrence of the factor is rare.[5–8]

- CROSSTABS
- /TABLES=malformations BY infant_mortality
- /FORMAT= AVALUE TABLES
- /STATISTIC=CHISQ
- /CELLS=COUNT ROW COLUMN
- /COUNT ROUND CELL

Once the syntax above is running, the output file in Figure 21 will be created.

Crosstabs

4. Multivariable Analysis

The reasons, ways of performing, and interpretations of multivariable analysis are all included in statistics books dealing generally with medical research [9, 10] and particularly perinatology [11]. There are four major reasons for performing multivariable analysis, all of which are detailed in the chapter "The importance of multivariable analysis for conducting and evaluating research in perinatology" in this book.

Stratification Using Mantel-Haenszel Procedure

One of the reasons for conducting stratified analysis is to determine the unique contributions of a single variable on a single outcome while holding other variables constant, thereby eliminating confounding [5–8, 11]. For example, in the bivariable analysis we found that congenital malformations are a significant risk factor for low birth weight (LBW). As seen in Figure 22, the risk for LBW of infants with congenital malformations is 3.72-fold that of infants with normal birth weight (95% CI 2.35–5.89, p < 0.001).

lbw * Congenital malformations Crosstabulation

			Congenital malformations		Total
			No	Yes	
lbw	.00	Count	1043	86	1129
		% within lbw	92.4%	7.6%	100.0%
		% within Congenital malformations	91.2%	73.5%	89.5%
	1.00	Count	101	31	132
		% within lbw	76.5%	23.5%	100.0%
		% within Congenital malformations	8.8%	26.5%	10.5%
Total		Count	1144	117	1261
		% within lbw	90.7%	9.3%	100.0%
		% within Congenital malformations	100.0%	100.0%	100.0%

Chi-Square Tests

	Value	df	Asymp. Sig. (2-sided)	Exact Sig. (2-sided)	Exact Sig. (1-sided)
Pearson Chi-Square	35.350[b]	1	.000		
Continuity Correction[a]	33.490	1	.000		
Likelihood Ratio	27.094	1	.000		
Fisher's Exact Test				.000	.000
Linear-by-Linear Association	35.322	1	.000		
N of Valid Cases	1261				

a. Computed only for a 2x2 table

b. 0 cells (.0%) have expected count less than 5. The minimum expected count is 12.25.

Risk Estimate

	Value	95% Confidence Interval	
		Lower	Upper
Odds Ratio for lbw (.00 / 1.00)	3.722	2.353	5.888
For cohort Congenital malformations = No	1.207	1.097	1.329
For cohort Congenital malformations = Yes	.324	.224	.469
N of Valid Cases	1261		

Figure 22. Crosstabulation and Risk Estimate Output.

lbw * preterm37 Crosstabulation

			preterm37		Total
			.00	1.00	
lbw	.00	Count	1098	29	1127
		% within lbw	97.4%	2.6%	100.0%
		% within preterm37	95.6%	26.4%	89.5%
	1.00	Count	51	81	132
		% within lbw	38.6%	61.4%	100.0%
		% within preterm37	4.4%	73.6%	10.5%
Total		Count	1149	110	1259
		% within lbw	91.3%	8.7%	100.0%
		% within preterm37	100.0%	100.0%	100.0%

Chi-Square Tests

	Value	df	Asymp. Sig. (2-sided)	Exact Sig. (2-sided)	Exact Sig. (1-sided)
Pearson Chi-Square	512.182[b]	1	.000		
Continuity Correction[a]	504.835	1	.000		
Likelihood Ratio	300.726	1	.000		
Fisher's Exact Test				.000	.000
Linear-by-Linear Association	511.775	1	.000		
N of Valid Cases	1259				

a. Computed only for a 2x2 table

b. 0 cells (.0%) have expected count less than 5. The minimum expected count is 11.53.

Risk Estimate

	Value	95% Confidence Interval	
		Lower	Upper
Odds Ratio for lbw (.00 / 1.00)	60.134	36.159	100.004
For cohort preterm37 = .00	2.522	2.033	3.127
For cohort preterm37 = 1.00	.042	.029	.062
N of Valid Cases	1259		

Figure 23. Crosstabulation and Risk Estimate Output.

As we know, one of the important risk factors for LBW is gestational age. The risk for LBW of infants born in preterm delivery is significantly greater than in infants born in term delivery. The results shown in Figure 23 are based on the definition of preterm delivery of < 37 weeks of gestational age. These results show that the risk is OR=60.13-fold (95% CI 36.16–100.00, p < 0.001).

Since there is an association between congenital malformation and gestational age, the possibility that gestational age may be a confounder should be tested (few epidemiology textbooks can give you further explanations for the concept of confounding) [5–8].

In order to resolve this question, one of the well-known adjustment procedures can be performed, for example, the Mantel-Haenszel procedure [5–8]. This procedure is designed to test the independence between a dichotomous factor variable and a dichotomous response variable, conditional upon covariate patterns defined by one or more layer (control) variable.

We will use the same Crosstabs procedure, adding the 3rd variable – preterm delivery, which is the layer variable (Figure 24, 1) [1–3]. Next, we will click on "statistics" and check the Mantel-Haenszel statistic (Figure 24, 2).

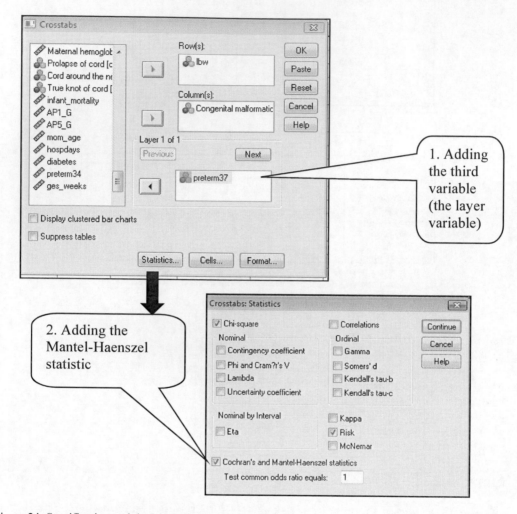

Figure 24. Stratification and the Mantel-Haenszel Procedure.

Once the following syntax is running, the output file shown in Figure 25A will be created.

- CROSSTABS
- /TABLES=lbw by malformations by preterm37
- /FORMAT=AVALUE TABLES
- /STATISTIC=CHISQ RISK CMH(1)
- /CELLS=COUNT ROW COLUMN
- /COUNT ROUND CELL.

Crosstabs

The first two tables (Figure 25A) are the stratification by preterm delivery; the first includes newborns born within term delivery, while the second includes newborns born within preterm delivery. We are able to look at each stratum separately, as well as each of their chi-square tests. Following, is another part of the output, in which the test of homogeneity of the odds ratio and the Mantel-Haenszel statistic is presented (Figure 25B). The test of homogeneity of the odds ratio (Breslow-Day test) is not statistically significant (p = 0.41), meaning we did not reject the null hypothesis of homogeneity of the two ORs. When looking at the last table of Figure 25B, we can notice that the Mantel-Haenszel statistic is significant (p = 0.016) and the adjusted OR is 2.51 95% CI 1.27–4.95.

lbw * Congenital malformations * preterm37 Crosstabulation

preterm37				Congenital malformations No	Congenital malformations Yes	Total
.00	lbw	.00	Count	1015	83	1098
			% within lbw	92.4%	7.6%	100.0%
			% within Congenital malformations	95.8%	92.2%	95.6%
		1.00	Count	44	7	51
			% within lbw	86.3%	13.7%	100.0%
			% within Congenital malformations	4.2%	7.8%	4.4%
	Total		Count	1059	90	1149
			% within lbw	92.2%	7.8%	100.0%
			% within Congenital malformations	100.0%	100.0%	100.0%
1.00	lbw	.00	Count	26	3	29
			% within lbw	89.7%	10.3%	100.0%
			% within Congenital malformations	31.3%	11.1%	26.4%
		1.00	Count	57	24	81
			% within lbw	70.4%	29.6%	100.0%
			% within Congenital malformations	68.7%	88.9%	73.6%
	Total		Count	83	27	110
			% within lbw	75.5%	24.5%	100.0%
			% within Congenital malformations	100.0%	100.0%	100.0%

Chi-Square Tests

preterm37		Value	df	Asymp. Sig. (2-sided)	Exact Sig. (2-sided)	Exact Sig. (1-sided)
.00	Pearson Chi-Square	2.567[b]	1	.109		
	Continuity Correction[a]	1.784	1	.182		
	Likelihood Ratio	2.154	1	.142		
	Fisher's Exact Test				.111	.097
	Linear-by-Linear Association	2.565	1	.109		
	N of Valid Cases	1149				
1.00	Pearson Chi-Square	4.288[c]	1	.038		
	Continuity Correction[a]	3.010	1	.083		
	Likelihood Ratio	4.866	1	.027		
	Fisher's Exact Test				.045	.030
	Linear-by-Linear Association	4.249	1	.039		
	N of Valid Cases	110				

a. Computed only for a 2x2 table

b. 1 cells (25.0%) have expected count less than 5. The minimum expected count is 3.99.

c. 0 cells (.0%) have expected count less than 5. The minimum expected count is 7.12.

Figure 25A. Stratification and the Chi Square Test Output.

Risk Estimate

preterm37		Value	95% Confidence Interval	
			Lower	Upper
.00	Odds Ratio for lbw (.00 / 1.00)	1.946	.850	4.454
	For cohort Congenital malformations = No	1.071	.959	1.197
	For cohort Congenital malformations = Yes	.551	.268	1.130
	N of Valid Cases	1149		
1.00	Odds Ratio for lbw (.00 / 1.00)	3.649	1.008	13.213
	For cohort Congenital malformations = No	1.274	1.056	1.537
	For cohort Congenital malformations = Yes	.349	.114	1.073
	N of Valid Cases	110		

Tests of Homogeneity of the Odds Ratio

	Chi-Squared	df	Asymp. Sig. (2-sided)
Breslow-Day	.691	1	.406
Tarone's	.658	1	.417

Tests of Conditional Independence

	Chi-Squared	df	Asymp. Sig. (2-sided)
Cochran's	6.790	1	.009
Mantel-Haenszel	5.839	1	.016

Under the conditional independence assumption, Cochran's statistic is asymptotically distributed as a 1 df chi-squared distribution, only if the number of strata is fixed, while the Mantel-Haenszel statistic is always asymptotically distributed as a a 1 df chi-squared distribution. Note that the continuity correction is removed from the Mantel-Haenszel statistic when the sum of the differences between the observed and the expected is 0.

Mantel-Haenszel Common Odds Ratio Estimate

Estimate			2.505
ln(Estimate)			.918
Std. Error of ln(Estimate)			.347
Asymp. Sig. (2-sided)			.008
Asymp. 95% Confidence Interval	Common Odds Ratio	Lower Bound	1.268
		Upper Bound	4.949
	ln(Common Odds Ratio)	Lower Bound	.238
		Upper Bound	1.599

The Mantel-Haenszel common odds ratio estimate is asymptotically normally distributed under the common odds ratio of 1.000 assumption. So is the natural log of the estimate.

Figure 25B. Stratification and the Mantel-Haenszel Output.

The crude OR (Figure 22) estimates the risk for LBW of infants with congenital malformations when compared with infants with no congenital malformations. The risk is found to be 3.72 (95% CI 2.35–5.89, $p < 0.001$), as shown in Figure 22. However, the adjusted OR for LBW is slightly lower, meaning that even after controlling for preterm delivery, congenital malformation is still a risk factor for LBW.

The Mantel-Haenszel procedure is an important statistical procedure that tests the possibility of confounding; however, if the homogeneity test is significant ($p < 0.05$), the adjusted statistic cannot be used since we are facing an interaction or an effect modification.

Multiple Logistic Regression Model

Stratification works well only in situations in which there is only one confounder. However, usually in perinatology there are many potential confounders or risk factors that are associated with the dependent variable (outcome) [9–11]. In such a case, a multivariable analysis should be applied, which will enable determination of the independent contribution of each of the risk factors. The type of multivariable analysis depends on the outcome variable type. If the outcome variable is continuous, multiple linear regression would be the suitable model to use, although in the case of a dichotomous dependent variable or outcome, the logistic regression model should be applied, for instance, congenital malformations (yes/no) [10].

To illustrate how to perform and interpret multiple logistic regression we will use the previous example in which the outcome variable is LBW and the two risk factors are preterm delivery and congenital malformations. The result of the stratification and the Mantel-Haenszel statistic is the adjusted OR of congenital malformations, while controlling for preterm delivery. Moreover, we can perform another Mantel-Haenszel procedure in which the result will be an adjusted OR of preterm delivery while controlling for congenital malformations (stratification by congenital malformations). However, when using multiple logistic regression the results will include both of the adjusted ORs (for congenital malformations and preterm delivery).

Before performing multiple logistic regression a few rules should be emphasized [2, 10]. These rules concern the type of variables that are included in the model, in addition to the number of variables. When the dependent variable is dichotomous or binary, it is better if the format is 0/1 and not another format, such as 1/2. The latest SPSS versions recode these values to the format of 0/1, which will also be reported in the output explaining the way it was done (1 → 0; 2→ 1). The disadvantage of this method is that we cannot decide how to code the groups ourselves (which group will be coded as 1), since this decision will influence the way the ORs will be calculated. For example, if we are to perform a logistic regression for the outcome of LBW, we will code newborns with LBW as 1, and newborns with normal weight as 0. By doing so, the ORs in this model will be calculated for the risk of LBW, while being compared to normal birth weight, and not the other way around.

With regard to the independent variables (covariates) or the risk factors, the variables can be either continuous, dichotomous (yes/no), or categorical. We can enter the first two types of variables in the model in their original format. However, categorical variables with three or more groups should be entered in the model as dummy variables and not in their original format. As far as the number of covariates, the ratio of at least ten outcomes per independent variable is acceptable [9–11].

In order to perform a logistic regression, do as the following [1–3]:

- Analyze>Regression >Binary Logistic…

First, we will add the dependent variable (LBW) and the independent variables (preterm delivery and congenital malformations) (Figure 26, 1). Then we will choose the "Enter" method (Figure 26, 2), which forces the computer to include all the variables in the model. It is also possible to choose methods other than "Enter", such as "Forward" or "Backward" eliminations. These methods can be useful if we would like the computer to choose the included variables in this model. In most cases, we are interested in controlling for potential confounders, and should avoid using methods other than "Enter".

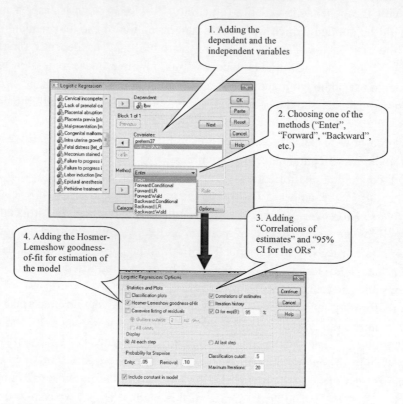

Figure 26. Multiple Logistic Regression Model procedure.

Next, click on "options", which will open the second screen shown in Figure 26, 2. There, check the confidence intervals and the estimation of correlations between variables included in the model (Figure 26, 3). By checking the "Correlations of estimates" we examine the correlation between covariates that are included in the model (multicollinearity). Try to avoid a high correlation between variables, because when two variables are highly correlated it is impossible for the model to identify the independent contribution of each of them. We can also add the Hosmer-Lemeshow goodness-of-fit (Figure 26, 4). Goodness-of-fit statistics are a measurement of how well an explanatory model predicts the outcome. This statistic compares the estimated to observed likelihood of outcome in the study. In a well-fitting model, the estimated likelihood will be close to that observed and the p value will not be significant (p > 0.05).

When running the following syntax, an output file will be created. Most of the output tables are shown in Figure 27A,B,C.

- LOGISTIC REGRESSION lbw
- /METHOD=ENTER preterm37 malformations
- /PRINT=GOODFIT CORR CI(95)
- /CRITERIA=PIN(.05) POUT(.10) ITERATE(20) CUT(.5).

Logistic Regression

In the first table of the Logistic Regresstion Model Output (Figure 27A) there is information about the number of participants included in the analysis and the missing cases percentage. Note that the percentage of missing cases is relatively low (2%). In cases of high percentages of missing cases, we need to compare the participants who were included in the analysis to the participants who were not. This comparison is done to indicate whether there is a selection bias [8]. The next table informs us about the recoding of the dependent variable; in our example the values remain the same because the original values were 0/1.

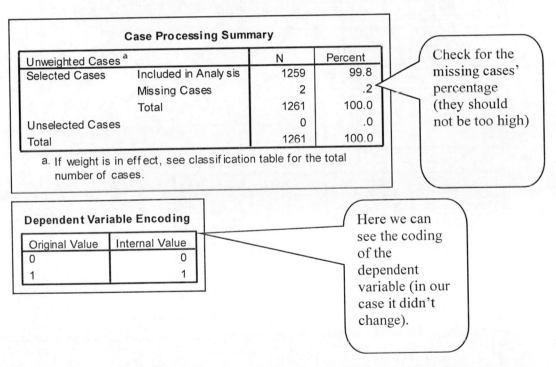

Case Processing Summary

Unweighted Cases [a]		N	Percent
Selected Cases	Included in Analysis	1259	99.8
	Missing Cases	2	.2
	Total	1261	100.0
Unselected Cases		0	.0
Total		1261	100.0

a. If weight is in effect, see classification table for the total number of cases.

Check for the missing cases' percentage (they should not be too high)

Dependent Variable Encoding

Original Value	Internal Value
0	0
1	1

Here we can see the coding of the dependent variable (in our case it didn't change).

Figure 27A. Part A of the Logistic Regression Model Output—Case Processing and the Dependent Variable.

Block 1: Method = Enter

The second part of the Logistic Regression Output (Figure 27B) presents information about the goodness-of-fit statistics. These statistics are a measurement of how well an explanatory model predicts the outcome. When looking at the -2LL and the Nagelkerke R square, notice that 44% of the variance of the dependent variable (LBW) can be explained due to the covariates included in the model (preterm delivery and congenital malformations). The Hosmer-Lemeshow goodness-of-fit is not statistically significant; in addition, according to the classification table there is a total prediction of 93.6%. In conclusion, according to all the statistics above, the model goodness-of-fit is fine.

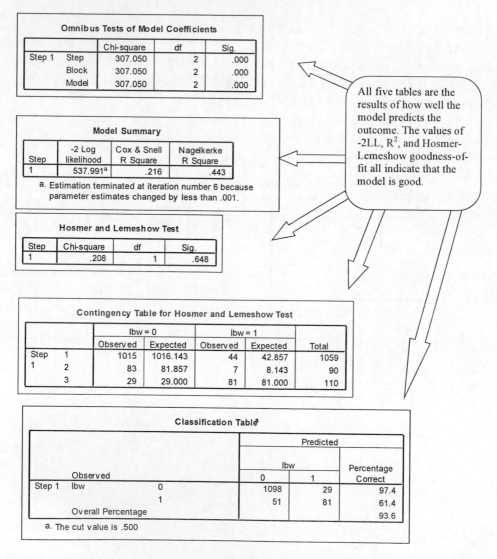

Omnibus Tests of Model Coefficients

		Chi-square	df	Sig.
Step 1	Step	307.050	2	.000
	Block	307.050	2	.000
	Model	307.050	2	.000

Model Summary

Step	-2 Log likelihood	Cox & Snell R Square	Nagelkerke R Square
1	537.991[a]	.216	.443

a. Estimation terminated at iteration number 6 because parameter estimates changed by less than .001.

Hosmer and Lemeshow Test

Step	Chi-square	df	Sig.
1	.208	1	.648

Contingency Table for Hosmer and Lemeshow Test

		lbw = 0		lbw = 1		Total
		Observed	Expected	Observed	Expected	
Step 1	1	1015	1016.143	44	42.857	1059
	2	83	81.857	7	8.143	90
	3	29	29.000	81	81.000	110

Classification Table[a]

			Predicted		
			lbw		Percentage Correct
Observed			0	1	
Step 1	lbw	0	1098	29	97.4
		1	51	81	61.4
	Overall Percentage				93.6

a. The cut value is .500

All five tables are the results of how well the model predicts the outcome. The values of -2LL, R^2, and Hosmer-Lemeshow goodness-of-fit all indicate that the model is good.

Figure 27B. Part B of the Logistic Regression Model Output—Goodness-of-Fit.

The third part of the Logistic Regresstion Output (Figure 27C) depicts information regarding the relationship between each of the independent variables (covariate) with the dependent variable. The most important results are the adjusted ORs and their 95% CIs. According to the first table (Figure 27C), infants born with congenital malformations are at a 2.4-fold risk (OR=2.4 95% CI 1.2–4.5) for LBW compared to infants without congenital malformations. Also, the risk for LBW of infants born in preterm delivery is 55.5-fold greater compared to infants born in term delivery. Both of these risks are adjusted for the other. In fact, the results of the stratification and the Mantel-Haenszel statistic, which we performed previously, are very similar to the adjusted OR originating from the logistic regression model. One of the important advantages of the regression model is being able to control for several variables at the same time. When several independent variables are included in the model, pay attention to the sample size, hence a sufficient number of LBW infants.

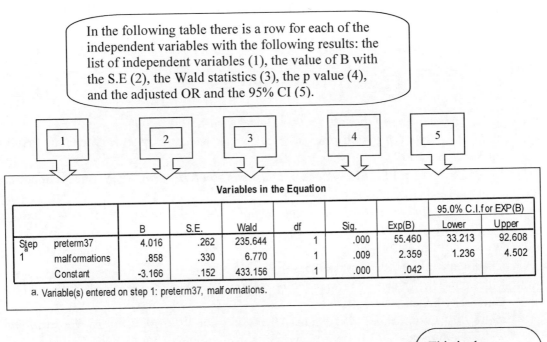

Figure 27C. Part C of the Logistic Regression Model Output—The Relationship between the Independent Variables and the Dependent Variable.

In the last table (Figure 27C) there is information about the correlations between the independent variables. Try to avoid a situation of high correlation between covariates included in the model (multicollinearity). In the case of a high correlation, change the model, for example, by removing one of the variables [9–11].

Summary

Although performing data analysis with SPSS® for Windows would be considered relatively friendly and simple, in the case of a perinatal study we should be very careful in the process of choosing a suitable statistical test.

Start with the descriptive statistics followed by the bivariable analysis; perform the multivariable analysis only at the end of the process.

In the field of perinatal epidemiology, the multivariable analysis models are a very important tool due to their ability to control for potential confounders. However, by performing all of the data analysis steps mentioned in this chapter, one will have better knowledge of the data, hence a better statistical analysis resulting in an improved ability to reach correct conclusions.

References

[1] *SPSS for Windows, 14.0: User's guide.* Chicago: SPSS Inc.; 2005.

[2] *Field A. Discovering statistics using SPSS for windows. 2nd ed.* London: SAGE Publications; 2005.

[3] Landau S, Everitt BS. *A Handbook of Statistical Analysis using SPSS.* Boca Raton, FL: Chapman & Hall/CRC Press; 2004.

[4] Stevens J. *Statistical analysis of epidemiology data. 2nd ed.* New York: Oxford University Press; 1996.

[5] Woodward M. *Epidemiology study design and data analysis. 2nd ed.* Boca Raton, FL: Chapman & Hall/CRC Press; 2005.

[6] Lilienfeld DE, Stolley PD. *Foundations of Epidemiology. 3rd ed.* New York: Oxford University Press; 1994.

[7] Kelsey JL, Whittemore AS, Evans AS, Thompson WD. *Methods in Observational Epidemiology. 2nd ed.* New York: Oxford University Press; 1996.

[8] Szklo M, Nieto FJ. *Epidemiology: beyond the basics. 2nd ed.* Sudbury, MA: Jones and Bartlett Publishers; 2007.

[9] Stevens J. *Applied multivariate statistics for the social sciences.* Mahwah, NJ: Lawrence Erlbaum Associates, Inc.; 2001.

[10] Hosmer DW, Lemeshow S. *Applied logistic regression.* New York: John Wiley & Sons, Inc.; 1989.

[11] Katz MH. *Multivariable analysis: a practical guide for clinicians. 2nd ed.* New York: Cambridge University Press; 2006.

In: Textbook of Perinatal Epidemiology
Editor: Eyal Sheiner, pp. 111-125

ISBN: 978-1-60741-648-7
© 2010 Nova Science Publishers, Inc.

Chapter IX

Meta-Analyses

Hairong Xu [*] *and William D. Fraser*

Department of Obstetrics and Gynecology, Hôpital Sainte-Justine,
Université de Montréal, QC, Canada

Definition

Meta-Analysis: A study which combines the results of several studies that address a set of related research hypotheses.

Introduction

Clinicians are increasingly required to guide their practice based on the best available evidence. Synthesis of the available evidence therefore remains essential for good clinical practice. One of important approaches to handling a vast array of data is systematic review. A systematic review is a form of research that provides a summary of medical reports, using explicit methods to search, critically appraise and synthesize the published or unpublished evidence concerning a specific clinical question. Quantitative systematic review, or meta-analysis, combine different studies to produce an overall effect estimate of a specific treatment using explicit statistical techniques. The role of systematic review and meta-analysis has been increasingly endorsed in evidence-based decision making. The present chapter provides an overview of basic and quantitative methods and issues needed to be considered for the conduct of meta-analysis.

[*] For Correspondence: Hairong Xu, MD, MSc, PhD Candidate, Department of Obstetrics and Gynecology and Social and Preventive Medicine, Université de Montréal hairongxx@yahoo.ca

History of Meta-Analysis

In 1904, Karl Pearson - a pioneering biostatistician, was probably the first to use formal techniques to combine data from different studies when investigating the preventive effect of serum inoculations against enteric fever.[1] Although meta-analysis is widely used in epidemiology and evidence-based medicine today, a meta-analysis of a medical treatment was not published until 1955. In 1976, the psychologist Gene Class first introduced the term 'meta-analysis' in a paper entitled 'primary, secondary, and meta-analysis of research'.[2] In the 1980s, meta analysis became more popular in medicine, in particular in the clinical trials of cardiovascular disease, oncology, and perinatal care.

In the 1980s, the Oxford Database of Perinatal Trials (ODPT) was founded and initially sought to create a registry of perinatal trials to "provide a resource for reviews of the safety and efficacy of interventions used in perinatal care".[3,4] In 1993, the Cochrane Pregnancy and Childbirth Database (CCPC) was published by reissuing the systematic reviews contained in the ODPT.[5] With the success of CCPC, the Cochrane Collaboration - an international network of health care professionals who prepare and regularly update systematic reviews ('Cochrane Reviews') - was established to facilitate the conduct of meta analysis in all fields of health care.[6] Since 1996, systematic reviews prepared and maintained through the Cochrane Collaboration have been published in The Cochrane Library. The Cochrane Database of Systematic Reviews, a component of the Cochrane Library, is periodically updated by professionals as more information becomes available and in response to comments and criticism.

Study Identification

Before commencing a meta-analysis, the first step is to determine 'what is your research question', including the definition of the principal exposure of interest and the outcome(s). For instance, one may be interested in investigating the effects of calcium supplementation during pregnancy (exposure) on the risk of preeclampsia (outcome). Then, a difficult but crucial task is to identify studies that are relevant to addressing the question. The reviewer must decide which type of study design should be included. For instance, one may decide to include only randomized trials or all relevant studies, including both observational studies and clinical trials. This decision will depend on the exposure under investigation and potential for bias in nonrandomized studies. A search of computerized databases (e.g. MEDLINE, PUBMED) may provide a reasonable start, but is often insufficient because not all studies are included in such databases. Some studies, particularly ones with negative results, may go unpublished and some may be published but only as abstracts or in journals not captured in electronic databases. One should manually search through references of each identified report in order to identify all relevant studies. In addition, databases that include information on graduate study theses may yield additional unpublished studies. One may also contact researchers who are experts in the field to see if they are aware of any unpublished data on such topics. In the end, it should be realized that the results may be biased due to systematic failure of other investigators to publish or report certain data (e.g. null results). Restricting the analysis to include only published data may aggravate such bias.

Study Quality

The validity of systematic reviews or meta-analyses depends heavily on the validity of the individual studies included. In some sense, the quantitative methods used to pool the results from several studies in a meta-analysis is of less importance than the qualitative methods employed to assess which studies should be aggregated.

To date, several approaches have been developed for assessing study quality, including the validity framework by Cook and Campbell,[7] scales and checklists by Moher et al.[8] and Deeks et al.[9] Although quality assessment scales may provide an overall estimate of quality, the validity of these scales has been questioned. It has been noted that most scales have been developed in an arbitrary fashion and serve better to evaluate the adequacy of reporting of a study rather than the quality of design and conduct of the study. The scales differ considerably in terms of dimensions covered, size, complexity and the weight assigned to the key domains most relevant to the control of bias such as randomization, blinding, and loss to follow up. In order to assess whether the types of scales used for assessing the quality of trials affects the conclusions of meta-analytic studies, Jüni et al. repeated a published meta analysis using different quality assessment scales.[10] The result indicated that none of the 25 scales yielded a statistically significant association between summary scores and effect sizes, and the effect size either increased or decreased with increasing trial quality depending on the scales used. The authors concluded that although the use of a summary score to identify trials of high quality is problematic, the relevant methodological aspects (e.g. concealment of treatment allocation, blinding of outcome assessment or double blinding, and handling of withdrawals and dropouts) should be always identified a priori, and assessed individually.[10] Greenland also pointed out that quality dimensions are highly application specific and therefore hard to measure from published information and the use of quality scores to weight studies in a meta-analysis could produce biased effect estimates.[11]

There appears to be little consensus concerning the optimum approach to dealing with study quality in meta-analysis. However, there is general agreement that a critical evaluation of studies included in the meta-analysis is essential for the interpretation of the results. Efforts to standardize the unbiased conduct and reporting of both randomized trials and meta-analyses should be enhanced.

Definition of Outcome Measures

Outcome measures in meta-analysis include measures such as odds ratio (OR), relative risk (RR), risk difference (RD), number needed to treat (NNT), mean difference, and standardized mean difference. Before combining the studies, one needs to choose a measure to use, based on consideration of whether it is statistically appropriate and convenient to work with, and whether it is clinically meaningful. For example, 'Number needed to treat' has been increasingly used in reporting clinical trials as it may provide a more useful and meaningful approach for clinical decision making. If the outcome of interest is rare, one may ignore the distinctions between odds ratios and rate ratios. However, this distinction can be important when studying outcomes that are frequent, especially in case-control design and analysis. Studies can be combined directly using the reported measures in each study if each study uses the same scale to measure the same parameter. Otherwise, it is common practice to transform data into the same standardized scale if different scales are used in each study if such transformation is possible.

Expressing the Effects across Studies (Fixed and Random Effects Models)

The decision as to whether to utilize a statistical technique to summarize the effects across studies is based on several considerations, including statistical heterogeneity and clinical heterogeneity.

These questions are addressed in more detail in the following section. The use of standard univariate fixed- and random-effects models in meta-analysis has become well known in the last 20 years. A fixed effects model to combine treatment effects assumes no heterogeneity between studies and assumes that the true treatment effect is the same in all studies. The overall treatment effect then is estimated as a weighted average-

$$\hat{\theta} = \frac{\sum_{i=1}^{k} w_i \hat{\theta}_i}{\sum_{i=1}^{k} w_i}, \text{ where } \hat{\theta}_i \text{ is observed effect estimate in } i\text{th study, k is the number of studies}$$

included in the meta-analysis, w_i is the weight of the ith study ($w_i = 1/v_i$). The $\hat{\theta}_i$ is assumed to have an approximate normal distribution of $N(\theta, v_i)$. Other fixed effect methods have been developed to combine the effect estimates (e.g. odds ratios) including Mantel-Haenszel method,[12] Peto's method[13] and maximum likelihood techniques[14].

Compared to the fixed effect model, the random effects model assumes that the effects between studies are different and vary at random. An additional variance component which accounts for the between study variance (σ^2_B) is therefore added in random effects models to incorporate heterogeneity. The overall random effects estimate is given by

$$\hat{\theta} = \frac{\sum_{i=1}^{k} w_i^* \hat{\theta}_i}{\sum_{i=1}^{k} w_i^*}, \text{ where } w_i^* = 1/(v_i + \hat{\sigma}_B^2), \quad \hat{\theta}_i \quad \text{estimates the individual treatment effects}$$

with a distribution of $N(\theta_i, v_i)$, and the true treatment effects in each study θ_i (random effects) is assumed to have a distribution of $N(\theta, \sigma^2_B)$. Generally, the between study variance (σ^2_B) can be estimated using either a moment estimate (weighted or unweighted least square) or maximum or restricted maximum likelihood methods.[15,16,17] Likelihood based approaches [15] yield, in general, wider confidence intervals than those generated with the standard random effects models (e.g. the approach of DerSimonian and Laird).[16]

It is worth noting that the confidence intervals for point estimates of treatment effects derived from a random effects model are wider than those from the corresponding fixed effect model. Different analytical models may lead to the different, or even opposite conclusions.[17-19] There is much debate on policies for choosing fixed versus random effects models.[17,20,21] Some researchers have advocated the use of random effects model even if there is no evidence of statistical heterogeneity.[22] As fixed and random effects models address different questions, it has been suggested to employ the random effects model as a way of performing a sensitivity analysis to check the robustness of conclusions derived from the fixed effects model whenever the estimate of between study heterogeneity is positive.[15,23,24]

Study Heterogeneity

Investigation of heterogeneity remains a key issue in the conduct of meta-analysis. Heterogeneity, in general, can be broadly categorized into three types: clinical, methodological and statistical.[25] Clinical heterogeneity reflects differences between studies in patient populations or in the context in which care was provided. Methodological heterogeneity reflects differences between studies in design, conduct or analysis (e.g. high versus low quality studies) that may be associated with results. Statistical heterogeneity relates to variation in effects and reflects the probability that differences observed between studies are consistent with chance variation. Statistical heterogeneity can be a consequence of clinical or methodological heterogeneity, or can be due to chance alone. Numerous factors could cause heterogeneity, including differences in inclusion and exclusion criteria, patients' baseline risk profile, outcome measures (e.g. definition, follow-up time), intervention (e.g. dose, timing, brand), or variability in methodological quality (e.g. analysis to handle withdrawals, blinding of assessment of outcomes).[26-29]A variety of approaches have been introduced to explore heterogeneity in meta-analyses.

The simplest and most frequently used approach to test for heterogeneity is the Cochrane Chi-square heterogeneity test (the Q statistic).[30] Heterogeneity can be quantified using the index of heterogeneity-I^2, which describes the percentage of total variation across the studies due to heterogeneity rather than random variation (I^2=100% *(Q-df)/Q (df=degrees of freedom), with I^2 ranging between 0% and 100%). The I^2 values of 25%, 50%, and 75% suggest low, moderate and high degree of heterogeneity.[31] It should be noted that the Q statistic can yield falsely negative results for heterogeneity, particularly when the number of patients in the meta analysis is small or the variance of the outcome varies significantly across studies.[32,33] Setting the critical-alpha at the 10% level has been suggested as a conservative method to compensate for this problem.[34,35] Other statistical tests have been developed to investigate the heterogeneity within and between studies, including the test proposed by Breslow and Day,[36] likelihood ratio tests based on the marginal likelihood of individual trial,[15] an exact test proposed by Zelen,[37] or the interaction test of study and treatment if linear or logistic regression are used to combine studies.[38] Compared with the Q statistic, these analytical methods are infrequently used in investigating heterogeneity. For the evaluation the presence of heterogeneity, the principle should be to explore or investigate potential influences of the specific clinical differences between studies rather than to merely rely on an overall statistical test of heterogeneity.

Other than standard statistical tests for heterogeneity, several graphical methods have been introduced as adjuncts for the investigation of heterogeneity in meta-analyses. Visual inspection of data using these plots can assist in the decision as to how to proceed with data synthesis, even in the absence of a statistically significant test for heterogeneity. Forest plots are the most frequently used graphic method to present the summary results of meta-analyses. For each study, the effect estimate and respective confidence interval, as well as the pooled effect estimates with their confidence intervals are plotted on a single dimension. The variability between estimates on the plot highlights the heterogeneity of trials. One example of such plots is given: Figure1 displays the results of the meta analysis of calcium in the prevention of preeclampsia.[39] The variability between estimates can be seen on the plot, indicating the presence of heterogeneity. However, the Forest plot is not very informative in identifying the trials that contribute most to the measured heterogeneity.

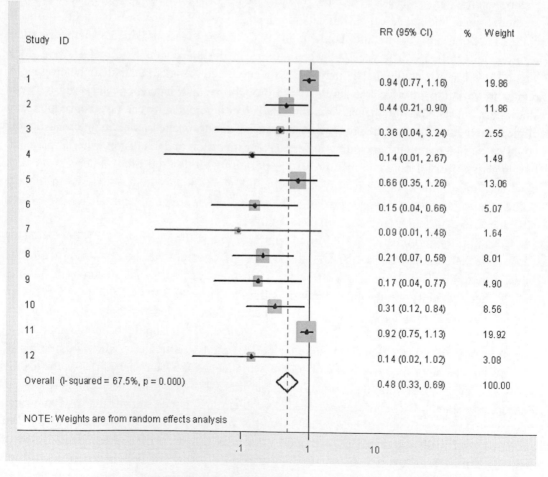

Figure1. Forest plot for relative effect of calcium supplementation during pregnancy on the risk of preeclampsia.

Galbraith proposed an alternative diagram for detecting heterogeneity, on which the z statistic (the ratio of the log RR-relative risk or log OR-odds ratio to its standard error) is plotted against the reciprocal of the standard error.[40] Hence, the least precise results from small trials appear near the origin of the plot, whereas the results of the larger trials appear towards the right. The pooled effect estimate is represented by the slope of the line that through the origin. The 95% confidence limits are positioned 2 units above and below of the line of original line (line of pooled effect estimate). In the absence of significant heterogeneity, the points representing studies will scatter with constant variance along the original line. Points outside of those two 95% limit lines indicate the studies that contribute most to heterogeneity. (Figure2)

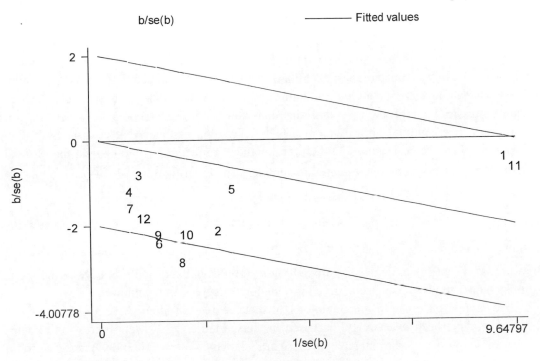

Source: reprint with permission of Paediatr Perinat Epidemiol. 2008, Suppl 1:18-28.

Figure 2. Galbraith plots for the rates of preeclamsia in the calcium and placebo groups.

L'Abbé and colleagues suggested a graphical means for exploring variation across studies by plotting the event rate in the treatment group (vertical axis) versus that of the control group (horizontal axis).[41] If the trials are fairly homogeneous, the points would lie around a line and the gradient of which corresponds to the pooled treatment effect. Large deviations from the line indicate possible heterogeneity.[41] A line of equal rates between groups, and hence of no treatment effect, can be added to the graph. Points below the line indicate that the experimental treatment is superior to that received by controls. Conversely, points above the line signify that the results are in favour of the control or placebo group. It has been suggested that the L'Abbé plot should be standardized before making comparisons for exploring clinical and methodological heterogeneity.[42] A further feature of L'Abbé's method is that it can address the question "Is the treatment effect size related to the baseline risk levels?" A non-consistent band of data points on the scatter-plot indicates a differential treatment effect related to baseline risk factors.

Some researchers would simply exclude the identified "outliers" to reduce the heterogeneity. However, the simple exclusion of outlying studies does not always improve the credibility of the meta-analysis. Furthermore, such exclusions further reduce the power of statistical tests for heterogeneity. Such a practice has been proven to be dangerous in some cases.[43] It is often the case that different methods may identify different "outliers" and therefore the conclusions of meta analysis may change considerably.[44] Thus, it may be practical to consider the exclusion of "outliers" as a part of sensitivity analysis.

Meta-Regression

Meta-regression remains an important means to explore sources of heterogeneity in meta-analysis and allows simultaneous examination of multiple characteristics. As with non-regression meta-analysis, fixed and random effects regression models are available. A fixed effect regression model assumes that the considered covariates completely account for variations across studies, while random effects regression assumes that covariates capture only a part of the heterogeneity and therefore includes a random term to explain the residual heterogeneity. The simple meta-regression model can be written as $y_i \sim N(\alpha + \beta\chi_i, v_i)$, where y_i is the observed log-odds ratio of study i (θ_i), v_i is the variance of log-odds ratio for study i, χ_i-covariate (e.g. baseline calcium intake). The model that incorporates the residual heterogeneity is then $y_i \sim N(\alpha + \beta x_i, v_i + \tau^2)$, where τ^2 reflects the additive between-study variance. Regression modelling is not a trivial task and it is beyond the scope of this chapter to give a comprehensive introduction of regression techniques.

The issues related to the methodology of meta regression along with its strengths and limitations have been extensively discussed in the literature.[32,44-47] Meta-regression remains an essential approach to investigate whether particular covariates explain the heterogeneity of treatment effects between studies. For instance, it can be used to investigate the relationship between the baseline risk (i.e. the observed risk of events in the control group, or the average risk in the control and treatment group) and treatment effect, which could be clinically important. It should be noted that, in the presence of misclassification of baseline risk, more complex models addressing measurement errors are required to obtain valid results for the relationship between the baseline risk and treatment effect.[26,47,48] It is appropriate to use meta-regression to explore the sources of heterogeneity even if the overall statistical test for heterogeneity (e.g. Q test) is not significant.

Meta regression faces similar challenges related to bias as do observational studies in general (e.g. confounding) and a causal interpretation is therefore difficult to derive from the results of meta regression models.[26,48] Similar to the situation in subgroup analysis, pre-specification of potential covariates is essential to reduce the likelihood of the false positive conclusions when conducting a meta-regression. Furthermore, one requires the effect estimate of treatment, its variance, and covariate values for each study in the systematic review to conduct a meta regression. Such data are not always available and reported in all included studies. Thus, analysis may be only based on the subgroup studies that provide such information, which introduce the potential bias. It has been reported that analyses based on individual patient data would be less prone to bias compared with the analyses based on study level characteristics, although such data is difficult to obtain for the conduct of meta analysis.[45,49] It worth pointing out that the potential for robust conclusions from meta – regression models is very limited and such analysis is most useful when the number of studies is large.[50]

Stratification (Subgroup) Analysis

Subgroup analysis is frequently used by researchers as a means of explaining or reducing heterogeneity that is often observed in the overall analysis. One can stratify either by study or patient characteristics. For instance, studies can be stratified with respect to many factors such as treatment assignment, control group, patient inclusion criteria, quality control, study conduct, and follow-up maturity. It is important that subgroups used for analysis should be specified before the analysis is commenced. The number of candidates for effect modifiers should be "kept to a minimum" as the likelihood of false positive (spurious) findings increases with the number of effect modifiers. Inappropriate conduct of subgroup analysis could be very misleading and therefore could change the conclusion of a systematic review.[51,52] Nevertheless, appropriate conduct of subgroup analysis, with increased sample size, can help to understand whether treatment effects differ systematically across patients, settings, and treatment variations (e.g. dose), which is difficult to address with a single trial.

Publication Bias

The results of meta-analysis may be seriously distorted if the included studies are biased samples. The classic form of this problem is publication bias: an editorial pre-selection for publishing particular findings, e.g., positive results, which could lead to the failure of authors to submit negative findings for publication.[53] If such bias is present, a meta analysis that includes only published reports will yield results biased away from the null effect. Meta analytic approaches for correction of such bias may not be sufficient for bias removal. Nevertheless, various methods have been developed and useful for detecting such biases. A simple informal visual way to detect publication bias is the funnel plot. A plot of sample size versus treatment effect from individual studies should be shaped like a funnel in the absence of publication bias. It has been suggested that the shape of funnel plot is largely determined by the arbitrary choice of the method to construct the plot. When a different definition of precision and/ or effect measure is used, the conclusion about the shape of the plot can be altered.[55] Therefore, asymmetrical funnel plots should be interpreted cautiously in the absence of a consensus on how the plot should be constructed.[54] Other statistical methods, including the rank correlation test,[55] Egger's method,[56] Begg's method,[57] maximum likelihood approach[58], and Rosenthal's "fail-safe N"[59] have also been developed.

Some investigators have also attempted to exclude studies under a certain size in order to minimize the problem of publication bias, as small studies tend to display more publication bias. However, the choice of the exact size is rather arbitrary, which may in fact aggravate the bias. The optimum way to eliminate publication bias may be to prevent it from occurring in the first place, either by prospective registration of every trial undertaken, or by publishing all studies, regardless of their outcome. However, these solutions will be difficult to achieve in the near future. Thus, researchers should always be aware of the potential for publication bias and make efforts to assess to what extent publication bias may affect their results.

Sensitivity Analysis

A sensitivity analysis remains an important approach for reviewers to test how robust the results of the review are, relative to key decisions and assumptions that were made in the process of conducting a review.[60] Several approaches to sensitivity analysis have been proposed in the Cochrane Collaboration handbook, including 1) changing the inclusion criteria, 2)including or excluding studies where there is some ambiguity as to whether they meet the inclusion criteria, 3) including or excluding unpublished studies, 4) including or excluding studies with low methodological quality, 5) re-analysing the data where uncertainties concerning values extracted exist, 6) re-analysing the data where missing values exist, and 7) simulation of extra trials. In addition, as mentioned earlier, it has been recommended to analyze data using different statistical approaches, namely fixed and random effects models, which serves a means of conducting a sensitivity analysis to check the robustness of results. The importance of sensitivity analysis should be emphasized and such analysis should be routinely done when conducting a meta-analysis.

Meta Analysis of Survival Data

There is a tendency in the literature to use survival curves for the outcome analysis, especially when the time to the event is of interest. Performing a meta-analysis on this kind of data requires special statistical techniques and has been extensively discussed in literature. The simplest way to carry out such as a meta analysis would be to extract data as the (log) hazard ratio and its variance from each study and then combine them using standard methods of meta analysis as fixed or random effects models. However, published reports seldom provide such data. Fortunately, the log hazard ratio and its variance can be estimated either directly from the observed number of events and the logrank expected number of events or indirectly from the p-value for the logrank, Mantel-Haenszel, or chi-square test. In addition, if none of these is possible, the statistics can be estimated from survival curves. Given the fact that there is often censoring in survival data, the ideal way to perform a meta-analysis of survival data may be to use individual patient data.

Bayesian Methods in Meta Analysis

A Bayesian model describes the structural relationship between data and unknown parameters, whereby both data and parameters are considered random variables with uncertainty. Bayesian modeling can efficiently incorporate all sources of variability and relevant quantifiable external information and it provides a more informative summary of the likely value of parameters than non-Bayesian approaches. The model can be simply written as $y_i \sim N(\xi_i, \psi_i)$, $\xi_i = \alpha + \beta x_i$, and $\psi_i = v_i + \tau^2$. Previous evidence is expressed through prior distributions about quantity of interest (e.g. log OR). Current data are expressed through the likelihood, on the basis of the appropriate model. Posterior distribution for the quantity of interest then can be obtained. The derived posterior distributions, in particular full posterior distribution, borrow strength from all studies and enable direct inference regarding probabilities about expectations, and give substantially more information than single point estimates.

Role and Limitation of Meta Analysis

The role of systematic review and meta-analysis has been increasingly endorsed in evidence-based decision making. Clinicians and researchers should consider the results of meta-analysis before recommending a clinical practice. They can be used to ascertain whether scientific findings are consistent and generalizable across populations, settings, and treatment variations or whether findings vary significantly by particular subgroup. Nevertheless, meta-analyses have inherent limitations because of their retrospective nature. For instance, pooling results does not overcome the epidemiological biases present in the original studies. New biases could even be introduced into meta-analyses by inappropriately pooling heterogeneous studies. For those reasons, the clinical interpretation of meta-analysis must be performed with appropriate caution. Variables that can account for the heterogeneity and which are candidates for stratified or 'influence' analysis should always be identified in the protocols of systematic reviews. Strong recommendation should not be solely based on a meta-analysis. Findings derived from meta-analysis must be primarily considered as hypothesis generating rather than hypothesis testing. On the other hand, data from large trials are not necessarily definitive for patients. A large trial may still be underpowered if the event studied is rare or the treatment effect is small, but clinically meaningful to detect. Expected power in a large trial may be still compromised by missing data, loss to follow up, and null bias. We should view evidence from small and large trials and meta-analyses as offering a complementary, evolving continuum of information. Comparison of large trials and meta-analysis may reach different conclusions depending on how trials and meta-analyses are selected and how end points and agreement are defined. Scrutiny of these two research methods and critical evaluation of evidence derived from both are essential for guiding medical practice.

Reference

[1]   Pearson K. Report on certain enteric fever inoculation statistics. *Br Med J* 1904; 3:1243-6.

[2]   Glass GV. Primary, secondary, and meta-analysis of research. *Educ Res* 1976; 5:3-8.

[3]   Chalmers I, editor. Oxford Database of Perinatal Trials. Oxford: *Oxford University Press.* 1988 – 1992.

[4]   Chalmers I, Hetherington J, Newdick M, Mutch L, Grant A, Enkin M, Enkin E, Dickersin K. The Oxford Database of Perinatal Trials: developing a register of published reports of controlled trials. *Control Clin Trials.* 1986;7: 306-24.

[5]   Chalmers I. The Cochrane Collaboration: preparing, maintaining, and disseminating systematic reviews of the effects of health care. *Ann N Y Acad Sci.* 1993; 703:156-65.

[6]   Bero L, Rennie D. The Cochrane Collaboration. Preparing, maintaining, and disseminating systematic reviews of the effects of health care. *JAMA* 1995; 274: 1935-8.

[7]   Cook TD, Campbell DT. 1979. Quasi-experimentation: *Design & Analysis Issue for Field Settings*. Boston: Houghton Mifflin.

[8]   Moher D, Jadad AR, Nichol G, Penman M, Tugwell P, Walsh S. Assessing the quality of randomized controlled trials:an annotated bibliography of scales and checklists. *Control Clin Trials* 1995; 16: 62-73.

[9]   Deeks J, Glanville J, Sheldon T. Undertaking systematic reviews of research on effectiveness: CRD guidelines for those carrying out or commissioning reviews CRD Report *Number 4, 2nd edn. In: Khan K., Riet G.,* Glanville J.*, Sowden A. & Kleijnen, J., eds CRDCentres for Reviews and Dissemination.* York: York Publishing Services Ltd; 2001.

[10]   Jüni P, Witschi A, Bloch R, Egger M. The hazards of scoring the quality of clinical trials for meta-analysis. *JAMA.* 1999;282 :1054-60.

[11]   Greenland S, O'Rourke K. On the bias produced by quality scores in meta-analysis, and a hierarchical view of proposed solutions. *Biostatistics.* 2001;2:463-71.

[12]   Mantel N, Haenszel W. Statistical aspects of the analysis of data from retrospective studies of disease. *J Natl Cancer Inst.* 1959; 22: 719-48.

[13]   Peto R, Pike MC, Armitage P, Breslow NE, Cox DR, Howard SV, Mantel N, McPherson K, Peto J, Smith PG. Design and analysis of randomized clinical trials requiring prolonged observation of each patient. II: analysis and examples. *Br J Cancer* 1977; 35: 1-39.

[14]   Hasselblad V, McCrory DC. Meta-analytic tools for medical decision making: a practical guide. *Med Decis Making* 1995; 15: 81-96.

[15]   Hardy RJ, Thompson SG. A likelihood approach to meta-analysis with random effects. *Stat Med.*1996; 15: 619-29.

[16]   DerSimonian R, Laird N. Meta analysis in clinical trials. *Control Clin Trials.* 1986;7: 177-88.

[17]   Dempster AP, Laird NM, Rubin DB. Maximum likelihood from incomplete via the EM algorithm. *Journal of the Royal Statistical Society* 1977; B39: 1-38.

[18]   Berlin JA, Laird NM, Sacks HS, Chalmers TC. A comparison of statistical methods for combining event rates from clinical trials. *Stat Med* 1989; 8: 141-51.

[19]   Mengersen KL, Tweedie RL, Biggerstaff BJ. The impact of method choice in meta-analysis. *Austral J Statist* 1995; 37: 19-44.

[20]   Villar J, Mackey ME, Carroli G, Donner A. Meta-analyses in systematic reviews of randomized controlled trials in perinatal medicine: comparison of fixed and random effects models. *Stat Med.* 2001; 20: 3635-47.

[21]   Greenland S. Quantitative methods in the review of epidemiologic literature. *Epidemiol Rev.* 1987; 9:1-30.

[22]   Peto R. Why do we need systematic overviews of randomized trials? *Stat Med.* 1987; 6: 233-244.

[23]   Thompson SG, Pocock SJ. Can meta-analyses be trusted? *Lancet* 1991; 338: 1127-30.

[24]   Spector TD, Thompson SG. The potential and limitations of meta analysis. *J Epidemiol Community Health.* 1991; 45: 89-92.

[25]   Thompson SG. Why sources of heterogeneity in meta-analysis should be investigated. *BMJ* 1994; 309: 1351-5.

[26]   Thompson SG, Smith TC, Sharp SJ. Investigating underlying risk as a source of heterogeneity in meta-analysis. *Stat Med.* 1997; 16: 2741-58.

[27]   Brand R, Kragt H. Importance of trends in the interpretation of an overall odds ratio in the meta-analysis of clinical trials. *Stat Med* 1992; 11: 2077-82.

[28]   Davey Smith G, Egger M. Commentary on the cholesterol papers: statistical problems. *BMJ.* 1994; 308: 1025-7.

[29]   Gelber R D, Goldhirsch A. Interpretation of results from subset analyses within overviews of randomized clinical trials. *Stat Med* 1987;6:371-8.

[30]   Cochran WG. The combination of estimates from different experiments. *Biometrics* 1954; 10: 101-29.

[31]   Higgins JP, Thompson SG, Deeks JJ, Altman DG. Measuring inconsistency in meta-analysis. *BMJ.* 2003; 327: 557-60.

[32]   Hardy RJ, Thompson SG. Detecting and describing heterogeneity in meta-analysis. *Stat Med.* 1998; 17: 841-56.

[33]   Jones MP, O'Gorman TW, Lemke JH, Woolson RF. A Monte Carlo investigation of homogeneity tests of the odds ratio under various sample size configurations. *Biometrics* 1989; 45: 171-81.

[34]   Fleiss JL. Analysis of data from multiclinic trials. *Control Clin Trials.* 1986; 7: 267-75.

[35]   Jackson D. The power of the standard test for the presence of heterogeneity in meta analysis. *Stat Med.* 2006; 25: 2688-99.

[36]   Breslow, N.E. and Day, N.E. The analysis of case-control studies. *In: Davis W. Lyon, eds. Statistical Methods in Cancer Research, Volume1.* IARC Scientific Publications, 1980: pp 142-3.

[37]   Zelen M. The analysis of several 2×2 contingency tables. *Biometrika* 1971; 58: 129-37.

[38]   Rosenthal R. Parametric measures of effect size. In: Copper H, Hedges LV, eds. *The handbook of Research Synthesis.* New York: Russell Sage Foundation; 1994; pp.231-44.

[39] Hofmeyr GJ, Atallah AN, Duley L. Calcium supplementation during pregnancy for preventing hypertensive disorders and related problems. *Cochrane Database Syst Rev* 2006; 3:CD001059.

[40] Galbraith RF. A note on graphical presentation of estimated odds ratios from several clinical trials. *Stat Med.*1988; 7: 889-94.

[41] L'Abbé KA, Detsky AS, O'Rourke K. Meta-analysis in clinical research. *Ann Intern Med.* 1987; 107:224-33.

[42] Song F. Exploring heterogeneity in meta-analysis: is L'Abbé plot useful? *J Clin Epidemiol.*1999; 52: 725-30.

[43] Berlin JA, Antman EM. Advantages and limitations of meta-analytic regressions of clinical trial data. *Online Journal of Clinical Trials* 1994; 3: Doc. No. 134.

[44] Sharp SJ, Thompson SG, Altman DG. The relation between treatment benefit and underlying risk in meta-analysis. *BMJ* 1996; 313:735-8.

[45] Arends LR, Hoes AW, Lubsen J, Grobbee DE, Stijnen T. Baseline risk as predictor of treatment benefit: three clinical meta-re-analyses. *Stat Med.* 2000;19:3497-518.

[46] Schmid CH. Exploring heterogeneity in randomised trials via meta-analysis. *Drug Information Journal* 1999; 33: 211-24.

[47] Greenwood CM, Midgley JP, Matthew AG, Logan AG. Statistical issues in a metaregression analysis of randomized trials: impact on the dietary sodium intake and blood pressure relationship. *Biometrics* 1999; 55: 630-6.

[48] Thompson SG, Higgins JP. How should meta-regression analyses be undertaken and interpreted? *Stat Med.* 2002; 21: 1559-73.

[49] Begg CB, Pilote L. A model for incorporating historical controls into a meta analysis. *Biometrics* 1991; 47: 899-906.

[50] Smith TC, Spiegelhalter DJ, Thomas A. Bayesian approaches to meta analysis: a comparative study. *Stat Med.* 1995; 14: 2685-99.

[51] Higgins J, Thompson S, Deeks J, Altman D. Statistical heterogeneity in systematic reviews of clinical trials: a critical appraisal of guidelines and practice. *J Health Serv Res Policy.* 2002; 7:51-61.

[52] Oxman AD, Guyatt GH. A consumer's guide to subgroup analysis. *Ann Intern Med.*1992;116: 78-84.

[53] Last JM, editor. A Dictionary of Epidemiology. Oxford: *Oxford University Press,1983.*p.12.

[54] Tang JL, Liu JL. Misleading funnel plot for detection of bias in meta-analysis. *J Clin Epidemiol.* 2000; 53: 477-84.

[55] Begg CB. Publication bias. *In: Cooper H, Hedges LV, eds. The handbook of Research Synthesis.* New York: Russell Sage Foundation, 1994. pp. 399-409.

[56] Egger M, Davey Smith G, Schneider M, Minder C. Bias in meta-analysis detected by a simple, graphical test. *BMJ* 1997; 315:629-34.

[57] Begg CB. A measure to aid in the interpretation of published clinical trial. *Stat Med.*1985;4:1-9.

[58] Rust RT, Lehmann DR, Farley JU. Estimating publication bias in meta-analysis. *J Market Res.* 1990; XXVII:220-6.

[59] Rosenthal R. The 'file drawer problem' and tolerance for null results. *Psychol Bull* 1979; 86:638-41.

[60] Oxman AD, editor. The Cochrane Collaboration handbook: preparing and maintaining systematic reviews. Second ed. *Oxford: Cochrane Collaboration.* 1996;p83.

In: Textbook of Perinatal Epidemiology
Editor: Eyal Sheiner, pp. 127-141

ISBN: 978-1-60741-648-7
© 2010 Nova Science Publishers, Inc.

Chapter X

Decision Analysis in Perinatal Medicine

William A. Grobman[*]

Definitions

- Decision analysis: A quantitative analysis that combines information, using a formal stepwise process, in an attempt to aid decision making.
- Decision tree: A model that illustrates the choices and probabilistic events that are relevant for a given decision analysis, and which also can be used to calculate outcomes of interest for the decision analysis.
- Markov model: A methodology that is used in decision analysis to allow for the inclusion of recursive processes, such as the moving back and forth between events, and complex changing of the values of input variables during the analytical timeframe.
- Quality-adjusted life year: Health effectiveness measure which represents the quality of health achieved during a year of life
- Sensitivity analysis: A process whereby the stability of results and corresponding conclusions are assessed through alterations in the input variables.

Decision Analysis: Advantages and Limitations

Physicians increasingly depend upon evidence-based medicine to aid in their decision making. Randomized controlled trials, which often provide the basis for the identification of a treatment's beneficial effect or adverse consequences, are considered to provide the "gold

---

[*] For Correspondence: William A. Grobman, MD, MBA, 250 East Superior Street, Suite 05-2175, Chicago, IL 60611, 312-472-4685, 312-472-4687 fax, w-grobman@northwestern.edu

standard" of medical evidence. Yet, although the information provided by these trials is quite powerful, not all questions are amenable to being answered by this type of study design.

In some cases, for example, an outcome of interest may be relatively uncommon. For example, a permanent brachial plexus injury occurs in approximately 0.01% of cases, making it difficult to randomize women to different regimens (such as with regard to estimated fetal weight assessment by ultrasound) to assess if this outcome can be significantly reduced. Alternatively, an outcome can take so long to develop that a randomized trial focusing on that outcome is not feasible. Such a circumstance may exist with regard to the screening for and the development of cervical cancer. Although women with no cervical dysplasia could be randomized to different screening strategies (e.g. routine Pap smear vs. Pap smear with the addition of HPV testing), the length of time until cervical cancer develops, and the corresponding follow-up that would be necessary, would be so long that a trial may be too difficult and expensive to perform.

Observational studies, such as those with a cohort or case control design, may provide helpful information in such cases, as they can be accomplished with less use of time and resources. However, even these types of studies cannot provide answers for all types of outcome assessments. For example, two treatments may have similar benefits but different types of undesirable consequences. In this circumstance, a randomized trial may not be able to define which treatment is "better". Also, even if an interventional or observational trial can be performed to answer a given clinical question, the results may not give insight into public health ramifications, such as the cost effectiveness of a medical intervention. In such settings, another type of study design may be necessary to inform the decision making of both caregivers and patients.

Decision analysis is one type of study design that can provide useful insights, and is particularly helpful in circumstances when an interventional or observational study design cannot provide the required information that is needed to differentiate between different tests or therapies. Some examples of decision analyses from the obstetrical and gynecological literature can help to illustrate this point. The best management strategy after identification of ASCUS on a Pap smear has been debated. The different screening intervals (e.g. 1 or 3 years) and many types of testing (e.g. liquid-based Pap smear, HPV DNA testing) that can be utilized result in many different potential strategies that need to be assessed. Moreover, as noted earlier in the chapter, the primary outcome of interest, namely cervical cancer, occurs relatively infrequently and may take years to develop. Theoretically, many different strategies could be compared in a randomized trial over many years, but the logistics of such a trial are overwhelming and the results may not allow a comprehensive assessment of all costs and benefits of different strategies. Using decision analysis, on the other hand, Kim et al were able to assess the outcomes of multiple different ASCUS triage strategies and make recommendations regarding the best strategy.[1] Thus, decision analysis provided a methodology to explicitly compare a multitude of treatment approaches and suggest the optimal one.

Another medical intervention that has been controversial is the need for routine thromboembolic prophylaxis at the time of cesarean delivery. Although a randomized trial of different treatment strategies is theoretically possible, many thousands of women would need to be randomized to discern a difference between treatments. Investigators who have attempted such a trial have had difficulty randomizing even several hundred women.[2] Observational studies also have not been able to provide an adequate answer, as ascertainment of women who have received prophylaxis, of women who have had a complication of prophylaxis, and of women who have had a thromboembolic event has been problematic.[3] Using decision analysis, however, Quinones et al were able to account for both the benefits and risks of different thromboprophylactic strategies and illustrate that intermittent pneumatic compression, compared to other thromboprophylactic treatments, would result in the fewest adverse events.[4] Other investigators also demonstrated that under certain circumstances, the use of intermittent pneumatic compression is cost-effective compared to no prophylaxis at all.[5]

Even though there are many circumstances in which decision analysis may be helpful, it is not a tool that can be used to answer all clinical questions. For example, it is best utilized when individual components of a larger decision are known and can be explicitly organized into an analytical model. Conversely, if the pieces of data needed to construct a reasonable analysis are not known, a decision model will be of little help in determining an optimal strategy. For example, Rouse et al undertook an analysis to better understand whether the use of ultrasound to diagnose macrosomia, and thereby indicate the need for cesarean, was a cost-effective strategy. For this question, the investigators were able to discern and use the relevant data they needed to obtain outcome measures.[6] Conversely, if the sensitivity of ultrasound for macrosomia or the probability of shoulder dystocia at different birth weights were unknown, a decision analysis could not have been used to arrive at a reliable outcome assessment, as these individual pieces of data are seminal in calculating the frequency of the primary health outcome of interest, namely, permanent brachial plexus palsy. Also, despite the contribution a decision analysis can make to an evidence-based assessment, it is important that the analysis be considered in the context of other available data and study outcomes. Caution should be applied in using a decision analytical model alone to define the most preferred test or treatment strategy; instead, a decision analysis is best used as one component in a body of evidence that can provide additional perspective to the question at hand.

The Analytic Structures
Underlying Decision Analyses

Decision Trees

Decision models are often represented using a decision "tree". This "tree" is an explicit and graphical depiction of the decisions under consideration, and the chance events that can occur after different decisions are made. For example, several investigators have studied the extent to which the introduction into a labor and delivery unit of a rapid HIV test for parturients with unknown HIV status at their admission for delivery reduces the number of perinatal HIV infections.[7,8] A partial and simplified tree for this analysis is shown in Figure 1. The initial choice in this analysis would be whether or not to use a rapid HIV test for the population under consideration. Typically, the point at which different decisions are made is represented in a decision tree as a square. Subsequent to that initial decision, there are several events that may or may not occur in the "HIV test available arm" – these probabilistic events are commonly represented by a circle. In the illustrated scenario, a woman may accept (probability "A") or decline ("1-probability A") the rapid HIV test. If she declines the test then her HIV status remains unknown, whereas if she accepts the test then she may have a positive ("probability B") or negative ("1-probability B") result. In contrast, if the test is not available, all women will have unknown status and be treated accordingly.

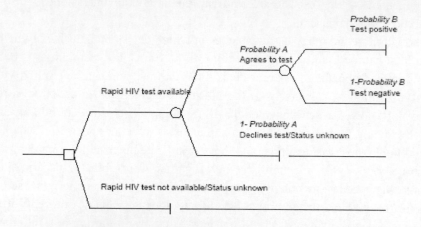

Figure 1. Simplified decision tree for an investigation to discern whether rapid HIV testing in labor and delivery for women with unknown HIV serostatus is a cost-effective strategy.

Markov Models

For many analyses, a simple decision tree will be sufficient to calculate the outcomes of interest. In some cases, however, a tree may not easily allow events that have changing probabilities of occurring during the course of the analysis to be depicted or incorporated into the calculations. In such a case, other analytic approaches are needed. Markov analysis is one type of methodology that is frequently used in the circumstance when a single event may occur with different probabilities, often contingent on other probabilistic events and when these events occur, during the timeframe of the analysis. [9-11] One analysis that demonstrates the usefulness of Markov analysis is that performed by Plunkett et al, who studied perinatal transmission of hepatitis C.[12] Once a person is chronically infected by hepatitis C, several different health states, including remission, cirrhoses, carcinoma, and death may arise. Moving from one health state to another does not always occur after a single length of time or via a single path of health states. In such a circumstance, a simple decision tree without Markov modeling could not have efficiently or accurately represented the dynamically complex life events experienced by a woman with hepatitis C. The use of Markov modeling, however, enabled these complex health state transitions to be incorporated into the analysis. Rather than being represented by a linear tree-like schematic, the complex relationships of variables in a Markov model are often represented by the use of a figure with arrows, depicting the different transitions that can be made between health states. Such a schematic is presented in Figure 2.

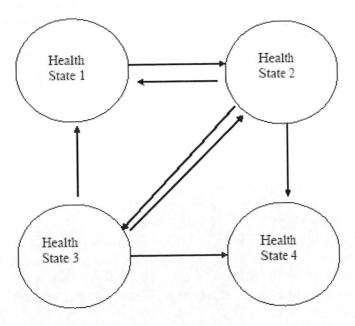

Figure 2. Schematic of the events incorporated in a Markov analysis. The arrows indicate which health states can transition to one another. For example, an individual may move from health state 1 to 2 or from 3 to 2; alternatively, after being in health state 2, the individual may move to health state 1 or 3 or 4.

Approach to a Decision Analysis

Type of Analysis

Before undertaking a decision analysis, investigators need to decide several important approaches to that analysis. First, investigators need to determine the outcomes of interest. In some cases, investigators may choose to compare strategies only on the basis of clinical outcomes, and not incorporate any other outcomes, such as economic ones. One example of this approach is provided by Quinones et al, who compared 4 strategies of thromboprophylaxis at the time of cesarean.[4] Outcomes assessed in this study included heparin-induced thrombocytopenia (HIT), HIT-related thrombosis, major maternal bleeding, and venous thromboembolism. They concluded that intermittent pneumatic compression was preferred to anticoagulation for prevention of thromboembolism because the former was associated with the lowest number of adverse events. Similarly, in trying to arrive at a recommendation with regard to the use of recurrent antenatal corticosteroids, Caughey and Parer compared different dosing regimens on the basis of neonatal morbidity and mortality events.[13] Analyses limited to only health states can help to answer specific clinical questions, such as "Which type of thromboprophylaxis leads to the fewest complications?" Yet, unless costs among the different strategies are essentially equivalent, analyses that examine only health outcomes cannot provide guidance as to the most preferred strategy from a cost-effectiveness perspective. In essence, even though one strategy may improve the health outcome, it is important to understand at what cost that improved outcome is obtained.

Analyses that incorporate costs may be of several different types. In a cost-minimization analysis, the investigators assess only cost as an outcome, and the decision of choice is the one that leads to the lowest costs incurred. One example of this type of analysis is that of Lavin et al, who compared one-tiered and two-tiered screening protocols for gestational diabetes mellitus and concluded that the 2-tiered approach was associated with lower costs.[14] If this type of analysis is going to identify a preferred strategy, the underlying assumption is that health outcomes are essentially equivalent. If not, even if one strategy is cheaper, it is not clear that it would be preferred, as the impact of that cost savings on health outcomes would remain unknown.

Since most alternate strategies have neither equivalent health nor cost outcomes, many investigators choose to incorporate both health and economic measures into the assessed outcome of their decision analyses. In the obstetric and gynecologic literature, the most common analysis of this type is the cost-effectiveness analysis. In this type of analysis, the outcome is a ratio that is composed of a numerator of a cost measure and a denominator of a health-effectiveness measure. For example, in evaluating whether cesarean delivery without labor for women infected with HIV was a desirable strategy, Chen et al performed a cost-effectiveness analysis in which they utilized "United States dollars" as their cost measure and "cases of perinatal HIV" as their health-effectiveness measure.[15] Each strategy, (i.e. labor vs. cesarean without labor), therefore, was associated with a certain number of dollars spent and neonates who had perinatally-acquired HIV. The cost-effectiveness of the cesarean delivery strategy was represented by the marginal expense required to prevent an HIV-infected neonate. Although the type of effectiveness measure used in this analysis is "case of illness averted", there are many other types of effectiveness measures, including number of lives saved, years of life saved, and quality-adjusted life years saved. These will be further discussed below.

Choice of Perspective

Another important consideration is the perspective that informs the analysis. Analyses may be from the perspective of the individual, the hospital, the third-party payer, or society as a whole. The perspective of the analysis is crucial to consider so that the proper costs and health outcomes can be included in the decision model. In the previously noted article by Quinones et al, for example, the perspective is that of the individual.[4] Thus, the health outcomes that are included are only those that occur in the context of thromboprophylaxis, and the chosen strategy is the one that results in an individual having the least chance of an adverse outcome. If an analysis from the perspective of the individual assesses costs, only those costs borne by the individual should be considered. Yet, in a health system that involves many economic stakeholders, an economic analysis from the perspective of an individual will give little guidance as to the best allocation of resources among members. A better understanding of resource allocation can be obtained by examining higher-order perspectives. The analysis by Chen et al, for example, utilized the perspective of a third-party payer, given that the entity responsible for paying for additional cesareans and benefitting from savings due to fewer cases of perinatal HIV infection can be a health care organization.[15] As illustrated by these examples, there is not one perspective that is unequivocally best, but different perspectives that enable investigators to achieve different objectives. It should be noted, though, that if an investigator wishes to choose a strategy based upon its ability to optimally allocate resources among members of a society, then a societal perspective need be chosen.[16]

Choice of Inputs

Costs

In order to determine a preferred strategy, several different types of information need to be known for an analysis to be possible. From a qualitative perspective, all the different strategies and the probabilistic events that can occur as a consequence of each strategy need to be determined. From a quantitative perspective, the probability that each event occurs needs to be established. Furthermore, if costs and measures of health effectiveness (such as quality-adjusted life years) are being assessed, the value of these measures associated with each event and health state need to be ascertained.

The quantitative information can be obtained in several ways. First, a thorough review of the literature should be performed to identify pre-existing estimates of the relevant probabilities, costs, and measures of health effectiveness. This review, moreover, should not just accumulate estimates, but choose the best estimates based on a critical review of the available studies. In their analysis on thromboprophylaxis, Quinones et al not only list their chosen estimates and the references from which these estimates were derived, but also provide a level of evidence designation to indicate the strength of the methodology in the investigation from which the estimate is based.[4]

Several other types of resources may be particularly helpful for cost assessment. Visco et al, in their study of universal cystoscopy to identify ureteral injury at hysterectomy, have illustrated the use of government reimbursement databases to derive cost estimates.[17] Other investigators have turned to local institutional data to obtain estimates of cost for particular medical procedures.[18,19]

Regardless of the source, estimates of economic variables should adhere to several standards. One should strive to ensure that the estimate is of costs and not of charges. The latter are not representative of the actual economic consequences of an event and any estimates that are obtained as charges should be converted to costs.[20] Most simply, this can be done with a single cost:charge ratio (e.g. 0.6). In actuality, however, charges are related to costs by different proportions in different settings (e.g. laboratory, pharmacy), and all attempts should be made to obtain the most relevant and specific cost:charge ratios for a given analysis.[21] Also, all costs should be expressed in equivalent units, such as the same type of currency, and be valued at equivalent times. If, for example, one estimate was available as "2004 US dollars" and one as "2007 US dollars", the "2004 US dollars" should be updated to "2007 US dollars" using the medical care component of the US Consumer Price Index (www.bls.gov). Lastly, costs that will accrue into the future should be discounted, as a given amount of money in the future has less value than that same amount in the present. Essentially, it is better to have $10 today than to be given $10 in five years. The Panel on Cost-Effectiveness has recommended that a discount rate of 3% be used as a baseline in cost-effectiveness analyses, although changes in the economic environment could lead to changes in this recommendation.[20]

Health-Effectiveness Measures

Health effectiveness may be expressed by several different measures. When Randolph et al attempted to determine whether acyclovir prophylaxis in late pregnancy was a cost-effective strategy to prevent neonatal herpes infection, they chose the number of infants with either neurodevelopmental disability or death as a measure of effectiveness.[22] The choice of an explicit health state as a measure of effectiveness often can simplify the analysis, as the health state can be easily defined and its probability of occurrence in each strategy can be derived from the basic probabilities that are embedded within the decision tree. Nevertheless, this type of effectiveness measure has some drawbacks. The final cost-effectiveness ratio will not account for the ramifications of other potentially relevant health outcomes on the overall health effectiveness of a given strategy. Indeed, the focus upon a single health outcome is a particular problem if the strategies that are being compared could result in differences in other types of health outcomes. Moreover, even if there were to be no other important health outcomes to consider, the final cost-effectiveness result from the analysis is difficult to compare within the context of a more general resource allocation. What is the benchmark, for example, to decide the number of dollars it would be reasonable to spend to avoid one case of neurodevelopmental disability or death due to perinatal HSV infection?

Other types of measures of health effectiveness can avoid these potential drawbacks. Kulasingham et al, who attempted to determine the most cost-effective screening interval for pap smears among low-risk women, used the number of life-years saved as their measure of health effectiveness.[23] A measure such as this allows the contribution of multiple different health states to be incorporated into the health-effectiveness measure of the analysis. Additionally, it allows the straightforward comparison of the results of this analysis with the results of other analyses that use the same health-effectiveness measure, even if those analyses examine very different health states and strategies. The study by Tengs et al demonstrates the many different medical (e.g. beta-blocker use for myocardial infarction) and non-medical (e.g. seat belt use) interventions that can be compared once the type of outcome measure is the same.[24]

Because some medical interventions may not result in a change in life expectancy, but may alter the quality of life, other measures of effectiveness, such as quality-adjusted life years (QALY), allow both survival and quality of survival to be incorporated into a single outcome measure.[25] Indeed, because of these advantages, QALY's are frequently used as a measure of health effectiveness in cost-effectiveness analyses.[26] QALY's can be calculated as a product of the number of years spent at a given "quality of life". This "quality of life" is typically represented by a "utility" value, which is a number between 0 and 1. Most commonly, a utility value of 1 represents full health while a utility value of 0 represents death. Thus, if a health state was considered to have a utility of 0.5, and an individual spent three years in that health state, he or she would have accumulated 1.5 (i.e. 3 * 0.5) QALY's.

Nevertheless, a measure such as a QALY adds some complexity to the analysis, as all health states within the analysis need to be converted to their QALY equivalent. In some cases, the reduction in quality of life associated with particular health states can be found in other cost-effectiveness analyses or in compilations of effectiveness measures.[26] If this estimate is not readily available in the literature, however, investigators need to determine it. De novo determination of a QALY for a given health state may involve the input of an expert panel, as was demonstrated in a study of the cost-effectiveness of routine hepatitis C screening in pregnancy.[27] Alternatively, investigators may use one of several methodologies to determine these effectiveness measures from a population of patients. Methodologies that have been used to obtain utilities include the time tradeoff and standard gamble techniques.[25] In the obstetrics literature, both Kuppermann et al and Grobman et al have used these types of methodologies to determine the utilities for the health states associated with the decision to proceed with prenatal diagnosis for the detection of Down Syndrome.[28,29]

Determining the Difference in Cost-Effectiveness Between Strategies

The comparison of the cost-effective outcomes between two different strategies is best, and typically, represented by the marginal difference of the two ratios. For example, consider 2 strategies. Strategy 1 costs $700 to implement, and yields a gain of 10 QALY's for a given patient, while strategy 2 costs $1200 to implement but results in 12 QALY's for a given patient. One method to calculate the difference in the two strategies would be 1200/12 − 700/10, yielding a result of $30/QALY. This result, however, is not the marginal difference, which instead, would be calculated as (1200 − 700) / (12-10), or a cost-effectiveness of $250/QALY. It should be noted that if one strategy is both less costly and more effective than another strategy, the former strategy is said to "dominate" the latter.

Sensitivity Analysis

The process whereby inputs are changed and the outcomes are re-assessed is commonly called "sensitivity analysis". Given that the results of a decision analytical model are based on inputs that have been chosen by the investigators, it is extremely important to assess the extent to which the results may be altered by changes in those inputs. For example, if small alterations in the inputs cause a strategy to change from being considered "cost effective" to "not cost effective", there should be less confidence that the model can clearly provide guidance as to the preferred strategy. Conversely, if the results of the model remain unchanged despite changes in the input variables (in which case the results of the model are called "stable" or "robust"), an investigator will have more confidence in the conclusions. Examining the effects engendered by changing the inputs can be further useful to the investigator, as the process can help to determine which particular circumstances are necessary in order for a strategy to be preferred. One particular use of sensitivity analysis is to alter the input variable (or variables) in such a way as to discern the value (or values) at which a given strategy changes from "cost effective" to "not cost effective". Such an analysis is called a "threshold analysis."

The range over which the variable is changed in a sensitivity analysis is determined by the investigator, who may use different methods to determine this range. In some cases, the investigator may base the range upon the range of different estimates for a given variable that is present in the literature. When less data is available, the investigator may choose to derive a range using other methods, such as the 95% confidence interval of a single proportion. In still other cases, for data such as costs or utilities, investigators may choose to use reasonable estimates, such as multiples of the baseline estimate, that are derived from their own judgment. The basis of the range that is chosen should be specified.

In one - way sensitivity analysis, the investigator changes one variable at a time, and assesses the resulting change in the outcome for each variable alteration. The results of this analysis may be presented in tabular format, in which the respective results for each "high" and "low" input are presented. Alternatively, graphical depictions may sometimes help a reader to more easily conceive which variable changes are associated with the greatest magnitude of outcome changes. One such depiction, presented in figure 3, is called a "tornado" diagram, for reasons obviously related to its shape.

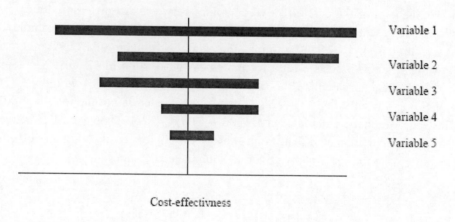

Figure 3. Tornado diagram. Each bar represents the range of results for cost effectiveness that are obtained when each respective variable is varied over its own range of inputs. The vertical line represents the cost-effectiveness value which is obtained when the baseline estimates are placed into the model.

A one-way sensitivity analysis is relatively easy to perform, but because only one variable at a time is changed, the one-way analysis cannot allow an investigator to understand to what extent the model's results are altered under more varied circumstances. One method to overcome this limitation is to perform a "best case" and "worst case" scenario, in which all variables are simultaneously changed to the values that favor or do not favor, respectively, a certain strategy. Certainly, if these changes in all the variables do not alter the basic conclusion of the analysis (e.g. that a given strategy is cost-effective), the model is very robust. Yet, many models will not be so robust, and a more nuanced assessment of the exact circumstances under which a strategy is cost effective will be desired. For example, an investigator may want to examine whether a strategy is cost-effective at different prevalences of illness and at different costs of treatment. In order to assess these circumstances, a two-way sensitivity analysis, in which multiple combinations of two variables are entered into the model and used to calculate the respective outcomes, can be performed. Often presented graphically, this analysis can demonstrate the combinations that are required to result in a cost-effective strategy. An example of the graphic of a two-way sensitivity analysis is presented in Figure 4. If more than two variables are altered at one time, then the sensitivity analysis continues to be characterized by the number of variables that are being simultaneously altered – thus, if three variables are being changed, the appellation for the process would be a "three-way" sensitivity analysis.

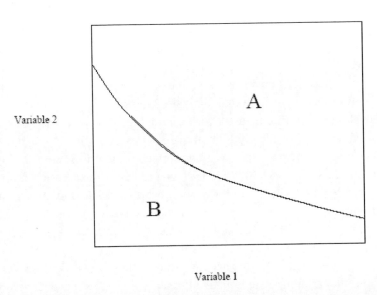

Figure 4. Graphical depiction of two-way sensitivity analysis for a model with two possible strategies. At all combinations of variables in sector "A", one strategy is preferred, while all combinations of variables in sector "B" will result in the other strategy being preferred.

In the sensitivity analyses described so far, one or several inputs simultaneously may be altered along their chosen ranges. One type of sensitivity analysis that is less restrictive and adds a further level of complexity is called a "Monte Carlo" analysis. In this analysis, not only the ranges for each variable, but also the distribution patterns within these ranges (e.g. Gaussian, logarithmic) are specified. Subsequently, all variables that are being assessed have a value simultaneously and probabilistically (according to the specified distribution) chosen from within the range, and placed into the model. This process is subsequently repeated many times (e.g. 10,000), and the distribution of consequent results assessed. In this way, an investigator may discern the distribution of possible results, which provides further information, such as the percent of simulated runs that lead to a strategy being cost-effective. One example of Monte Carlo simulation is provided by Cahill et al, who used decision analysis to assess whether magnesium sulfate should be used for seizure prophylaxis in women with mild preeclampsia.[30]

Further Considerations

When is a Strategy Cost-Effective?

A strategy need not save both money and health to be considered cost-effective. In fact, most strategies that are used as well as accepted as reasonable allocations of resources improve health but at a cost.[24] Accordingly, it is important to consider the amount of expenditure that is acceptable, from a societal perspective, to obtain improved health. Those strategies that are less costly than this threshold are considered "cost effective".

For many years, a cost-effectiveness ratio less than $50,000 (United States dollars) per QALY saved has been used as a benchmark to indicate that a strategy is cost effective. Recently, however, the reasonableness of this benchmark has been questioned.[31] First, the benchmark is essentially arbitrary, as it is based upon the cost effectiveness of a US governmental entitlement, namely renal dialysis. Correspondingly, others have suggested replacement benchmarks. Laupacis et al, for example, have recommended a system whereby results of the analysis are not merely dichotomized (i.e. cost-effective or not cost-effective) but categorized into several grades: a grade A intervention is cost saving, a grade B intervention costs less than $20,000/QALY, a grade C intervention costs $20,000 to $100,000/QALY, a grade D intervention costs more than $100,000/QALY, and a grade E intervention is both no more effective and more costly.[32] Also, the $50,000/QALY benchmark, despite being established approximately one-quarter of a century ago, has not been adjusted for inflation. Ubel has argued that whatever cost-effective threshold is used needs to be adjusted regularly to account for inflation as well as other changing circumstances in the economic and medical realms.[31] Others have contended that cost-effectiveness thresholds, rather than being based on governmental benchmarks, should be more directly based upon patients' actual willingness to pay for additional QALY's.[33] Attempting to discern the exact value of this willingness to pay, however, has proven difficult.[34] Thus, at this point, many authors continue to use $50,000/QALY as a cost-effective threshold, although thresholds ranging up to $100,000/QALY, given the adjustment for inflation, are utilized as well.

Summary

Decision analysis is a type of study design that can help to explicitly compare different medical strategies and provide additional perspective to information provided by observational and interventional studies. Depending on the metrics that are used, decision analysis allows comparison of medical strategies according to health outcomes alone, costs alone, or a combined cost-effectiveness measure. Moreover, depending on the input data that are used, individuals, third-party payers, and society as a whole can better understand the most desirable choices from each of their perspectives. In an effort to achieve proper and consistent methodology, investigators should adhere to the consensus guidelines promulgated by the Panel on Cost-Effectiveness in Health and Medicine. [15,19]

References

[1]   Kim JJ, Wright TC, Goldie SJ. Cost-effectiveness of alternative triage strategies for atypical squamous cells of undetermined significance. *JAMA* 2002;287:2382-90.

[2]   Gates S, Brocklehurst P, Ayers S, Bowler U. Thromboprophylaxis in Pregnancy Advisory Group. Thromboprophylaxis and pregnancy: two randomized controlled pilot trials that used low-molecular-weight heparin. *Am J Obstet Gynecol* 2004 191:1296-303.

[3]   Drife J. *Brit Med Bulletin* 2003;67:177-90.

[4]   Quinones JN, James DN, Stamilio DM, Cleary KL, Macones GA. Thromboprophylaxis after cesarean delivery: a decision analysis. *Obstet Gynecol* 2005;106:733-40.

[5]   Casele H, Grobman WA. Cost effectiveness of thromboprophylaxis with intermittent pneumatic compression at cesarean delivery. *Obstet Gynecol* 2006;108:535-40.

[6]   Rouse DJ, Owen J, Goldenberg RL, Cliver SP. The effectiveness and costs of elective cesarean delivery for fetal macrosomia diagnosed by ultrasound. *JAMA* 1996;276:1480-6.

[7]   Stringer JS, Rouse DJ. Rapid testing and zidovudine treatment to prevent vertical transmission of human immunodeficiency virus in unregistered parturients: a cost-effectiveness analysis. *Obstet Gynecol* 1999;94:34-40.

[8]   Grobman WA, Garcia PM. The cost-effectiveness of voluntary intrapartum rapid human immunodeficiency virus testing for women without adequate prenatal care. *Am J Obstet Gynecol* 1999;181:1062-71.

[9]   Detsky AS, Naglie G, Krahn MD, Redelmeier DA, Naimark D. Primer on medical decision analysis: Part 2 – building a tree. *Med Decis Making* 1997;17:126-35.

[10]   Krahn MD, Naglie G, Naimark D, Redelmeier DA, Detsky AS. Primer on medical decision analysis: Part 4 – analyzing the model and interpreting the results. *Med Decis Making* 1997;17:142-51.

[11]   Sonnenberg FA, Beck JR. Markov models in medical decision making: a practical guide. *Med Decis Making* 1993;13:322-38.

[12]   Plunkett BA, Grobman WA. Elective cesarean delivery to prevent perinatal transmission of hepatitis C virus: a cost-effectiveness analysis. Am J Obstet Gynecol 2004;191:998-1003.

[13]   Caughey AB, Parer JT. Recommendations for repeat courses of antenatal corticosteroids: a decision analysis. *Am J Obstet Gynecol* 2002;186:1221-9.

[14]   Lavin JP, Lavin B, O'Donnell N. A comparison of costs associated with screening for gestational diabetes with two-tiered and one-tiered testing protocols. *Am J Obstet Gynecol* 2001;184:363-7.

[15]   Chen KT, Sell RL, Tuomala RE. Cost-effectiveness of elective cesarean delivery in human immunodeficiency virus-infected women. *Obstet Gynecol* 2001;97:161-8.

[16]   Weinstein MC, Siegel JE, Gold MR, Siegel JE, Daniels N, Weinstein MC,et al. Recommendations of the panel on cost-effectiveness in health and medicine. *JAMA* 1996;276:1172-7.

[17] Visco AG, Taber KH, Weidner AC, Barber MD, Myers ER. Cost-effectiveness of universal cystoscopy to identify ureteral injury at hysterectomy. *Obstet Gynecol* 2001;97:685-92.

[18] Cowett AA, Golub RM, Grobman WA. Cost-effectiveness of dilation and evacuation versus the induction of labor for second-trimester pregnancy termination. *Am J Obstet Gynecol* 2006;194:768-73.

[19] Grable IA. Cost-effectiveness of induction after preterm premature rupture of the membranes. *Am J Obstet Gynecol* 2002;187:1153-8 .

[20] Gold MR, Siegel JE, Russel LB, et al, eds. *Cost-effectiveness in health and medicine.* New York:Oxford University Press, 1996.

[21] Rogowski J. Measuring the cost of neonatal and perinatal care. *Pediatrics* 1999;103:329-35.

[22] Randolph AG, Hartshorn RM, Washington AE, Acyclovir prophylaxis in late pregnancy to prevent neonatal herpes: a cost-effectiveness analysis. *Obstet Gynecol* 1996;88:603-10.

[23] Kulasingham SL, Myers ER, Lawson HW, McConnell KJ, Kerlikowske K, Washington AE, et al. Cost-effectiveness of extending cervical cancer screening intervals among women with prior normal pap tests. *Obstet Gynecol* 2006;107:321-8.

[24] Tengs TO, Adams ME, Pliskin JS, Safran DG, Siegel JE, Weinstein MC, et al. Five-hundred life-saving interventions and their cost-effectiveness. *Risk Analysis.* 1995;15:369-90.

[25] Giesler RB, Ashton CM, Brody B, Byrne MM, Cook K, Geraci JM, et al. Assessing the performance of utility techniques in the absence of a gold standard. *Med Care* 1999;37:580-88.

[26] Tengs TO, Wallace A. One thousand health-related quality-of-life estimates. *Med Care* 2000;38:583-637.

[27] Plunkett BA, Grobman WA. Routine hepatitis C virus screening in pregnancy: a cost-effectiveness analysis. *Am J Obstet Gynecol* 2005;192:1153-61 .

[28] Kuppermann M, Nease RF, Learman LA, Gates E, Blumberg B, Washington AE. Procedure-related miscarriages and Down syndrome-affected births: implications for prenatal testing based on women's preferences. *Obstet Gynecol* 2000;96:511-6.

[29] Grobman WA, Dooley SL, Welshman EE, Pergament E, Calhoun EA. Preference assessment of prenatal diagnosis for Down syndrome: is 35 years a rational cutoff? *Prenatal Diagnosis* 2002;22:1195-200.

[30] Cahill AG, Macones GA, Odibo AO, Stamilio DM. Magnesium for seizure prophylaxis in patients with mild preeclampsia. *Obstet Gynecol* 2007;110:601-7.

[31] Ubel PA. What is the price of life and why doesn't it increase at the rate of inflation? *Arch Intern Med* 2003;163:1637-41.

[32] Laupacis A, Feeny D, Detsky AS, Tugwell PX. How attractive does a new technology have to be to warrant adoption and utilization? Tentative guidelines for using clinical and economic evaluations. *Can Med Assoc J* 1992;146:473-81.

[33] Johannesson M, Meltzer D. Some reflections on cost-effectiveness analysis. *Health Econ* 1998;7:1-7.

[34] Hirth RA, Chernew ME, Miller E, Fendrick M, Weissert WG. Willingness to pay for a quality-adjusted life year: in search of a standard. *Med Decis Making* 2000;20:332-42.

Section II: Clinical Aspects in Perinatal Epidemiology

Preconception and Early Pregnancy

In: Textbook of Perinatal Epidemiology
Editor: Eyal Sheiner, pp. 147-172

ISBN: 978-1-60741-648-7
© 2010 Nova Science Publishers, Inc.

Chapter XI

Epidemiology of Fertility, Pregnancies and Abortions

Brady E. Hamilton[*] *and Stephanie J. Ventura*
Division of Vital Statistics, National Center for Health Statistics
Centers for Disease Control and Prevention

Definitions

- Live Births – The complete expulsion or extraction from its mother of a product of human conception, irrespective of the duration of pregnancy, which, after such expulsion or extraction, breathes, or shows any other evidence of life, such as beating of the heart, pulsation of the umbilical cord, or definite movement of voluntary muscles, whether or not the umbilical cord has been cut or the placenta is attached.
- General Fertility Rate – The number of live births (regardless of the age of mother) during a year per 1,000 women aged 15-44 years in a specified group.
- Age-Specific Birth Rate – The number of births to women in a designated age range during a year per 1,000 women in the same age range.
- Total Fertility Rate – The average number of births expected for a hypothetical cohort of 1,000 women during their childbearing years, assuming the age-specific birth rates for a given period are representative of the whole of the childbearing time. The total fertility rate is the sum of the age-specific birth rates for 5-year age groups multiplied by 5.
- Mean Age – The arithmetic average of the age of women at the time of the birth, computed directly from the frequency of birth by age of mother.

[*] For Correspondence: Brady E. Hamilton, Ph.D, Centers for Disease Control & Prevention, National Center for Health Statistics, Division of Vital Statistics, 3311 Toledo Road, Rm. 7416, Hyattsville, MD 20782, USA. E-mail: BHamilton@cdc.gov

- Birth rate for married women – The number of live births to married women (regardless of the age of mother) during a year per 1,000 married women aged 15-44 years in a specified group.

- Birth rate for unmarried women – The number of live births to unmarried women (regardless of the age of mother) during a year per 1,000 unmarried women aged 15-44 years in a specified group.

- Pregnancy – The state of carrying of one or more developing embryos or fetuses within the female body between conception and either birth, induced termination, or loss.

- Pregnancy Rate – The number of pregnancies (regardless of the age of mother) during a year per 1,000 women aged 15-44 years in a specified group.

- Age-Specific Pregnancy Rate – The number of pregnancies to women in a designated age range during a year per 1,000 women in the same age range.

- Total Pregnancy Rate – The average number of pregnancies expected for a hypothetical cohort of 1,000 women during their childbearing years, assuming the age-specific pregnancy rates for a given period are representative of the whole of the childbearing time. The total pregnancy rate is the sum of the age-specific pregnancy rates for 5-year age groups multiplied by 5.

- Induced Abortion – A suspected or known pregnancy terminated by a licensed physician or someone acting under the supervision of a licensed physician, intended to produce a nonviable fetus irrespective of the duration of pregnancy.

- Induced Abortion Rate – The number of induced abortions (regardless of the age of mother) during a year per 1,000 women aged 15-44 years in a specified group.

- Age-Specific Abortion Rate – The number of abortions to women in a designated age range during a year per 1,000 women in the same age range.

- Total Abortion Rate – The average number of abortions expected for a hypothetical cohort of 1,000 women during their childbearing years, assuming the age-specific abortion rates for a given period are representative of the whole of the childbearing time. The total abortion rate is the sum of the age-specific abortion rates for 5-year age groups multiplied by 5.

- Fetal Loss – A death before the complete expulsion or extraction from its mother of a product of conception, irrespective of the duration of pregnancy; the death is indicated by the fact that after such separation, the fetus does not breathe or show any other evidence of life, such as beating of the heart, pulsation of the umbilical cord, or definite movement of voluntary muscles.

- Fetal Loss Rate – The number of fetal losses (regardless of the age of mother) during a year per 1,000 women aged 15-44 years in a specified group.

- Age-Specific Fetal Loss Rate – The number of fetal losses to women in a designated age range during a year per 1,000 women in the same age range.

- Total Fetal Loss Rate – The average number of fetal losses expected for a hypothetical cohort of 1,000 women during their childbearing years, assuming the age-specific fetal loss rates for a given period are representative of the whole of the childbearing time. The total fetal loss rate is the sum of the age-specific fetal loss rates for 5-year age groups multiplied by 5.

Introduction

Since the mid 20th century, U.S. fertility patterns have changed dramatically. Factors shaping the change in fertility patterns include, in part, trends in marriage and family formation, new contraceptive methods and abortion, which became legal throughout the U.S. in 1973, as well as, changes in the population and the substantial increases in immigration (particularly for Hispanics). This chapter provides a general overview of the long-term and recent changes in birth and fertility patterns important to understanding changes in the health and morbidity of the newborn population in the United States. The discussion is based in most cases on 2006 data or the most recently published data.

The number of births, general fertility rates, and total fertility rates are presented for 1960 to 2006, age specific birth rates are presented for 1980 to 2006, and by race and Hispanic origin of mother for the three largest groups in the U.S. (non-Hispanic white, non-Hispanic black, and Hispanic women) for 1990 to 2006. In addition to birth and fertility rates, this chapter also presents the mean age of mother at first birth for 1968 to 2006 and birth rates for married women and the percentage of births to and birth rates for unmarried women from 1980 to 2006. Also presented are the general pregnancy and abortion rates from 1976 to 2004, age specific and total pregnancy, abortion, and fetal loss rates from 1980 to 2004, and by race and Hispanic origin of mother for the three largest groups for 1990 to 2004.

The birth statistics presented in this chapter are taken from the latest available data (as of the writing of this chapter) from the Centers for Disease Control and Prevention's (CDC) National Center for Health Statistics (NCHS). The most recent detailed fertility data are for 2006. The data are based on 100 percent of birth certificates filed in all states and the District of Columbia and are provided to NCHS through the National Vital Statistics System (NVSS). Detailed technical information on birth certificate data is presented in the NCHS reports.[1-5] The abortion data presented in this chapter are also taken from the latest available data and are based on abortion surveillance information collected from most states by CDC's National Center for Chronic Disease Prevention and Health Promotion (NCCDPHP). These data are adjusted to national totals compiled by the Guttmacher Institute from their surveys of all known abortion providers.[6,7] The most recent detailed abortion data are for 2004 (more recent data on abortion were not available as of the writing of this chapter).

Number of Births

The most basic measure of trends and variations in childbearing is the number of children born. The number of births registered in the United States in 2006 was 4,265,555. This is the largest number of births since 1961, 4,268,326 (Table 1; Figure 1).[1,8] Births began to decline in 1958, after peaking in 1957 (at 4.3 million) during the postwar "baby-boom" (1946 to 1964). Between 1957 and 1973, the number of births fell by 27 percent to 3,136,965.

Table 1. Live births, general fertility rates, total fertility rates, and mean age of mother, United States, 1960-2006, by race and Hispanic origin, 1990-2006, and pregnancy and abortion rates, United States, 1976-2004, by race and Hispanic origin, 1990-2004

[Rates per 1,000 women in specified group. Population for general and total fertility rates enumerated as of April 1 for 1960, 1970, 1980, 1990 and 2000, and estimated as of July 1 for all other years. Population for married and unmarried birth rates estimated as of July 1 for all years]

Race and Hispanic origin of mother and year	Number of births	General fertility rate [1]	Total fertility rate [2]	Mean age of mother at first birth	Birth rate for married women [3]	Percentage of births to unmarried women	Birth rate for unmarried women [4]	Pregnancy rate [5]	Induced abortion rate [6]
					All races and origins [7]				
2006	4,265,555	68.5	2,100.5	25.0	88.0	38.5	50.6	---	---
2005	4,138,349	66.7	2,053.5	25.2	87.3	36.9	47.5	---	---
2004	4,112,052	66.3	2,045.5	25.2	87.6	35.8	46.1	103.0	19.7
2003	4,089,950	66.1	2,042.5	25.2	88.1	34.6	44.9	103.2	20.2
2002	4,021,726	64.8	2,013.0	25.1	86.3	34.0	43.7	101.9	20.5
2001	4,025,933	65.3	2,034.0	25.0	86.7	33.5	43.8	102.9	20.9
2000	4,058,814	65.9	2,056.0	24.9	87.4	33.2	44.1	104.1	21.3
1999	3,959,417	64.4	2,007.5	24.8	84.8	33.0	43.3	102.2	21.4
1998	3,941,553	64.3	1,999.0	24.7	84.2	32.8	43.3	102.2	21.5
1997	3,880,894	63.6	1,971.0	24.7	82.7	32.4	42.9	101.6	21.9
1996	3,891,494	64.1	1,976.0	24.6	82.3	32.4	43.8	102.8	22.4
1995	3,899,589	64.6	1,978.0	24.5	82.6	32.2	44.3	103.5	22.5
1994	3,952,767	65.9	2,001.5	24.4	82.9	32.6	46.2	106.1	23.7
1993	4,000,240	67.0	2,019.5	24.4	86.1	31.0	44.8	108.8	25.0
1992	4,065,014	68.4	2,046.0	24.4	88.5	30.1	44.9	111.1	25.7
1991	4,110,907	69.3	2,062.5	24.2	89.6	29.5	45.0	112.7	26.2
1990	4,158,212	70.9	2,081.0	24.2	93.2	28.0	43.8	115.8	27.4
1989	4,040,958	69.2	2,014.0	24.2	91.9	27.1	41.6	111.8	26.8
1988	3,909,510	67.3	1,934.0	24.1	90.8	25.7	38.5	110.0	27.4
1987	3,809,394	65.8	1,872.0	24.0	90.0	24.5	36.0	106.8	26.9
1986	3,756,547	65.4	1,837.5	23.8	90.7	23.4	34.2	106.7	27.4
1985	3,760,561	66.3	1,844.0	23.7	93.3	22.0	32.8	108.3	28.0
1984 [8]	3,669,141	65.5	1,806.5	23.5	93.1	21.0	31.0	107.4	28.1

Table 1. (Continued)

Year									
1983 [8]	3,6?8,933	65.7	1,799.0	23.3	93.6	20.3	30.3	108.0	28.5
1982 [8]	3,6?0,537	67.3	1,827.5	23.1	96.2	19.4	30.0	110.1	28.8
1981 [8]	3,6?9,238	67.3	1,812.0	22.9	96.0	18.9	29.5	110.5	29.3
1980 [8]	3,6?2,258	68.4	1,839.5	22.7	97.0	18.4	29.4	111.9	29.4
1979 [8]	3,4?4,398	67.2	1,808.0	22.6	96.4	17.1	27.2	109.9	28.8
1978 [8]	3,3?3,279	65.5	1,760.0	22.4	93.6	16.3	25.7	106.7	27.7
1977 [8]	3,3?6,632	66.8	1,789.5	22.2	94.9	15.5	25.6	107.0	26.4
1976 [8]	3,1?7,788	65.0	1,738.0	22.0	91.6	14.8	24.3	102.7	24.2
1975 [8]	3,1?4,198	66.0	1,774.0	21.8	92.1	14.3	24.5	---	---
1974 [8]	3,1?9,958	67.8	1,835.0	21.7	94.2	13.2	23.9	---	---
1973 [8]	3,1?6,965	68.8	1,879.0	21.5	94.7	13.0	24.3	---	---
1972 [8]	3,2?8,411	73.1	2,010.0	21.4	100.8	12.4	24.8	---	---
1971 [9]	3,5?5,970	81.6	2,266.5	21.4	113.2	11.3	25.5	---	---
1970 [9]	3,7?1,386	87.9	2,480.0	21.4	121.1	10.7	26.4	---	---
1969 [9]	3,6?0,206	86.1	2,455.5	21.4	118.8	10.0	24.8	---	---
1968 [9]	3,5?1,564	85.2	2,464.2	21.4	116.6	9.7	24.3	---	---
1967 [10]	3,5?0,959	87.2	2,557.7	---	118.7	9.0	23.7	---	---
1966 [9]	3,6?6,274	90.8	2,721.4	---	123.6	8.4	23.3	---	---
1965 [9]	3,7?0,358	96.3	2,912.6	---	130.2	7.7	23.4	---	---
1964 [9]	4,0?7,490	104.7	3,190.5	---	141.8	6.9	23.0	---	---
1963 [9]	4,0?8,020	108.3	3,318.8	---	145.9	6.3	22.5	---	---
1962 [9]	4,1?7,362	112.0	3,461.3	---	150.8	5.9	21.9	---	---
1961 [9]	4,2?8,326	117.1	3,620.3	---	155.8	5.6	22.7	---	---
1960 [9]	4,2?7,850	118.0	3,653.6	---	156.6	5.3	21.6	---	---
Non-Hispanic White									
2006	2,308,?40	59.5	1,863.5	26.0	86.5	26.6	32.0	---	---
2005	2,279,?68	58.3	1,839.5	26.2	85.8	25.3	30.1	---	10.5
2004	2,296,?83	58.4	1,847.0	26.2	85.9	24.5	29.4	84.3	10.8
2003	2,321,?04	58.5	1,856.5	26.2	86.4	23.6	28.6	84.8	10.9
2002	2,298,?56	57.4	1,828.5	26.1	84.4	23.0	27.8	83.4	11.3
2001	2,326,378	57.7	1,843.0	26.0	84.1	22.5	27.8	84.2	11.7
2000	2,362,?68	58.5	1,866.0	25.9	85.0	22.1	28.0	85.6	11.9
1999	2,346,?50	57.7	1,838.5	25.8	82.9	22.1	27.9	84.8	12.5
1998	2,361,?62	57.6	1,825.0	25.7	82.1	21.9	27.9	85.2	

Table 1. (Continued)

Year								
1997	2,333,363	56.8	1,785.5	25.6	80.2	21.5	27.5	84.8	13.2
1996	2,358,989	57.1	1,781.0	25.6	79.6	21.5	28.2	85.6	13.6
1995	2,382,638	57.5	1,777.5	25.4	79.8	21.2	28.1	86.6	14.2
1994	2,438,855	58.2	1,782.5	25.4	80.5	20.8	28.4	88.0	14.8
1993	2,472,031	58.9	1,786.0	25.3	---	19.5	---	90.0	16.1
1992 [11]	2,527,207	60.0	1,803.5	25.2	---	18.5	---	92.0	16.7
1991 [11]	2,589,878	60.9	1,822.5	25.1	---	18.0	---	94.4	18.1
1990 [12]	2,626,500	62.8	1,850.5	25.0	---	16.9	24.4	98.3	19.7

Non-Hispanic Black

Year								
2006	617,247	70.6	2,115.0	22.7	---	70.7	---	---	---
2005	583,759	67.2	2,019.0	22.7	---	69.9	---	---	---
2004	578,772	67.0	2,020.0	22.7	---	69.3	---	139.3	52.1
2003	576,033	67.1	2,027.5	22.7	---	68.5	---	140.4	53.1
2002	578,335	67.4	2,047.0	22.6	---	68.4	---	141.9	54.2
2001	589,917	69.1	2,104.5	22.4	---	68.6	---	145.5	55.5
2000	604,346	71.4	2,178.5	22.3	---	68.7	---	150.2	57.4
1999	588,981	69.9	2,134.0	22.2	---	69.1	---	148.0	57.2
1998	593,127	70.9	2,164.0	22.2	---	69.3	---	148.7	56.5
1997	581,431	70.3	2,137.5	22.1	---	69.4	---	148.9	57.5
1996	578,099	70.7	2,140.0	22.0	---	70.0	---	150.5	58.6
1995	587,781	72.8	2,186.5	21.9	---	70.0	---	151.3	56.7
1994	619,198	77.5	2,314.5	21.8	---	70.7	---	161.7	61.1
1993	641,273	81.5	2,412.5	21.8	---	68.9	---	170.6	65.0
1992 [11]	657,450	84.5	2,482.5	21.8	---	68.3	---	175.2	65.9
1991 [11]	666,758	87.0	2,532.0	21.7	---	68.2	---	177.9	65.5
1990 [12]	661,701	89.0	2,547.5	21.7	---	66.7	---	181.8	67.0

Hispanic [13]

Year								
2006	1,039,077	101.5	2,959.5	23.1	97.3	49.9	106.1	---	---
2005	985,505	99.4	2,885.0	23.1	98.6	48.0	100.3	---	---
2004	946,349	97.8	2,824.5	23.1	99.7	46.4	95.7	145.7	27.8
2003	912,329	96.9	2,785.5	23.1	101.2	45.0	92.2	145.4	28.7
2002	876,642	94.4	2,748.0	23.0	100.1	43.5	87.9	143.1	29.3
2001	851,851	96.0	2,748.5	22.8	103.1	42.5	87.8	145.4	29.8
2000	815,868	95.9	2,730.0	22.7	101.8	42.7	87.2	146.1	30.6
1999	764,339	93.0	2,649.0	22.6	100.0	42.2	84.9	143.5	31.4
1998	734,661	93.2	2,652.5	22.6	102.3	41.6	82.8	143.9	31.6

Table 1. (Continued)

1997	709,767	94.2	2,680.5	22.5	103.7	40.9	83.2	144.3	30.7
1996	701,335	97.5	2,772.0	22.5	107.2	40.7	86.2	149.4	31.9
1995	679,768	98.8	2,798.5	22.4	107.1	40.8	88.8	151.2	32.2
1994	665,026	100.7	2,839.0	22.4	104.7	43.1	95.8	156.6	35.4
1993	654,418	103.3	2,894.5	22.4	113.0	40.0	91.4	160.6	36.4
1992[11]	643,271	106.1	2,957.5	22.4	117.0	39.1	92.8	166.2	38.8
1991[11]	623,085	106.9	2,963.5	22.4	118.5	38.5	92.5	164.1	35.8
1990[12]	595,073	107.7	2,959.5	22.4	120.0	36.7	89.6	164.2	35.1

--- Data not available.

[1] General fertility rates are the number of live births per 1,000 women aged 15–44 years.

[2] Total fertility rates are the sums of birth rates for 5-year age groups multiplied by 5.

[3] Rates for married women are the number of live births to married women per 1,000 married women aged 15–44 years.

[4] Rates for unmarried women are the number of live births to unmarried women per 1,000 unmarried women aged 15–44 years.

[5] Pregnancy rates are the number of pregnancies (live births, induced abortions, and fetal losses) per 1,000 women aged 15–44 years.

[6] Induced abortion rates are the number of induced abortions per 1,000 women aged 15–44 years.

[7] Includes race and Hispanic origin groups other than non-Hispanic white, non-Hispanic black, and Hispanic.

[8] Based on 100 percent of births in selected States and on a 50 percent sample of births in all other States; see reference 1.

[9] Based on a 50 percent sample of births; see reference 1.

[10] Based on a 20 to 50 percent sample of births; see reference 1.

[11] Excludes data for New Hampshire, which did not report Hispanic origin.

[12] Excludes data for New Hampshire and Oklahoma, which did not report Hispanic origin.

[13] Includes all persons of Hispanic origin of any race.

SOURCES: See references 1, 4, 5, 6, 7, 8, 14, and 15.

From 1974 to 1990, the number increased by 32 percent (more than one million births) to 4,158,212. The increase in the number of births until 1990 was due largely to the concomitant increase in the number of women of reproductive age; the "baby-boom" generation (representing women born during 1946-64) accounted for a 23-percent jump in this population between 1975 and 1990.[9,10] After a downward trend from 1990 to 1997, the number of births has generally increased, with the number of births in 2006 surpassing the number of births in 1990.

Trends in the number of births for the three largest race and Hispanic origin groups in the U.S. differed markedly between 1990 and 2006. Births to non-Hispanic white and non-Hispanic black women decreased 12 and 7 percent, respectively, whereas births to Hispanic women increased 75 percent between 1990 and 2006, exceeding one million, or one in every four births in 2006. The steep growth of the Hispanic population and the higher fertility of Hispanic women have been the major factors in the increased number of births since 1990.

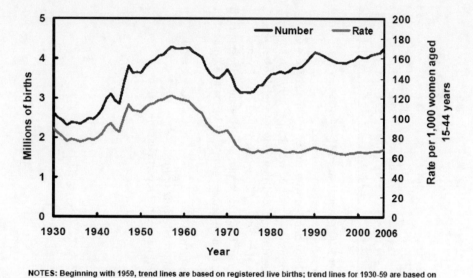

NOTES: Beginning with 1959, trend lines are based on registered live births; trend lines for 1930-59 are based on live births adjusted for underregistration.
SOURCE: CDC/NCHS, National Vital Statistics System.

Figure 1. Live births and fertility rates: United States, 1930-2006.

General Fertility Rate

The general fertility rate is the key summary measure that describes trends and variations in childbearing. The rate is defined as the number of live births (regardless of the age of mother) during a year per 1,000 women of reproductive age (women aged 15-44 years). The rate was 68.5 for the United States in 2006, 42 percent lower compared with 1960 (118.0) (Tables 1 and 2; Figure 1). The general fertility rate has declined for the most part since peaking in 1957.[1,8] The trends in the fertility rate and the number of births were essentially parallel until the mid 1970s and have since diverged. The rate fell substantially (45 percent) from 1960 to 1976, when it reached the low point to that date, 65.0 births per 1,000 women. However, between 1976 and 1990, the most recent peak, the rate rose by 9 percent. Between

1990 and 1997, the general fertility rate decreased substantially, reaching an historic low for the United States (63.6 births to women in 1997). However, the rate has generally increased since, nearly reaching the level set in 1991.

Table 2. Total pregnancy, induced abortion, and fetal loss rates and pregnancy, induced abortion, and fetal loss rates by age of mother, United States, 1980-2004, by race and Hispanic origin, 1990-2004, and total fertility rates and birth rates by age of woman, United States, 1980-2006, by race and Hispanic origin, 1990-2006

[Rates per 1,000 women in specified group. Population enumerated as of April 1 for 1980, 1990 and 2000, and estimated as of July 1 for all other years.]

Race and Hispanic origin of mother, pregnancy outcome and year	Total rate [1]	15-44 years [2]	Under 15 years [3]	15-19 years Total	15-17 years	18-19 years	20-24 years	25-29 years	30-34 years	35-39 years	40-44 years [4]
					Age of woman						
					All races and origins [5]						
					All pregnancies						
2004	3,173.5	103.0	1.6	72.2	41.5	118.6	163.7	169.1	135.2	75.8	17.1
2003	3,186.5	103.2	1.6	73.7	42.7	120.7	166.4	170.0	135.3	73.5	16.8
2002	3,159.0	101.9	1.7	76.0	44.1	124.4	169.0	168.1	130.9	70.0	16.1
2001	3,201.5	102.9	1.8	80.4	46.7	130.5	174.0	168.2	131.5	68.7	15.7
2000	3,243.5	104.1	2.0	84.8	50.8	134.5	179.9	168.6	130.6	67.4	15.4
1999	3,186.0	102.2	2.1	86.9	53.1	136.6	177.8	166.0	125.1	64.7	14.6
1998	3,180.5	102.2	2.3	90.1	56.7	140.3	178.9	164.7	122.4	63.3	14.4
1997	3,155.5	101.6	2.4	92.7	59.5	144.3	178.7	162.5	119.5	61.4	13.9
1996	3,179.5	102.8	2.7	97.0	63.4	149.0	180.5	163.2	118.4	60.6	13.5
1995	3,179.0	103.5	2.9	101.1	67.4	153.4	179.8	162.8	117.0	59.1	13.1
1994	3,241.5	106.1	3.2	106.1	71.1	159.6	184.8	166.1	116.7	58.5	12.9
1993	3,297.5	108.8	3.2	109.4	72.7	164.1	190.4	169.8	116.6	57.7	12.4
1992	3,345.0	111.1	3.3	112.3	73.5	169.3	194.3	173.1	116.6	57.4	12.0
1991	3,378.5	112.7	3.3	116.4	76.1	172.1	196.8	174.9	116.2	56.8	11.3
1990	3,424.0	115.8	3.4	116.8	77.1	167.7	198.5	179.0	118.8	56.9	11.4
1989	3,278.5	111.8	3.4	113.0	76.9	159.3	190.8	173.0	114.2	51.0	10.3
1988	3,188.0	110.0	3.4	109.9	74.1	158.7	186.3	169.0	110.8	48.4	9.8
1987	3,063.0	106.8	3.5	104.8	70.9	154.8	178.9	163.6	107.7	45.1	9.0
1986	3,020.0	106.7	3.6	104.7	69.8	157.1	178.2	161.6	105.0	42.4	8.5
1985	3,034.0	108.3	3.6	106.9	71.1	158.3	179.4	163.0	103.7	41.8	8.4
1984 [6]	2,981.0	107.4	3.5	105.8	70.4	154.4	177.2	160.2	101.1	40.1	8.3
1983 [6]	2,971.5	108.0	3.3	107.2	72.2	153.5	177.8	160.0	98.4	39.0	8.6
1982 [6]	3,002.0	110.1	3.1	107.8	72.1	155.7	182.4	163.4	97.3	37.6	8.8
1981 [6]	2,985.0	110.5	3.1	109.2	72.6	159.6	180.0	164.3	94.8	36.8	8.8
1980 [6]	3,014.5	111.9	3.2	110.0	73.2	162.2	183.5	165.7	95.0	36.4	9.1
					Live births						
2006	2,100.5	68.5	0.6	41.9	22.0	73.0	105.9	116.7	97.7	47.3	10.

Table 2(Continued).

2005	2,053.5	66.7	0.7	40.5	21.4	69.9	102.2	115.5	95.8	46.3	9.7
2004	2,045.5	66.3	0.7	41.1	22.1	70.0	101.7	115.5	95.3	45.4	9.5
2003	2,042.5	66.1	0.6	41.6	22.4	70.7	102.6	115.6	95.1	43.8	9.2
2002	2,013.0	64.8	0.7	43.0	23.2	72.8	103.6	113.6	91.5	41.4	8.7
2001	2,034.0	65.3	0.8	45.3	24.7	76.1	106.2	113.4	91.9	40.6	8.5
2000	2,056.0	65.9	0.9	47.7	26.9	78.1	109.7	113.5	91.2	39.7	8.4
1999	2,007.5	64.4	0.9	48.8	28.2	79.1	107.9	111.2	87.1	37.8	7.8
1998	1,999.0	64.3	1.0	50.3	29.9	80.9	108.4	110.2	85.2	36.9	7.7
1997	1,971.0	63.6	1.1	51.3	31.4	82.1	107.3	108.3	83.0	35.7	7.4
1996	1,976.0	64.1	1.2	53.5	33.3	84.7	107.8	108.6	82.1	34.9	7.1
1995	1,978.0	64.6	1.3	56.0	35.5	87.7	107.5	108.8	81.1	34.0	6.8
1994	2,001.5	65.9	1.4	58.2	37.2	90.2	109.2	111.0	80.4	33.4	6.6
1993	2,019.5	67.0	1.4	59.0	37.5	91.1	111.3	113.2	79.9	32.7	6.3
1992	2,046.0	68.4	1.4	60.3	37.6	93.6	113.7	115.7	79.6	32.3	6.1
1991	2,062.5	69.3	1.4	61.8	38.6	94.0	115.3	117.2	79.2	31.9	5.7
1990	2,081.0	70.9	1.4	59.9	37.5	88.6	116.5	120.2	80.8	31.7	5.6
1989	2,014.0	69.2	1.4	57.3	36.4	84.2	113.8	117.6	77.4	29.9	5.3
1988	1,934.0	67.3	1.3	53.0	33.6	79.9	110.2	114.4	74.8	28.1	5.0
1987	1,872.0	65.8	1.3	50.6	31.7	78.5	107.9	111.6	72.1	26.3	4.6
1986	1,837.5	65.4	1.3	50.2	30.5	79.6	107.4	109.8	70.1	24.4	4.2
1985	1,844.0	66.3	1.2	51.0	31.0	79.6	108.3	111.0	69.1	24.0	4.1
1984 [6]	1,806.5	65.5	1.2	50.6	31.0	77.4	106.8	108.7	67.0	22.9	4.0
1983 [6]	1,799.0	65.7	1.1	51.4	31.8	77.4	107.8	108.5	64.9	22.0	4.0
1982 [6]	1,827.5	67.3	1.1	52.4	32.3	79.4	111.6	111.0	64.1	21.2	4.1
1981 [6]	1,812.0	67.3	1.1	52.2	32.0	80.0	112.2	111.5	61.4	20.0	4.0
1980 [6]	1,839.5	68.4	1.1	53.0	32.5	82.1	115.1	112.9	61.9	19.8	4.1
Induced abortions											
2004	607.0	19.7	0.7	19.8	11.8	31.9	39.9	29.7	18.2	9.8	3.3
2003	625.0	20.2	0.7	20.7	12.5	33.0	41.5	30.4	18.5	9.8	3.4
2002	638.0	20.5	0.7	21.3	12.8	34.1	42.9	31.0	18.6	9.7	3.4
2001	656.0	20.9	0.8	22.6	13.5	36.3	44.7	31.4	18.7	9.7	3.3
2000	672.0	21.3	0.9	24.0	14.5	37.7	46.3	31.6	18.7	9.7	3.2
1999	674.5	21.4	0.9	24.7	15.2	38.6	46.4	31.7	18.3	9.7	3.2
1998	680.5	21.5	1.0	25.8	16.4	40.0	47.0	31.7	17.9	9.5	3.2
1997	692.0	21.9	1.0	27.1	17.2	42.6	48.1	31.9	17.7	9.5	3.1
1996	708.5	22.4	1.1	28.6	18.6	44.0	49.3	32.1	17.7	9.7	3.2
1995	708.0	22.5	1.2	29.4	19.5	44.8	49.1	31.5	17.5	9.7	3.2
1994	740.5	23.7	1.3	31.6	21.0	47.8	51.9	32.1	18.1	9.9	3.2
1993	777.0	25.0	1.4	33.9	22.2	51.2	54.9	33.2	18.6	10.2	3.2
1992	792.0	25.7	1.4	35.2	22.9	53.3	55.9	33.5	18.9	10.3	3.2
1991	805.0	26.2	1.4	37.4	24.2	55.7	56.4	33.4	19.0	10.4	3.0
1990	830.5	27.4	1.5	40.3	26.5	57.9	56.7	33.9	19.7	10.8	3.2
1989	806.5	26.8	1.6	42.0	28.0	60.0	53.8	32.2	18.6	10.1	3.0
1988	811.0	27.4	1.7	43.5	30.2	62.0	53.6	32.0	18.4	10.0	3.0
1987	788.0	26.9	1.8	41.8	29.6	59.8	52.0	31.0	18.2	9.9	2.9

1986	788.5	27.4	2.0	42.3	29.9	60.8	51.8	31.1	18.0	9.7	2.8
1985	795.5	28.0	2.0	43.5	30.6	62.0	52.0	31.1	17.9	9.7	2.9
1984	789.5	28.1	2.0	42.9	29.9	60.8	51.6	31.0	17.9	9.6	2.9
1983	787.5	28.5	1.9	43.2	30.7	59.9	50.9	31.0	17.8	9.5	3.2
1982	786.5	28.8	1.6	42.7	30.0	59.7	51.1	31.5	17.8	9.3	3.3
1981	789.5	29.3	1.7	42.9	30.1	60.6	51.4	31.3	17.7	9.5	3.4
1980	785.5	29.4	1.7	42.7	30.1	60.6	51.6	31.0	17.2	9.4	3.5

Fetal losses

2004	520.5	17.0	0.2	11.3	7.7	16.7	22.1	23.9	21.7	20.6	4.3
2003	517.5	16.9	0.2	11.4	7.8	16.9	22.3	23.9	21.6	19.9	4.2
2002	508.0	16.6	0.2	11.8	8.1	17.4	22.5	23.5	20.8	18.8	4.0
2001	513.0	16.7	0.3	12.4	8.6	18.2	23.1	23.5	20.9	18.5	3.9
2000	517.0	16.9	0.3	13.1	9.4	18.7	23.9	23.5	20.7	18.1	3.8
1999	504.5	16.5	0.3	13.5	9.8	18.9	23.5	23.0	19.8	17.2	3.6
1998	501.5	16.4	0.3	14.0	10.4	19.4	23.6	22.8	19.3	16.8	3.5
1997	494.0	16.2	0.4	14.3	10.9	19.6	23.3	22.4	18.8	16.2	3.4
1996	495.0	16.3	0.4	15.0	11.6	20.3	23.4	22.5	18.6	15.9	3.2
1995	495.5	16.3	0.5	15.7	12.3	21.0	23.3	22.6	18.4	15.5	3.1
1994	499.5	16.6	0.5	16.3	12.9	21.6	23.7	23.0	18.2	15.2	3.0
1993	503.0	16.7	0.5	16.5	13.0	21.8	24.2	23.5	18.1	14.9	2.9
1992	508.0	17.0	0.5	16.8	13.0	22.4	24.7	24.0	18.1	14.7	2.8
1991	511.0	17.1	0.5	17.2	13.4	22.5	25.1	24.3	18.0	14.5	2.6
1990	513.0	17.4	0.5	16.6	13.0	21.2	25.3	24.9	18.3	14.4	2.6
1989	460.5	15.7	0.5	13.7	12.6	15.2	23.3	23.3	18.3	11.0	2.0
1988	445.0	15.4	0.4	13.5	10.3	16.8	22.5	22.7	17.7	10.4	1.8
1987	402.5	14.1	0.4	12.4	9.6	16.5	19.0	21.0	17.4	8.8	1.5
1986	394.5	13.9	0.4	12.3	9.3	16.7	19.0	20.7	16.9	8.2	1.4
1985	395.0	14.0	0.4	12.4	9.4	16.7	19.1	20.9	16.7	8.1	1.4
1984	387.0	13.8	0.4	12.3	9.5	16.2	18.9	20.5	16.2	7.7	1.4
1983	383.5	13.8	0.3	12.5	9.7	16.2	19.0	20.4	15.7	7.4	1.4
1982	388.0	14.1	0.3	12.7	9.8	16.7	19.7	20.9	15.5	7.1	1.4
1981	384.5	13.9	0.4	14.1	10.5	19.0	16.5	21.6	15.7	7.2	1.4
1980	389.5	14.1	0.4	14.3	10.6	19.5	16.9	21.8	15.8	7.2	1.5

Non-Hispanic White

All pregnancies

2004	2,658.5	84.3	0.6	45.2	22.4	79.3	122.8	148.9	128.4	70.9	14.9
2003	2,680.5	84.8	0.6	47.1	23.9	82.2	125.7	150.1	129.3	68.7	14.6
2002	2,648.5	83.4	0.6	49.0	25.0	85.2	126.8	148.5	125.6	65.2	14.0
2001	2,679.5	84.2	0.6	52.4	27.0	90.6	131.9	148.2	125.5	63.7	13.6
2000	2,723.5	85.6	0.7	56.3	29.8	95.4	138.0	149.5	124.3	62.5	13.4
1999	2,697.5	84.8	0.8	59.0	32.4	98.2	137.7	148.9	119.9	60.3	12.9
1998	2,699.0	85.2	0.9	61.8	35.4	101.8	139.8	148.3	117.3	59.1	12.6
1997	2,672.5	84.8	1.0	64.5	37.9	106.1	140.0	146.0	114.0	57.0	12.0
1996	2,679.5	85.6	1.0	67.2	40.3	109.1	141.1	146.6	112.3	56.0	11.7
1995	2,690.5	86.6	1.2	70.6	43.0	113.7	142.4	147.4	110.9	54.4	11.2

Table 2(Continued).

1994	2,713.5	88.0	1.2	73.4	44.7	117.4	144.9	149.2	109.7	53.4	10.9
1993	2,751.5	90.0	1.3	75.9	46.0	120.8	149.5	152.3	108.7	52.2	10.4
1992 [7]	2,788.5	92.0	1.3	78.3	46.6	125.3	152.8	155.6	108.2	51.5	10.0
1991 [7]	2,852.0	94.4	1.3	83.8	50.1	130.4	157.6	158.9	108.2	51.3	9.3
1990 [8]	2,930.0	98.3	1.4	86.8	52.5	129.8	162.1	164.0	110.9	51.4	9.4
Live births										
2006	1,863.5	59.5	0.2	26.6	11.8	49.3	83.4	109.1	98.1	46.3	9.0
2005	1,839.5	58.3	0.2	25.9	11.5	48.0	81.4	109.1	96.9	45.6	8.8
2004	1,847.0	58.4	0.2	26.7	12.0	48.7	81.9	110.0	97.1	44.8	8.8
2003	1,856.5	58.5	0.2	27.4	12.4	50.0	83.5	110.8	97.6	43.2	8.6
2002	1,828.5	57.4	0.2	28.5	13.1	51.9	84.3	109.3	94.4	40.9	8.1
2001	1,843.0	57.7	0.3	30.3	14.0	54.8	87.1	108.9	94.3	39.8	7.9
2000	1,866.0	58.5	0.3	32.6	15.8	57.5	91.2	109.4	93.2	38.8	7.7
1999	1,838.5	57.7	0.3	34.1	17.1	59.4	90.6	108.6	89.5	37.3	7.3
1998	1,825.0	57.6	0.3	35.3	18.3	60.9	91.2	107.4	87.2	36.4	7.1
1997	1,785.5	56.8	0.4	36.0	19.3	62.1	90.0	104.8	84.3	34.8	6.8
1996	1,781.0	57.1	0.4	37.6	20.6	64.0	90.1	104.9	82.8	33.9	6.5
1995	1,777.5	57.5	0.4	39.3	22.0	66.2	90.2	105.1	81.5	32.8	6.1
1994	1,782.5	58.2	0.5	40.4	22.7	67.6	90.9	106.6	80.2	32.0	5.9
1993	1,786.0	58.9	0.5	40.7	22.7	67.7	92.2	108.2	79.0	31.0	5.6
1992 [7]	1,803.5	60.0	0.5	41.7	22.7	69.8	93.9	110.6	78.3	30.4	5.3
1991 [7]	1,822.5	60.9	0.5	43.4	23.6	70.6	95.7	112.1	77.7	30.2	4.8
1990 [8]	1,850.5	62.8	0.5	42.5	23.2	66.6	97.5	115.3	79.4	30.0	4.8
Induced abortions										
2004	329.5	10.5	0.3	11.4	6.2	19.0	22.1	14.8	9.4	5.8	2.1
2003	342.5	10.8	0.3	12.4	7.2	20.2	23.1	15.0	9.7	5.8	2.2
2002	347.0	10.9	0.3	12.7	7.3	20.9	23.3	15.3	9.9	5.7	2.2
2001	362.5	11.3	0.3	13.9	8.1	22.7	24.9	15.6	9.9	5.8	2.1
2000	378.5	11.7	0.3	14.8	8.5	24.1	26.0	16.2	10.2	6.0	2.2
1999	386.5	11.9	0.4	15.5	9.4	24.6	26.3	16.6	10.2	6.1	2.2
1998	407.0	12.5	0.4	16.9	10.7	26.3	27.7	17.5	10.4	6.3	2.2
1997	430.5	13.2	0.5	18.6	11.8	29.1	29.4	18.3	10.7	6.4	2.2
1996	443.5	13.6	0.5	19.3	12.6	29.8	30.3	18.8	10.8	6.7	2.3
1995	460.5	14.2	0.6	20.5	13.4	31.6	31.6	19.3	11.1	6.7	2.3
1994	476.0	14.8	0.6	21.8	14.1	33.7	33.2	19.2	11.4	6.7	2.3
1993	512.5	16.1	0.6	24.0	15.4	36.9	36.2	20.4	11.9	7.1	2.3
1992 [7]	530.0	16.7	0.7	25.3	16.0	38.9	37.5	20.8	12.2	7.2	2.3
1991 [7]	571.5	18.1	0.7	28.7	18.3	43.0	40.0	22.2	13.0	7.5	2.2
1990 [8]	613.5	19.7	0.8	32.5	21.1	46.8	41.9	23.4	13.8	7.9	2.4
Fetal losses										
	482.0	15.5	0.1	7.2	4.2	11.6	18.8	24.0	21.9	20.4	4.0
2003	482.0	15.5	0.1	7.4	4.3	12.0	19.1	24.2	22.0	19.7	3.9
2002	473.0	15.2	0.1	7.7	4.6	12.4	19.3	23.9	21.3	18.6	3.7
2001	475.0	15.2	0.1	8.2	4.9	13.1	19.9	23.8	21.3	18.1	3.6
2000	479.5	15.4	0.1	8.8	5.5	13.8	20.9	23.9	21.0	17.7	3.5

1999	471.5	15.2	0.1	9.3	5.9	14.2	20.8	23.7	20.2	16.9	3.3
1998	467.5	15.1	0.1	9.6	6.4	14.6	20.9	23.5	19.7	16.5	3.2
1997	457.0	14.9	0.1	9.9	6.7	14.9	20.6	22.9	19.0	15.8	3.1
1996	454.5	14.9	0.1	10.3	7.2	15.3	20.6	22.9	18.7	15.4	2.9
1995	453.5	14.9	0.2	10.8	7.6	15.8	20.6	23.0	18.4	14.9	2.8
1994	454.5	15.0	0.2	11.2	7.9	16.2	20.8	23.3	18.1	14.6	2.7
1993	453.0	15.1	0.2	11.2	7.9	16.2	21.1	23.7	17.8	14.1	2.5
1992 [7]	456.0	15.2	0.2	11.4	7.9	16.7	21.5	24.2	17.7	13.8	2.4
1991 [7]	459.0	15.4	0.2	11.8	8.2	16.9	21.9	24.5	17.5	13.7	2.2
1990 [8]	465.5	15.8	0.2	11.6	8.1	16.0	22.4	25.2	17.9	13.6	2.2

Non-Hispanic Black

All pregnancies

2004	4,200.5	139.3	4.4	128.0	80.1	202.9	259.0	211.5	141.1	76.3	19.8
2003	4,243.5	140.4	4.6	131.6	83.7	206.2	264.7	212.7	141.3	74.7	19.1
2002	4,309.5	141.9	5.0	138.0	87.8	215.5	272.8	215.0	139.2	72.9	19.0
2001	4,427.0	145.5	5.5	147.2	93.9	228.0	285.1	216.5	139.9	72.8	18.4
2000	4,581.0	150.2	6.1	158.8	104.8	237.8	302.6	217.9	140.0	72.5	18.3
1999	4,519.0	148.0	6.4	161.9	106.4	242.9	298.9	214.6	134.8	70.3	16.9
1998	4,537.5	148.7	7.0	168.4	114.5	247.8	299.1	213.4	133.5	69.1	17.0
1997	4,529.5	148.9	7.6	174.7	121.3	257.3	296.7	210.2	132.0	68.0	16.7
1996	4,557.5	150.5	8.6	182.2	129.7	264.0	297.1	209.3	130.9	67.1	16.3
1995	4,545.5	151.3	9.6	189.6	139.4	268.4	291.7	205.3	130.8	66.3	15.8
1994	4,825.0	161.7	10.9	207.3	152.9	292.2	313.3	215.4	134.7	67.6	15.8
1993	5,051.5	170.6	11.1	219.0	161.9	305.1	331.5	224.7	139.3	68.9	15.8
1992 [7]	5,145.5	175.2	11.5	226.0	165.2	314.8	339.3	228.8	139.6	68.7	15.2
1991 [7]	5,181.5	177.9	11.7	231.8	170.5	316.0	342.1	228.8	139.2	67.6	15.1
1990 [8]	5,214.0	181.8	12.2	232.7	172.0	312.6	340.2	232.7	141.7	68.0	15.3

Live births

2006	2,115.0	70.6	1.6	63.7	36.2	108.4	133.2	107.1	72.6	36.0	8.8
2005	2,019.0	67.2	1.7	60.9	34.9	103.0	126.8	103.0	68.4	34.3	8.7
2004	2,020.0	67.0	1.6	63.1	37.1	103.9	126.9	103.0	67.4	33.7	8.3
2003	2,027.5	67.1	1.6	64.7	38.7	105.3	128.1	102.1	67.4	33.4	8.1
2002	2,047.0	67.4	1.9	68.3	41.0	110.3	131.0	102.1	66.1	32.1	7.9
2001	2,104.5	69.1	2.1	73.5	44.9	116.7	137.2	102.1	66.2	32.1	7.6
2000	2,178.5	71.4	2.4	79.2	50.1	121.9	145.4	102.8	66.5	31.8	7.5
1999	2,134.0	69.9	2.6	81.0	51.7	123.9	142.1	99.8	63.9	30.6	6.8
1998	2,164.0	70.9	2.9	85.7	56.8	128.2	142.5	99.9	64.4	30.4	6.9
1997	2,137.5	70.3	3.2	88.3	60.7	131.0	138.8	97.2	63.6	29.6	6.8
1996	2,140.0	70.7	3.6	91.9	64.8	134.1	137.0	96.7	63.2	29.1	6.4
1995	2,186.5	72.8	4.2	97.2	70.4	139.2	137.8	98.5	64.4	28.8	6.3
1994	2,314.5	77.5	4.6	105.7	77.0	150.4	146.8	104.1	66.3	29.1	6.2
1993	2,412.5	81.5	4.6	110.5	81.1	154.6	154.5	109.2	68.1	29.4	6.1
1992 [7]	2,482.5	84.5	4.8	114.7	82.9	161.1	160.8	112.8	68.4	29.1	5.8
1991 [7]	2,532.0	87.0	4.9	118.2	86.1	162.2	164.8	115.1	68.9	28.7	5.7
1990 [8]	2,547.5	89.0	5.0	116.2	84.9	157.5	165.1	118.4	70.2	28.7	5.8

Table 2(Continued).

					Induced abortions					
2004	1,571.0	52.1	2.2	47.3	30.2	74.2	99.9	83.4	50.5	23.9	7.0
2003	1,604.5	53.1	2.4	48.8	31.6	75.7	104.0	85.7	50.8	22.7	6.5
2002	1,649.5	54.2	2.5	50.7	32.5	78.7	108.5	87.9	50.5	23.0	6.8
2001	1,693.0	55.5	2.7	53.2	33.4	83.3	112.9	89.4	51.0	22.9	6.5
2000	1,753.5	57.4	2.9	57.4	37.3	86.8	120.2	89.9	50.7	23.0	6.6
1999	1,751.0	57.2	3.0	58.1	36.7	89.4	120.8	90.3	49.0	22.7	6.3
1998	1,731.0	56.5	3.2	58.6	38.0	89.0	120.3	89.0	47.0	21.9	6.2
1997	1,756.5	57.5	3.2	61.3	39.5	95.0	122.7	89.3	46.6	22.0	6.2
1996	1,782.5	58.6	3.8	64.1	42.4	97.9	125.3	88.9	46.1	21.9	6.4
1995	1,710.0	56.7	3.9	64.6	44.6	96.0	118.9	82.8	44.3	21.4	6.1
1994	1,825.5	61.1	4.6	71.2	49.1	105.8	129.2	85.9	45.7	22.3	6.2
1993	1,927.5	65.0	4.8	76.9	52.6	113.5	137.7	88.8	47.9	23.1	6.3
1992 [7]	1,935.0	65.9	5.1	78.6	53.5	115.2	137.6	88.4	47.7	23.4	6.2
1991 [7]	1,909.0	65.5	5.1	80.0	54.5	115.0	135.4	85.4	46.8	22.9	6.2
1990 [8]	1,924.0	67.0	5.4	83.5	57.7	117.4	133.1	85.4	47.5	23.5	6.4
					Fetal losses					
2004	610.0	20.2	0.6	17.5	12.9	24.8	32.3	25.2	23.1	18.7	4.6
2003	612.0	20.3	0.6	18.0	13.4	25.2	32.6	25.0	23.1	18.6	4.5
2002	614.0	20.3	0.7	19.0	14.2	26.4	33.3	25.0	22.6	17.8	4.4
2001	629.0	20.8	0.7	20.5	15.6	27.9	34.9	25.0	22.7	17.8	4.2
2000	649.5	21.4	0.8	22.2	17.4	29.1	37.0	25.2	22.8	17.7	4.2
1999	634.0	20.9	0.9	22.7	18.0	29.6	36.1	24.4	21.9	17.0	3.8
1998	643.5	21.3	1.0	24.1	19.7	30.7	36.2	24.5	22.1	16.9	3.9
1997	636.5	21.1	1.1	25.1	21.1	31.3	35.3	23.8	21.8	16.4	3.8
1996	636.5	21.2	1.3	26.2	22.5	32.1	34.8	23.7	21.6	16.2	3.5
1995	650.0	21.8	1.5	27.9	24.4	33.3	35.0	24.1	22.0	16.0	3.5
1994	685.5	23.1	1.6	30.4	26.8	36.0	37.3	25.5	22.7	16.2	3.4
1993	712.0	24.1	1.6	31.7	28.2	37.0	39.3	26.7	23.3	16.4	3.4
1992 [7]	728.5	24.8	1.7	32.7	28.8	38.5	40.9	27.6	23.4	16.2	3.2
1991 [7]	741.5	25.4	1.7	33.7	29.9	38.8	41.9	28.2	23.6	16.0	3.2
1990 [8]	744.0	25.8	1.7	33.0	29.5	37.7	42.0	29.0	24.0	15.9	3.2
					Hispanic					
					All pregnancies					
2004	4,219.0	145.7	2.5	132.8	82.9	210.0	244.8	206.3	148.4	86.2	22.8
2003	4,189.0	145.4	2.5	132.1	82.8	207.5	243.4	205.9	146.9	83.9	23.1
2002	4,128.5	143.1	2.7	134.7	84.8	210.1	247.2	200.3	138.9	79.8	22.1
2001	4,172.5	145.4	3.0	139.2	88.1	213.6	245.7	201.6	142.6	80.3	22.1
2000	4,171.0	146.1	3.3	142.1	93.3	211.6	244.0	202.4	142.3	78.4	21.7
1999	4,095.5	143.5	3.5	143.2	97.0	209.6	241.1	198.6	136.4	75.9	20.4
1998	4,104.5	143.9	3.8	146.3	100.3	214.5	243.2	199.1	133.7	74.2	20.6
1997	4,115.5	144.3	4.0	147.7	102.6	215.5	245.8	199.9	131.6	73.6	20.5
1996	4,258.0	149.4	4.4	157.1	109.4	228.4	256.5	204.4	134.0	74.9	20.3
1995	4,297.5	151.2	4.7	163.3	115.5	234.2	259.6	203.2	133.4	74.8	20.5
1994	4,431.0	156.6	4.9	169.0	120.3	240.7	270.1	208.8	136.5	75.8	21.1

1993	4,518.0	160.6	4.9	170.3	117.8	247.9	277.3	213.8	139.9	76.6	20.8
1992 [7]	4,653.5	166.2	4.9	174.0	119.7	253.9	286.6	219.3	144.1	80.1	21.7
1991 [7]	4,570.0	164.1	4.6	173.7	117.4	254.3	279.5	217.0	141.3	77.3	20.6
1990 [8]	4,534.0	164.2	4.4	167.4	113.0	242.4	271.2	219.3	145.4	78.1	21.0

Live births										
2006	2,959.5	101.5	1.3	83.0	47.9	139.7	177.0	152.4	108.5	55.6	13.9
2005	2,885.0	99.4	1.3	81.7	48.5	134.6	170.0	149.2	106.8	54.2	13.6
2004	2,824.5	97.8	1.3	82.6	49.7	133.5	165.3	145.6	104.1	52.9	13.0
2003	2,785.5	96.9	1.3	82.3	49.7	132.0	163.4	144.4	102.0	50.8	12.8
2002	2,718.0	94.4	1.4	83.4	50.7	133.0	164.3	139.4	95.1	47.8	12.1
2001	2,748.5	96.0	1.6	86.4	52.8	135.5	163.5	140.4	97.6	47.9	12.1
2000	2,730.0	95.9	1.7	87.3	55.5	132.6	161.3	139.9	97.1	46.6	12.0
1999	2,649.0	93.0	1.9	86.8	56.9	129.5	157.3	135.8	92.3	44.5	11.1
1998	2,652.5	93.2	1.9	87.9	58.5	131.5	159.3	136.1	90.5	43.4	11.3
1997	2,680.5	94.2	2.1	89.6	61.1	132.4	162.6	137.5	89.6	43.4	11.2
1996	2,772.0	97.5	2.4	94.6	64.2	140.0	170.2	140.7	91.3	43.9	11.2
1995	2,798.5	98.8	2.6	99.3	68.3	145.4	171.9	140.4	90.5	43.7	11.2
1994	2,839.0	100.7	2.6	101.3	69.9	147.5	175.7	142.4	91.1	43.4	11.1
1993	2,894.5	103.3	2.6	101.8	68.5	151.1	180.0	146.0	93.2	44.1	11.1
1992 [7]	2,957.5	106.1	2.5	103.3	68.9	153.9	185.2	148.8	94.8	45.3	11.4
1991 [7]	2,963.5	106.9	2.4	104.6	69.2	155.5	184.6	150.0	95.1	44.7	11.1
1990 [8]	2,959.5	107.7	2.4	100.3	65.9	147.7	181.0	153.0	98.3	45.3	11.4

Induced abortions										
2004	805.5	27.8	0.8	27.1	15.9	44.6	54.8	37.8	23.0	12.8	4.8
2003	825.0	28.7	0.8	26.9	15.8	44.0	55.6	38.8	24.0	13.5	5.4
2002	847.0	29.3	0.8	28.0	16.5	45.3	58.4	39.0	24.2	13.6	5.4
2001	853.0	29.8	0.9	28.7	16.9	45.8	57.8	39.1	25.0	13.8	5.3
2000	872.0	30.6	1.0	30.3	18.4	47.3	58.6	40.5	25.2	13.8	5.0
1999	896.0	31.4	1.0	32.1	20.2	49.1	60.3	41.5	25.2	14.1	5.0
1998	900.5	31.6	1.1	33.7	21.5	51.6	60.1	41.6	24.6	14.0	5.0
1997	877.0	30.7	1.1	32.7	20.3	51.4	58.8	40.8	23.7	13.4	4.9
1996	911.5	31.9	1.2	35.7	22.9	54.9	60.9	41.6	24.1	14.0	4.8
1995	918.0	32.2	1.2	35.8	23.5	54.0	62.1	40.8	24.4	14.3	5.0
1994	1,004.0	35.4	1.4	39.0	26.1	58.0	68.2	44.1	26.8	15.6	5.7
1993	1,024.5	36.4	1.4	39.7	25.5	60.7	70.4	45.0	27.6	15.4	5.4
1992 [7]	1,086.5	38.8	1.5	41.6	26.8	63.3	73.9	47.3	29.9	17.2	5.9
1991 [7]	997.0	35.8	1.4	39.6	24.2	61.7	67.4	43.6	26.8	15.4	5.2
1990 [8]	970.0	35.1	1.1	39.1	24.3	59.5	63.4	42.6	27.2	15.4	5.2

Fetal losses										
2004	588.0	20.1	0.4	23.0	17.3	31.9	24.7	22.8	21.3	20.4	5.0
2003	579.5	19.8	0.5	22.9	17.3	31.6	24.4	22.7	20.9	19.6	4.9
2002	564.5	19.3	0.5	23.3	17.6	31.8	24.5	21.9	19.5	18.5	4.7
2001	571.0	19.6	0.5	24.1	18.3	32.4	24.4	22.0	20.0	18.5	4.7
2000	568.5	19.6	0.6	24.4	19.3	31.7	24.1	22.0	19.9	18.0	4.7
1999	551.0	19.0	0.6	24.4	19.8	31.0	23.5	21.3	18.9	17.2	4.3

Table 2(Continued).

1998	552.0	19.1	0.7	24.8	20.3	31.4	23.8	21.4	18.5	16.8	4.4
1997	557.5	19.3	0.7	25.4	21.2	31.7	24.3	21.6	18.4	16.8	4.3
1996	575.5	20.0	0.8	26.8	22.3	33.5	25.4	22.1	18.7	17.0	4.3
1995	582.5	20.2	0.9	28.2	23.7	34.8	25.7	22.0	18.5	16.9	4.3
1994	590.0	20.5	0.9	28.7	24.3	35.3	26.3	22.3	18.7	16.8	4.3
1993	599.5	20.9	0.9	28.8	23.8	36.1	26.9	22.9	19.1	17.0	4.3
1992 [7]	611.5	21.4	0.9	29.1	23.9	36.8	27.7	23.3	19.4	17.5	4.4
1991 [7]	612.0	21.5	0.8	29.4	24.0	37.2	27.6	23.5	19.5	17.3	4.3
1990 [8]	609.5	21.5	0.8	28.1	22.9	35.3	27.0	24.0	20.1	17.5	4.4

[1] Total pregnancy rates are the sums of pregnancy rates for 5-year age groups multiplied by 5. Total fertility rates are the sums of birth rates for 5-year age groups multiplied by 5. Total abortion rates are the sums of abortion rates for 5-year age groups multiplied by 5. Total fetal loss rates are the sums of fetal loss rates for 5-year age groups multiplied by 5.

[2] Rates computed by relating the number of events to women of all ages to women aged 15-44 years.

[3] Rates computed by relating the number of events to women under 15 years to women aged 10-14 years.

[4] Rates computed by relating the number of events to women aged 40 years and over to women aged 40-44 years.

[5] Includes race and Hispanic origin groups other than non-Hispanic white, non-Hispanic black, and Hispanic.

[6] Based on 100 percent of births in selected States and on a 50 percent sample of births in all other States; see reference 1.

[7] Excludes data for New Hampshire, which did not report Hispanic origin.

[8] Excludes data for New Hampshire and Oklahoma, which did not report Hispanic origin.

SOURCES: See reference 1, 6, and 7.

Table 3. General fertility rates and total fertility rates by Hispanic origin, 1990 and 2006

[Rates per 1,000 women in specified group. Population for general and total fertility rates enumerated as of April 1 for 1990 and estimated as of July 1, 2006]

Hispanic origin of mother	General fertility rate [1]		Total fertility rate [2]	
	1990 [3]	2006	1990 [3]	2006
Total	107.7	101.5	2,959.5	2,959.5
Mexican	118.9	109.0	3,214.0	3,107.5
Puerto Rican	82.9	74.0	2,301.0	2,167.0
Cuban	52.6	49.3	1,459.5	1,601.5
Other Hispanic [4]	102.7	98.6	2,877.0	3,014.0

[1] General fertility rates are the number of live births per 1,000 women aged 15-44 years.

[2] Total fertility rates are the sums of birth rates for 5-year age groups multiplied by 5.

[3] Excludes data for New Hampshire and Oklahoma, which did not report Hispanic origin.

[4] Rates for other Hispanic population include unknown Hispanic and Central and South American.

SOURCE: See reference 1.

The general fertility rates differed considerably by race and Hispanic origin. The rate for Hispanic women in 2006, 101.5 births per 1,000, was 44 percent higher than the rate for non-Hispanic black women (70.6) and 71 percent higher than the rate for non-Hispanic white women (59.5). Among the specified Hispanic groups, however, there is a comparable range of differences in fertility as well, with the rates ranging from 49.3 for Cuban women to 109.0 for Mexican women (Table 3). The general fertility rates for the three largest race and Hispanic origin groups are generally lower in 2006 compared with 1990. However, a comparison of these declines reveals important differences. Rates decreased 5 percent for non-Hispanic white women and 6 percent for Hispanic women, whereas the rate for non-Hispanic black women declined by 21 percent. Rates decreased from 4 percent for other Hispanic (which include Central and South American) women to 11 percent for Puerto Rican women.

Age-Specific Birth Rates

Teenage childbearing is problematic because it is associated with a variety of maternal and infant health and social risks. Teenage mothers are less educated, are more likely to be unmarried, have fewer financial resources and more limited social support.[1,11] Babies born to teenagers are more likely to be low birthweight and preterm, and are at greater risk of infant morbidity and mortality.[1,12] Birth rates at the younger ages have generally fallen since the late 1950s, except for a brief upward spike in the late 1980s (Figure 2). Rates for teenagers 15-19 years had been on a steady downward trend during 1991-2005, but then increased 3 percent in 2006.[1] Nonetheless, the teenage birth rate in 2006, 41.9 births per 1,000 women aged 15-19 years, was less than half the peak rate reported for 1957 (96.3).[1,8] Partly as a result of the generally falling teenage birth rate, the proportion of all births that are to teenagers has fallen sharply in the U.S., from a high of 19 percent in 1975 to 10 percent in 2006.

The birth rate for the youngest teenagers was 0.6 births per 1,000 females aged 10-14 years in 2006, less than half the level recorded in 1994 (1.4). The number of births to this age group has dropped more than 50 percent, from an historic peak of 12,901 in 1994 to 6,396 in 2006.[1]

Among teenagers 15-19 years, the steepest declines in childbearing from 1991 to 2005 were for young adolescents 15-17 years. Their birth rate dropped by 45 percent between 1991 and 2005, from 38.6 to 21.4 per 1,000 females; the rate increased 3 percent between 2005 and 2006, to 22.0. Within that age group, the rate for non-Hispanic black teenagers fell the most between 1991 and 2005, by 59 percent, from 86.1 to 34.9 per 1,000; this rate increased 4 percent in 2006 to 36.2. Rates for older teenagers 18-19 years overall dropped by 26 percent from 94.0 per 1,000 in 1991 to 69.9 in 2005. The rate in 2006 was 73.0.[1]

While the U.S. teenage birth rate dropped considerably in the last decade, it still remains one of the highest among the developed countries of the world.[13] Comparing the most recent data, the U.S. rate in 2006 (41.9 per 1,000) was substantially higher than the rates in 2005 for the United Kingdom (26.7) and France (7.8) and in 2006 for Japan (5.6), for example. Later in this chapter we will describe trends in teenage *pregnancy* (including births, induced abortions, and fetal losses).

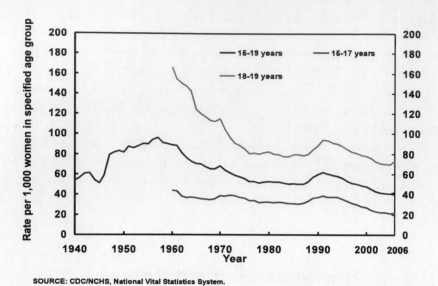

SOURCE: CDC/NCHS, National Vital Statistics System.

Figure 2. Birth rates for teenagers by age of mother: United States, 1940-2006.

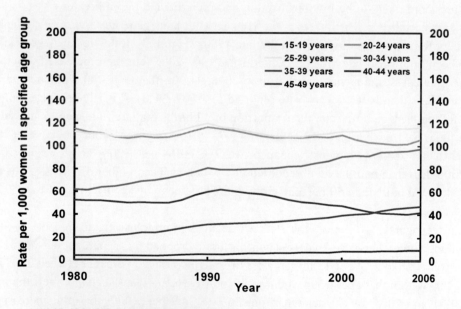

SOURCE: CDC/NCHS, National Vital Statistics System.

Figure 3. Birth rates by selected age of mother: United States, 1980-2006.

The birth rates for women in the principal childbearing ages, the twenties, were higher than any other group, with the rate for women aged 25-29 years at 116.7 births per 1,000 women and the rate for women aged 20-24 years at 105.9 in 2006 (Table 2). The rates for women aged 25-29 years have been higher than any other age groups since 1983 (Figure 3).

Prior to this, the rates were higher for women aged 20-24 years.[1,8] This shift shows the general trend in which birth rates for women less than 25 years of age have generally declined over the last fifteen years, with continuous declines through 2005 for teenagers. The rate for women aged 20-24 years has generally decreased too, down 9 percent since the 1990 peak. However, the rate for women aged 25-29 years has generally fluctuated between 108.3 and 120.2 during the period from 1980 to 2006, whereas the rates for women 30 years or more have increased between 1980 and 2006. Births per 1,000 women aged 30-34 years rose 21 percent between 1990 and 2006 and births per 1,000 women aged 35-39 years increased each year since 1978, rising 46 percent between 1990 and 2006. Finally, the rate for women aged 40-44 years has more than doubled between 1981 and 2006, rising 65 percent since 1990 alone, whereas, the birth rate for women aged 45-49 years has more than tripled between 1990 and 2006.

Total Fertility Rate

Another way to compare fertility patterns is to examine variations in the total fertility rate (TFR), a measure of lifetime fertility. This rate estimates the average number of births to a hypothetical cohort of 1,000 women, if they experienced throughout their childbearing years the age-specific birth rates observed in a given year, summarizing the potential impact of current fertility patterns on completed family size.[1,8] The total fertility rate is computed by summing the rates for the five-year age groups and multiplying the total by 5. Because it is based on age-specific birth rates, the TFR is not affected by differences or changes in the age composition of a population and can be used to compare the fertility of different populations or to compare the fertility of a population with an age structure that changes over time.[1,8]

Between 1960 and 2006, the TFR declined 43 percent, from 3,653.6 births per 1,000 women in 1960 to 2,100.5 in 2006 (Tables 1 and 2). The rate fell substantially from 1960 to 1976, 1,738.0, to reach the lowest point in the last four decades.[1,8] Between 1976 and 1990, the rate rose to 2,081.0, an increase of almost 20 percent. From 1990 to 1997, the rate decreased again (5 percent, from 2,081.0 to 1,971.0), but has generally increased since 1998, rising 5 percent by 2006. The total fertility rate in 2006 was above "replacement" for the first time in the U.S. since 1971. Replacement is the level at which a given generation can exactly replace itself, generally considered to be 2,100 births per 1,000 women.[1,8] Before 1972, the TFR had never fallen below replacement.

Differences in the total fertility rate for the three largest race and Hispanic origin groups in the U.S. are substantial. The rate for Hispanic woman was above "replacement" for every year between 1990 and 2006. The rate for non Hispanic black woman was again above "replacement" in 2006, having fallen below between 2002 and 2005, whereas the rate for non-Hispanic white women were consistently below "replacement" during that time (1990-2006). Likewise, changes in the total fertility rate for the three largest race and Hispanic origin groups differed substantially between 1990 and 2006. The rate for non-Hispanic white women increased slightly (1 percent) between 1990 and 2006, whereas the rate for non-Hispanic black women decreased 17 percent, generally declining throughout the period. The rate for Hispanic women, which was above "replacement" for every year, generally declined from 1992 to 1999 and then rose from 2000 to 2006, with the 1990 rate similar to the 2006 rate.

Mean Age of Mother

Another useful measure in interpreting childbearing patterns by age of mother is the mean age of mother. It is the arithmetic average of the age of women at the time of birth, computed directly from the frequency of birth by age of mother. The impact of the changes in birth rates for women under 30 years of age compared with women 30 years of age and over is clearly seen by examining the mean age at first birth. The mean age at first birth of mother in the U.S. was 25.0 years in 2006, down from 25.2 in 2005. This is the first decline in the mean age at first birth since the measure has been available in 1968 (Table 1).[1,8,14] However, this decline in the mean age of first-time mothers reflects the large increase in first birth rates for women aged 15-19 and 20-24 years compared with women aged 25 years and over between 2005 and 2006.[1] Prior to this decrease, the mean age at first birth of mother in the U.S. was generally increasing, up 3.8 years from 21.4 years in 1968 to 25.2 years in 2005, reflecting a delay in childbearing, that is, the rise in the first time birth rates for older women.

Among the three largest race and Hispanic origin population groups in the U.S., a substantial range and variation in age at first birth exists. In 2006, age at first birth ranged from 22.7 years for non-Hispanic black, 23.1 years for Hispanic, and 26.0 years for non-Hispanic white women. Between 1990 and 2006, the mean age of mother at first birth generally increased for the three population groups with the greatest increase for non-Hispanic white and non-Hispanic black women (1 year). The mean age for first-time non-Hispanic white mothers did decline between 2005 (26.2) and 2006, the only group of the three to do so. The age of first-time Hispanic mothers increased slightly less than 1 year during this period (2005-2006).

Births to Married and Unmarried Women

Nearly two-thirds of U.S. births are to married women. The overall birth rate for married women dropped substantially in the last half of the 20th century, with sustained declines from 1960 until the mid 1990s (Table 1). Birth rates for *married* women in their twenties have changed relatively little since 1990.[8] In contrast, rates increased considerably for married women 30 and older, especially women 35 years and older. Increases in rates for *unmarried* women have been widespread among women aged 20 and older.[1,8]

One of the striking trends of the last decades of the 20th century was the tremendous increase in childbearing among unmarried women.[1,8,15] The birth rate for unmarried women in 2006 (50.6 per 1,000 aged 15-44) was more than seven times the rate in 1940 (7.1 per 1,000) (Table 1).[1,8] The rate tripled from 1940 to 1960 (21.6 per 1,000), moderated its increase for the next two decades, reaching 29.4 in 1980, and then resumed steep increases from 1980 to 1994, when the rate increased 57 percent, or more than 3 percent per year. The rate was fairly level from 1995 to 2002; since 2002, the rate rose rapidly – by 16 percent –

reaching 50.6 per 1,000 in 2006.[1] The number of births to unmarried women in 2006 was a record high for the nation, 1,641,946.[1]

Another critical trend was the explosion in the size of the unmarried female (and male) population of reproductive age. The impact on the "baby-boom" generation's declining marriage rates was dramatic. A growing proportion of a growing population was delaying marriage, with the result that the number of unmarried women of reproductive age increased substantially. The total number of unmarried women aged 15-44 years rose more than 2.5 times from the mid 1960s to 2006.[16,17] The number of unmarried women aged 25-29 years rose more than six-fold, from 750,000 in 1965 to nearly 4.9 million in 2006; the number of unmarried women aged 30-34 rose six times, from about 527,000 in 1965 to 3.2 million in 2006.[16,17]

These changes in marriage and fertility among married and unmarried women have led to a steep rise in the proportion of all births that are to unmarried women, from 4 percent in 1940 to 39 percent in 2006.[1,15] This upward trend was across the board – in terms of large increases among women in all age, race, and ethnicity groups. Until the mid 1990s, the proportion of births to unmarried women rose because births and birth rates for unmarried women were increasing while childbearing among married women was declining. More recently, births to married women have declined modestly, although there was a slight increase in 2006, but increases in nonmarital births are accelerating, so the overall proportion of out-of-wedlock births has continued to climb.

While differentials in overall fertility by race and ethnicity have narrowed over the last quarter century, racial disparities persist in rates by marital status. Among married women, rates are highest for Hispanic women (97.3 per 1,000 in 2006) followed by non-Hispanic white women (86.5 per 1,000), and black women (73.5 per 1,000) (data for *non-Hispanic* black women are not available).[18] Among unmarried women, the birth rates were highest for Hispanic women (106.1 per 1,000), followed by black women (71.5 per 1,000) and non-Hispanic white women (32.0 per 1,000).[1]

Pregnancy and Abortion Patterns

Not all pregnancies end in live births, the focus of most of this chapter. In this section recent trends and variations in *pregnancy* and *abortion* rates will be briefly reviewed. Pregnancies include live births, induced abortions, and fetal losses (that is, miscarriages or stillbirths). Public policy interventions in recent years have focused on preventing teen *pregnancy*.[19] According to the most recent estimates, 57 percent of pregnancies among teenagers 15-19 in 2004 ended in live births, 27 percent in induced abortions, and 16 percent in fetal losses (including miscarriages or stillbirths).[6] A consistent series of pregnancy estimates is available from NCHS for 1976 through 2004 (Table 1).[6,7]

Teenage pregnancy rates have fallen considerably since 1990, by about 38 percent overall. The rate for 1990, 116.8 pregnancies per 1,000 females aged 15-19 years, was a record high for the nation; by 2004 the rate fell to 72.2 per 1,000, an historic low. The teen birth rate fell 31 percent and the teen abortion rate dropped 51 percent during the period 1990-2004.[6,7] As noted earlier in this chapter, the teenage *birth* rate increased in 2006 following continuous declines from 1991 through 2005.[1] We do not have the necessary information as yet to determine if the downward trend in the teenage *pregnancy* rate has also reversed.

Looking at pregnancy rates among adult women, rates are consistently highest among women in their twenties with rates of 163.7 and 169.1 per 1,000 for women aged 20-24 and 25-29 years in 2004 (Table 2; Figure 4).[6] The rate for women aged 30-34 was 135.2 per 1,000 in 2004. Compared with pregnancies among teenagers, pregnancies among women in their twenties and thirties are much more likely to end in live birth and less likely to end in induced abortion.[6,7] The likelihood of a fetal loss outcome rises with maternal age through the late thirties. This pattern is reflected in higher levels of impaired fecundity among older women.[20]

Total pregnancy rates are, methodologically, extensions of the better-known total fertility rates (TFR) (discussed above). The TFR suggests the number of births per 1,000 women implied by the current age-specific birth rates. Expanding this approach, a total abortion rate and a total fetal loss rate can also be calculated. Summing these rates yields a total pregnancy rate and answers the question: "How many pregnancies would a hypothetical group of 1,000 women have in their lifetime if they experience the age-specific pregnancy rates observed in the current year?" As shown in table 2, non-Hispanic black and Hispanic women experienced 4,200 and 4,219 pregnancies per 1,000 women, respectively, as of 2004, compared with 2,659 per 1,000 for non-Hispanic white women. Rates declined for all groups between 1990 and 2004.

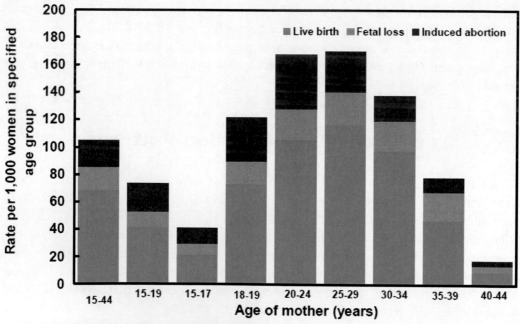

SOURCE: CDC/NCHS, National Vital Statistics System.

Figure 4. Pregnancy, live birth, abortion, and fetal loss rates by selected age of mother: United States, 2004.

Pregnancy rates and outcomes also vary considerably by marital status. Overall pregnancy rates are about 30 percent higher for married than for unmarried women. These patterns differ considerably by pregnancy outcome. Birth rates for married women are about double the rates for unmarried women (88 per 1,000 compared with 51, respectively), while abortion rates for unmarried women are more than four times the rates for married women.[6]

Pregnancy rates vary considerably by race and Hispanic origin. In 2004, the rates were 84.3 per 1,000 for non-Hispanic whites, 139.3 for non-Hispanic blacks, and 145.7 for Hispanic women.[6] While overall pregnancy rates for non-Hispanic black and Hispanic women are similar, rates by outcome are quite different; birth rates are lower and abortion rates are higher for non-Hispanic black than for Hispanic women, regardless of age (Table 2).

Pregnancies were less likely to end in induced abortion in 2004 compared with 1990: nineteen percent of pregnancies, overall, ended in induced abortion in 2004, down from 24 percent in 1990 (data not shown).[6] Pregnancies among teenagers and women in their early twenties continue to be more likely than pregnancies among older women to end in induced abortion. In 2004, 25 percent of pregnancies among women under 25 years ended in abortion, compared with 15 percent among women 25 years and older.

Generally abortions and abortion rates have fallen considerably, since peaking in 1990. The estimated number of abortions fell from 1,609,000 in 1990 to 1,222,000 in 2004, and the abortion rate (per 1,000 women aged 15-44 years) fell from 27.4 in 1990 to 19.7 in 2004 (Table 2).[6] According to a recent study, abortions continued to decline in 2005, to an estimated 1,210,000.[21] Declines through 2004 have been widespread across age groups and race and Hispanic origin population groups.[6] The steepest declines were reported for teenagers and women in their early twenties; rates fell by 30 to 55 percent between 1990 and 2004. Abortion rates dropped sharply for non-Hispanic white women, by 47 percent, during 1990-2004, and fell 21 and 22 percent, respectively, for Hispanic and non-Hispanic black women.

Looking Ahead

As we consider some of the possible birth and pregnancy trends in the next few years, several factors should be considered. Based on the period of increased births that occurred in the late 1980s through the early 1990s, the largest growth in the female population in the childbearing ages is expected to be among women who will be aged 25-34 years in 2020.[22] (Population projections from the Census Bureau assume the continuation of recent patterns of fertility, mortality, and immigration.[23]). Women aged 25-34 accounted for 32 percent of women aged 15-44 years in 2006, but 50 percent of the births in that year.[1,24] By 2020, it is projected that they will account for 35 percent of women in the reproductive ages. Even though the total number of women aged 15-44 is projected to increase 3 percent, the number aged 25-34 will rise by 13 percent.[22] Assuming that birth rates by age remain at their 2006 levels throughout the next two decades, the number of births could be expected to rise by about 6 percent, from 4.27 million in 2006 to 4.53 million in 2020. Thus substantial shifts in the number of women in the peak years of childbearing alone will account for a sizeable increase in the number of births and pregnancies, even if birth rates by age remain unchanged. The projected drop in the number of women born before the period of increased births in the late 1980s through the early 1990s is expected to keep the total number of births from increasing more, but these projections could also be conservative, in part, because they do not take account of the impact of the growing Hispanic population with accompanying higher fertility levels.[4,24]

Pregnancies and births to unmarried women may be expected to rise as well because of the growth of the population in the ages where rates of out-of-wedlock childbearing are rising most rapidly (25-34 years), unless there are compensating increases in marriage rates.[25] Given the steep increases in nonmarital births since 2002, largely concentrated among women in their twenties, the ongoing trends are likely to continue, especially if the unexpected increase in teenage birth rates in 2006 continues over the next few years. Pregnancies and births that occur in the teenage years are much more likely to take place out of wedlock than those to older women.

Fundamental changes in behavior and attitudes as well as societal trends may play important roles. For example, birth rates for teenagers have likely been affected by changing attitudes about premarital sex. The large array of public and private initiatives at the Federal, state, and local levels have focused teenagers' attention on the importance of pregnancy prevention through abstinence and responsible behavior.[19] While large proportions of teenagers are sexually experienced, teenage sexual activity has leveled off according to several national surveys.[26,27] Also important has been the introduction of effective new birth control methods (implant and injectable contraceptives), especially for sexually active teenagers and adult unmarried women. To the extent that young peoples' educational and career aspirations continue to grow, they may be deterred from early and out-of-wedlock childbearing, and encouraged to begin their families when they are ready for the emotional, physical and economic responsibilities of parenthood.[28] However, the upturn in 2006 in teenage birth rates and increases in nonmarital births among adult women may reflect new changes in attitudes that may impact fertility and family formation trends.[29]

References

[1]   Martin, JA, Hamilton, BE, Sutton, PD, Ventura, SJ, Menacker F, Kirmeyer S, Mathews TJ. Births: Final data for 2006 *National vital statistics reports;* Hyattsville, Maryland: National Center for Health Statistics (NCHS). 2009;57(7).

[2]   National Center for Health Statistics. Technical Appendix. *Vital Statistics of the United States, 2006.* Volume 1, Natality. Hyattsville, *Maryland:* National Center for Health Statistics, 2009.

[3]   National Center for Health Statistics. Technical Appendix. *Vital Statistics of the United States, 1999.* Volume 1, Natality. Hyattsville, Maryland: National Center for Health Statistics, 2001.

[4]   Martin JA, Hamilton BE, Sutton, PD, Ventura SJ, Menacker F, Kirmeyer S, Munson ML. Births: Final Data for 2005. *National Vital Statistics Reports;* Hyattsville, Maryland: National Center for Health Statistics (NCHS). 2007;56(6).

[5]   Martin JA, Hamilton BE, Sutton, PD, Ventura SJ, Menacker F, Kirmeyer S. Births: Final Data for 2004. *National Vital Statistics Reports;* Hyattsville, Maryland: National Center for Health Statistics (NCHS). 2006;55(1).

[6]   Ventura SJ, Abma JC, Mosher WD, Henshaw SK. Estimated pregnancy rates by outcome for the United States, 1990-2004. *National vital statistics reports;* Hyattsville, Maryland: National Center for Health Statistics. 2008;56(15).

[7]   Ventura, SJ, Mosher, WD, Curtin, SC, Abma, JC, Henshaw, S. Highlights of trends in pregnancies and pregnancy rates by outcome: Estimates for the United States, 1976-96. *National vital statistics reports;* Hyattsville, Maryland: National Center for Health Statistics. 1999;47(29).

[8]   National Center for Health Statistics. *Vital Statistics of the United States, 2003, Volume I, Natality.* Hyattsville, Maryland: National Center for Health Statistics, 2008.

[9]   U.S. Bureau of the Census. Preliminary estimates of the population of the United States, by age, sex, and race: 1970 to 1981. *Current Population Reports.* P-25(917). Washington, DC: U.S. Department of Commerce, 1982.

[10] Hollmann FW. U.S. population estimates, by age, sex, race, and Hispanic origin: 1980 to 1991. *Current Population Reports.* P-25(1095). Washington, DC: U.S. Bureau of the Census, 1993.

[11] Maynard R, ed. *Kids Having Kids: Economic costs and social consequences of teen pregnancy.* Washington, DC: The Urban Institute, 1997.

[12] Mathews TJ, MacDorman MF. Infant Mortality Statistics from the 2005 Period Linked Birth/Infant Death Data Set. *National Vital Statistics Reports;* Hyattsville, Maryland: National Center for Health Statistics (NCHS). 2008;57(2).

[13] *Department of Economic and Social Affairs, Statistical Office,* United Nations. Demographic Yearbook, 2006. New York, NY: United Nations, 2008. Accessed December 31, 2008.

[14] Mathews, T.J., Hamilton, B.E. Mean age of mother, 1970-2000. *National vital statistics reports.* Hyattsville, Maryland: National Center for Health Statistics. 2002;51(1).

[15] Ventura SJ, Bachrach CA. Nonmarital Childbearing in the United States. 1940-99. *National Vital Statistics Reports;* Hyattsville, Maryland: National Center for Health Statistics (NCHS). 2000;48(16).

[16] U.S. Bureau of the Census. Marital Status and Family Status: March 1965. *Current Population Reports.* P-20(144). Washington, DC: U.S. Department of Commerce, 1965.

[17] U.S. Census Bureau. Unpublished data from the March 2006 *Current Population Survey. U.S. Census Bureau.* 2006.

[18] National Center for Health Statistics. *Vital Statistics of the United States, 2006, Volume I, Natality.* Hyattsville, Maryland: National Center for Health Statistics. In preparation.

[19] National Campaign to Prevent Teen Pregnancy. Various reports. Available at: *http://www.thenationalcampaign.org/.*

[20] Chandra A, Martinez GM, Mosher WD, Abma JA, Jones J. Fertility, Family Planning and Reproductive Health of U.S. Women: Data from the 2002 National Survey of Family Growth. *Vital Health Stat* 23(25). National Center for Health Statistics.

Available at: http://www.cdc.gov/nchs/data/series/sr_23/sr23_025.pdf (Accessed December 31, 2008).

[21] Jones RK, Zolna MRS, Henshaw SK, and Finer LB. Abortion in the United States: Incidence and Access to Services, 2005. *Perspectives on Sexual and Reproductive Health* 40(1):6-16. 2008.

[22] Population Projections Program, Population Division, U.S. Census Bureau. State Interim Population Projections by Age and Sex: 2004 – 2030 (Interim State Projections of Population by Single Year of Age and Sex: July 1, 2004 to 2030). U.S. Department of Commerce. Release April 21, 2005. Available at: *http://www.census .gov/population/projections/DownldFile4.xls and http://www.census.gov/population/ projections/DownldFile4.csv.*

[23] U.S. Census Bureau. Methodology Summary: Interim Population Projections for States by Age and Sex: 2004 to 2030. April 21, 2005. Available at: *http://www. census.gov/population/www/projections/InterimShortMethod.doc.*

[24] National Center for Health Statistics. Postcensal estimates of the resident population of the United States as of July 1, 2006, by year, state and county, age, bridged race, sex, and Hispanic origin (vintage 2005). File pcen_v2006.zip. Released August 16, 2007. Available at: *http://www.cdc.gov/nchs/about/major/dvs/popbridge/datadoc.htm# vintage2006*

[25] Fields J. America's Families and Living Arrangements: 2003. *Current Population Reports.* P-20(553). Washington, DC: U.S. Department of Commerce, 2004.

[26] Abma JC, Martinez GM, Mosher WD, and Dawson BS. Teenagers in the United States: Sexual Activity, Contraceptive Use, and Childbearing, 2002. *Vital and Health Statistics* 23(24). Hyattsville, Maryland: National Center for Health Statistics, 2004.

[27] Eaton DK, Kann L, Kinchen S, et al. Youth Risk Behavior Surveillance – United States, 2005. In: *Surveillance Summaries* 55(SS-5):1-108. 2006.

[28] The National Campaign to Prevent Teen Pregnancy. Linking Teen Pregnancy Prevention to Other Critical Social Issues. Available at: *http://www. teenpregnancy.org/wim/default.asp. 2007.*

[29] Moore KA. Teen Births: Examining the Recent Increase. *The National Campaign to Prevent Teen and Unplanned Pregnancy. 2008.*

In: Textbook of Perinatal Epidemiology
Editor: Eyal Sheiner, pp. 173-195

ISBN: 978-1-60741-648-7
© 2010 Nova Science Publishers, Inc.

Chapter XII

Epidemiology of Ectopic Pregnancy

Avi Harlev[*]*, Arnon Wiznitzer and Eyal Sheiner*

Department of Obstetrics & Gynecology, Soroka University Medical Center, Faculty of
Health Sciences, Ben-Gurion University of the Negev, Beer-Sheva, Israel

Definitions

- Ectopic pregnancy: an implantation of a fertilized ovum outside the uterus.
- Heterotopic pregnancy: coexisting intrauterine and extrauterine pregnancies.

Introduction

Ectopic pregnancy is defined as an implantation of a fertilized ovum outside the uterus. Ectopic pregnancies are considered a major cause of pregnancy-related death during the first 20 weeks of pregnancy. The complications of ectopic pregnancy are a main cause of maternal mortality in the United States and were the leading reason of maternal death during the first trimester of pregnancy in 1970–89 [2].

Total costs associated with ectopic pregnancy in the United States for 1990 were estimated at $1.1 billion [3], with 64,000 women hospitalized for ectopic pregnancy in that year [4].

[*] For Correspondence: Avi Harlev, M.D., Department of Obstetrics and Gynecology, Soroka University Medical Center, P.O. Box 151, Beer Sheva 84101, Israel. Tel: +972-8-640-3762; Fax: +972-8-640-3057; e-mail: harlev@bgu.ac.il

Incidence

The reported incidence of ectopic pregnancy varies widely, especially since different methods are used to determine incidence. The three commonly-used denominators are the number of births, the number of pregnancies, and the number of women of reproductive age (15–44 years). A reliable calculation of the incidence of ectopic pregnancy is necessary, since accurate information on the rate of this condition is vital in planning health policies [5].

Assessing the accurate incidence of ectopic pregnancy is difficult for two main reasons. First, the rate of ectopic pregnancy is usually calculated as the number of cases per reported pregnancies, which might or might not include data for pregnancies that terminate or end in early miscarriage as well as for those that result in live births. Second, available data does not include conditions handled in out-patient clinics, and therefore the true incidence is most likely underestimated [6]. One study estimated that 108,000 ectopic pregnancies may have occurred in 1992, with only 58,000 of these, or about half, involving hospitalization [4].

The annual incidence of ectopic pregnancy in the U.S. in 1948 was reported as 0.4% of pregnancies, but is now nearly 2% [7,8]. An interesting trend in ectopic pregnancy incidence rate was observed worldwide over the last three decades. The ectopic pregnancy incidence increased rapidly and then, over the last decade, either slowed or declined [9-11]. Possible reasons for the increase of ectopic pregnancy incidence include the change in the use of intrauterine devices [7,8,11], earlier diagnosis of pelvic inflammatory disease resulting in tubal damage, the rise in the number of ectopic pregnancies resulting from assisted reproductive technologies (ART), and early detection of ectopic pregnancies due to technological advances such as higher resolution ultrasound scanners and sensitive hCG hormone test kits. The slowing or even declining incidence of ectopic pregnancy rates can be explained by the decrease of *chlamydia* infection as a result of the effect of prevention. All factors mentioned above may account for the change in ectopic pregnancy incidence over the years [12].

Mortality rate declined from 35.5 to 3.8 deaths per 10,000 women between 1970 and 1989 in the U.S. [13] and from 16 to three deaths per 10,000 pregnancies between 1973 and 1993 in the U.K. [9]. In the developing world, however, mortality remains high, e.g., 100–300 deaths per 10,000 in Cameroon [14].

Etiology and Risk Factors

Many studies have investigated the risk factors for ectopic pregnancy. The strongest association to ectopic pregnancy was found in conditions which impaired migration of the fertilized ovum to the uterus. These conditions include prior pelvic inflammatory disease, history of ectopic pregnancy and previous surgery for tubal obstruction and injury [15]. It is postulated that with more damage to the fallopian tube, there is a greater risk for developing an ectopic pregnancy [16].

Ankum and colleagues published a meta-analysis in 1996 reviewing 36 prior studies. The strongest risk factor for ectopic pregnancy was previous ectopic pregnancy with an odds ratio of 6.6 (95% CI, 5.2–8.4). This finding of previous ectopic pregnancy as the strongest risk factor associated with recurrent ectopic pregnancy was confirmed by Barnhart and colleagues [17]. A history of one previous ectopic pregnancy presented an odds ratio of 2.98 (95% CI, 1.88–4.73) and a history of two ectopic pregnancies increased the risk to 16% overall (odds ratio 16.04; 95% CI, 5.39–47.72). Moreover, past history of ectopic pregnancy is an important risk factor for rupture [18]. The incidence of rupture of the ectopic pregnancy sac in women with past history of ectopic pregnancy was 75%, whereas the incidence of women with free history was 59%; slight though this difference is, it was statistically significant and correlates with the study by Latchaw et al. [19].

Previous pelvic inflammatory disease, especially those caused by *Chlamydia trachomatis*, is a major risk factor for ectopic pregnancy [20]. The adjusted odds ratio (OR) for previous pelvic infectious disease was recently found to be 3.4 (95% confidence interval [CI]: 2.4–5.0) [2]. Hillis and colleagues [21] reported that repeated *Chlamydia* infections increased the risk for ectopic pregnancy. The odds ratio after two infections was 2.1 and rose to 4.5 after three infections. In a prospective study of 1,204 patients followed until first pregnancy after infection, 47 of 746 (6%) women with laparoscopically documented PID had a tubal gestation, which is significantly higher than the 0.9% incidence that occurred in the control group [22].

Other factors associated with an increased risk of ectopic pregnancy include a history of infertility (and specifically *in vitro* fertilization), prior tubal surgery, diethylstilbestrol exposure (which alters fallopian tube morphology) with a nine-fold increase of the risk for ectopic pregnancy [23] and advanced maternal age.

Cigarette smoking is a known risk factor for ectopic pregnancy, causing alterations in tubal motility and ciliary activity. Waylen et al. performed a meta-analysis comparing the success rate and clinical outcomes of assisted reproductive technologies between women who actively smoke cigarettes at the time of treatment and those who do not. Beside the poor outcome of the procedure, significantly greater odds of ectopic were obtained pregnancy (OR 15.69, 95% CI 2.87–85.76) [24].

A number of studies have concluded that surgical abortion in the first trimester does not increase the risk of ectopic pregnancy [25,26]. In a retrospective, case-control study, Smith et al. concluded that women with an adverse obstetric history that included interrupted pregnancies were more likely to have ectopic pregnancies [27]. Controversy exists regarding the association between ectopic pregnancy and medical abortions. While Bouyer et al. [2] found prior medical induced abortions to be associated with an increased risk of ectopic pregnancy (adjusted OR = 2.8, 95% CI: 1.1–7.2), no such association was observed by Shannon and co-authors [28]. Nevertheless, Jasveer et al. reported in 2007 [29] in a population-based cohort study, that no associations between medical abortions and ectopic pregnancy were found, as opposed to Bouyer's results. This study differs in several aspects from Bouyer's study. Jasveer used a population-based cohort, whereas the previous findings reported by Bouyer and colleagues were from population-based case patients and controls. In addition, the abortion information was obtained from a clinical registry, whereas abortion information was self-reported in Bouyer's study. Jasveer included a large number of women who had had a medical abortion, providing 90% power to detect a minimal relative risk of 1.5 and almost 100% power to detect the relative risk of 2.8 that was reported in the previous study for ectopic pregnancy. However, the previous study included data from in-depth personal interviews that were unavailable to Jasveer et al.

Inert and copper-containing IUDs prevent both intrauterine and extrauterine pregnancies [30-32]. Nevertheless, if a woman who has been sterilized or is a current user of an IUD or progesterone-only contraceptives becomes pregnant, her risk for an ectopic pregnancy is increased 6–10-fold, since these methods of contraception provide greater protection against intrauterine pregnancies than ectopic pregnancy [30-32]. The frequency of ectopic pregnancies in women hospitalized yearly in relation to IUD insertions and number of live births, possible associated variables, and characteristics of diagnosis and treatment were investigated by Fernandes and colleagues [33]. In their cohort cross-sectional study, the frequency of ectopic pregnancy did not increase during the five years studied. Only the percentage of women with a previous ectopic pregnancy was associated with prevalence of ectopic pregnancy.

Tubal ligation failures also confer a high risk for ectopic pregnancy. The U.S. Collaborative Review of Sterilization prospectively followed 10,863 women electing tubal sterilization. Thirty-three percent of post-sterilization pregnancies occurring in this population (47 of 143 pregnancies) were ectopic. The risk was highest in patients who had a tubal ligation using bipolar cautery, probably as a result of a fistula formed in the fallopian tube, and in women sterilized under the age of 30. The risk of ectopic pregnancy in these patients was 31.9 per 1000 procedures compared with 1.2 per 1000 procedures in patients who had a postpartum salpingectomy [34]. The first two years after sterilization carry the greatest risk for pregnancy in general, and ectopic pregnancy in particular [35]. Sterilization reversal, alternatively, increases the risk for ectopic pregnancy due to possible obstruction and abnormal tube anatomy.

The risk of ectopic pregnancy is increased among women undergoing assisted reproductive technology (ART) and specifically *in vitro* fertilization (IVF). The risk is particularly high for women with underlying tubal disease. Hormone alterations during ovulation induction can cause alteration in tubal function and peristalsis [36]. Other possible explanations include placement of the embryo high in the uterine cavity during embryo transfer (deep fundal transfer), and fluid reflux into the tubes [37]. Stepwise logistic regression analysis shows that tubal-factor infertility and previous myomectomy account for 85% of ectopic pregnancies in women who receive fertility treatment [38].

Other less common causes for ectopic pregnancy include salpingitis isthmica nodosa (anatomic thickening of the fallopian tube with epithelium, leading to multiple lumen diverticula), and multiple sexual partners (leading to higher risk for pelvic infections) [15,39].

Signs and Symptoms

A wide spectrum of clinical manifestations from asymptomatic to hemodynamic shock makes the diagnosis of ectopic pregnancy difficult. The clinical presentation is mainly dependent on whether rupture has occurred. The classic symptom triad of ectopic pregnancy includes amenorrhea, irregular bleeding, and lower abdominal pain.

Sudden severe abdominal pain is the most common complaint. Pain, however, is present in more than 90% of patients, but the severity and nature of the pain vary widely. The triad is present in only half of patients and most commonly when rupture has occurred [40]. The non-specific symptoms have also been associated with spontaneous miscarriage, cervical irritation or trauma, and infection, thus patients' complaints to their physician may be delayed [12].

Measurements of vital signs are important in the physical examination. Abdominal and pelvic tenderness, especially cervical motion tenderness, are common when rupture has occurred (and present in about 75% of patients). Hypotension and tachycardia with rebound tenderness and guarding should alert the clinician to the possibility of tubal rupture with immediate need for surgical intervention. However, pelvic examination before rupture is commonly non-specific. Palpable pelvic mass on bimanual examination is established in less than half of the cases. Barnhart and colleagues reported an increased odds ratio for ectopic pregnancy in patients presenting with first-trimester symptoms if moderate to severe bleeding (odds ratio 1.42; 95% CI, 1.04–1.93) and pain (odds ratio 1.42; 95% CI, 1.06–1.92) were present [17].

Evaluating a patient with a non-ruptured ectopic pregnancy is not accurate and additional tests are required to differentiate ectopic pregnancy from early intrauterine pregnancy. The next diagnostic steps after taking the medical history and the physical examination are performing a transvaginal ultrasound and a serum human chorionic gonodatropin (hCG) level measurement. The sensitivity and specificity of combining these tests has been reported to range from 95% to 100% [41,42].

Laboratory Assessment

The initial evaluation of a patient with signs and symptoms of suspected ectopic pregnancy is to determine if the patient is pregnant. The human chorionic gonadotropin (hCG) enzyme immunoassay, with a sensitivity of 25 mIU/mL, is an accurate screening test for ectopic pregnancy; it is positive in nearly all ectopic pregnancy cases [43].

The level of hCG rises during the beginning of the pregnancy and reaches a peak of approximately 100,000 mIU/mL at 6–10 weeks. During the next weeks the levels decrease and remain stable at approximately 20,000 mIU/mL. In normal pregnancies, the hCG is expected to double every 1.4–2.1 days [44]. The rising pattern of the hCG is termed "doubling time". There is wide agreement that the expected rise in serial hCG measurements is different from the slow rise or plateau of an ectopic pregnancy [43-48]. The established minimal hCG rate of increase for a normal intrauterine pregnancy is 24% at 1 day and 53% at 2 days. Approximately 15% of normal pregnancies demonstrate less than a 66% increase in hCG, and 17% of ectopic pregnancies have normal doubling times [43]. An abnormal rising pattern of hCG is highly suggestive of an abnormal pregnancy, although it cannot discriminate an ectopic pregnancy from a miscarried intrauterine pregnancy. Moreover, a normal hCG increase pattern does not exclude ectopic pregnancy. In addition, a decline in hCG levels is suggestive for an abnormal pregnancy, but the presence of an ectopic pregnancy should be highly suspected when the hCG level does not fall by 21–35% in 2 days

[44]. A recently published study by Silva et al. follwed the hCG levels of 200 patients diagnosed with ectopic pregnancy. The rise in hCG for women with ectopic pregnancies (0.28; 75% increase in 2 days) was slower than the mean increase reported for a viable intrauterine pregnancy. The decline in hCG for women with ectopic pregnancies (-0.225; 27% decline in 2 days) was slower than the mean reported for completed spontaneous abortion. However, 20.8% of women presented with a rise in hCG values similar to the minimal rise for women with a viable gestation, and 8% of women presented with a fall in hCG values similar to women with a completed spontaneous abortion. The conclusion of the study was that hCG profile in women with ectopic pregnancy can mimic that of an intrauterine pregnancy or a completed spontaneous abortion in approximately 29% of cases and therefore there is no definitive way to characterize the pattern of hCG for women with an ectopic pregnancy [49].

The serial hCG level surveillance is required when initial ultrasound fails to demonstrate either intra- or extrauterine pregnancy. If the hCG level does not decline by 15% after uterine curettage due to suspected miscarried intrauterine pregnancy, the possibility of ectopic pregnancy emerges and treatment is indicated [50].

Serum Progesterone

In normal intrauterine pregnancy, the serum progesterone level increases [51]. A serum progesterone level of <20nmol/L may be used to recognize an abnormal pregnancy with a PPV of ≥95% [52]. Of pregnant patients with serum progesterone values of less than 5nmol/L, 85% have spontaneous abortions, 0.16% have viable intrauterine pregnancies and 14% have ectopic pregnancies [53]. Thus, serum progesterone level inspections have been shown to be useful in evaluating the probability of early pregnancy failure [54,55]. Most ectopic pregnancies are associated with serum progesterone levels lower than 20nmol/L [56].

As noted, serum progesterone levels cannot differentiate ectopic pregnancy from intrauterine non-viable pregnancy [55]. In 1998, a meta-analysis of 26 studies concluded that progesterone alone is not sufficient to diagnose ectopic pregnancy with good reliability [57].

Ultrasonography

As a result of the technical improvements in ultrasound equipment, earlier diagnosis of intra- and extrauterine pregnancies is achieved (Fig. 1a,1b). Direct visualization of the gestational sac is the best method for the diagnosis of ectopic pregnancy, only it is not seen in all cases. About 90% of the cases may be visualized using transvaginal sonography within 5 weeks of the last menstrual period [58-60].

The discriminatory zone is defined as the hCG level from which an intrauterine pregnancy should be directly visualized by an ultrasound scan. Abdominal ultrasound can detect all intrauterine pregnancies at hCG levels above 6500 mIU/mL; using transvaginal ultrasound, at hCG levels between 1000 and 2000 mIU/mL, or at 5.5 weeks of gestation, a viable intrauterine pregnancy should be detected [61,62]. The sensitivity of the ultrasound to detect a normally developing intrauterine pregnancy comes up to almost 100% [61-64]. The sensitivity of transvaginal ultrasonography to identify ectopic pregnancy varies from 20.1% to 84% and specificity from 98.9% to 100% [65]. The combination of positive hCG and transvaginal ultrasound has a positive predictive value of 95% for an ectopic pregnancy [66].

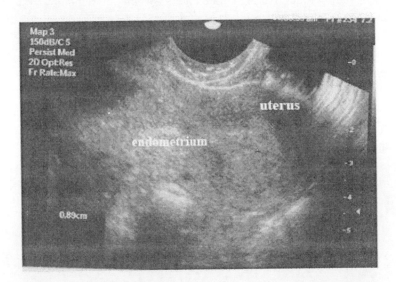

Figure 1a. Normal uterine US scan. A thin endometrial line can be observed.

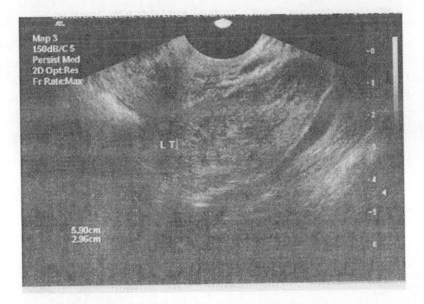

Figure 1b. A mass in the left adnexa diagnosed as left ectopic pregnancy.

An early sign for normal intrauterine pregnancy is the double decidual sac sign, i.e., two concentric echogenic rings separated by a hypoechogenic space. This sign is believed to be the decidua capsularis and parietalis. In the presence of an hCG level higher than 2,000 mIU/mL or when the mean sac diameter is equal to or greater than 3 mm, the sensitivity of the diagnosis of an intrauterine pregnancy based on the double decidual sac sign increases

[67]. Visualizing a yolk sac within the gestational sac is superior to the double decidual sac sign in verifying an intrauterine pregnancy [68].

Heterotopic pregnancy coexists with intra and extrauterine pregnancies. This is an uncommon finding in a spontaneous pregnancy, with an incidence of 1 in 30,000 [1]. Conceiving by assisted reproductive techniques increases the incidence by up to 1% [69].

Intrauterine fluid or blood collection, called a pseudo-sac, may be mistakenly diagnosed as an intrauterine pregnancy. The pseudo-sac lacks the double decidual ring or a yolk sac and is located centrally. Clots within the sac may imitate the fetal pole. Discrimination between intrauterine pregnancy miscarriage and an ectopic pregnancy solely using the diagnosis of a pseudo-sac is not possible [70]. The addition of color flow Doppler study improves the discrimination between pseudo-sac and normal intrauterine sac; however, better technical skills and technical equipment are required [71-73].

Laparoscopy is the gold standard for the diagnosis of ectopic pregnancy. Generally, the fallopian tubes are easily visualized and evaluated, although the diagnosis of ectopic pregnancy is missed in 3% to 4% of patients who have very small ectopic gestations [74].

Dilatation and Curettage

When hCG levels are above the discrimination zone and an intrauterine pregnancy is not visualized or when the hCG levels point toward an abnormal pregnancy, uterine evacuation using dilatation and curettage is recommended. An incorrect diagnosis of an ectopic pregnancy was found in 40% of the women with hCG levels above the discrimination zone with no evidence of an intrauterine sac in the ultrasound scan [75]. The presence of villi in the tissue sample obtained by the curettage confirms the diagnosis of intrauterine abnormal pregnancy. Ancillary hCG level surveillance is indicated after the curettage. Decreasing hCG levels of 15% or more 12 hours after the curettage indicates a complete abortion. A plateau or a rise in the hCG levels is diagnostic for an ectopic pregnancy and medical or surgical treatment for ectopic pregnancy is mandatory [50, 75-78].

Treatment of Ectopic Pregnancy

Ectopic pregnancy can be treated by three main strategies: surgical treatment, i.e., laparoscopy/laparotomy, medical treatment by methotrexate, or by expectant management. The small number of patients (less than 10%) who appear in an unstable hemodynamic state, e.g., hypovolemic shock, or show peritoneal signs[79] do not present a treatment dilemma as they require immediate fluid and blood resuscitation and emergency surgical treatment. Postponement of treatment can end in maternal mortality that was reported to be nearly 1% during 2000 [80,81]. When an early diagnosis of a patient in a clinically stable state is achieved, an option for either minimally invasive surgery or medical therapy is possible [12].

Surgical Treatment

In a hemodynamically stable patient, surgical treatment will be offered to patients who do not meet the criteria for medical treatment as discussed below. After deciding to operate on the patient, several other dilemmas arise determining the preferred surgical method and whether to preserve or remove the fallopian tube.

Laparotomy Versus Laparoscopy

In a hemodynamically stable patient, the superior surgical technique in most aspects is the laparoscopy (Figure 2). The advantages of laparoscopy include decreased surgical blood loss, a decrease in the amount of analgesia, and shorter postoperative hospital stay [82-85]. Not only has the laparoscopic approach been shown to be safe and effective, it is also less costly [86].

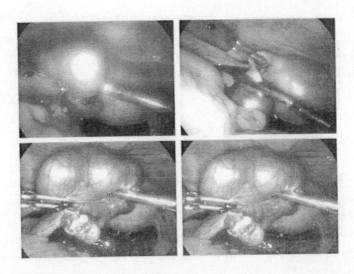

Figure 2. Laparoscopy of left tubal ectopic pregnancy.

Laparotomy and salpingectomy were, in the past, the treatment and diagnostic procedure for ectopic pregnancy. The advances of earlier diagnosis of the ectopic pregnancy, along with the advances in the minimally invasive procedure of laparoscopy, made the laparoscopy the favored treatment of ectopic pregnancy [12]. Odejinmi et al. reported a progressive rise in the proportion of ectopic pregnancies managed by operative laparoscopy. A total of 34% of women were managed laparoscopically between 2000 and 2002, increasing to 90% between 2003 and 2006, a statistically significant change [87].

Laparotomy is still the treatment in the hemodynamically unstable patient due to extensive blood loss or in hypovolemic shock. In such cases when quick good visualization and access of the ectopic pregnancy is required, the Pfannenstiel incision is superior to laparoscopy. The benefits of laparoscopic treatment include less blood loss, less analgesia, less postoperative pain, shorter recovery period, and decreased hospital costs [82,83]. In a meta-analysis, the average laparoscopy resolution rate was above 90%, with an average of 2% for intra-operative complications and 9% for post-operative complications [88].

Salpingostomy Versus Salpingectomy

Surgical removal of the ectopic pregnancy can be performed either by resecting the fallopian tube, a procedure termed salpingectomy, or by removing the trophoblast tissue alone through an incision in the tube, a procedure termed salpingostomy. In a ruptured uncontrolled bleeding ectopic pregnancy, as well as in cases of recurrent EP in the same tube and for sterilization, the salpingectomy is the preferred procedure [89]. In a review of nine studies [90], Yao et al. reported a similar rate of 50% subsequent intrauterine pregnancies in patients treated by salpingostomy and those treated with salpingectomy. Nevertheless, the rate of a subsequent ectopic pregnancy appeared higher in the salpingostomy group (15% versus 10%). Thus, laparoscopic salpingectomy is the favored surgical procedure for a tubal, enraptured ectopic pregnancy [83].

Laparotomy is still considered the chosen surgical procedure in cases of most ovarian and abdominal pregnancies, cornual or interstitial pregnancies, although laparoscopic management has been described [91]. In cases of known or suspected severe intraabdominal adhesions, laparotomy should be considered in order to avoid abdominal or pelvic organ injury.

Medical Treatment with Methotrexate

Methotrexate is a folic acid antagonist that inhibits dehydrofolate reductase, interrupting DNA synthesis and repair and cell replication. Methotrexate affects actively proliferating tissues such as bone marrow, malignant cells, and trophoblastic tissue [92]. The rapidly dividing trophoblast cells are most vulnerable to the methotrexate action [93]. In a meta-analysis, Morlock et al. reported that methotrexate is a cost-saving non-surgical fallopian tube sparing treatment [88]. Thus, in hemodynamically stable patients, who meet the methotraxate treatment criteria, it is considered the treatment of choice for ectopic pregnancy [1,94].

Candidates for Medical Therapy

Indications and contraindications for methotrexate treatments are presented in Table 1. Two regimens of treatment are commonly used. The first is the multiple dose methotrexate regimen, which includes 1 mg per kg methotrexate intramuscularly on alternate days (days 1, 3, 5, 7) and administration of leucovorin 0.1 mg per kg intramuscularly on alternate days 2, 4, 6, 8 [94,95]. The hCG levels should be monitored during the treatment course and decreasing levels of hCG are expected. The other, newer, medical treatment regimen is a single dose of methotrexate of 50 mg/m^2 of body surface area, without leucovorin rescue. The levels of hCG are monitored, and if hCG concentrations do not fall by 15% between days 4 and 7, weekly repeated doses are required. In this regimen 13% of women need two doses and 1% need more than two doses [96]. Defining treatment successes as avoidance of surgery, both protocols have been demonstrated to have good success rates in the treatment of ectopic pregnancy [95-102]. The single dose regimen is easier to manage, and results in fewer side effects. Comparison of the two treatment regimens in a randomized trial of 108 patients, found a non-statistically significant difference in the success rate between the single dose and multidose treatment (88.9% vs. 92.6%, respectively, odds ratio 0.64; 95% CI, 0.17–2.1). No differences in side effect profiles were reported [103]. Nonetheless, a systematic meta-analysis comparing the treatment options reported the single dose protocol was associated with a higher failure rate. The crude OR was 1.7; 95%CI 1.04–2.82, and the OR adjusted for hCG value and for the presence of fetal cardiac activity was 4.7; 95%CI 1.77–12.62 [104].

Table 1. Indications and contraindications to medical treatment.

Absolute indications
Hemodynamically patient
General anesthesia poses a significant risk
No contraindications to methotrexate

Relative indications
Unruptured mass <3.5 cm at its greatest dimension
No fetal cardiac motion
hCG level < 6,000-15,000 mIU/mL
Non tubal pregnancy e.g pregnancy in scar

Absolute contraindications
Breastfeeding
Overt or laboratory evidence of immunodeficiency
Alcoholism, alcoholic liver disease, or other chronic liver disease
bone marrow hypoplasia, leukopenia, thrombocytopenia, or significant anemia
Sensitivity to methotrexate
Active pulmonary disease
Peptic ulcer disease
Hepatic, renal, or hematologic impaired function

The success of the medical treatment is primarily dependent on the selection of the patients. The presence of fetal cardiac activity, the size of the ectopic pregnancy, the initial levels of β-hCG, progesterone levels, free peritoneal blood in the cul-de-sac, and endometrial thickness are factors reported to be important in forecasting methotrexate treatment success [105-107]. A history of a previous ectopic pregnancy is an independent risk factor for methotrexate failure [108,109]. An important factor in the treatment regimen selection is the initial level of β-hCG. In a systematic review of several observational studies, Menson et al. described a failure rate of 14.3% or higher with single-dose methotrexate when initial hCG levels were more than 5,000 mIU/mL, compared with a 3.7% failure rate for hCG levels were below 5,000 mIU/mL [110]. Thus, when hCG levels are higher than 5,000 mIU/mL, multiple doses should be considered [111].

Surveillance

The medically conservative treatment of ectopic pregnancy necessitates close monitoring for treatment success. The elimination of trophoblastic activity is monitored by serial hCG levels. The hCG levels during the first days of treatment may increase and peak 4 days following injection to levels above those prior to the treatment, but then a gradual progressive decrease is expected [95]. A decline of hCG of more than 15% weekly points toward a response to the treatment and indicates weekly monitoring of hCG levels until documentation of non-detectable levels [112,113]. Failure of the hCG level to decrease by at least 15% from day 4 to day 7 after methotrexate administration is considered treatment failure [92]. If hCG levels plateau or increase in one week, an additional methotrexate administration is possible [95,114,115]. Persistent ectopic pregnancy, hemoperitoneum, or patient hemodynamic instability imposes the surgical treatment consideration.

Any change in clinical status such as vaginal or intra-abdominal bleeding, augmented pelvic pain, or an insufficient decline of hCG levels mandates repeated ultrasound evaluation. Blood type should be determined since all patients with ectopic pregnancy who are Rh negative require Rh (D) immune globulin, 50 micrograms [95,114-117].

Side Effects

The majority of side effects during medical oral treatment for ectopic pregnancy are minor and self-limited. There is a correlation between the drug toxicity and the amount and duration of treatment.

The most common side effects of methotrexate are gastrointestinal, such as nausea, vomiting, and stomatitis. Hence, women treated with methotrexate should be advised not to use alcohol and nonsteroidal anti-inflammatory drugs (NSAIDs). Abdominal pain 2–3 days after administration, apparently from the cytotoxic effect of the drug on the trophoblast tissue, causing tubal abortion is common. In the absence of signs for tubal rupture, the abdominal pain can be managed expectantly [92].

Liver enzyme elevation may be inspected, especially with multidose regimens, and resolves after methotrexate cessation or increasing the rescue dose of folinic acid [118]. Pulmonary fibrosis alopecia and photosensitivity were also described as un-common side effects [119-120]. The use of the single-dose regimen is associated with fewer side effects than the multidose regimen [104].

A patient treated with methotrexate for an ectopic pregnancy has a constant risk of tubal rupture. Therefore, besides instructing the patient of the possible side effects of the treatment, it is important to educate patients about symptoms of tubal rupture and to emphasize the need to seek immediate medical attention if these symptoms occur [92].

The patient should be advised during therapy not to use folic acid supplements, NSAIDs, or alcohol, to avoid sunlight exposure, and to abstain from sexual intercourse or vigorous physical activity [118].

Fertility after an Ectopic Pregnancy

After treating an ectopic pregnancy with methotrexate, the intrauterine pregnancy rate was 66.9% after 2 years. The cumulative ectopic pregnancy rate was 15.4% after 1 year and 23.7% after 2 years [121]. Conception rates within the first year after treatment ranged between 57.5% and 79.6%. Following laparoscopic treatment, the intrauterine pregnancy rate was 54% with a recurrent ectopic pregnancy rate of 13% [122].

Interestingly, in a mean follow-up period of 28 months, in women who had an initial ectopic pregnancy with an IUD there were no repeat ectopic pregnancies and 87% conceived within one year. Conversely, women who had had an ectopic pregnancy without an IUD *in situ* had a much lower rate of conception (44%), and repeat ectopic pregnancy was more likely (28%) [123].

The studies of fertility after ectopic pregnancy treatment are all non-randomized. Therefore, there are various difficulties in the interpretation of these studies because of their observational nature [92]. It seems that fertility depends more on the patient's previous medical history (i.e., a history of infertility) than on her treatment for ectopic pregnancy [124].

Expectant Management

In a selected group of patients with asymptomatic unruptured early ectopic pregnancy, an expectant management approach is optional and is successful in 50–70% of the patients [52,125-128]. A serum hCG of less than 1000 IU/mL accompanied by a small adnexal mass (<4 cm) predicts spontaneous resolution in 75% of the cases, while falling levels of hCG predict resolution in about 90% of ectopic pregnancies [125,126]. Unquestionably, fetal cardiac activity, adnexal mass greater than 4 cm, and hCG levels greater than 2000 IU/mL are considered contraindications for expectant management. Suspected tubal rupture warrants immediate intervention, and persistent levels of hCG mandates active treatment as a replacement of the expectant management [124].

In a prospective observational study of expectantly managed patients with ectopic pregnancies on an outpatient basis, a total of 107/179 (59.8%) tubal ectopic pregnancies were treated with expectant management. Ectopic pregnancy resolved spontaneously in 75/107 (70%) women. Initial serum hCG level was the best predictor of the outcome of expectant management [128]. When hCG concentrations were 175 IU/L or less, treatment was successful in 96% of cases; whereas in those with hCG concentration of 175–1500 IU/L, expectant management was only effective in 66%. The threshold for treatment remains unclear and is a decision to be taken after discussion between the patient and her doctor [129].

Persistent Ectopic Pregnancy

Trophoblastic tissue remaining after surgical treatment of ectopic pregnancy causes persistent ectopic pregnancy, resulting in continued non-decreasing hCG levels. This condition is more common after laparoscopic surgeries than after laparotomies [130-133]; the reported frequency after laparoscopic surgery is 5–15% [134-137]. The size of the ectopic pregnancy and the preoperative hCG levels are considered to be risk factors for persistent ectopic pregnancy. Women with a small ectopic pregnancy size (8 mm or less), identified by pre-operative ultrasound, were at an increased risk for persistent ectopic pregnancy [138,139].

Non-Tubal and Heterotopic Ectopic Pregnancies

As many as 95% of ectopic pregnancies are tubal, 2% are either interstitial or corneal, 2% are ovarian, and the remainder are cervical or abdominal [129]. Another reported location of ectopic pregnancies is the scar of a previous cesarean (Figure 3). Until 2005, a total of 38 cases of ectopic pregnancy in cesarean scars were reported, half of them after two or more prior cesarean deliveries, suggesting an increasing rate of this kind of ectopic pregnancy as the cesarean delivery rate increases [129].

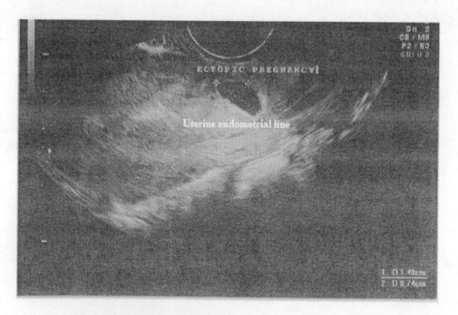

Figure 3. Pregnancy in previous cesarean delivery scar. Notice the endometrial line and the ectopic pregnancy observed at the low segment of the uterus.

Heterotopic pregnancy is defined as coexisting intrauterine and extrauterine pregnancies [140]. The occurrence of a heterotopic pregnancy following spontaneous cycles is rare, with an estimated incidence of 1 in 30,000 [1]. This incidence was calculated by multiplying the rate of ectopic pregnancy (0.37%) by that of dizygous twinning (0.8%), thus producing a hypothetical approximation. However, the incidence is increased to about 1% by the use of assisted reproductive techniques [69], especially in women undergoing ovulation induction with gonadotropins and among women undergoing *in vitro* fertilization, since it has become standard practice to transfer at least two embryos [141]. This kind of ectopic pregnancy is difficult to diagnose. It has been reported that 50% of patients had a late diagnosis, hence admission to the hospital after rupture [142]. Management of heterotopic pregnancy is surgical. In hemodynamically unstable patients, an explorative laparotomy should be performed. Since hCG levels cannot be monitored accurately due to the intrauterine pregnancy, expectant management is irrelevant. The prognosis for the intrauterine pregnancy is superb, and the majority are carried to term [143]. Most women who have fertility treatment and who conceive are reviewed in the early weeks of pregnancy; the diagnosis of ectopic pregnancy and heterotopic pregnancy should be considered [129].

Summary

Ectopic pregnancy is the primary cause of maternal death in the first half of the pregnancy. Moreover, ectopic pregnancy is a major cause of maternal morbidity due to infertility, hemodynamic instability and its consequences, anesthesia and surgical complications, etc. The annual incidence of ectopic pregnancy in the U.S. is now nearly 2%. The main risk factors associated with ectopic pregnancy include prior pelvic inflammatory disease, history of ectopic pregnancy and previous surgery for tubal obstruction and injury. Sudden severe abdominal pain is the most common complaint, and a classic symptom triad of ectopic pregnancy includes amenorrhea, irregular bleeding, and lower abdominal pain. Diagnosis is based on sonographic or laparoscopic direct visualization with an optional diagnostic support via serial hCG levels measurements. Other optional diagnosis options such as progesterone or other hormonal serial level measurements are debatable. Treatment options include medical or surgical therapy. Surgical treatment is mandatory for hemodynamically ustable patients. Patients with small ectopic pregnancies characterized by low hCG levels are candidates for medical treatment. Conditions that present surgical difficulties include pregnancy in previous cesarean delivery or corneal pregnancy, which may also be initially treated conservatively.

References

[1]   *ACOG Practice Bulletin:* Clinical management guidelines for obstetrician—gynecologists: Medical management of tubal pregnancy. Number 3, December 1998.

[2]   Bouyer J, Coste J, Shojaei T, Pouly JL, Fernandez H, Gerbaud L, Job-Spira N. Risk factors for ectopic pregnancy: a comprehensive analysis based on a large case-control, population-based study in France. *Am J Epidemiol*. 2003;157:185-94.

[3]   Washington AE, Katz P. Ectopic pregnancy in the United States: Economic consequences and payment source trends. *Obstet Gynecol* 1993;81:287–92.

[4]   CDC. Ectopic pregnancy–United States, 1990–1992. *MMWR Morb Mortal Wkly Rep*. 1995;44:46-8.

[5]   Salman G, Irvine LM. Ectopic pregnancy, the need for standardisation of rate. *J Obstet Gynaecol*. 2008;28(1):32-5.

[6]   Zane S, Kieke B, Kendrick J, Bruce C. Surveillance in a time of changing health care practices: estimating ectopic pregnancy incidence in the United States. *Mat Child Health J*. 2002;6:227-36.

[7]   Centers for Disease Control and Prevention. Ectopic pregnancy—United States, 1990-1992. *MMWR Morb Mortal Wkly Rep*. 1995;44:46-48.

[8]   Coste J, Bouyer J, Job-Spira N. Epidemiology of ectopic pregnancy: incidence and risk factors. *Fertil Contracept Sex*. 1996;24:135-9.

[9]   Lewis G, Drife JO. Why mothers die 1997–1999. The fifth report of the confidential enquiries into maternal deaths in the United Kingdom 1997–1999. London: RCOG Press; 2001.

[10]   Kamwendo F, Forslin L, Bodin L, Danielsson D. Epidemiology of ectopic pregnancy during a 28 year period and the role of pelvic inflammatory disease. *Sex Transm Infect*. 2000;76:28-32.

[11]   Ory SJ. New options for diagnosis and treatment of ectopic pregnancy. *JAMA*. 1992;267:534-7.

[12]   Seeber BE, Barnhart KT. Suspected Ectopic Pregnancy. *Obstet Gynecol*. 2006;107:399-413.

[13]   Goldner TE, Lawson H, Xia Z, Atrash H. Surveillance for ectopic pregnancy—United States, 1970–1989. *MMWR Morb Mortal Wkly Rep*. 1993;42:73-85.

[14]   Nathalie G, Robert L, Namory K, Patrick T. Ectopic pregnancy in African developing countries. *Acta Obstet Gynecol Scand*. 2003; 82: 305-312

[15]   Ankum WM, Mol BWJ, Van der Veen F, Bossuyt PM. Risk factors for ectopic pregnancy: a meta-analysis. *Fertile steril*. 1996;65:1093-9.

[16]   Mukul LV, Teal SB. Current Management of Ectopic Pregnancy. *Obstet Gynecol Clin N Am*. 2007;34:403-19.

[17]   Barnhart KT, Sammel MD, Gracia CR, Chittams J, Hummel AC, Shaunik A. Risk factors for ectopic pregnancy in women with symptomatic first-trimester pregnancies. *Fertil Steril*. 2006;86(1):36-43.

[18]   Sindos M, Togia A, Sergentanis TN, Kabagiannis A, Malamas F, Farfaras A, Sergentanis IN, Bassiotou V, Antoniou S. Ruptured ectopic pregnancy: risk factors for a life-threatening Condition. *Arch Gynecol Obstet* 2008 Sep 2 [Epub ahead of print].

[19]   Latchaw G, Takacs P, Gaitan L, Geren S, Burzawa J. Risk factors associated with the rupture of tubal ectopic pregnancy. *Gynecol Obstet Invest*. 2005;60:177-80.

[20]   Chow WH, Daling JR, Cates W Jr, Greenberg RS. Epidemiology of ectopic pregnancy. *Epidemiol Rev*. 1987;9:70-94.

[21]   Hillis SD, Owens LM, Marchbanks PA, Amsterdam LF, MacDenzie WR. Recurrent chlamydial infections increase the risks of hospitalization for ectopic pregnancy and pelvic inflammatory disease. *Am J Obstet Gynecol*. 1997;176:103-7.

[22] Coste J, Job-Spira N, Fernandez H, Papiernik E, Spira A. Risk factors for ectopic pregnancy: a case-control study in France, with special focus on infectious factors. *Am J Epidemiol* 1991;133:839-49.

[23] Goldberg JM, Falcone T. Effect of diethylstilbestrol on reproductive function. *Fertil Steril*. 1999;72(1):1-7.

[24] Waylen AL, Metwally M, Jones GL, Wilkinson AJ, Ledger WL. Effects of cigarette smoking upon clinical outcomes of assisted reproduction: a meta-analysis. *Hum Reprod Update*. 2009;15:3-44. Epub 2008 Oct 15.

[25] Atrash HK, Hogue CJ. The effect of pregnancy termination on future reproduction. *Baillieres Clin Obstet Gynaecol*. 1990;4:391-405.

[26] Frank PI, McNamee R, Hannaford PC, Kay CR, Hirsch S. The effect of induced abortion on subsequent pregnancy outcome. *Br J Obstet Gynaecol*. 1991;98:1015-24.

[27] Smith C, Bush J, Sutija VG. Adverse obstetric history and ectopic pregnancy. *J Reprod Med*. 2007;52(9):801-4.

[28] Shannon C, Brothers PL, Philip NM, Winikoff B. Ectopic pregnancy and medical abortion. *Obstet Gynecol*. 2004;104:161-7.

[29] Virk J, Zhang J, Olsen J. Medical Abortion and the Risk of Subsequent Adverse Pregnancy Outcomes. *N Engl J Med*. 2007;357:648-53.

[30] Ory HM. The women's health study. Ectopic pregnancy and intrauterine contraceptive devices: new perspectives. *Obstet Gynecol*. 1981;57:137-44.

[31] Westrom L, Bengtsson LP, Mardh PA. Incidence, trends and risks of ectopic pregnancy in a population of women. *Br Med J*. (Clin Res Ed) 1981;282(6257):15-8.

[32] World Health Organization, Task Force on Intrauterine devices for fertility Regulation. A multinational case-control study of ectopic pregnancy. *Clin Reprod Fertil*. 1985;3:131-43.

[33] Fernandes AM, Moretti TB, Olivotti BR. Epidemiological and clinical aspects of ectopic pregnancies at a university service between 2000 and 2004. *Rev Assoc Med Bras*. 2007;53(3):213-6.

[34] Peterson HB, Xia Z, Hughes JM, Wilcox LS, Tylor LR, Trussell J. The risk of ectopic pregnancy after tubal sterilization. U.S. Collaborative Review of Sterilization Working Group. *N Engl J Med*. 1997;336(11):762-7.

[35] Cheng MC, Wong YM, Rochat RW, Ratnam SS. Sterilization failure in Singapore: an examination of ligation techniques and failure rates. *Stud Fam Plann*. 1977;8:109-15.

[36] Karande VC, Flood JT, Heard N, Veek L, Muasher SJ. Analysis of ectopic pregnancies resulting from in vitro fertilization and embryo transfer. *Hum Reprod*. 1991;6:446-9.

[37] Nazari A, Askari HA, Check JH, O'Shaughnessy AO. Embryo transfer techniques as a cause for ectopic pregnancy in in-vitro fertilization. *Fertil Steril*. 1993;60:919-21.

[38] Strandell A, Thorburn J, Hamberger L. Risk factors for ectopic pregnancy in assisted reproduction. *Fertil Steril*. 1999;71:282-86.

[39] Homm RJ, Holtz G, Garvin AJ. Isthmic ectopic pregnancy and salpingitis isthmica nodosa. *Fertil Steril*. 1987;48:756-60.

[40] Weckstein LN, Boucher AR, Tucker H, Gibson D, Rettenmaier MA. Accurate diagnosis of early ectopic pregnancy. *Obstet Gynecol*. 1985;65:393-7.

[41] Aleem FA, DeFazio M, Gintautas J. Endovaginal sonography for the early diagnosis of intrauterine and ectopic pregnancies. *Hum Reprod.* 1990;5(6):755-8.

[42] Ankum WM, Van der Veen F, Hamerlynck JV, Lammes FB. Laparoscopy: a dispensable tool in the diagnosis of ectopic pregnancy? *Hum Reprod.* 1993;8(8):1301-6.

[43] Kadar N, Caldwell BV, Romero R. A method of screening for ectopic pregnancy and its indications. *Obstet Gynecol.* 1981;58:162-6.

[44] Barnhart KT, Sammel MD, Rinaudo PF, Zhou L, Hummel AC, Guo W. Symptomatic patients with an early viable intrauterine pregnancy: hCG curves redefined. *Obstet Gynecol.* 2004;104:50-5.

[45] Kadar N, Romero R. Observations on the log human chorionic gonadotropin-time relationship in early pregnancy and its practical implication. *Am J Obstet Gynecol.* 1987;157:73-8.

[46] Kadar N, Freedman M, Zacher M. Further observation on the doubling time of human chorionic gonadotropin in early asymptomatic pregnancy. *Fertil Steril.* 1990;54:783-7.

[47] Romero R, Kadar N, Copel JA, Jeanty P, DeCherney AH, Hobbins JC. The value of serial human chorionic gonadotropin testing as a diagnostic tool in ectopic pregnancy. *Am J Obstet Gynecol.* 1986;155:392-4.

[48] Shepherd RW, Patton PE, Novy MJ, Burry KA. Serial beta-hCG measurements in the early detection of ectopic pregnancy. *Obstet Gynecol.* 1990;75:417-20.

[49] Silva C, Sammel MD, Zhou L, Gracia C, Hummel AC, Barnhart K. Human chorionic gonadotropin profile for women with ectopic pregnancy. *Obstet Gynecol.* 2006;107(3):605-10.

[50] Carson SA, Buster JE. Ectopic pregnancy. *N Engl J Med.* 1993;329:1174-81.

[51] Stern JJ, Voss F, Coulam CB. Early diagnosis of ectopic pregnancy using receiver-operator characteristic curves of serum progesterone concentrations. *Hum Reprod.* 1993;8:775-9.

[52] Banerjee S, Aslam N, Woelfer B, Lawrence A, Elson J, Jurkovic D. Expectant management of early pregnancies of unknown location: a prospective evaluation of methods to predict spontaneous resolution of pregnancy. *Br J Obstet Gynaecol.* 2001;108:158-63.

[53] McCord ML, Muram D, Buster JE, Arheart KL, Stovall TG, Carson SA. Single serum progesterone as a screen for ectopic pregnancy: exchanging specificity and sensitivity to obtain optimal test performance. *Fertil Steril.* 1996;66:513-6.

[54] Condous G, Lu C, Van Huffel SV, Timmerman D, Bourne T. Human chorionic gonadotrophin and progesterone levels in pregnancies of unknown location. *Int J Gynaecol Obstet.* 2004;86:351-7.

[55] Stovall TG, Ling FW, Carson SA, Buster JE. Serum progesterone and uterine curettage in differential diagnosis of ectopic pregnancy. *Fertil Steril.* 1992;57:456-7.

[56] Gelder MS, Boots LR, Younger JB. Use of a single random serum progesterone value as a diagnostic aid for ectopic pregnancy. *Fertil Steril.* 1991;55:497-500.

[57] Mol BW, Lijmer JG, AnkumWM, van der Veen F, Bossuyt PM. The accuracy of single serum progesterone measurement in the diagnosis of ectopic pregnancy: a meta-analysis. *Hum Reprod.* 1998;13(11):3220-7.

[58] Shalev E, Yarom I, Bustan M, Weiner E, Ben-Shlomo I. Transvaginal sonography as the ultimate diagnostic tool for the management of ectopic pregnancy: experience with 840 cases. *Fertil Steril.* 1998;69:62-5.

[59] Cacciatore B, Stenman UH, Ylostalo P. Diagnosis of ectopic pregnancy by vaginal ultrasonography in combination with a discriminatory serum hCG level of 1000 IU/l (IRP). *Br J Obstet Gynaecol.* 1990;97:904-8.

[60] Condous G, Okaro E, Khalid A, Lu C, Van Huffel S, Timmerman D, Bourne T. The accuracy of transvaginal ultrasonography for the diagnosis of ectopic pregnancy prior to surgery. *Hum Reprod.* 2005;20(5):1404-9.

[61] Fossum GT, Davajam V, Kletzky OA. Early detection of pregnancy with transvaginal ultrasound. *Fertil Steril.* 1988;49:788-91.

[62] Goldstein SR, Snyder JR, Watson C, Danon M. Very early pregnancy detection with endovaginal ultrasound. *Obstet Gynecol.* 1988;72:200-4.

[63] Timor-Tritsch IE, Yeh MN, Peisner DB, Lesser KB, Salvik BS. The use of transvaginal ultrasound in the diagnosis of ectopic pregnancy. *Am J Obstet Gynecol.* 1988;161:157-61.

[64] Barnhart KT, Kamelle SA, Simhan H. Diagnostic accuracy of ultrasound, above and below the beta-hCG discriminatory zone. *Obstet Gynecol.* 1999;94:583-7.

[65] Brown DL, Doubilet PM. Transvaginal sonography for diagnosing ectopic pregnancy: positivity criteria and performance characteristics. *J Ultrasound Med.* 1994;13:259-66.

[66] Ankum WM, Hajenius PJ, Schrevel LS, Van der Veen F. Management of suspected ectopic pregnancy. *J Reprod Med.* 1996;41:724-8.

[67] Chiang G, Levine D, Swire M, McNamara A, Mehta T. The intradecidual sign: is it reliable for diagnosis of early intrauterine pregnancy? *Am J Roentgenol.* 2004;183:725-31.

[68] Nyberg DA, Mack LA, Harvey D. Value of the yolk sac in evaluating early pregnancies. *J Ultrasound Med* 1988;7:129-35.

[69] Svare J, Norup P, Grove Thomsen S, Hornnes P, Maigaard S, Helm P, Petersen K, Nyboe Andersen A. Heterotopic pregnancies after in-vitro fertilization and embryo transfer—a Danish survey. *Hum Reprod.* 1993;8:116-8.

[70] Ahmed AA, Tom BD, Calabrese P. Ectopic pregnancy diagnosis and the pseudo-sac. *Fertil Steril.* 2004;81:1225-8.

[71] Dillon EH, Feyock AL, Taylor KJW. Pseudogestational sacs: Doppler US differentiation from normal or abnormal intrauterine pregnancies. *Radiology* 1990;176:359-64.

[72] Kirchler HC, Seebacher S, Alge AA, Muller-Holzner E, Fessler S, Kolle D. Early diagnosis of tubal pregnancy: changes in tubal blood flow evaluated by endovaginal color Doppler sonography. *Obstet Gynecol.* 1993;82:561-5.

[73] Pellerito JS, Troiano RN, Quedens-Case C, Taylor KJ. Common pitfalls of endovaginal color Doppler flow imaging. *Radiographics* 1995;15:37-47.

[74] Stovall TG. Early Pregnancy Loss and Ectopic Pregnancy. In: Berek JS, ed. *Berek & Novak's Gynecology*, 14th ed. Philadelphia, PA: Lippincott William & Wilkins; 2006:882-931.

[75] Barnhart KT, Katz I, Hummel A, Gracia CR. Presumed diagnosis of ectopic pregnancy. *Obstet Gynecol*. 2002;100:505-10.

[76] Barnhart K, Mennuti MT, Benjamin I, Jacobson S, Goodman D, Coutifaris C. Prompt diagnosis of ectopic pregnancy in an emergency department setting. *Obstet Gynecol*. 1994;84:1010-5.

[77] Kaplan BC, Dart RG, Moskos M, Kuligowska E, Chun B, Adel Hamid M, Northern K, Schmidt J, Kharwadkar A. Ectopic pregnancy: Prospective study with improved diagnostic accuracy. *Ann Emerg Med*. 1996;28:10-7.

[78] Gracia CR, Barnhart KT. Diagnosing ectopic pregnancy in the emergency room setting: A decision analysis comparing six diagnostic strategies. *Obstet Gynecol*. 2001;97:464-70.

[79] Maruri F, Azziz R. Laparoscopic surgery for ectopic pregnancies: technology assessment and public health implications. *Fertil Steril*. 1993;59:487-98.

[80] Dorfman SF. Maternal mortality in New York City, 1981–1983. *Obstet Gynecol*. 1990;76:317-23.

[81] De Swiet M. Maternal mortality: confidential enquiries into maternal deaths in the United Kingdom. *Am J Obstet Gynecol*. 2000;182:760-6.

[82] Tintara H, Choobun T. Laparoscopic adnexectomy for benign tubo-ovarian disease using abdominal wall lift: a comparison to laparotomy. *Int J Gynaecol Obstet*. 2004;84:147-55.

[83] Tulandi T, Saleh A. Surgical management of ectopic pregnancy. *Clinical Obstet Gynecol*. 1999;42:31-8.

[84] Vermesh M, Silva PD, Rosen GF, Stein AL, Fossum GT, Sauer MV. Management of unruptured ectopic gestation by linear salpingostomy: a prospective, randomized clinical trial of laparoscopy versus laparotomy. *Obstet Gynecol*. 1989;73:400-4.

[85] Murphy AA, Nager CW, Wujek JJ, Kettel LM, Torp VA, Chin HG. Operative laparoscopy versus laparotomy for the management of ectopic pregnancy: a prospective trial. *Fertil Steril*. 1992;57:1180-5.

[86] Hajenius PJ, Mol BW, Bossuyt PM, Ankum WM, van der Veen F. Interventions for tubal ectopic pregnancy. *Cochrane Database Syst Rev*. 2007;(1):CD000324.

[87] Odejinmi FO, Rizzuto MI, Macrae RE, Thakur V. Changing trends in the laparoscopic management of ectopic pregnancy in a London district general hospital: 7-years experience. *J Obstet Gynaecol*. 2008;28:614-7.

[88] Morlock RJ, Lafata JE, Eisenstein D. Cost-effectiveness of single-dose methotrexate compared with laparoscopic treatment of ectopic pregnancy. *Obstet Gynecol*. 2000;95:407-12.

[89] Brezinski A, Schenker JG. Current status of endoscopic surgical management of tubal pregnancy. *Eur J Obstet Gynecol Reprod Biol*. 1994;54:43-53.

[90] Yao M, Tulandi T. Current status of surgical and nonsurgical management of ectopic pregnancy. *Fertil Steril*. 1997;67:421-33.

[91] Hill GA, Segars JH Jr, Herbert CM III. Laparoscopic management of interstitial pregnancy. *J Gynecol Surg*. 1989;5:209-12.

[92] *ACOG Practice Bulletin:* Medical Management of Ectopic Pregnancy. Number 94, June 2008.

[93] Hertz R. Folic acid antagonists: Effects on the cell and the patient. Clinical staff conference at NIH. *Ann Intern Med*. 1963;59:931-56.

[94] Stovall TG, Ling FW, Gray LA, Carson SA, Buster JE. Methotrexate treatment of unruptured ectopic pregnancy: a report of 100 cases. *Obstet Gynecol*. 1991;77:749-53.

[95] Stovall TG, Ling FW. Single-dose methotrexate: an expanded clinical trial. *Am J Obstet Gynecol*. 1993;168:1759-65.

[96] Saraj AJ, Wilcox JG, Najmabadi S, Stein SM, Johnson MB, Paulson RJ. Resolution of hormonal markers of ectopic gestation: A randomized trial comparing single-dose intramuscular methotrexate with salpingostomy. *Obstet Gynecol*. 1998;92:989-94.

[97] Thoen LD, Creinin MD. Medical treatment of ectopic pregnancy with methotrexate. *Fertil Steril*. 1997;68:727-30.

[98] Jimenez-Caraballo A, Rodriguez-Donoso G. A 6-year clinical trial of methotrexate therapy in the treatment of ectopic pregnancy. *Eur J Obstet Gynecol Reprod Biol*. 1998;79:167-71.

[99] Lecuru F, Robin F, Bernard JP, Maizan de Malartic C, Mac-Cordick C, Boucaya V, Taurelle R. Single-dose methotrexate for unruptured ectopic pregnancy. *Int J Gynaecol Obstet*. 1998;61:253-9.

[100] Lipscomb GH, Bran D, McCord ML, Portera JC, Ling FW. Analysis of three hundred fifteen ectopic pregnancies treated with single-dose methotrexate. *Am J Obstet Gynecol*. 1998;178:1354-8.

[101] Sauer MV, Gorrill MJ, Rodi IA, Yeko TR. Nonsurgical management of unruptured tubal pregnancy: An extended clinical trial. *Fertil Steril*. 1987;48:752-5.

[102] Fernandez H, Bourget P, Ville Y, Lelaidier C, Frydman R. Treatment of unruptured tubal pregnancy with methotrexate: Pharmacokinetic analysis of local versus intramuscular administration. *Fertil Steril*. 1994;62:943-7.

[103] Alleyassin A, Khademi A, Aghahosseini M, Safdarian L, Badenoosh B, Hamed FA. Comparison of success rates in the medical management of ectopic pregnancy with single-dose and multiple-dose administration of methotrexate: a prospective, randomized clinical trial. *Fertil Steril*. 2006;85(6):1661-6.

[104] Barnhart KT, Gosman G, Ashby R, Sammel M. The medical management of ectopic pregnancy: a meta-analysis comparing "single dose" and "multidose" regimens. *Obstet Gynecol*. 2003;101:778-84.

[105] Costa Soares R, Elito J, Han KK, Camano L. Endometrial thickness as an orienting factor for the medical treatment of unruptured tubal pregnancy. *Acta Obstet Gynecol Scand*. 2004;83:289-92.

[106] Elito J Jr, Reichmann AP, Uchiyama MN, Camano L. Predictive score for the systemic treatment of unruptured ectopic pregnancy with a single dose of methotrexate. *Int J Gynecol Obstet*. 1999;67:75-9.

[107] Lipscomb G, McCord M, Stovall T, Huff G, Portera SG, Ling FW. Predictors of success of methotrexate treatment in women with tubal ectopic pregnancies. *N Engl J Med*. 1999;341:1974-8.

[108] Laibl V, Takacs P, Kang J. Previous ectopic pregnancy as a predictor of methotrexate failure. *Int J Gynecol Obstet*. 2004;85:177-8.

[109] Lipscomb GH, Givens VA, Meyer NL, Bran D. Previous ectopic pregnancy as a predictor of failure of systemic methotrexate therapy. *Fertil Steril*. 2004;81:1221-4.

[110] Menon S, Colins J, Barnhart KT. Establishing a human chorionic gonadotropin cutoff to guide methotrexate treatment of ectopic pregnancy: a systematic review. *Fertil Steril*. 2007;87:481-4.

[111] Alleyassin A, Khademi A, Aghahosseini M, Safdarian L, Badenoosh B, Hamed EA. Comparison of success rates in the medical management of ectopic pregnancy with single-dose and multiple-dose administration of methotrexate: a prospective, randomized clinical trial. *Fertil Steril*. 2006;85:1661-6.

[112] Corsan GH, Karacan M, Qasim S, Bohrer MK, Ransom MX, Kemmann E. Identification of hormonal parameters for successful systemic single-dose methotrexate therapy in ectopic pregnancy. *Hum Reprod*. 1995;10:2719-22.

[113] Wolf GC, Nickisch SA, George KE, Teicher JR, Simms TD. Completely nonsurgical management of ectopic pregnancies. *Gynecol Obstet Invest*. 1994;37:232-5.

[114] Gross Z, Rodriguez JJ, Stalnaker BL. Ectopic pregnancy: nonsurgical, outpatient evaluation and single-dose methotrexate treatment. *J Reprod Med*. 1995;40:371-4.

[115] Stika CS, Anderson L, Frederiksen MC. Single-dose methotrexate for the treatment of ectopic pregnancy: Northwestern Memorial Hospital three-year experience. *Am J Obstet Gynecol*. 1996;174:1840-6; discussion 1846-8.

[116] Glock JL, Johnson JV, Brumsted JR. Efficacy and safety of single-dose systemic methotrexate in the treatment of ectopic pregnancy. *Fertil Steril*. 1994;62:716-21.

[117] Yao M, Tulandi T, Falcone T. Treatment of ectopic pregnancy by systemic methotrexate, transvaginal methotrexate, and operative laparoscopy. *Int J Fertil*. 1996;41:470-5.

[118] Pisarska MD, Carson SA, Buster JE. Ectopic pregnancy. *Lancet* 1998;351:1115-20.

[119] Schoenfeld A, Mashiach R, Vardy M, Ovadia J. Methotrexate pneumonitis in nonsurgical treatment of ectopic pregnancy. *Obstet Gynecol*. 1992;80:520-1.

[120] Isaacs JD, Mcgehee RP, Cowan BD. Life threatening neutropenia following methotrexate treatment of ectopic pregnancy: A report of two cases. *Obstet Gynecol*. 1996;88:694-6.

[121] Gervaise A, Masson L, de Tayrac R, Frydman R, Fernandez H. Reproductive outcome after methotrexate treatment of tubal pregnancies. *Fertil Steril*. 2004;82:304-8.

[122] Vermesh M. Conservative management of ectopic gestation. *Fertil Steril*. 1990;53:382-7.

[123] Bernoux A, Job-Spira N, Germain E, Coste J, Bouyer J. Fertility outcome after ectopic pregnancy and use of an intrauterine device at the time of the index ectopic pregnancy. *Hum Reprod*. 2000;15:1173-77.

[124] Wiznitzer A, Sheiner E. Ectopic and heterotopic pregnancies. In: Reece EA, Hobbins J, eds. *Clinical obstetrics: The fetus and mother*. Blackwell Publishing; 2007:161-76.

[125] Trio D, Strobelt N, Picciolo C, Lapinski RH, Ghidini A. Prognostic factors for successful expectant management. *Fertil Steril*. 1995;63:469-72.

[126] Shalev E, Peleg D, Tsabari A, Romano S, Bustan M. Spontaneous resolution of ectopic tubal pregnancy: natural history. *Fertil Steril*. 1995;63:15-9.

[127] Korhonen J, Stenman UH, Ylöstalo P. Serum human chorionic gonadotropin dynamics during spontaneous resolution of ectopic pregnancy. *Fertil Steril*. 1994;61:632-6.

[128] Elson J, Tailor A, Banerjee S, Salim R, Hillaby K, Jurkovic D. Expectant management of tubal ectopic pregnancy: prediction of successful outcome using decision tree analysis. *Ultrasound Obstet Gynecol*. 2004;23:552-6.

[129] Farquhar CM. Ectopic pregnancy. *Lancet* 2005;366:583-91.

[130] Vermesh M, Silva PD, Sauer MV, Vargyas JM, Lobo RA. Persistent tubal ectopic gestation: patterns of circulating beta-human chorionic gonadotropin and progesterone, and management options. *Fertil Steril*. 1988;50:584.

[131] Popp LW, Colditz A, Gaetje R. Management of early ectopic pregnancy. *Int J Gynaecol Obstet*. 1994;44:239-44.

[132] Seifer DB, Gutmann JN, Grant WD, Kamps CA, DeCherney AH. Comparison of persistent ectopic pregnancy after laparoscopic salpingostomy versus salpingostomy and laparotomy for ectopic pregnancy. *Obstet Gynecol*. 1993;81:378-82.

[133] Hajenius PJ, Mol BW, Ankum WM, van der Veen F, Bossuyt PM, Lammes FB. Clearance curves of serum human chorionic gonadotrophin for the diagnosis of persistent trophoblast. *Hum Reprod*. 1995;10:683-7.

[134] Hoppe DE, Bekkar BE, Nager CW. Single-dose systemic methotrexate for the treatment of persistent ectopic pregnancy after conservative surgery. *Obstet Gynecol*. 1994;83:51-4.

[135] Bengtsson G, Bryman I, Thorburn J, Lindblom B. Low-dose oral methotrexate as second-line therapy for persistent trophoblast after conservative treatment of ectopic pregnancy. *Obstet Gynecol*. 1992;79:589-91.

[136] Pouly JL, Mahnes H, Mage G, Canis M, Bruhat MA. Conservative laparoscopic treatment of 321 ectopic pregnancies. *Fertil Steril*. 1986;46:1093-7.

[137] Lundorff P, Hahlin M, Sjoblom P, Lindblom B. Persistent trophoblast after conservative treatment of tubal pregnancy: prediction and detection. *Obstet Gynecol*. 1991;77:129-33.

[138] Nathorst-Böös J, Hamad RR. Risk factors for persistent trophoblastic activity after surgery for ectopic pregnancy. *Acta Obstet Gynecol Scand*. 2004;83:471-5.

[139] Seifer DB, Gutmann JN, Doyle MB, Jones EE, Diamond MP, DeCherney AH. Persistent ectopic pregnancy following laparoscopic linear salpingostomy. *Obstet Gynecol*. 1990;76:1121-5.

[140] Reece EA, Petrie RH, Sirmans MF, Finster M, Todd WD. Combined intrauterine and extrauterine gestations: a review. *Am J Obstet Gynecol*. 1983;146:323-30.

[141] Laband SJ, Cherny WB, Finberg HJ. Heterotopic pregnancy: report of four cases. *Am J Obstet Gynecol*. 1988;158:437-8

[142] Rojansky N, Schenker JG. Heterotopic pregnancy and assisted reproduction: an update. *J Assist Reprod Genet*. 1996;13:594-601.

[143] Beckmann CR, Tomasi AM, Thomason JL. Combined interstitial and intrauterine pregnancy: corneal resection in early pregnancy and cesarean delivery at term. *Am J Obstet Gynecol*. 1984;149:83-5.

In: Textbook of Perinatal Epidemiology
Editor: Eyal Sheiner, pp. 197-236

ISBN: 978-1-60741-648-7
© 2010 Nova Science Publishers, Inc.

Chapter XIII

Reproductive Environmental Epidemiology

Joanna Jurewicz[*]*, Kinga Polańska and Wojciech Hanke*
Unit of Reproductive Environmental Epidemiology, Nofer Institute of Occupational
Medicine, 91-348 Lodz, Poland

Definition

- Reproductive environmental epidemiology: a study that identifies and quantifies exposures to environmental contaminants; conducts risk assessments and risk communication; provides medical evaluation and surveillance for adverse developmental and reproductive health effects; and provides health-based guidance on levels of exposure to such contaminants.

Introduction

Interest in the application of epidemiology to the study of environmental stressors present in our environment is increasing, since epidemiologic studies can validate the models used in predicting hazards and can characterize the actual and potential health effects of such exposures. Reproductive environmental epidemiology identifies and quantifies exposures to environmental contaminants, conducts risk assessments and risk communication, provides medical evaluation and surveillance for adverse developmental and reproductive health effects, and provides health-based guidance on levels of exposure to such contaminants.

The major strength of reproductive epidemiological studies is their ability to assess the relationship between environmental exposures and wide-scope developmental and

[*] For Correspondence: Joanna Jurewicz, PhD, Unit of Reproductive Environmental Epidemiology, Nofer Institute of Occupational Medicine, 91-348 Lodz, Poland. Phone +48 42 6134-569; E-mail: joannaj@imp.lodz.pl

reproductive outcomes in humans under real-life conditions. However, this is a difficult task. A relationship between an exposure and developmental and reproductive outcomes recognised as causative has to fulfill several conditions: (a) relationship in time, (b) strength of association, (c) dose-response relationship, (d) replication of the findings, (e) biologic plausibility, (f) cessation of exposure, (g) specificity of the association and (h) consistency with other knowledge and validity of the measurements of exposure and biological outcomes. Identification of possible socio-economic confounders and correction of risk estimates for their effects is of major importance.

This chapter explores pregnancy outcomes and exposure to environmental and occupational hazards including pesticides, air pollution, PCBs and dioxins, smoking, noise, trihalomethanes, stress at work and stressful live events and heavy physical work during pregnancy. Among the overarching themes are increased time to pregnancy, poor sperm quality, infertility, spontaneous abortion, birth weight, preterm delivery and intrauterine growth restriction (IUGR) and assessment of small for gestational age (SGA). Additionally, each hazard is supported by the status of knowledge of the biological mechanism of exposure and a conclusion that illustrates limitations of the studies.

Air Pollution and Pregnancy

The major air pollutants in Europe and North America are sulphur dioxide (SO_2), nitrogen oxides (NO_x), ozone (O_3), and particulate matter (PM). SO_2 is mainly produced from the burning of fossil fuels while most NO_x comes from motor vehicle exhaust (about 80%). Ozone is produced when NO_x and volatile organic compounds react under the action of light.

PM, sometimes referred to as airborne particles, include dust, dirt, soot, smoke, and liquid droplets. PM is emitted directly into the air from a variety of sources. That which is related to human activity includes motor vehicle emissions, industrial processes, unpaved roads and woodheaters. Particles can be classified on the basis of their size, referred to as their "aerodynamic diameter". "Coarse particles" are those between 10 and 2.5 micrometres (μm) in diameter, "fine particles" are smaller than 2.5 μm and "ultrafine particles" are smaller than 0.1 μm. For comparison, the diameter of a human hair is 70 μm. An amount of PM_{10} is related to the amount in the air.

Most epidemiological studies gather information on birth weight or gestation duration from birth certificate records and correlate it to exposure data from monitoring stations closest to the the home address of the parturients. Only a few studies used data from birth cohorts [1, 2, 3], gathered data on socioeconomic confounders (not available from birth certificates) [4, 5] or utilized ultrasound measurements during pregnancy [6].

Fetal growth was typically measured as the risk of SGA (small-for-gestational age), IUGR (intrauterine growth restriction) or term low birth weight infants (LBW). The effect on gestational duration was assessed by the risk preterm delivery (PD). Several studies selected "birth weight" or "low birth weight" as the outcome variables. The interpretation of the results is difficult as both growth restriction and shortened gestational duration influence the actual birth weight. The overview of current evidence regarding the impact of air pollutants on human reproduction was summarized by Slama et al. [7].

Fetal growth: A first study to report an increased risk of term LBW in relation to third trimester CO, total suspended particulates (TSP) and SO_2 exposure was done in China [8]. The results, in relation to the effect of exposure to CO, were confirmed by a study in southern California. Infants of mothers with third trimester exposure levels above 5.5 ppm were at an increased risk of LBW [9]. However, two following studies conducted in California were not consisted regarding the effect of CO on fetal growth. While Salam et al. [10] reported a negative effect of CO and PM (first trimester exposure) on intrauterine growth, Parker et al. [11] found association with the SGA only for $PM_{2.5}$. To some extent, differences in methods of CO measurements and data analysis can be responsible for the inconsistency.

In a recent study of more than 70,000 singleton births in Vancouver, British Columbia, residence within 50m from highways was associated with 26% increase in SGA. Exposures to all pollutants except O_3 were associated with SGA. Despite a very large sample size, given high correlations between NO, CO, SO_2, it was not possible to differentiate impacts of specific pollutant [12].

Race and related cultural and socioeconomic factors may influence the susceptibility to air pollution. In a project carried out in six north-eastern cities of the United States, the impact of CO, and SO_2 on the risk of term LBW infants was reported [13]. However, when the data was stratified by maternal race, it was found that the association of CO with term LBW appeared to be limited to African-American infants, while the effects of SO_2 were more consistent in white infants.

An association between the risk of intrauterine growth restriction (diagnosed as birth weight below the 10th percentile) and exposure to PM_{10} and $PM_{2.5}$ during the first month of pregnancy was analyzed in Czech Republic [14]. Based on studies of two populations (with low and high exposure to PM_{10}), the authors concluded that exposure to c-PAHs in early gestation may be associated with poor growth [15].

In case of exposure to PM, similarly to gaseous pollutants, the maternal race might be a risk (or protective) factor. In a small cohort of African American and Dominican women in New York City, an increase in prenatal PAH was associated with increase of SGA children of only African American women. Similar results were found when fetal growth ratio <85% or increased cephalisation index (head size/birth weight) were selected as pregnancy outcomes [1].

In accordance with the hypothesis that air pollutants negatively affect fetal growth are the results of studies reporting a decline in term birth weigh (or adjusted for pregnancy duration) with increasing maternal exposure to fine particles smaller than 10 μm ($PM_{2.5}$) 2, 16, 17]. For example, in a cohort study in Poland among 362 non-smoking women an association between personal $PM_{2.5}$ levels and birth weight adjusted for gestational duration and passive smoking has been reported. A decrease of 140g in mean birth weight was observed when exposure to $PM_{2.5}$ increased from a level of 10ug/m3 to 50ug/m3 [2]. In a cohort of more than 1000 full term births in Munich increased risk for birth <3000g at term was associated with increase of $PM_{2.5}$ [3].

Gestational duration: Association between PD and air pollutants was examined in studies in China [18], Czech Republic [19], Southern California [20, 21, 22, 23], Pennsylvania, U.S. [24], Georgia, U.S. [25, 26], Vancouver, Canada [12], and Republic of Korea [27]. Xu et al. reported a dose-response relation between environmental TSP and SO_2

exposure and preterm delivery [18]. Women in two residential areas of Beijing, China were observed to have shortened gestational periods after high exposures to TSP and SO_2. The effect was more pronounced in younger mothers. Likewise, prematurity was associated with SO_2 and less strongly with TSP in a study from Czech Republic [19].

More detailed information about PD risk assessment was provided by the study of Ritz et al. [20]. A 20% increase in preterm birth per 50 μg increase in ambient fine particles smaller than 10 μm (PM_{10}) levels averaged over 6 weeks before birth was reported as well as a 16% increase when averaging over the first month of pregnancy. CO exposure 6 weeks before birth consistently exhibited an effect only during the first month of pregnancy [20]. Clear dose-response pattern of PD with distance weighted traffic density (DWTD) primarily for women who delivered in the winter or fall (more stagnant air conditions) were documented in further studies of this group [21].

Ritz et al. provided detailed information on PD risk assessment in relation to different air pollutants [5]. The risk of preterm birth increased with increasing CO exposures (last 6 weeks of pregnancy) and $PM_{2.5}$. After adjustment for socio-demographic covariates the OR of preterm birth increased in 11–17% for women with average CO levels of 0.59 –1.25 ppm and as much as 21–25% for women with CO exposure greater then 1.25 ppm. When analyses were restricted to women who did not change residence throughout the pregnancy, the effects of first trimester CO exposures strengthened. Parous women who did not work outside the house experienced an increased odd for PD [5].

In Georgia, US, increased risk of very low birth weight (VLBW <1500g) was observed with exposure to PM_{10} , although both cases and controls were appropriate for gestational age [26].

As indicated by a study covering a large number of births in Vancouver, British Columbia, Canada, residency within 50m of highways was clearly a risk factor for PD [12]. Even relatively low concentrations of CO under current air quality standards (10.4mg/m^3) may contribute to an increased risk of PD [27].

Birth weight: More than 30 years ago, Williams documented an adverse effect of air pollutants (CO,NO_2, SO_2) on birth weight in Los Angeles [28]. Several studies have reported associations between TSP and PM_{10} in place of living during pregnancy with infant's birth [29, 30, 31]. In general, the increase of 1μg/m3 in $PM_{2.5}$ was related to 3–7g of birth weight [22, 17].

Low birth weight (LBW): Ambient levels of TSP, SO_2 and CO have been examined in relation to the risk of LBW in several studies, but no consistent pattern was established. In the Czech Republic, the relationship between average annual LBW in the country districts and the levels of SO_2, TSP and NO_x was investigated [32]. A small increase in the risk was observed in districts with high exposures to SO_2, but not to other contaminants.

In two other studies, no relationships between single indicators of air pollution and LBW were reported. Alderman et al. studied the relation between LBW and ambient levels of CO during the last trimester of pregnancy [33]. An insignificant increase in the risk of LBW was observed among infants exposed to CO levels equal to or greater than 3 pm. Likewise, Dolk and colleagues did not find an association between LBW and residence near coke works [34].

The supportive information for the negative effect of air pollutants on the risk of LBW was reported in Massachusetts where gestational exposure to NO_x, PM_{10}, $PM_{2,5}$ was associated with an increased risk of LBW after adjustment for several socioeconomic covariates including smoking [17].

Ultrasound measurements: In more than 15,000 women studied in South East Queensland and Northern New South Wales (Australia), a reduction in several ultrasound measures [such as AC (abdominal circumference), BPD (bipartial diameter) and Fl (femur length)] was associated with exposures to O_3, SO_2, and PM $_{2,5}$ during the first trimester [6].

Windows of susceptibility: Results across studies have not consistently identified specific periods of exposures that are most closely linked to adverse pregnancy outcome [12]. In the study in Connecticut and Massachusetts, LBW was associated with second- and third-trimester PM2,5 levels [17], while in Munich LBW was associated with first- and third trimester exposures to PM2,5 [3]. Difficulties in identification of critical exposure windows for IUGR were discussed by Slama et al. [7].

Confounding variables: Socioeconomic confounding variables including maternal active and passive smoking are major threats to studies relating pregnancy outcomes to air pollutants. When data on smoking status of study participants were available it was used to adjust the risk estimates [5, 12, 13, 14, 17]. In other situation authors restricted study participants to nonsmokers [1, 2] or validated an argument that maternal smoking is not related to exposure to air pollutants [19].

Prematurity may be related to the season of year (e.g., as an effect of respiratory infectious diseases). However, adjustment for season of delivery may underestimate the risk parameters. Thus it was advised to adjust for season of conception rather then to the season of delivery [7].

Status of research on biological mechanisms: The biological mechanism by which air pollution might cause growth restriction has not been established. Several lines of evidence support the plausibility of a negative effect of CO trans-placental exposure on birth weight. Fetal hemoglobin has greater affinity for binding CO than adult hemoglobin, and accordingly O2 delivery to fetal tissues compromise. The resulted tissue hypoxia has the potential to reduce fetal growth [10].

The role of hematologic factors (increased blood viscosity influencing the blood perfusion of the placentas) has also been postulated [5, 19]. A biologic mechanisms through oxidative pathways and alternation of maternal host-defence mechanisms through increased prostaglandin levels triggered by inflammatory mediators during exposure periods has been postulated [5, 27]. Engel et al. suggested that the common genetic variants in the proinflammatory cytokine genes could influence the risk for spontaneous PD [35].

Interestingly, exposure to polycyclic aromatic hydrocarbons (PAHs) absorbed to airborne particles may influence fetal growth [36]. The role of PAHs as a major source of genotoxic and embryotoxic activity of organic mixtures related to air pollution was supported by the results of in vitro cellular assay coupled with 32P-postlabelling of DNA adducts and chick embryotoxicity screening tests [37].

Conclusions

The Atmospheric Pollution and Human Reproduction group (gathered in 2007 in Munich) agreed that "given the heterogeneous chemical and physical nature of pollutants such as PM, there is no reason to believe in the existence of unique biological mechanism likely to explain PM effects on complex events such as fetal growth and premature birth". The group made several recommendations regarding future studies. It was emphasized that in addition to the already broadly targeted reproductive outcomes; other perinatal end points may be sensitive to air pollutant exposures and could be considered in future studies. Standard set points to report (size of population, reproductive outcomes, exposure assessment, socio-economic covariates, and statistical analysis) would facilitate comparisons across studies on air pollution and human reproduction. As the spatial resolution of exposure models is often inadequate, the ways of their improvement should be investigated. The development of biomarkers of exposure to traffic-related air pollutants reflecting the dose absorbed by relevant target organs such as the feto-placental unit should be also encouraged. It was recommended to promote studies investigating the short-term effects of air pollution on endothelial function, inflammatory response, and blood pressure of pregnant women, which could help understanding if these are possible pathways for air pollutants effects on reproductive outcomes. It was also stressed that in addition to epidemiological studies, animal experiments are needed to help identify relevant biological mechanisms.

Studies that collect detailed exposure and covariate information and biological samples, possibly in nested subgroups of larger populations, should be further encouraged.

Study designs that have proven useful in assessing air pollution impacts on other health outcomes (e.g., time-series, case-crossover designs) could be further explored in the context of reproductive outcomes

Environmental Tobacco Smoke Exposure

Fetal exposure to tobacco smoke compounds can be the consequence of maternal active smoking or maternal exposure to environmental tobacco smoke (ETS) during pregnancy. Based on the data from epidemiological studies, about 20–30% of women actively smoke during pregnancy. In addition, about half of the non-smokers can be exposed to passive smoking. Taking into account the high prevalence and serious health consequences of exposure, active and passive smoking in preconception period and during pregnancy is a significant public health problem.

Delay conception and infertility: Studies evaluating the effect of smoking on pregnancy rates indicated that tobacco smoking can be related to delayed conception (low probability of conception per menstrual cycle) [38, 39]. Epidemiological studies reported dose-response trends between smoking and increased time to conception although the effect of cigarette smoking appears to be reversible. Current cigarette smoking was associated with increased risk for primary or secondary female infertility (failure to conceive after unprotected sexual intercourse over a period of 12 months) [38, 40].

Many studies suggested that cigarette smoking was associated with alerted semen quality, but conclusions about the extent of its deleterious effects on variable including motility, sperm density, total sperm count, semen volume and morphology are widely varied [41, 42, 43, 44, 45].

Pregnancy complications: Preconception smoking or smoking during pregnancy is a significant and preventable factor increasing the risk of ectopic pregnancy, placental abruption, placenta praevia, preterm premature rupture of the membranes (PPROM) and spontaneous abortion [46, 38, 40]. The relative risk for ectopic pregnancy after adjustment for confounding factors ranged from 1.5 to 2.5 for smokers comparing to non-smokers [46] Abruptio placenta estimated to cause 15–25% of perinatal deaths was also related to smoking during pregnancy [46]. Placenta previa can predispose the women for caesarean section, fetal mal-presentation and postpartum hemorrhage. Epidemiological data indicated RR for placenta previa of 1.5–3.0 among women who smoke during pregnancy (compared to those who did not) [46]. A metaanalysis study noted almost two fold increase risk of PPROM among smokers [46]. Another metaanalysis indicated two folds increased risk of spontaneous abortion for smoking women comparing to non-smokers [47]. However, the evidence for the effects of ETS on the risk of spontaneous abortions is inconclusive [48]. In a Swedish prospective study an excess risk of intrauterine death (spontaneous abortion and fetal death) was observed among working women spending most of their time at work in rooms with smokers [49]. Exposure at home was not related to abortion. Windham observed an increased risk of spontaneous abortion among non-smokers, for ETS exposure of 1 hour or more per day [50]. In a more recent prospective study by the same author no evidence was found for an association between spontaneous abortions and exposure to ETS [51]. In some studies the risks were increased among exposed women who also consumed alcohol and caffeine in moderate to high amounts. Two studies confirmed the increased risk of spontaneous abortion [52, 53]. An odds ratio of 3.4 was documented for fetal death in the highest cotinine quintile (0.236–10 ng/mL), compared with the lowest quintile (<0.026 ng/mL). The association could reflect an effect of ETS exposure on the mother and fetus, but also a direct effect of smoking on the sperm (if losses were due to fetal abnormalities) [52].

Stillbirth or fetal death: Tobacco smoking during pregnancy can increase the risk of stillbirth (fetal death after 28 weeks of gestation). A moderate increase in the risk for stillbirth has been found with increasing cigarette consumption [38].

Birth weight: Since 1957 when Simpson has reported an adverse effect of maternal smoking on birth weight, several studies have demonstrated a direct dose-response effect [54]. Currently, cigarette smoking in pregnancy is the single most important factor affecting birth weight in developed countries [55]. Active smoking during pregnancy reduces birth weight by 10–15 g per cigarette smoked daily (average 250g) [56]. Eliminating smoking during pregnancy improves infant birth weight. Studies on ETS show weight decrement from 25 to 100 grams and pooled weight decrement was -24.9g (-33.7g to -16.1g) and even -82g (-126g to -37g) in studies that were based on cotinine measurements (saliva, serum) and were adjusted for at least one confounder [57, 58, 59, 60, 48].

The relative risk for SGA among smoking women comparing to nonsmokers in published epidemiological studies ranged from 1.5 do 10.0 and in most studies dose-response effect was observed. ETS exposure of pregnant women also adversely affects fetal growth. The pooled

OR for IUGR or LBW at term (based on 11 studies) was 1.2 (95%CI: 1.1-1.3) [61]. Kharrazi et al. found a linear dose-dependent effect of log cotinine on mean infant length (-0.84 cm) over a wide range of serum cotinine concentrations, while body mass index declined with exposures above 0.5 ng/mL [53].

Preterm delivery: Preterm delivery is associated with increased risk of perinatal mortality. In a metaanalysis of 20 prospective studies, Shah and Bracken found 30% increased risk for PD for smokers as compared with nonsmokers [62]. The dose-response relationship between prenatal expose to smoking compounds was not consistent. Smoking cessation during pregnancy seems to reduce the risk of PD. A higher risk has been associated with greater number of hours of ETS exposure [63, 64]. In a study in which ETS exposure assessment was based on nicotine concentration in maternal hair sampled after delivery, the risk of PD (<37 weeks) was increased in the high- and medium-exposure categories compared with the low one [65].

Status of research on biological mechanisms: Clinical and laboratory data on the mechanisms by which smoking may affect female fertility indicate adverse effect of smoking compounds (nicotine and PAHs) on the release of gonadotropins, formation of the corpus luteum, gamete interaction, tubal function and implementation of fertilized ova. Those effects can lead to dysfunction of the fallopian tubes, delayed conception, infertility, spontaneous abortion or ectopic pregnancy. The mechanism by which cigarette smoking affects semen quality is not fully understood. The increased risk of stillbirth is believed to be caused by IUGR and/or placental complications. Other postulated mechanism is that nicotine induces change in central respiratory control mechanism that may elicit fetal hypoxia-isochemia, leading to stillbirth [38]. Nicotine may impair fetal growth by affecting uterine blood flow. Fetal hypoxia due to elevated carboxyhemoglobin levels from the CO in cigarette smoke may also restrict fetal growth. Another mechanism to the reduced birth weight may be related to less weight-gain of smokers as compared to non-smoking mothers. The association between smoking in pregnancy and PD is biologically plausible; however nicotine can induce vasoconstriction in placentas which could initiate delivery. Also, higher levels of circulating catecholamines may initiate premature labor.

Conclusions

While the association between active cigarette smoking during pregnancy and LBW is well established, some improvement may be added by prospective studies with well documented smoking status, confirmed by biochemical verification, and controlling for confounders. Little is known about the impact of ETS on the risk of spontaneous abortion, birth defects, infertility and male reproductive health.

Pesticides

Pesticides are a broad group of heterogeneous chemicals, which are used to kill insects, weed, fungi and rodents. Several classes of compounds are used for this purpose. These substances have a significant public health benefit by increasing food production productivity and decreasing diseases. On the other hand, public concern has been raised about the potential health effects of exposure to pesticides on the developing fetus. Pesticides may enter the body by dermal, inhalation or oral absorption. In addition to residues found in food as a result of agricultural use, pesticides are also found at home, in schools and recreational areas, creating many possible exposure sources and a potential risk for cumulative exposure. Concern has been expressed about co-exposure to multiple pesticides, especially when the substances share a common mechanism of toxicity (e.g., acetylcholine esterase inhibition induced by carbamates or organophosphates).

Increased interval to pregnancy: The data on the effect of employment in agriculture on time to pregnancy are unequivocal. While some suggest that there is a relationship between decreased fecundability ratio and pesticide exposure [66, 67, 68, 69, 70, 71, 72], others did not find such an association [73, 74, 75]. The following pesticides were linked to decreased fecundability ratio: cynazine, carbamates, pyretroids, benzimidazoles, thiocarbamate and organophosphates [69].

Poor sperm quality: A number of male infertility cases were first discovered among workers exposed to 1,2-dibromo-3-chloropropane (DBCP) at a California pesticide factory. Azospermia, oligospermia and elevated levels of serum follicle stimulating hormone (FSH) and luteinizing hormone (LH) were observed among workers exposed to DBCP [76]. The results of the most recent studies performed in Hawaii [77], Denmark [78], China [79] and Mexico [80] also indicated that employment in agriculture increased the risk of specific morphological abnormalities of the sperm [77, 79, 80, 81] decreased sperm count per ejaculate [78, 77] and the percentage of viable sperm [77]. The first study, which demonstrates links between specific biomarkers of environmental exposure to pesticides and biomarkers of male reproduction in humans, was performed in the United States. Men with high exposure level of alachlor (>0.15 µg/g creatinine) had lower semen parameters (concentration, percentage sperm with normal morphology, percentage of motile sperm) [82]. The exposure to herbicide 2,4-D, metolachlor and atrazine was also associated with poorer sperm quality [82].

Female infertility: Several epidemiological studies of the effects of pesticide exposure on infertility were based on couples attending infertility clinics [83, 84, 85]. The findings indicate that agricultural work related to pesticide exposure might be a significant risk for female infertility [83, 84, 85]. In studies in the U.S., infertile women were observed to be three times more likely to be exposed to pesticides [86] and nine times more likely to work in agriculture [83]. On the other hand, in study in Canada, no correlation between female infertility and self-reported overall pesticide exposure was found [87].

Sex ratio: The studies of offspring sex ratio in families with occupational exposure to pesticides found increased likelihood of conceiving girls than boys [88]. The reduction in the number of male infants was noticed also for children born to workers using dibromochloropropane (DBCP) and organochlorine pesticides [89]. Garry et al. in a study of male pesticide applicators in Minnesota also noticed a deficit in the number of male children born to the spouses of fungicide applicator [90]. On the other hand, study of female workers revealed that pesticide exposure seemed to increase the chance to conceive a boy [91], whereas Savitz et al. did not find an association between sex ratio and chemical activities (OR = 1.0 95%CI (0.8–1.2) [92].

Spontaneous abortions: An increased risk for spontaneous abortions has been found among women in agricultural occupations and among gardeners using pesticides in Canada [92, 93], Columbia [94], Norway [95], Italy [96, 97], the U.S. [98], the Netherlands [99] and the Philippines [100]. In Ontario, parental preconception exposure to phenoxy herbicides was associated with the risk of early (< 12 weeks) spontaneous abortions [101, 102]. However, in a study carried out in West Sumatra, Indonesia, the number of spontaneous abortions among female spraying operators was not significantly increased compared to female rice farmers [103].

Stillbirth: The rate of stillbirth (excluding birth defects) was increased among women who worked in agriculture or horticulture more than 30h/week [104]. Among farmers in California, occupational exposure to pesticides during the first two months of pregnancy was positively associated with stillbirth due to congenital anomalies, while during the first and second trimesters with stillbirth due to all causes of death [105].

The data on the risk for adverse reproductive effects in a population of residents (nonfarmers) exposed to pesticides via drift from agriculture fields are lacking. An increased risk of fetal death was observed for women who during the second trimester of pregnancy resided near the application of: carbamates in general, estrogenic pesticides (endocrine disruptors), and carbamate acetylcholinoesterase inhibitors [106]. In Indonesia the number of stillbirths was slightly higher among the rice farmers but the difference was not significant [103], while the study of the Norwegian grain farmers did not reveal an excess of risk of stillbirth in grain farmers as compared to non-farmers [95].

Preterm delivery: Working in agriculture is not related to an increased risk of preterm delivery [93, 107]. However, in one study, preterm delivery was associated with mixing or applying atrazine and 4-[2,4-dichlorophenoxy] butric acid within a three-months period prior to conception [92]. Similar association was found for wives of male workers exposed to pesticides in floriculture [94]. No significant effect of grain farming was documented in the Norwegian study [95].

Birth weight and small-for-gestational-age: No increased risk for LBW and SGA was found among women working in agricultural occupations in Scotland, Norway and Canada [92, 93, 95, 107]. Despite the most negative results on the risk of LBW, there are some indications for further research in this area. In Northeast Brazil, the mean birth weight of infants born to women who worked in agriculture was lower by 190 g than that in the non-exposed group [108].

Maternal exposure to pesticides in the 1st or the 2nd trimesters of pregnancy affected infant birth weight in a population of Polish female farmers who had infants with birth weight lower by 100 g than that of infants born to non-exposed women [109]. Another study, carried out in Poland showed that involvement in field work delivered infants with a significantly higher birth weight than mothers not reporting such activities in the 1st or 2nd trimester of pregnancy. Also maternal exposure to synthetic pyrethroids in the 1st or the 2nd trimesters was associated with a decreased birth weight [110].

Status of research on biological mechanisms: Some pesticides are now suspected of being endocrine disrupting chemicals (EDCs). These chemicals might cause an adverse effect by interfering in some way with the body's hormones or chemical messengers. Many of these endocrine disrupters have been linked to adverse effects on either embryonic development or reproductive function in humans and wildlife [111, 112, 113].

The effects that can be seen in an organism exposed to EDC depend on which hormone system it is targeted. The mechanisms of endocrine disruption focused on sex hormone disrupters include: (1) binding and activating the estrogen receptor (therefore acting as an estrogen); (2) binding but not activating the estrogen receptor (therefore acting as an anti-estrogen); (3) binding other receptors; (4) modifying the metabolism of natural hormones; (5) modifying the number of hormone receptors in a cell; (6) modifying the production of natural hormones [111, 112, 113].

Conclusions

The epidemiological methods employed so far have not significantly contributed to the assessment of adverse reproductive and developmental toxicity of pesticides. Although several pesticides were associated with wide range of reproductive disorders, the results of the presented studies are inconsistent and have several limitations. The exposure to pesticides was in general evaluated only with the use of qualitative indicators and only in few studies it was possible to distinguish groups of different level of exposure. Only some of these studies provided an evidence for dose-response relationship. Biological monitoring of exposure was used rarely. Standard protocols for biological monitoring of the most prevalent pesticides should be developed to achieve progress in assessing the risk of adverse reproductive outcomes in the population of rural area residents exposed to drifts of pesticides from agriculture fields. Systematic studies addressing the risk of each adverse reproductive outcome should be undertaken.

Organochlorine Contaminants, Dioxins and Polychlorinated Biphenyls

Organochlorines were widely used worldwide from 1940 through the 1970s, but most have been eliminated or restricted in use after recognition of their persistence in the environment, bioaccumulation in animals and humans and toxicity in laboratory animals and wildlife.

Dioxins may be formed as unwanted byproducts in a variety of industrial and combustion processes, as well as household fires. Dioxins and polychlorinated biphenyls (PCBs) from these various sources may be released in small quantities to air, water or land. These compounds have no immediate effect on health, even at the highest levels found in foods. The potential risks to health come from long-term exposure. They have been shown to cause a wide range of effects, including cancer and damage to the immune and reproductive systems.

Increased interval to pregnancy: An increased time to getting pregnant was found only among heavy smokers in the east cost cohort of fishermen's wives in Sweden as compared to west cost cohort [114]. East cost fishermen and their wives were a group with a relatively high exposure to PCBs and dioxins because of their consumption of fish contaminated with these chemicals. An East Coast cohort also showed an increased risk for infertility (reported time to pregnancy of 12 months or longer and no children). However, the results of the New York State Angler Cohort Study did not imply that the consumption of PCB-contaminated sport fish from Lake Ontario was a significant risk factor for either resolved (time to pregnancy > 12 cycles) or unresolved infecundity (no pregnancy). An insignificantly increased risk of infecundity was found for women with the highest duration of fish consumption [115]. Weak and inconclusive results were also documented by other studies [116].

Poor sperm quality: The studies on exposure to organochlorine compounds and semen quality suggested association between PCBs exposure and poor sperm quality. In a study of 170 semen samples that were screened for PCBs and p,p'-DDE (DDT metabolite) an inverse relationship was found between sperm motility and the concentration of PCBs congeners 153, 118 and 138 which are rather ubiquitous in the human population [117].

The findings of the pilot study carried out in the Boston area population were also indicative of an association between PCBs and p,p'-DDE and abnormal sperm count, motility and morphology. [118] The total motile sperm counts were inversely proportional to the PCBs concentrations and were significantly lower among infertile male than those of the controls [119]. Also, in a study performed by Dallinga et al among 65 males with fertility problems, sperm count and motility were inversely related to sum of PCB congeners [120].

A strong and monotonically increasing DNA fragmentation index with increasing serum levels of 2,2',4,4',5,5'- hexachlorobiphenyl (CB-153) was found in a study performed by Spanò et al. [121]. In a study of young Swedish men statistically significant, negative correlations between CB-153 levels and biologically active free testosterone fraction and sperm motility were observed. No statistically significant association with other seminal, hormonal, or clinical markers of male reproductive function was found [122].

On the other hand, the international cross-sectional study of semen quality and serum concentration of CB-153 and p,p'-DDE showed that sperm concentration was not impaired with increasing serum CB-153 or p,p'-DDE levels. Similarly, the proportion of morphologically normal sperm was not associated with either CB-153 or p,p'-DDE blood concentration. However, sperm motility was inversely related to CB-153 concentration in Greenland and the Swedish fishermen population. The concentration of p,p'-DDE was negatively associated with sperm motility in the Greenlandic population [123].

Sex ratio: Studies have reported that high paternal PCB concentrations affected sex ratio [124], but others found no effect of maternal PCB intake on the sex ratio of the offspring [125, 126]. Unintentional contaminations of PCBs have been reported from two separate accidents. The first was in 1968 in west Japan, but there was no excess of births of girls over boys [127, 128].

Spontaneous abortion and stillbirth: In one early study, blood PCB levels among women with miscarriages were found to be higher than in women with normal deliveries [129]. However the analysis did not include adjustments for several confounding factors. The results were not confirmed in further studies. Exposure to PCBs did not increase the risk of spontaneous abortion among women living near Great Lakes [130, 131, 132] and in Japan [133]. Two studies which have measured fetal exposure to PCBs by maternal fish intake from contaminated waters also did not find an association between high intake of PCBs and stillbirth [114, 134].

Preterm delivery: Studies on preterm delivery and exposure to organochlorine compounds provided inconsistent results. The decrease in the length of gestation was found in cohort of 385 women in Salinas Valley, an agricultural community in California [135]. Preterm delivery was associated with increasing levels of lipid-adjusted hexachlorobenzene (HCB). Also higher HCB serum levels in preterm deliveries compared with term births were reported in a birth cohort study [136] but not in a case-control study [137]. Additionally, Bjerregaard and Hansen did not find a significant association between HCB levels in cord blood and gestational duration [138]. The literature on β-hexachlorocyclohexane (β-HCCH) and risk of preterm delivery is also conflicting. One study reported a possible elevated risk for preterm delivery with increasing maternal serum β-HCCH levels [137], whereas other studies did not find such an association [136].

Birth weight and small-for-gestational-age: Most studies found an association between exposure to PCBs and the risk for SGA infants. Fein et al examined the size of the newborn, gestational age, and maturity in relation to maternal consumption of fish from Lake Michigan. PCBs were measured in cord serum [139]. Detectable levels of PCBs in cord serum were associated with lower birth weight (160 to 190 grams lighter than controls), smaller head circumference (average 0.6 centimeters smaller than controls) and shorter gestational age (on average 4.9 days less than controls). There was also a consistent dose-response relationship between overall fish consumption and birth weight, head circumference and gestational age.

Studies concerning the wives of the Baltic Sea fishermen have also shown an association between high dietary intake of Baltic Sea fish contaminated with persistent organochlorine compounds and low birth weight [140, 141, 142, 134]. Likewise, in a general Dutch population, a negative correlation has been observed between plasma levels of dioxins and PCB and the birth weight [143].

Bjerregaard and Hansen examined the relationship of HCB hexachlorobenzene measured in cord blood and birth weight in a sample of 120 births in Greenland [138]. After controlling for confounders they did not find a significant relationship between HCB levels and birth weight. A lack of association between HCB levels and birth weight was also found in the Spanish population [136] and in a Ukrainian one [144].

Occupational exposure to PCBs has been associated with a decrease in birth weight in babies born to women working in the areas of high PCB exposure [145]. In Chapayevsk, Russia, where the town was contaminated with dioxins from a chemical plant, an increased risk of low birth weight was also observed [146].

Some evidence about the mother's residence near hazardous waste sites increasing the risk of having low birth weight births has been reported [147], although in these studies there was a possibility of exposure to other chemicals or risk factors. In the study performed in Seveso, Italy, where explosion at trichlorophenol plant took place, no association was found between the exposure to TCDD (2,3,7,8-tetrachlorodibenzo-para-dioxin) and birth weight or with births that were SGA. However, the associations with birth weight and with SGA were stronger for pregnancies within the first 8 years after exposure [148].

On the other hand, birth weight and head circumference were unrelated to average plasma PCB levels in a study of more than 900 North Carolina infants [149]. The cohort was a sample from the general population and had no history of occupational exposure, or specific dietary exposure to PCBs. Similarly, Khanjani et al. did not find any association between maternal PCB contamination and low birth weight and small for gestational age [126]. No significant association between the concentration of PCBs in milk samples and birth weight was found in two other studies [149, 150].

Status of research on biological mechanisms: PCBs and DDT are well known chemicals with estrogen-like characteristics and are referred to as estrogen disrupters. Animal studies suggest that these chemicals readily penetrate the blood-testis barrier and can directly affect spermatogenesis. It was also documented that PCB metabolites bind to estrogen receptors. Jansen hypothesized that adverse reproductive affects of PCBs may result from PCB congeners increasing gonadotropin-releasing hormone or affecting the production and release of luteinizing hormone from the pituitary [151]. Kelce et al. showed that p,p'-DDE has an antiandrogenic activity [152].

Conclusions

There is little scope for removal of dioxins and PCBs from foods once they have entered the food chain. It is generally agreed that the best method of preventing dioxins and PCBs from entering the food chain is to control release of these chemicals to the environment.

The results of the presented studies are inconsistent, although most suggest that there is an association between exposure and adverse pregnancy outcome, especially poor sperm quality, lower birth weight or small-for-gestational age. Some studies measured fetal exposure to PCBs by maternal fish intake from contaminated waters [134,131,139], and several studies measured the level of PCBs in maternal milk samples [149, 150]. The latter is a stronger method than indirect measures of exposure, such as fish consumption, because of the possible contamination of fish with other chemicals (e.g., methyl mercury).

There is a need for better understanding the relationship between environmental exposures to dioxins and PCBs and pregnancy outcome after controlling for potential confounders. Further research on the relationship between the dietary intake of organochlorine-contaminated food (mostly fish) and pregnancy outcome should be perused.

Trihalomethanes in Drinking Water

Chlorination by-products in drinking water come from the reaction of chlorine with organic material in the water. This reaction occurs naturally or originates from municipal, agricultural, and industrial wastes. Trihalomethanes (THMs) such as chloroform, bromoform, chlorodibromomethane, bromodichloromethane, are the most prevalent and routinely measured class of disinfection by-products (DBPs) found in the water [153]. Routes of exposure to THMs include dermal absorption during hand washing and bathing, inhalation during showering and ingestion of drinking water. Owing to high prevalence of exposure, potential adverse health effects attributable to exposure to these chemicals have important public health implications [153, 154, 155].

Delay conception and infertility: Few studies examined the relationship between THMs and delay conception and/or infertility. A population of 157 healthy men from couples without a known risk of infertility were examined in California and their exposure to THMs was assessed based on water utility measurements taken during 90 days preceding semen collection [156]. Only for one motility parameter, a small decrease for every unit increase in bromodichloromethane exposure level was found. A more recent study conducted by Luben et al. supported an association between exposure to levels of DBPs near or below regulatory limits and adverse sperm outcomes in humans [157].

Windham et al. suggested that THMs exposure may affect ovarian function including decrease in mean cycle length and reduced follicular phase length [158]. Nevertheless, MacLehose et al. found no evidence of an increased time to pregnancy among women who were exposed to higher levels of drinking water DBPs [159].

Spontaneous abortions: Some studies suggest a positive association between exposure to THMs and spontaneous abortions although serious limitations exist in those studies including lack of adjustments for confounding factors [160]. Exposure to THMs and the risk of spontaneous abortion was examined in a prospective study of more than 5,000 pregnant women in California [161]. The exposure to individual THMs as well as total THMs (TTHMs) was calculated by averaging all measurements taken by the subject's water utility during her first trimester of pregnancy. Women who drank $\geq$ 5 glasses/day of cold tapwater containing $\geq$ 75 µg/l of TTHMs were at an increased risk for spontaneous abortions. Of the four individual THMs, only high bromodichloromethane exposure was associated with an increased risk for spontaneous abortions. Swan et al. concluded that the associations with cold tapwater and bottled water with increased risk of spontaneous abortion could not be explained by exposure to chlorination by-products, because the association was seen in the absence of high levels of these chemicals. The grounds for such reasoning were observations that in one of the examined regions, the association appeared stronger in women who let the water stand before drinking [162]. Savitz et al. found that pregnancy loss was not associated with high personal THMs exposure ($\geq$75 µg/l and $\geq$5 glasses/day) [163].

Stillbirth or fetal death: The results of the studies examining the association between the exposure to THMs and the risk of stillbirth or fetal death are not consistent. Aschngrau et al. [160] and Bove et al. [166] showed no association whereas later studies conducted by Dodds et al. [167, 168] and King et al. [169] reported an association between stillbirths and high compared to low exposure to TTHMs. Small excess risk in areas with high TTHM concentrations was found for stillbirths in a study conducted in England [170].

Preterm delivery: While in the study conducted by Yang et al. [171] an association was found between exposure to TTHMs and PD (<37 weeks of gestation), in most studies no such an association was observed [166, 163, 172, 173, 167, 174, 175, 176]. Interestingly, several researchers found that THMs were associated with increased gestational duration and reduced risk of PD [177, 178].

Low and very low birth weight, intrauterine growth restriction and small for gestational age: Various toxicological and epidemiological studies pointed out an association between THMs and LBW (<2500g) although the evidence is not conclusive. The risk estimates were small or not significant and the assessment of exposure was rather limited [163, 172, 173, 167, 174, 170]. The significant LBW results were found by Gallagher et al. for high (≥61ppb) vs. low (≤20 ppb) THMs [173]. However, in that study few births were in the high exposure category. Similarly, in the study conducted in Massachusetts the authors observed reduction in mean birth weight for higher maternal THM exposure compared with lower one [177, 179]. On other hand, Kramer et al. did not find LBW effects for individual THM exposure [174]. Likewise, very low birth weight (<1500g) was not significantly associated with exposure to DBP in three other studies [155, 167, 170].

Increased risk of IUGR, and SGA was reported by several authors [174, 155, 173, 167, 179] but not by others [171, 175, 180, 181]. An increased risk of SGA births was found in Iowa among women living in communities with chloroform levels > 10 µg/l (based on finished water samples from municipal water survey) compared with a reference group with no detectable level of chloroform. One limitation of the exposure classification in this study was that individual exposures were based on samples taken from municipal water survey at least one year before the date of birth [174]. In New Jersey, THMs exposure was determined for each mother as the estimated monthly THM level in her town's water supply, based on a quarterly sampling for these chemicals [166]. Slightly elevated OR was found for term LBW for exposure categories above 40 ppb THMs. An increase in SGA births was reported, which was associated with THMs concentrations higher than 100 ppb. Gallagher et al. examined 1893 live singleton Colorado white births (28–42 week of gestation) for 1990–1993 and matched them to historical water sample data with respect to the time and location of maternal residence based on census information. A large increase in the risk of term LBW at highest level of exposure was found [173]. Dodds et al. observed small association between TTHMs (>=100ppb vs. <50 ppb) and SGA but the RR was not adjusted for factors such as smoking or socioeconomic status [167]. Wright et al. found higher frequency of SGA births among mothers with pregnancy average TTHM exposures greater than 80 µg/l [179].

In the study conducted by Infante-Rivard the exposure to THMs at the highest level affected fetal growth but only in genetically susceptible newborns (CYP2E1 variant) [182]. No association between exposure to THMs and SGA or IUGR was found by Yang et al. as well as in the recent studies conducted in Taiwan [175] and the U.S. [180, 181]. Hoffman et al. found an association between TTHM and SGA only for concentrations above the current regulatory standard [183].

Status of research on biological mechanisms: The biological mechanism by which THMs may influence intra-uterine development is not well understood. Many outcomes are complex to study and it is difficult to determine the extent by which chemicals in the water supply may affect the developing fetus and what is the critical gestational period. In laboratory animal models the association between exposure to THMs and pregnancy outcomes was observed when doses were sufficiently high to cause the symptoms of general toxicity in mothers. Such doses are much greater than those obtained by humans consuming chlorinated drinking water [153].

Conclusions

Studies examining the association between the exposure to THMs and its influence on pregnancy outcome are difficult to compare and to draw conclusions from. They analyze different levels of exposure: surface water vs. ground water, higher TTHM vs. low TTHM (defined differently), highest vs. lowest quintiles, etc. The studies also differ in the adverse pregnancy outcomes investigated. Exposure to disinfection by-products has been mostly made based on routine monitoring of public weather supplies matched to maternal residence. In order to determine that there is an association between the exposure to THMs and pregnancy outcome studies must consider THMs concentration and the quantity of the water actually consumed by pregnant women [184]. It is also important to remember about other (not only ingestion) exposures pathways such as inhalation or dermal contact during showering, bathing or swimming [185, 154, 155, 186, 187]. Furthermore, not all studies considered confounding factors including maternal age, ethnicity, education, employment, parity, maternal status, smoking and alcohol consumption which can influence pregnancy outcome. It is also important to notice that published papers may be subject to publication bias (papers published include only positive results since the total body of evidence including negative studies were not published). Taking into account the extent of THM exposures, the problem should be carefully examined in well-designed studies.

Environmental Noise Exposure

Most of the knowledge regarding the damage from noise comes from studies of persons with occupational exposure. In non-occupational settings environmental noise mostly originate from the transport including road-traffic and aircraft noise, industry and neighbours.

Birth weight and preterm delivery: Several studies examined the relationship between fetal growth and exposure to noise from airports in Amsterdam, Paris, Japan and the United States [188, 189, 190, 191, 192, 193]. Stronger association was noticed among female than male births.

The strongest evidence for an effect of airport noise on prenatal development is presented in studies of the residents of an area near Osaka Airport in Japan [192, 193]. Both reduced birth weight and higher frequency of SGA were more common in the communities with greater noise exposure from the airport [192]. In a study of changes in birth weight before and after the introduction of jet planes to the Osaka Airport, Ando found that the rate of births below 3000g increased dramatically as the frequency of jet flights increased [193].

Morrell et al. in a review article indicated that there is no strong evidence that aircraft noise has significant perinatal effects [194]. It was also confirmed in a more recent paper in which the authors suggest that in carefully controlled studies, noise exposure was not related to LBW [195]. Matsui et al. showed a significant dose-response relationship between LBW and noise exposure [196]. Significantly higher rates of preterm births were also found across the noise exposed municipalities. It is important to notice that in the above study the authors omitted important confounders like maternal smoking which may influence the results. The studies analysing the influence of noise on gestation duration concentrate mostly on occupational exposure rather than on environmental exposures and did not give conclusive results [197, 198, 199, 188, 200, 201, 202].

Birth defects: There are inconsistent findings on the role of noise exposure in the development of birth defects. In a study of 1475 Finnish mothers who delivered infants with structural defects, the frequency of self-reported noise exposure in the first trimester was not higher in the mothers of children with birth defects [203]. Nowell-Jones and Tauscher, using data from birth certificates, found a significantly higher incidence of birth defects in census tracts under the landing pattern at Los Angeles International Airport [204]. However, Edmonds et al. were not able to replicate these findings with data from the Metropolitan Atlanta Congenital Defects Program (MACDP) [205]. Stansfeld et al. postulated that after adjustment for confounding factors, noise exposure did not increase the risk of congenital birth defects [195].

The inconsistencies between the latter two studies may be due to differences in the definitions of noise exposure, or to differences in the ascertainment of birth defects.

Status of research on biological mechanisms: A plausible biological mechanism for the causal relationship between noise exposure and reduction in prenatal growth may be the development of the stress reaction. Another explanation could be that the auditory pathways of the central nervous system include direct pathways to the auditory cortex and indirect ones to the reticular endothelial activating system, thereby involving the limbic system, the autonomic nervous system and the neuroendocrine system [206]. Responses of the autonomic nervous system and the neuroendocrine system which include components that may impair growth, e.g., by frequent release of corticosteroids, were documented both in animal [207] and human experiments [208]. Nicolic et al. analysed hormone reactions to aircraft noise in pregnant women. Women in the first three months of pregnancy were exposed to aircraft noise of 75–85 dB/A during 60 minutes. The level of cortisone, cortisol, testosterone and prolaction were analysed in urine samples before and after the exposures. The results suggested that aircraft noise modified the hormonal reaction [209].

Conclusions

Several epidemiological studies described the relationship between noise exposure and reduction in growth. The potential confounding factors should be carefully controlled study designs and/or analyses. The role of individual susceptibility should be investigated. Gender-related differences in response should be a subject to further studies in order to verify the hypothesis that females fetuses are more sensitive than male fetuses to noise.

Heavy Work during Pregnancy

An increasing proportion of women are employed during pregnancy and continuing employment later into pregnancy. Maternal work during pregnancy involving high work-related physical exertion is considered a risk factor of adverse pregnancy outcome: heavy work is thought to reduce the blood volume available to the fetus and, consequently, the amount of oxygen and nutrients [210].

Increased time to pregnancy interval: Female occupational exposure seems to have only a small effect on time to pregnancy interval. The regression analysis showed that the most important determinants of longer time to pregnancy were: the age of women, parity, smoking and coffee consumption in an Italian study [211].

Sex ratio: Women working during pregnancy have a decrease chance to have a son compared to women not working during pregnancy [212].

Spontaneous abortion: Evidence obtained thus far indicates that there is an association between heavy work during pregnancy and spontaneous abortion. For women with a history of two or more spontaneous abortions, standing at work more than 7 hours per day increased the risk of spontaneous abortion. Women without such a history who stood more than 7 hours at work had an adjusted OR near unity [213]. The adjusted risk ratio for spontaneous abortions for women who reported physical stain higher than the average at day 6 to 9 after the estimated date of ovulation was 2.5 (95%CI [1.3–1.4]) [214].

Preterm delivery: Studies of maternal involvement in heavy work during pregnancy suggest that it may have impact on preterm delivery [215, 216, 217, 218]. Florack et al. found that work with a high intensity score and less extent work with a high fatigue scores had the strongest effect (up to 18 days shorter) on pregnancy duration [215]. Climbing stairs ≥ 10 times per day and purposive walking ≥ 4 days per week was associated with preterm delivery as well [219]. Women who reported more than five hours of both standing and walking had an increased risk of preterm delivery compared with women who reported two or less on both exposures [220]. The exposure to medium or high level physical workload increased the risk of preterm birth in studies performed in Spain and in the U.S. [221, 222]. On the contrary, no differences in pregnancy duration between the housewife and the employees were observed among 517 pregnant Sudanese women [223]. Likewise, while preterm delivery was significantly increased among women who worked throughout pregnancy in Egypt, after adjustment for confounders the risk of preterm delivery was not significant [224].

Birth weight and small-for-gestational-age: Heavy physical effort at work during pregnancy is often considered as a risk factor of SGA. Such findings were reported by majority of investigators [225, 213, 226, 227] although not all [228]. A negative correlation was found between physical workload and growth restriction in newborns of working women in Finland [213]. The more than two folds increased risk of SGA babies was calculated for mothers performing work with a moderate physical load in the third trimester, compared with that for mothers at sedentary work. Two studies conducted in Poland demonstrated an increased risk of SGA for moderate energy expenditure during work [229, 226]. Assessment of physical exertion based on job title, using an established catalogue of occupational characteristics performed by Homer et al showed that women in job characterised by high physical exertion experienced a higher rate of low birth weight [230]. The number of standing hours per day at work was found to be significantly associated with reduced birth weight [231]. Also climbing, lifting, long working hours and the combination of prolonged standing with a lengthy work week was associated with the fetal growth reduction [232].

Status of research on biological mechanisms: The adverse pregnancy outcomes associated with heavy work load are probably due to reduced blood flow from the uterus to the placenta [233, 234]. Under-perfusion can restrict fetal growth [235]. Mothers performing heavy physical work may also use calories that are needed for fetal growth, particularly if they are undernourished [236]. It is also possible that occupational tasks such as bending or lifting may increase intra-abdominal pressure, predisposing to premature birth [237].

Conclusions

Despite years of interest the effects of maternal heavy activity on the pregnancy are still uncertain, although most studies suggest that there is an association between heavy work in pregnancy and low birth weight, spontaneous abortions or preterm deliveries. Studies on maternal activity during pregnancy have several limitations. They were carried out in different settings, and working conditions vary over time and from place to place. Apparently, different job characteristics may entail different risks. Moreover, the determination of job characteristics was often based only on the job title and could potentially lead to an under or overestimation of the effect. The definitions and categories of exposures differed between studies as did the reference groups. Some authors focused on a single job characteristic and thus failed to take into account the possible confounding or modifying effects of other occupational factors. Also only few studies have considered non-occupational physically demanding activities. Despite the still limited evidence it should be recommended that pregnant women should avoid extremely heavy physical exertion during pregnancy. Continuous standing or walking during the whole workload should be avoided at least during late pregnancy. Pregnant women should not be exposed to manual handling involving risk of injury, awkward movements and posture, especially in confined spaces, work at heights, long periods spent handling loads or standing or sitting without regular exercise or movement to maintain healthy circulation.

Occupational and Stressful Life Events

The influence of stress at work and major life events on birth outcomes has been investigated for at least 38 years. The findings were not consistent and methodological concerns prevented definite conclusions to be reached [238, 239]. Studies relating the occupational stress and stressful life events to pregnancy outcome encounter several obstacles [240-245]. Most of the studies were cross-sectional and only a few were prospective cohorts [240, 241, 242]. The former introduced the possibility of recall bias [243]. The level of job strain was rarely defined [244]. Several confounders were identified, including socioeconomic status (income, education) marital status, ethnicity or race, parity, medical factors, complications of current or past pregnancies, smoking and use of alcohol [246].

The most often examined outcomes were birth weight, LBW or PD. The level of exposure to work stress was assessed by several methods; the two most popular were the Karasek model [247] or Mamele's (psychological factors and other strenuous conditions) [248].

Karasek identified two principal elements of work stress: demands and control [247]. Demands were described by number of tasks (work load, unpredictability of events, complex interpersonal relations) delegated to employee. Control involved the level of individual decision employee had in responding to challenges of work. Karasek proposed four types of work: relaxed (low demand, high control), active (high demand, high control), passive (low demands, low control), very demanding (high demands, low control). Mamelle et al. carried out an analytical breakdown of the job into its diverse components which led them to define five sources of fatigue and to construct an index capable of detecting the strenuous working conditions [248]. Several authors used jobs tittles as indicators of sources of stress [249, 250, 251, 252].

Stressful life events were usually measured by Modified Life Events Inventory using selected subsets of items. The events measured included legal conflicts, changes in relationships, financial difficulties, physical conflicts and family illness or death, etc. [253].

Spontaneous abortions: It is often believed that stress can cause spontaneous abortions. Two large prospective studies supported this belief [243, 254]. Brandt and Nielsen in a cohort of more than 200,000 Danish pregnant commercial and clerical workers found that women experiencing high job stress had significantly higher risk of spontaneous abortions (SA). Authors corrected for several possible confounders including smoking [243]. Fenster et al. examined prospectively almost 4,000 pregnant women in California employed in managerial jobs [254]. A small excess in the risk of SA was observed for women with stressful jobs (high demands, low control) who were above 32 years old, smokers, and primiparous. Low social support increased risk of SA in those working more than 40 hours a week. In a study in Finland, slightly increased risk of SA in flight attendants was noted [249].

The important finding supporting plausibility of biological mechanism on which stress may induce SA, was studied, reporting that SA at 11 weeks or greater was associated with more life events stress, whereas SA at other gestational age was not stress-associated, implying that life event stress increases the risk of chromosomally normal SA [255] Nepomnaschy et al. [256] examined miscarriages and levels of maternal urinary cortisol during the first weeks after conception. Pregnancies characterized by increased maternal cortisol during 3 weeks after conception were more likely to result in SA. [256].

Preterm delivery: The results of epidemiological studies indicated a rather modest effect of stress on the risk of PD. The associations were weak and usually limited only to high risk subpopulations. On the other hand, in few well designed studies no such effects were found [243, 257].

The influences of work-related psychosocial strain on the risk of PD seemed to be small in countries with highly developed social support systems. In Denmark, in study of more than 3500 women (worked at least 30 hours per week during 16 weeks of gestation) a work related psychological strain was modestly related to the risk of PD. Although a clear trend was seen for increase risk for PD with decreasing control and increasing demands, the relative risk estimates were not statistically significant [258]. Women working in very psychologically demanding job and those employed more than 40 hours a week or continue to work in advanced pregnancy were at a higher risk for PD. In the UK, in a study of almost 10,000 pregnant women, professionals had a lower risk of PD while those engaged in gardening, trading and production had the highest [250]. In Poland, in a study of more than 1,400 women, PD occurred more frequently in women who have accumulated the high number of negative psychosocial demands at work.[259] Similarly, women in military service, experiencing in second trimester sleep disturbance as result of high psychological demand of their jobs had increased risk of PD [260].

Africa-American women who continued to work in pregnancy after 24–26 week and had opportunities for rest had lower risk of PD compared with those who did not have such opportunities [251]. The risk of PD in women reporting high level psychosocial stress and who continued to work after 5 month of pregnancy in Poland was significantly higher than in women with less working load [259]. It was repeatedly found that Africa-American women were at an higher risk of PD due to high psychological demands at work [261, 262].

The Institute of Medicine concluded that the evidence between experiencing life events and PD was consistent but not uniform [263]. As summarized by Whitehead [253], three out of eight studies found no association [264, 265, 266] while five did, although they were often limited to the subgroup of examined population [241, 267, 268, 269, 270].

Several stressful life events were independently related to LBW or moderately LBW, e.g., experiencing major injury accident or illness as was pregnancy denial and unhappiness about pregnancy [271]. In a recent study, four out of 18 events examined were associated with PD: being in debt, being injured by a partner, having someone close attempting suicide and being divorced. One event, having a partner who lost his (her) job was associated with decreased risk of PD [253]. In another small-sized study, being widowed during pregnancy was not associated with gestational length [272]. Hedegaard et al. in group of more than 5,800 Danish pregnant women assessed the risk of PD in relation to stressful life events experienced during late pregnancy [258]. The modest association was found when life events were assessed as highly stressful. No evidence of protective effect of social support was also seen. It is in accordance with the negative results of several large scale intervention studies that have attempted to decrease the risk of PD by providing different kinds of social support [258, 241].

Smoking may explain at least some of the reported effects of stressful live events on pregnancy outcome. Women who experienced multiple risk factors (types of emotional stress) were more likely to deliver SGA infants, although the association was driven mostly by maternal smoking [274, 275].

Preeclampsia: The results of population-based studies of employed women in Norway suggested that women with low level of control at work (both manual and nonmanual workers) had slightly higher risk of preeclampsia [245]. The excess risk of preeclampsia was also reported in a case-control study in North Carolina [244].

Influence on fetal growth: The number of studies evaluating relationships between job strain/stress to intrauterine growth is limited. In a large study in Denmark, an increased risk of LBW was found in women experiencing stress at work (high demand, low control) [243]. Similarly, in another study in Denmark, a clear trend was noted for increased risk for SGA with decreasing control and increasing demands, yet it was not statistically significant [240, 258].

Further confirmation was provided by studies in Poland [276] and Thailand [277]. Makowska and Makowiec found that unfriendly interpersonal relations and low level of control at work had elevated the risk of SGA [276]. Likewise, in a group of almost 1,800 pregnant women, high psychological demands significantly increased the risk of SGA [277].

Status of research on biological mechanisms: Several mechanisms of the effect of maternal stress on pregnancy outcome have been postulated. Physical and psychological stress activates the hypothalamic-pituitary-adrenal (HPA) axis and the release of corticotrophin-releasing hormone (CRH) from the hypothalamus. CRH promotes prostaglandin production, and by priming the uterus to respond to oxytocin it may lead to cervical softening and uterine contractions [278, 253]. High-demand, low-control jobs have been found to increase the risk of hypertension [279] while hypertension itself appears to increase the risk of PD. Another possibility is that job strain may increase pregnant women's smoking, use of alcohol, drugs or be associated to unbalanced diet [262].

Conclusions

Stress at work was consistently found to be related to spontaneous abortions and restricted fetal growth. The modest effect was demonstrated for preterm delivery and LBW. On other hand, the evidence between experiencing life events and preterm delivery was not uniform [263].

Further progress in elucidation of the association of either stress at work or stressful life events will not take place unless researchers can set up large prospective cohort studies utilizing valid measures of exposure for stressful situations. Such studies are extremely difficult to perform, as it is difficult to recruit and follow women under stress in a prospective manner even if it were to be deemed ethically acceptable.

References

[1]   Choi H, Jedrychowski W, Spengler J, Camann DE, Whyatt RM, Rauh V. International studies of prenatal exposure to polycyclic aromatic hydrocarbons and fetal growth. *Environ Health Perspect* 2006; 114:1744–50

[2]   Jedrychowski W, Bendkowska I, Flak E, Penar A, Jacek R, Kaim I.. Estimated risk for altered fetal growth resulting from exposure to fine particles during pregnancy: an epidemiologic prospective cohort study in Poland. *Environ Health Perspect* 2004; 112:1398–1402

[3]   Slama R, Morgenstern V, Cyrys J, Zutavern A, Herbarth O, Wichmann HE. Traffic-related atmospheric pollutants levels during pregnancy and offspring's term birth weight: a study relying on a land-use regression exposure model. *Environ Health Perspect* 2007; 115:1283–1292.

[4]   Wilhelm M, Ritz B. Residential proximity to traffic and adverse birth outcomes in Los Angeles County, California, 1994–1996. *Environ Health Perspect* 2003; 111:207–216.

[5]   Ritz B, Wilhelm M, Hoggat K J, Ghosh J KC. Ambient Air Pollution and Preterm Birth in the Environment and Pregnancy Outcomes Study at the University of California, Los Angeles. *Am J Epidemiol* 2007; 166(9):1045-52

[6]   Hansen CA,. Barnett AG, Pritchard G. The Effect of Ambient Air Pollution during Early Pregnancy on Fetal Ultrasonic Measurements during Mid-Pregnancy. *Environ Health Perspect* 2008; 116:362–9

[7]   Slama R, Darrow L, Parker J, Woodruff T, Strickland M, Nieuwenhuijsen M. Meeting Report: Atmospheric pollution and human reproduction. *Environ Health Perspect* 2008; 116:791–798.

[8]   Wang X, Dung H, Ryan L, Xu X. Association between air pollution and low birth weight: a community-based study. *Environ Health Perpect* 1997; 1105, 514-21

[9]   Ritz B, Yu F. The effect of ambient carbon monoxide on low birth weight among children born in southern California between 1989 and 1993. *Environ Health Perspect* 1999; 107:17–25.

[10] Salam MT, Millstein J, Li YF, Lurmann FW, Margolis HG, Gilliland FD.. Birth outcomes and prenatal exposure to ozone, carbon monoxide, and particulate matter: results from The Children's Health Study. *Environ Health Perspect* 2005; 113:1638–1644.

[11] Parker JD, Woodruff TJ, Basu R, Schoendorf KC. 2005. Air pollution and birth weight among term infants in California. *Pediatrics* 115(1):121–128.

[12] Brauer M, Lencar C, Tamburic L, Koehoorn M, Demers P,Karr C. A cohort study of traffic-related air pollution impacts on birth outcomes. *Environ Health Perspect* 2008; 116:680–6.

[13] Maisonet M, Bush TJ, Correa A, Jaakkola J JK. Relation between ambient air pollution and low birth weight in the Norteastern United States. *Environ Health Perspect* 2001, 109 (suppl 3): 351-356

[14] Dejmek J, Selevan S, Benes I, Solansky I, Sram R. Foetal growth and maternal exposure to particulate matter during pregnancy. *Environ Health Perspect* 1999, 107, 475-80

[15] Dejmek J, Solansky I, Benes I, Lenicek J, Sram R. The impact of polycyclic hydrocarbons and fine particles on pregnancy outcome. *Environ Health Perspect* 2000; 109, 1159-1164

[16] Basu R, Woodruff TJ, Parker JD, Saulnier L, Schoendorf KC. Comparing exposure metrics in the relationship between $PM_{2.5}$ and birth weight in California. *J Expo Anal Environ Epidemiol* 2005; 14:391–6.

[17] Bell ML, Ebisu K, Belanger K. Ambient air pollution and low birth weight in Connecticut and Massachusetts. *Environ Health Perspect* 2007; 115:1118–25

[18] Xu X, Ding H, Wang X. Acute effects of total suspended particles and sulfur dioxides on preterm delivery: a community- based cohort study. *Arch Environ Health* 1995; 50:407–41

[19] Bobak M. Outdoor air pollution, low birth weight, and prematurity. *Environ Health Perspect* 2000; 108:173–6.

[20] Ritz B, Yu F, Chapa G, Fruin S. Effect of air pollution on preterm birth among children born in southern California between 1989 and 1993. *Epidemiology* 2000; 11(5):502–11.

[21] Wilhelm M, Ritz B. Residential proximity to traffic and adverse birth outcomes in Los Angeles County, California, 1994–1996. *Environ Health Perspect* 2006; 111:207–16.

[22] Parker JD, Woodruff TJ, Basu R, Schoendorf KC. Air pollution and birth weight among term infants in California. *Pediatrics* 2005; 115:121–8.

[23] Huynh M, Woodruff TJ, Parker JD, Schoendorf KC. Relationships between air pollution and preterm birth in California. *Paediatr Perinat Epidemiol* 2005; 20:454–61

[24] Sagiv SK, Mendola P, Loomis D, Herring AH, Neas LM, Savitz DA. A time-series analysis of air pollution and preterm birth in Pennsylvania, 1997–2001. *Environ Health Perspect* 2005; 113:602–6.

[25] Rogers JF, Thompson SJ, Addy CL, McKeown RE, Cowen DJ, Decoufle P. Association of very low birth weight with exposures to environmental sulphur dioxide and total suspended particulates. *Am J Epidemiol* 2000, 151, 602-13

[26] Rogers JF, Dunlop AL. Air pollution and very low birth weight infants: a target population? *Pediatrics* 2006; 118:156–64.

[27] Leem JH, Kaplan B M, Shim YK, Pohl HR, Gotway CA, Bullard SM, Rogers JF, Smith, Tylenda CA.Exposures to Air Pollutants during Pregnancy and Preterm Delivery. *Environ Health Perspect* 2006; 114: 905–10

[28] Williams L, Spence A, Tideman SC. Implications of the observed effects of air pollution on birth weight. *Soc Biol* 1977; 24(1):1–9.

[29] Glinianaia SV, Rankin J, Bell R, Pless-Mulloli T, Howel D. Particulate air pollution and foetal health: a systematic review of the epidemiologic evidence. *Epidemiology* 2004; 15(1):36–45

[30] Maisonet M, Correa A, Misra D, Jaakkola JJ. A review of the literature on the effects of ambient air pollution on foetal growth. *Environ Res* 2004; 95:106–115.

[31] Sram RJ, Binková B, Dejmek J, Bobak M. Ambient air pollution and pregnancy outcomes: a review of the literature. *Environ Health Perspect* 2005; 113:375–82.

[32] Bobak M, Leon DA. Pregnancy outcomes and outdoor levels of air pollution: an ecological study in districts of Czech republic 1986-1988. *Occup Med*. 1999, 56: 539-43

[33] Alderman BW, Baron AE, Savitz DA. Maternal exposure to neighbourhood carbon monoxide and risk of low infant birth weight. *Public Health Rep* 1987; 102: 410-4

[34] Dolk H, Pattenden S, Virjheld M, Thakrar B, Armstrong B: Perinatal and infant mortality and low birth weight among residents near cokeworks in Great Britain. *Arch Environ Health* 2000,55, 26-30

[35] Engel SA, Erichsen HC, Savitz DA, Thorp J, Chanock SJ, Olshan AF. Risk of spontaneous preterm birth is associated with common proinflammatory cytokine polymorphisms. *Epidemiology* 2005; 16:469–77.

[36] Sram RJ, Binkova B, Rossner P, Rubes J, Topinka J, Dejmek J. Adverse reproductive outcomes from exposure to environmental mutagens. *Mutat Res* 1999, 428, 203-15

[37] Binkova B, Vesely D, Vesela D, Jelnek R, Sram RJ: Genotoxicity and embryotoxicity of urban air particulate matter collected during winter and summer period in two different districts of the Czech Republic. *Mutat Res* 1999, 440, 45-58

[38] CDC (National Center for Chronic Disease Prevention and Health Promotion, 2001). Women and smoking: a report of the surgeon general. *http:// www.cdc. gov/tobacco/ sgr/sgr_forwomen/.*

[39] Waylen M, Metwally GL, Jones AJ, Wilkinson WL, Ledger. Effects of cigarette smoking upon clinical outcomes of assisted reproduction: a meta-analysis. *Human Reproduction Update* 2009;15(1):31-31.

[40] CDC (National Center for Chronic Disease Prevention and Health Promotion, 2004). The health consequences of smoking: a report of the surgeon general. *http://www.cdc.gov/tobacco/sgr/sgr_2004/index.htm.*

[41] Vine MF, Margolin BH, Morrison HI, Hulka BS. Cigarette smoking and sperm density: a meta-analysis. *Fertil Steril* 1994;61(1):35-43.

[42] Vine MF. Smoking and male reproduction: a review. *Int J Androl* 1996;19(6):323-37.

[43] Rubes J, Lowe X, Moore D, Perreault S, Slott V, Evenson D, Selevan SG, Wyrobek AJ. Smoking cigarettes is associated with increased sperm disomy in teenage men. *Fertil Steril* 1998;70(4):715-23.

[44] Chia, SE, Lim, STA, Tay, SK and Lim, ST. Factors associated with male infertility: a case-control study of 218 infertile and 240 fertile men. *Br J Obstet Gynaecol* 2000;107(1):55 – 61.

[45] Künzle R, Mueller MD, Hänggi W, Birkhäuser MH. Semen quality of male smokers and nonsmokers in infertile couples. *Fertility and Sterility* 2003;79(2):287-91.

[46] Castles A, Adams E, Melvin C, Kelsch C, Boulton M. Effects of smoking during pregnancy. Five meta-analyses. *Am J Prev Med* 1999;16(3):208-15.

[47] Waylen AL, Metwally M. Janes GL, Wilkinson AJ, Ledger WL. Effects of smoking upon clinical outcomes of assisted reproduction: a meta-analysis. *Human Reproduction Update* 2009;15(1):31-31.

[48] Lindbohm ML, Sallmen M, Taskinen H. Effects of exposure to environmental tobacco smoke on reproductive health. *Scand J Work Environ Health* 2002;28(2):84-96.

[49] Ahlborg G, Bodin L: Tobacco smoke exposure and pregnancy outcome among working women: a prospective study at prenatal care centers in Orebro County, Sweden. *Am J Epidemiol* 1991, 133, 338-47

[50] Windham GC, Swan SH, Fenster L. Parental cigarette smoking and the risk of spontaneous abortion. *Am J Epidemiol* 1992;135:1394–403.

[51] Windham GC, Von Behren J, Waller K, Fenster L. Exposure to environmental and mainstream tobacco smoke and risk of spontaneous abortion. *Am J Epidemiol* 1999;149:243–7.

[52] Venners SA, Wang X, Chen C, Wang L, Chen D. Paternal Smoking and Pregnancy Loss: A Prospective Study Using a Biomarker of Pregnancy. *Am J Epidemiol* 2004;159(10):993-1001.

[53] Kharrazi M, DeLorenze GN, Kaufman FL, Eskenazi B, Bernert JT, Graham S, Pearl M, Pirkle J. Environmental Tobacco Smoke and Pregnancy Outcome. *Epidemiology* 2004;15(6):660-70.

[54] Simpson WJ. A preliminary raport on cigarette smoking and the incidence of prematurity. *Am J Obstet Gyneacol* 1957;73:808-15.

[55] DiFranza JR, Aligne CA, Weitzman M. Prenatal and postnatal environmental tobacco smoke exposure and children's health. *Pediatrics* 2004;113 Suppl 4:1007-15.

[56] Anders RL, Day MC. Perinatal complications associated with maternal tobacco use. *Semin Neonatol* 2000;5:231-41.

[57] Windham GC, Eaton A, Hopkins B. Evidence for an association between environmental tobacco smoke exposure and birth weight: a meta-analysis and new data. *Paediatr Perinat Epidemiol* 1999;13:35-57.

[58] Rebagliato M, Floey CdV, Bolumar F. Exposure to environmental tobacco smoke in nonsmoking pregnant women in relation to birth weight. *Am J Epidemiol* 1995;142:531-7.

[59] Haddow JE, Knight GJ, Palomaki GE, McCarthy JE. Second-trimester serum cotinine levels in nonsmoking in relation to birth weight. *Am J Obstet Gynecol* 1988;159:481-4.

[60] Eskenazi B, Prehn AW, Christianson RE. Passive and active maternal smoking as measured by cotinine; the effect on birth weight. *Am J Public Health* 1995;85:395-8.

[61] California-EPA (1997). Health effects of exposure to environmental tobacco smoke. San Francisco, CA, California Environmental Protection Agency.

[62] Shah NR, Bracken MB. A systematic review and metaanalysis of prospective studies on the association between maternal cigarette smoking and preterm delivery. *American Journal of Obstetrics and Gynecology* 2000;182(2):465–72.

[63] Hanke W, Kalinka J, Florek E, Sobala W. Passive smoking and pregnancy outcome in central Poland. *Human & Experimental Toxicology* 1999;18(4):265-71.

[64] Windham GC, Hopkins B, Fenster L, Swan SH. Prenatal active or passive tobacco smoke exposure and the risk of preterm delivery or low birth weight. *Epidemiology* 2000;11:427-33.

[65] Jaakkola JJK, Jaakkola N, Zahlsen K. Fetal growth and length of gestation in relation to prenatal exposure to environmental tobacco smoke assessed by hair nicotine concentration. *Environ Health Prospect* 2001;109:557-61.

[66] Abell A, Juul S, Bonde JPE. Time to pregnancy among female greenhouse workers. *Scand J Work Environ Health* 2000; 26(2): 131–6.

[67] de Cock J, Westveer K, Heederik D, te Velde E, van Kooij R: Time to pregnancy and occupational exposure to pesticides in fruit growers in the Netherlands. *Occup Environ Med.* 1994; 51: 693-9

[68] Petrelli G, Figa-Talamanca I. Reduction in fertility in male greenhouse workers exposed to pesticides. *Europ J Epidemiol* 2001; 17: 675–7.

[69] Sallmén M, Liesivuori J, Taskinen H, Lindbohm M-L, Anttila A, Alto L, et al. Time to pregnancy among wives of Finnish greenhouse workers. *Scand J Work Environ Health* 2003; 29(2): 85–93.

[70] Bretveld R., Zielhuis GA., Roeleveld N.: Time to pregnancy among female greenhouse workers. *Scand J Work Environ Health* 2006; 32(5):359 67

[71] Lauria L., Settimi L., Spinelli A., Figa-Talamanca I.: Exposure to pesticides and time to pregnancy among female greenhouse workers. *Reprod Toxicol* 2006; 22(3): 425-30.

[72] Idrovo AJ, Sanin LH, Cole D, Chavarro J, Cáceres H., Narváez J, Restrepo M. Time to first pregnancy among women working in agricultural production. *Int Arch Occup Environ Health* 2005; 78(6): 493-500

[73] Larsen SB, Joffe M, Bonde JPE. Pesticides and time to pregnancy among Danish farmers (Abstract). *Ugeskrift Laeger* 1999; 161(47): 6480–4.

[74] Thonneau P, Abell A, Larsen SB, Bonde JPE, Joffe M, Clavert A, et al. Effect of pesticide exposure on time to pregnancy. Am J Epidemiol 1999; 150(2): 157–63.

[75] Curtis KM, Savitz DA, Weinberg CR, Arbuckle TE. The effect of pesticide exposure on time to pregnancy. *Epidemiology* 1999,10:103-105

[76] Whorton D, Krauss RM, Marshall S, Milby TH. Infertility in male pesticide workers. *Lancet* 1977; 2(8051): 1259–61.

[77] Ratcliffe JM, Schrader SM, Steenland K, ClappDE, Turner T, Hornung RW. Semen quality in papaya workers with long term exposure to ethylene dibromide. *Br J Ind Med* 1987; 44: 317–26.

[78] Abell A, Ernst E, Bonde JPE. Semen quality and sexual hormones in greenhouse workers. *Scand J Work Environ Health* 2000; 26(6): 492–500.

[79] Recio R, Robbins WA, Ocampo-Gómez G, Borja-Aburto V, Morán-Martinez J, Froines JR, et. al. Organophosphorous pesticide exposure increases the frequency of sperm sex null aneuploidy. *Environ Health Persp* 2001; 109(12): 1237–40.

[80] Levine RJ. Seasonal variation of semen quality and fertility. *Scand J Work Environ Health* 1999; 25 Suppl 1: 34–7.

[81] Larsen SB, Giwercman A, Span M, Bonde JPE. Seminal characteristics following exposure to pesticides among agricultural workers. *Scand J Work Environ Health* 1999; 25 Suppl 1: 74–5.

[82] Swan S., Kruse R., Liu F., Barr DB., Drobnis E., Redmon J., Wang C., Brazil C., Overstreet J.: Semen quality in relation to biomarkers of pesticide exposure. *Environ Health Perspect* 2003; 111(12): 1478-84

[83] Fuortes L, Clark MK, Krichner HL, Smith EM. Association between female infertility and agricultural work history. *Am J Ind Med* 1997; 31: 445–51.

[84] Tielemans E, van Kooij R, te Velde ER, Burdrof A, Heederik D. Pesticide exposure and decreased fertilisation rates in vitro. *Lancet* 1999; 354: 484.

[85] Kenkel S, Rolf C, Nieschlag E. Occupational risks for male fertility: an analysis of patients attending a tertiary referral centre. *Int J Androl* 2001; 24(6): 318–26.

[86] Smith EM, Hammonds-Ehlers M, Clark MK, Krichner HL, Fourtes L. Occupational exposures and risk of female infertility. *J Occup Environ Med* 1997; 39: 138-47

[87] Greenlee AR, Arbuckle TE, Chyou PH. Risk factors for female infertility in an agricultural region. *Epidemiology* 2003; 14: 429-36

[88] de Cock J, Heederik D, Tielemans E, te Velde E, von Kooij R. Author's reply to the letter: Offspring sex ratio as an indicator of reproductive hazards associated with pesticides. *Occup Environ Med* 1995; 52: 429–29.

[89] Davis DL, Gottlieb MB, Stampnitzky JR. Reduced ratio of male to female births in several industrial countries. *J Am Med Assoc* 1998; 279: 1018–23.

[90] Garry VF, Harkins ME, Erickson LL, Long-Simpson LK, Holland SE, Burroughs BL. Births defects, season of conception, and sex of children born to pesticide applicators living in the Red River Valley of Minnesota, USA. *Environ Health Perspect* 2002; 110 Suppl 3: 441–9.

[91] Taskinen HK, Kyyrönen P, Liesivuori J, Sallmén M. Greenhouse work, pesticides and pregnancy outcome (Abstract). *Epidemiol* 1995; 6 Suppl 109.

[92] Savitz DA, Arbuckle T, Kaczor D, Curtis KM: Male pesticide exposure and pregnancy outcome. *Am J Epidemiol* 1997, 146, 1025

[93] McDonald AD, McDonald JC, Armstrong B, Cherry N, Cote R, Lavoie J, et al. Fetal death and work in pregnancy. *Br J Ind Med* 1988; 4593): 148–57.

[94] Restrepo M, Munoz N, Day EN, Parra JE, Romero L, Nguyen-Dinh X. Prevalence of adverse reproductive outcomes in a population occupationally exposed to pesticides in Columbia. *Scand J Work Environ Health* 1990; 16: 232–8.

[95] Kristensen P, Ingens LM, Andersen A, Bye A, Sundheim L. Gestational age, birth weight, and perinatal death among births to Norwegian farmers, 1967–1991. *Am J Epidemiol* 1997; 146, 329–338.

[96] Petrelli G, Figa-Talamanca I, Tropeano R, Tangucci M, Cini C, Aquilani S. Reproductive male-mediated risk: Spontaneous abortion among wives of pesticide applicators. *Eur J Epidemiol* 2000; 16: 391–3.

[97] Settimi L., Spinelli A., Lauria L., Miceli G., Pupp N., Angotzi G., Fedi A., Donati S., Miligi L., Osborn J., Figa-Talamanca I.: Spontaneous abortion and maternal work in greenhouses. *Am J Ind Med* 2008; 51(4): 209-5

[98] Garry VF, Harkins M, Lyubimov A, Erickson L, Long L. Reproductive outcomes in the women of the Red River Valley of the North. The spouses of pesticide applicators: pregnancy loss, age at menarche and exposures to pesticides. *J Toxicol Environ Health* 2002; 65: 769–86.

[99] Bretveld RW., Hooiveld M., Zielhuis GA., Pellegrino A., van Rooij IALM., Roeleveld N.: Reproductive disorders among male and female greenhouse workers. *Repr Toxicol* 2008; 25(1): 107-14

[100] Crisostomo L, Molina VV. Pregnancy outcomes among farming householders of Nueva Ecija with conventional pesticide use versus integrated pest management. *Int J Occup Environ Health* 2002; 8(3): 232–42.

[101] Arbuckle TE, Savitz DA, Mery LS, Curtis KM: Exposure to phenoxy herbicides and the risk of spontaneous abortion. *Epidemiology* 1999, 10, 752-760

[102] Arbuckle T.E., Lin Z., Mery L.S.: An exploratory analysis of the effect of pesticide exposure on the risk of spontaneous abortion in an Ontario Farm Population. *Environ Health Persp* 2001, 109, 851-857

[103] Murphy HH, Sanusi A, Dilts DR, Djajadisastra M, Hirschhorn N, Yuliantiningsih S. Health effects of pesticide use among Indonesian Women Farmers. II: Reproductive health outcomes. *J Agromedicine* 2000; 6(4): 27–43.

[104] McDonald AD, McDonald JC, Armstrong B, Cherry N, Delorme C, Nolin AD, et al. Occupation and pregnancy outcome. *Br J Ind Med* 1987; 44: 521–9.

[105] Pastore LM., Hertz-Picciotto I, Beaumont JJ,; Risk of stillbirth from occupational and residential exposures. *Occup Environ Med.* 1997, 54, 511-518

[106] Bell EM, Hertz-Picciotto I, Beaumont JJ. Case-control analysis of agricultural pesticide applicators near maternal residence and selected causes of fetal death. *Am J Epidemiol* 2001; 154(8): 702–10.

[107] San Jose S, Roman E, Beral V: Low birth weight and preterm delivery, Scotland, 1981-84: effect of parent's occupation. *Lancet* 1991, 338,438-431

[108] Lima M., Ismail S., Ashworth A., Morris SS.: Influence of heavy agricultural work during pregnancy on birth weight in northeast Brazil. *Int J Epidemiol* 1999, 28, 469-74

[109] Dąbrowski S, Hanke W, Polańska K, Makowiec-Dąbrowska T, Sobala W. Pesticide exposure and birth weight: an epidemiological study in Central Poland. *Int J Occup Med Environ Health* 2003; 16(1): 31–9.

[110] Hanke W, Romitti P, Fuortes L, Sobala W, Mikulski M. The use of pesticides in Polish rural population and its effect on birth weight. *Int Arch Occup Environ Health* 2003; 76:614–20.

[111] Colborn T, Vom Saal FS, Soto AM. Developmental effects of endocrine-disrupting chemicals in wildlife and humans. *Environ Health Perspect* 1993; 101: 378–84.

[112] Tyler CR, Jobling S, Sumpter JP. Endocrine disruption in wildlife: a critical review of the evidence. *Crit Rev Toxicol* 1988; 28(4): 319–61.

[113] Anderson AM, Skakkebaek NE. Exposure to exogenous estrogens in food: possible impact on human development and health. *Eur J Endocrinol* 1999; 104(6): 477–85.

[114] Axmon A., Rylander L., Stromberg U., Hagmar L.: Miscarriages and stillbirths in women with a high intake of fish contaminated with persistent organochlorine compounds. *Int Arch Occup Environ Health* 2000; 73: 204-8

[115] McGuinness BM, Buck GM, Mendola P, Sever LE, Vena JE: Infecundity and consumption of polychlorinated biphenyl-contaminated fish. *Arch Environ Health* 2001, 56, 250-253

[116] Law DC., Klebanoff MA., Brock JW., Dunson DB., Langnecker MP.: Maternal serum levels of polychlorinated biphenyls and 1,1-dichloro-2,2-bis(p-chlorophenyl)ethylene (DDE) and time to pregnancy. *Am J Epidemiol* 2005; 162(6): 523-32

[117] Bush B, Bennett AH, Snow JT: Polychlorobiphenyl congeners, p.p'DDE, and sperm function in humans. *Arch Environ Contam Toxicol* 1986, 15, 333-341

[118] Hauser R et al.: Environmental organochlorines and semen quality: results of a pilot study. *Environmental Health Perspectives* 2002, 110, 229-233

[119] Rozati R., Reddy PP., Reddanna P., Mujtaba R.: Xenoestrogens and male fertility: myth or reality? *Asian J Androl* 2000; 2(4): 263-9

[120] Dallinga JW, Moonen EJ, Dumoulin JC, Evers JL, Geraedts JP, Kleinjans JC.: Decreased human semen quality and organochlorine compounds in blood. *Hum Reprod* 2002;17:1973–1979.

[121] Spanò M., Toft G., Hagmar L., Eleuteri P., Rescia M., Rignell-Hydbom A., Tyrkiel E., Zvyezday V., Bonde JP.: Exposure to PCB and p,p'-DDE in European and Inuit populations: impact on human sperm chromatin integrity. *Hum Reprod* 2005; 20(12): 3488-99

[122] Richthoff J., Rylander L., Jönsson BAG., Akesson H., Hagmar L., Nilsson-Ehle P., Stridsberg M., Giwercman A.: Serum levels of 2,2',4,4',5,5'-hexachlorobiphenyl (CB-153) in relation to markers of reproductive function in young males from the general Swedish population. *Environ Health Perspect.* 2003; 111 (4):409-13

[123] Toft G., Rignell-Hydbom A., Tyrkiel E., Shvets M., Giwercman A., Lindh Ch., Pedersen H., Ludwicki J., Lesovoy V., Hagmar L., Spanó M., Manicardi G, Bonefeld-Jorgensen E., Thulstrup A., Bonde J.: Semen Quality and Exposure to Persistent Organochlorine Pollutants. *Epidemiol.* 2006; 23

[124] Karamaus W., Huang S., Cameron L.: Paternal concentration of dichlorodiphenyl dichloroethene and polychlorinated biphenyls in Michigan fish easters and sex ratio in offspring. *J Occup Environ Med* 2002: 44: 8-13

[125] Schade G., Heinzow B.: Organochlorine pesticides and polychlorinated biphenyls in human milk of mothers living in northern Germany. Current extend of contamination, time trend from 1986-1997 and factors that influence the levels of contamination. *Sci Total Environ* 1998; 215: 31-9

[126] Khanjani N., Ross Sim M.: maternal contamination with PCBs and reproductive outcomes in an Australian population. *J Expo Sci Environ Epidemiol* 2007; 17: 191-5

[127] Yohimura T., Kaneko S., Hayabuchi H.: Sex ratio in offspring of those affected by dioxin and dioxin-like compounds: the Yusho, Seveso, and Yucheng incidents. *Occup Environ Med* 2001: 58: 540-1

[128] Rogan WJ., Gladen BC., Guo YL., Hsu C.: Sex ratio after exposure to dioxin like chemicals in Tajwan. *Lancet* 1999; 353: 206-7

[129] Leoni V, Fabiani L, Marinelli G, Puccetti G, Tarsitani GF, De Carolis A, Vescia N, Morini A, Aleandri V, Pozzi V, et al.: PCB and other organochlorine compounds in blood of women with or without miscarriage: a hypothesis of correlation. *Ecotoxicol Environ* 1989, 17, 1-11

[130] Dar E, Kanarek MS, Anderson HA, Sonzogini WC: Fish consumption and reproductive outcomes in Green Bay, Wisconsin, *Environ Res* 1992,59, 189-201

[131] Mandola P., Buck GM., Vena JE., Zielezny M., Sever LE.: Consumption of PCB contaminated sport fish and risk of spontaneous fetal death. *Environ Health Perspect* 1995; 103: 498-502

[132] Small C., Cheslack-Postava K., Terrell M., Blank HM., Henderson A., Marcus M.: Risk of spontaneous abortion among women exposed to polybrominated biphenyls. *Environ Res* 2007; 105(2): 247-55

[133] Tsukimori K., Tokunaga S., Shibata S., Uchi H., Nakayama D., Ishimaru T., Nakano H., Wake N., Yoshimura T., Furue M.: Long-term effects of polychlorinated biphenyls and dioxins on pregnancy outcomes in women affected by the Yusho Incident. *Environ Health Perspect* 2008; 116(5): 626-30

[134] Rylander L. Stromberg U., Hagmar L.: Lowered birth weight among infants born to women with a high intake of fish contaminated with persistent organochlorine compounds. *Chemosphere* 2000; 40: 1255-62

[135] Fenster L., Eskenazi B., Anderson M., Bradman A., Harley K., Hernandez H., Hubbard A., Barr DB.: Association of in utero organochlorine pesticide exposure and fetal growth and length of gestation in an agricultural population. *Environ Health Persp* 2006; 114(4): 597-602

[136] Ribas-Fito N., Sala M., Cardo E., Mazon C., De Muga ME., Verdu A et al.: Association of hexachlorobenzene and other organochlorine compounds with anthropometric measures at birth. *Pediatr Res* 2002; 52(2): 163-7

[137] Torres-Arreola L., Berkowitz G., Torres-Sanches L., Lopez-Cervantes M., Cebrian ME., Uriba M et al. Preterm birth in relation to maternal organochlorine serum levels. *Ann Epidemiol* 2003; 13(3): 158-62

[138] Bjerregaard P., Hansen JC.: Organochlorines and heavy metals in pregnant women from the Disko Bay area in Greenland. *Sci Total Environ* 2000; 245(1-3): 195-202

[139] Fein GG., Jacobson SW., Schwartz PM., Dowler JK.: Prenatal exposure to polychlorinated biphenyls: effects on birth size and gestational age. *J Pediatr* 1984; 105: 315-20

[140] Rylander L, Stromberg U, Hagmar L: Dietary intake of fish contaminated with persistents organochlorine compounds in relation to low birth weight. *Scan J Work Environ Health* 1996, 22, 260-6

[141] Rylander L, Stromberg U, Hagmar L: Decreased birth weight among infants born to women with a high dietary intake of fish contaminated with persistent organochlorine compounds. *Scand J Work Environ Health* 1995, 21, 368-75

[142] Rylander L., Stromberg U., Dyremark E., Ostman C., Nilsson-Ehle P., Hagmar L.: Polychlorinated biphenyls in blood plasma among swidish female fish consumers in relation to low birth weight. *Am J Epidemiol* 1998; 147: 493-502

[143] Petandin S., Koopman-Esseboom C., De Ridder MAJ., Weisglas-Kuperus N., Sauer PJJ.: Effects of environmental exposure to polychlorinated biphenyls and dioxins on birth size and growth in Dutch children. *Pediatr Res* 1998; 44: 538-45

[144] Gladen BC., Shkiryak-Nyzhnyk ZA., Chyslovska N., Zadorozhnaja TD., Little RE.: Presistent organochlorine compounds and birth weight. *Ann Epidemiol* 2003; 13(3): 151-7

[145] Taylor P., Stelma J., Lawrence C.: The relation of polychlorinated biphenyls to birth weight and gestational age of offspring of occupationally exposedmothers. *Am J Epidemiol* 1989: 129: 395-406

[146] Revich B, Aksel E, Ushakova T, Ivanova I, Zhuchenko N, Klyuev N, Brodsky B., Sotskov Y.: Dioxin exposure and public health in Chapaevsk, Russia. *Chemosphere* 2001; 43 (4-7): 951-966

[147] Baibergenova A., Kudyakov R., Zdeb M., Carpenter DO.: Low birth weight and residential proximity to PCB-contaminated waste site. *Environ Health Perspect* 2003; 111: 1352-6

[148] Eskenazi B., Mocarelli P., Warner M., Chee WY., Gerthoux PM., Samuels S., Needham LL., Patterson DG.: Maternal serum dioxin levels and birth outcomes in women of Sevesco, Italy. *Environ Health Perspect* 2003; 111(7): 947-53

[149] Rogan WJ., Gladen BC., McKinney JD., Carreras N., Hardy P., Thullen J., et al.: Neonatal effects of transplacental exposure to PCBs and DDE. *J Pediatr* 1986; 109: 335-41

[150] Vartiainen T., Jaakkola JJK., Saarikoski S., Tuomisto J.: Birth weight and sex of children and the correlation to the body burden of PCDDs/PCDFs and PCBs of the mother. *Environ Health Perspect* 1998; 106: 61-6

[151] Jensen HT, Cooke PS, Porcelli J, Liu TC, Hensen LG: Estrognic and antiestrogenic actions of pCBs in the female rat: in vitro studies. *Reprod Toxicol*, 1993, 7, 237-248, 1993

[152] Kelce WR et al: Persistent DDT metabolite p,p' DDE is a potent androgen receptor. *Nature* 1995, 375, 581-585

[153] Graves CG, Matanoski GM, Tardiff RG. Weight of evidence for an association between adverse reproductive and developmental effects and exposure to disinfection by-products: A critical review. *Regulatory Toxicology and Pharmacology* 2001; 34:103-24.

[154] Nieuwenhuijsen MJ, Toledano MB, Eaton NE, Fawell J, Elliott P. Chlorination disinfection byproducts in water and their association with adverse reproductive outcomes: a review. *Occup Environ Med* 2000;57:73-85.

[155] Bove F, Shim Y, Zeitz P. Drinking water contaminants and adverse pregnancy outcomes: a review. *Environ Health Perspect* 2002;110(1):61–74.

[156] Fenster L, Waller K, Windham G, Henneman T, Anderson M, Mendola P, Overstreet JW, Swan SH. Trihalomethane levels in home tap water and semen quality. *Epidemiology.* 2003;14(6):650-8.

[157] Luben TJ, Olshan AF, Herring AH, Jeffay S, Strader L, Buus RM, Chan RL, Savitz DA, Singer PC, Weinberg HS, Perreault SD. The healthy men study: an evaluation of exposure to disinfection by-products in tap water and sperm quality. *Environ Health Perspect.* 2007;115(8):1169-76.

[158] Windham GC, Waller K, Anderson M, Fenster L, Mendola P, Swan S. Chlorination by-products in drinking water and menstrual cycle function. *Environ Health Perspect* 2003;111(7): 935–41.

[159] MacLehose RF, Savitz DA, Herring AH, Hartmann KE, Singer PC, Weinberg HS. Drinking water disinfection by-products and time to pregnancy. *Epidemiology* 2008;19(3):451-8

[160] Aschengrau A, Zierler S, Cohen A. Quality of community drinking water and the occurrence of spontaneous abortion. *Arch Environ Health* 1989;44,5:283-90.

[161] Waller K, Swan SH, DeLorenze G, Hopkins B. Trihalomethans in drinking water and spontaneous abortion. *Epidemiology* 1998;9(2):134-40.

[162] Swan SH, Waller K, Hopkins B, Windham G, Fenster L, Schaefer C, Neutra RR. A prospective study of spontaneous abortion: relation to amount and source of drinking water consumed in early pregnancy. *Epidemiology* 1998;9:126–33.

[163] Savitz DA, Andrews KW, Pastore LM. Drinking water and pregnancy outcome in central North Carolina: source, amount, and trihalomethane levels. *Environ Health Perspect* 1995;103:592–6.

[164] Savitz DA, Singer PC, Herling AH, Hartmann KE, Weinberg HS, Makarushka Ch. Exposure to drinking water disinfection by-products and pregnancy loss. *Am J Epidemiol* 2006;164:1043-51.

[165] Aschengrau A, Zierler S, Cohen A. Quality of community drinking water and the occurrence of late adverse pregnancy outcomes. *Arch Environ Health* 1993;48(2):105-13.

[166] Bove FJ, Fulcomer MC, Klotz JB, Esmart J, Dufficy EM, Savrin JE. Public drinking water contamination and birth outcomes. *American Journal of Epidemiology* 1995;141(9):850-62.

[167] Dodds L, King W, Woolcott C, Pole J. Trihalomethanes in public water supplies and adverse birth outcomes. *Epidemiology* 1999;10(3):233–7.

[168] Dodds L, King W, Allen AC, Armson BA, Fell DB, Nimrod C. Trihalomethanes in public water supplies and risk of stillbirth. *Epidemiology* 2004;15(2):179-86.

[169] King WD, Dodds L, Allen A. Relation between stillbirth and specific chlorination by-products in public water supplies. *Env Health Perspect* 2000;108(9):883-6.

[170] Toledano MB, Nieuwenhuijsen MJ, Best N, Whitaker H, Hambly P, Hoogh C, Fawell J, Jarup L, Elliott P. Relation of Trihalomethane concentrations in public water supplies to stillbirth and birth weight in three water regions in England. *Environ Health Perspect* 2005;113(2):225–32.

[171] Yang ChY, Cheng BH, Tsai SS, Wu TN, Lin MCh, Lin KCh. Association between chlorination of drinking water and adverse pregnancy outcome in Taiwan. *Environ Health Perspect* 2000;108:765-8.

[172] Kanitz S, Franco Y, Patrone V, Caltabellotta M, Raffo E, Riggi C, Timitilli D, Ravera G. Association between drinking water disinfection and somatic parameters at birth. *Environ.Health Perspect* 1996;104(5):516–20.

[173] Gallagher MD, Nuckols JR, Stallones L, Savitz DA. Exposure to trihalomethanes and adverse pregnancy outcomes. *Epidemiology* 1998;9(5):484–9.

[174] Kramer MD, Lynch CF, Isacson P, Hanson JW. The association of waterborne chloroform with intrauterine growth retardation. *Epidemiology* 1992;3(5):407–13.

[175] Yang ChY, Ciao ZP, Ho SCh, Wu T N, Tsai SS. Association between trihalomethane concentrations in drinking water and adverse pregnancy outcome in Taiwan. *Environmental Research* 2007;104:390-5.

[176] Hoffman CS, Mendola P, Savitz DA, Herring AH, Loomis D, Hartmann KE, Singer PC, Weinberg HS, Olshan AF. Drinking water disinfection by-product exposure and duration of gestation. *Epidemiology* 2008;19(5):738-46.

[177] Wright JM, Schwartz J, Dockery DW. The effect of disinfection by-products and mutagenic activity on birth weight and gestational duration. *Environ Health Perspect* 2004;112(8):920–5.

[178] Lewis Ch, Suffet IH, Hoggatt K, Ritz B. Estimated Effects of Disinfection By-products on Preterm Birth in a Population Served by a Single Water Utility. *Environ Health Perspect* 2007;115(2):290-5.

[179] Wright JM, Schwartz J, Dockery DW. Effect of trihalomethane exposure on fetal development. *Occupational and Environmental Medicine* 2003;60:173-80.

[180] Hinckley F, Bachand AM, Reif JS. Late Pregnancy Exposures to Disinfection By-products and Growth-Related Birth Outcomes. *Environ Health Perspect* 2005;113:1808-13.

[181] Porter ChK, Putnam SD, Hunting KL Riddle MR. The effect of trihalomethane and haloacetic acid exposure on fetal growth in a Maryland County. *American Journal of Epidemiology* 2005;162(4):334-44.

[182] Infante-Rivard C. Drinking water contaminants, gene polymorphism, and fetal growth. *Environ Health Perspect* 2004;112(11):1213-6.

[183] Hoffman CS, Mendola P, Savitz DA, Herring AH, Loomis D, Hartmann KE, Singer PC, Weinberg HS, Olshan AF. Drinking water disinfection by-product exposure and fetal growth. *Epidemiology* 2008;19(5):729-37.

[184] Rothman K J. Disinfection by-products and adverse pregnancy outcomes: What is the agent and how should it be measured? *Epidemiology* 1998;9(5):479-81.

[185] Reif JS, Hatch MC, Bracken M, Holmes LB, Schwetz BA, Singer PC. Reproductive and developmental effects of disinfection by-products in drinking water. *Environ Health Perspect* 1996;104(10):1056-61.

[186] King WD, Dodds L, Armson BA, Allen AC, Fell DB, Nimrod C. Exposure assessment in epidemiologic studies of adverse pregnancy outcomes and disinfection byproducts *Journal of Exposure Analysis and Environmental Epidemiology* 2004;14:466–72.

[187] Villanueva CM, Gagniere B, Monfort C, Nieuwenhuijsen MJ, Cordier S. Sources of variability in levels and exposure to trihalomethanes. *Environ Res* 2007;103(2):211-20.

[188] Schell LM. Environmental noise and human prenatal growth. *American Journal of Phys Anthropol* 1981;56(1):63-70.

[189] Schell LM. Auxological epidemiology and the determination of the effects of noise on health. In : Susanne C. (ed.). *Genetic and environmental factors during the growth period*. New York: Plenum Press 1984:209-19.

[190] Schell LM, Hodges DC. Airport noise and human physical development. In : *Noise control in industry: Internoise Beijing: Acoustical Society of China* 1987;87(2):957-960

[191] Knipshild P, Meijer H, Salle H. Aircraft noise and birth weight. *Int Arch Occup Environ Health* 1981;48:131-6.

[192] Ando Y, Haattori H. Effects of noise on human placental lactogen (HPL) levels in maternal plasma. *Br J Obstet Gynecol* 1977; 84:115-8.

[193] Ando Y. Effects of daily noise on fetuses and cerebral hemisphere specialization in children. *J Sound Vibr* 1988;127:411-7.

[194] Morrell S, Taylor R, Lyle D. A review of health effects of aircraft noise. *Aust N Z J Public Health* 1997;21(2):221-36.

[195] Stansfeld S, Haines M, Brown B. Noise and Health in the urban environment. *Rev Environ Health*. 2000;15:43-82.

[196] Matsui T, Matsuno T, Ashimine K, Miyakita T, Hiramatsu K, Yamamoto T. Association between the rates of low birth-weight and/or preterm infants and aircraft noise exposure. Nippon Eiseigaku Zasshi 2003;58(3):385-94.

[197] Noise: A hazard for the fetus and newborn. American academy of pediatrics. *Pediatrics* 1997;100:724-7.

[198] Mamelle N, Laumon B, Lazar P. Prematurity and occupational activity during pregnancy. *Am J Epidemiol* 1984;119:309–22.

[199] McDonald AD, McDonald JC, Armstrong B, Cherry NM, Nolin AD, Robert D. Prematurity and work in pregnancy *Br J Ind Med* 1988;45:56–62.

[200] Luke B, Mamelle N, Keith L. The association between occupational factors and preterm birth: a United States nurses' study. *Am J Obstem Gynecol* 1995;173:849–62.

[201] Hartikainen AL, Sorri M, Anttonen H, Tuimala R, Laara E. Effect of occupational noise on the course and outcome of pregnancy. *Scand J Work Environ Health* 1994;20:444–450.

[202] Nurminen T, Kurppa K. Occupational noise exposure and course of pregnancy. *Scand J Work Environ Health*. 1989;15:117–24.

[203] Kurppa K, Rantala K, Nurminen T, Holmberg PC, Starck J. Noise exposure during pregnancy and selected structural malformations in infants. *Scand J Work Environ Health* 1989;15:111-6.

[204] Nowell-Jones F, Tauscher J. Residence under airport landing pattern as a factor in teratism. *Arch Environ Health* 1978;33:10-2.

[205] Edmonds LD, Layde PM, Erickson JD. Airport noise and teratogenesis. *Arch Environ Health* 1979;34:243-7.

[206] Cohen A. Extraauditory effects of acoustic stimulation. In: Lee D.H.K. (ed.) *Handbook of physiology-reactions to environmental agents*. Bethesda, Md.: American Physiology Society 1970.

[207] Welch BL, Welch AM. *Physiological effects of noise* . New York: Plenum Pressc 1970.

[208] Westman JC Walters JR : Noise and stress: A comprehensive approach. *Environ Health Perspect* 1981;41:291-309.

[209] Nicolic M, Gec M, Nicolic G, Sbutega-Milosevic G, Belojevic G, Neskovic B. Specific hormone reactions to aircraft noise in pregnant women. *Glas Srp Akad Nauka* 1991,41:81-5.

[210] Morris N, Osborn SB, Wright HP, Hart A (1956) Effective uterine blood flow during exercise in normal and pre-eclamptic pregnancies. *Lancet* ii: 481-84

[211] Spinelli A., Figa-Talamanca I., Osborn J.: Time to pregnancy and occupation in a group of Italian women. *Int J Epidemiol* 1997; 26(3): 601-9

[212] Hansen D., Moller H., Olsen J.: Severe periconceptional life events and the sex ratio in offspring: follow up study based on five national registers. *BMJ* 1999; 319(7209): 548-9

[213] Nurminen T., Lusa S., Ilmarinen J., Kurppa K.: Physical work load, fetal development and course of pregnancy. *Scand J Work Environ Health*. 1989, 15(6): 404-14

[214] Hjollund NHI., Jensen TK., Bonde JPE., Henriksen TB., Andersson AM., Kolstad HA., Ernst E., Giwercman A., Skakkebaek E., Olsen J.: Spontaneous abortion and physical stain around implantation: a follow-up study of first-pregnancy planners. *Epidemiol* 2000; 11(1): 18-3

[215] Florack EJM.: Influence of occupational physical activity on pregnancy duration and birth weight. *Scand J Work Environ Health* 1995; 21: 199-207

[216] Mozurkewich EL., Luke B., Avni M., Wolf FM.: Working conditions and adverse pregnancy outcome: a meta-analysis. *Obstet Gynecol*. 2000, 95(4): 623-35

[217] Teitelman AM., Welch LS., Hellenbrand KG., Bracken MB.: Effect of maternal work activity on preterm birth and low birth weight. *Am J Epidemiol* 1990; 131:104-13

[218] 96. Saurel-Cubizolles MJ., Zeitlin J., Lelong N., Papiernik E., Renzo GC., Breart G.: Employment, working conditions and preterm birth: results from the Europop case-control survey. *J Epidemiol Comm Health* 2004; 58: 395-401

[219] Misra DP., Strobino DM., Stashinko EE., Nagey DA., Nanda J.: Effects of physical activity on preterm birth. *Am J Epidemiol*. 1998, 147(7): 628-35

[220] Brink HT., Hedegaard M., Jorgen SN., Wilcox AJ.: Standing at work and preterm delivery. *Int J Gynecol Obstet* 1996; 52(1): 105

[221] Escriba-Aguir V., Perez-Hoyos S., Saurel-Cubizolles MJ.: Physical load and psychological demand at work during pregnancy and preterm birth. *Int Arch Occup Environ Health* 2001, 74(8): 583-8.

[222] Homer CJ., Beresford SA., James SA, Siegel E., Wilcox S.: Work-related physical exertion and risk of preterm, low birth weight delivery. *Paediatr Perinat Epidemiol.* 1990, 4(2): 161-74

[223] Sheikh MAA., Yasin M.: The effect of physical activity during pregnancy on preterm delivery and birth weight. *Yem Med J* 1999; 3(2): 1-8

[224] Arafa MA., Amine T., Fattah MA.: Association of maternal work with adverse perinatal outcome. *Can J Pub Health* 2007; 98(3): 217-21

[225] Koemeester AP., Broersen JP., Treffers PE.: Physical work load and gestational age at delivery. *Occup Environ Med.* 1995, 52(5): 313-5

[226] Hanke W, Kalinka J, Makowiec-Dąbrowska T, Sobala W (1999) Heavy physical work during pregnancy- a risk factor for small-for-gestational-age babies in Poland. *Am J Ind Med.* 36(1): 200-5

[227] Croteau A., Marcoux S., Brisson C.: Work activity in pregnancy, preventive measures and the risk of delivering a small-for-gestational-age infant. *Am J Public Health* 2006; 96(5): 846-55

[228] Fortier I., Marcoux S., Brisson J.: Maternal work during pregnancy and the risks of delivering a small-for-gestational-age or preterm infant. *Scand J Work Environ Health.* 1995, 21(6): 412-8.

[229] Makowiec-Dąbrowska T., Siedlecka J.: Wysiłek fizyczny w pracy zawodowej a przebieg i wynik ciąży. *Med Pr* 1996, 47 (6): 629-49

[230] Homer CJ., Beresford SA., James SA, Siegel E., Wilcox S.: Work-related physical exertion and risk of preterm, low birth weight delivery. *Paediatr Perinat Epidemiol.* 1990, 4(2): 161-74

[231] Ha E., Cho SI., Park H., Chen D., Chen C., Wang L., Xu X., Christiani DC.: Does standing at work during pregnancy result in reduced infant birth weight? *J Occup Environ Med* 2002, 44(9): 815-21

[232] Hatch M., Ji BT., Shu XO., Susser M.: Do standing, lifting, climbing, or long hours of work during pregnancy have an effect on fetal growth? *Epidemiology* 1997, 8(5): 530-6

[233] Lango LD., Hewitt CW., Lorijn RHW.: To what extent does maternal exercise affect fetal oxygenation and uterine blood flow? *Fed Proc* 1987; 37: 905

[234] Pomerance J., Gluck L., Lynch VA.: Maternal exercise as a screening test for uteroplacental insufficiency. *Obstet Gynecol* 1974; 44: 383

[235] Naeye RL.: Nutritional/nonnutritional interactions that affect the outcome of pregnancy. *Am J Clin Nutr* 1981; 34: 727

[236] Tafari N., Naeye RL., Gobezie A.: Effects of maternal undernutrition and heavy physical work during pregnancy on birth weight. *Br J Obstet Gynaecol* 1980; 87: 222

[237] Heyne CR.: Manual transport of loads by women. *Physiotherapy* 1981; 67: 431-42

[238] Newton RW, Webster PAC, Binu PS, Maskrey N, Philips AB. Psychosocial stress in pregnancy and its relation to the onset of premature labour. *BMJ* 1979, 2, 411-3

[239] Berkowitz GS, Kasl SV. The role of psychsocial factors in spontaneous preterm delivery. *J Psychsom Res.* 1983, 273, 283-290

[240] Henriksen B, Hedegaard M, Secher NJ. The relation between psychosocial job strain, and preterm delivery and low birth weight for gestational age. *Int J Epi.* 1994, 23, 764-73

[241] Nordentoft M, Lou HC, Hansen D, Nim J, Pryds O, Rubin P, et al. Intrauterine growth retardataion and premature delivery: the influence of maternal smoking and psychosocial factors. *Am J Public Health.* 1996;86(3):347-54.

[242] Copper RL, Goldenberg RL, Das A, Elder N, Swain M, Norman G, Ramsey R, Cotroneo P, Collins BA, Johnson F, Jones P, Meier AM. The preterm prediction study: maternal stress is associated with spontaneous preterm birth at less than thirty-five weeks' gestation *J Psychom Res.* 1996, 39, 563-95.

[243] Brandt LP, Nielsen CV. Job stress and adverse outcome of pregnancy: a casual link or recall bias? *Am. J Epidemiol.* 1992, 135 , 302-11.

[244] Klonoff-Cohen HS, Cross JL, Pieper CF. Job stress and preclampsia. *Epidemiology* 1996, 7, 245-249

[245] Wergeland E, Strand K. Work pace control pregnancy health in a population-based sample of employed women in Norway. *Scand J Work Environ Health* 1998, 24, 206-212.

[246] Dunker-Schetter C. Maternal stress and preterm delivery. *Prenat Neonat Med.* 1998, 3, 39-42.

[247] Karasek R. Job demands, job decision latitude, and mental strain. Implications for job redesign. *Adm Science Quart.* 1979, 24, 285-308

[248] Mamelle N, Laumon B, Lazar P. Prematurity and occupational activity during pregnancy. *Am. J Epidemiol.* 1984, 119, 309-322.

[249] Aspholm R, Lindbohm ML, Paakkulainen H, Taskinen H, Nurminen T, Tiitinen A.: Spontaneous Abortions Among Finnish Flight Attendants. *JOEM American College of Occupational and Environmental Medicine* 1996, 6, 486-491.

[250] Farrow A, Shea KK, Little RE. and the ALSPAC study team: Birth weight of term infants and maternal occupation in a prospective cohort of pregnant woman. *Occupational and Environmental Medicine* 1998, 55, 18-23.

[251] Hickey CA., Cliver SP., Mulvihill FX., McNeal SF., Hoffman HJ., Goldenberg RL.: Employment-Related stress and preterm delivery: a contextual examination. *Public Health Reports* 1995, 110, 410-8.

[252]   Fortier I, Marcoux S, Brisson J.: Maternal work during pregnancy and the risks of delivering a small-for-gestational-age or preterm infant. *Scand J Work Environ Health* 1995; 21(6):412-8.

[253] Whitehead N.: The relationship between individual life events and preterm delivery. RTI Press publication No. RR-0003-0809; 2008, Research Triangle Park, NC: RTI International Retrived (data) from http://www,rti.org/rtipress

[254] Fenster L., Schaefer C., Mathur A., Hiatt RA., Pieper C., Hubbard AE., Von Behren J., Swan SH.: Psychologic stress in the workplace and spontaneus abortion. *Am J of Epidemiology* 1995, 142, 1176-1183

[255] Boyles SH, Ness RB, Grisso JA, Markovic N, Bromberger J, CiFelli D. Life event stress and the association with spontaneous abortion in gravid women at an urban emergency department. *Health Psychol.* 2000, 19,510-4

[256] Nepomnaschy PA, Welch KB, McConnell DS, Low BS, Strassmann BI, England BG. Cortisol levels and very early pregnancy loss in humans. *PNAS*. 103, 3938-3942, 2006

[257] Escriba-Aguir V, Perez-Hoyos S, Saurel-Cubizolles MJ. Psychosocial load and psychological demand at work during pregnancy and preterm birth. *Int Arch Occup Environ Health* 2001, 74, 583-588

[258] Hedegaard M, Henriksen TB, Secher NJ, Hatch MC, Sabroe S. Do stressful life events affect duration of gestation and risk of preterm delivery? *Epidemiology*. 1996, 7, 339-45

[259] Biernacka J,B. Hanke W, Makowiec-Dąbrowska T, Makowska Z, Sobala W. Occupation-related psychosocial factors in pregnancy and risk of preterm delivery. *Medycyna Pracy* 2007, 58, 205-214

[260] Stinson JC, Lee KA. Premature labor and birth: influence of rank and perception of fatigue in active duty military woman. *Military Medicine* 2003, 168, 385-90.

[261] Orr ST, James SA, Miller CA, Barakat B, Daikoku N, Pupkin M, Engstrom K, Huggins G.: Psychosocial stressors and low birth weight in an urban population. *Am J Prev Med* 1996, 12: 459-66

[262] Brett KM, Strogatz D S, Savitz DA. Employment, job strain, and preterm delivery among women in North Carolina. *Am J Public Health* 1997, 87, 199-204

[263] Committee on Understanding Premature Birth and Assuring Healthy Outcomes. *Preterm birth: causes, consequences and prevention*. Washington, DC: The National Academic Press 2007.

[264] Goldenberg RL, Cliver SP, Mulvihill FX, Hickey CA, Hoffman HJ, Klerman LV, et al. Obstetrics: medical, psychosocial, and behavioral risk factors do not explain the increased risk for low birth weight among black women. *Am J Obstet Gynecol*. 1996;175(5):1317-24.

[265] Lobel M, Dunkel-Schetter C, Scrimshaw SCM. Prenatal maternal stress and prematurity: a prospective study of socioeconomically disadvantaged women. *Health Psychol*. 1992;11(1):32-40.

[266] Lu MC, Chen B. Racial and ethnic disparities in preterm birth: the role of stressful life events. *Am J Obstet Gynecol*. 2004;191(3):691-9.

[267] Dole N, Savitz DA, Hertz-Picciotto I, Siega-Riz AM, McMahon MJ, Buekens P. Maternal stress and preterm birth. *Am J Epidemiol*. 2003;157(1):14-24.

[268] Whitehead N, Hill HA, Brogan DJ, Blackmore- Prince C. Exploration of threshold analysis in the relation between stressful life events and preterm delivery. *Am J Epidemiol*. 2002;155(2):117-24.

[269] Dominguez TP, Schetter CD, Mancuso R, Rini CM, Hobel C. Stress in African American pregnancies: testing the roles of various stress concepts in prediction of birth outcomes. *Ann Behav Med*. 2005 Feb;29(1):12-21.

[270] Collins JW Jr, David RJ, Symons R, Handler A, Wall S, Andes S. African-American mothers' perception of their residential environment, stressful life events, and very low birth weight. *Epidemiology* 1998 May;9(3):286-9.

[271] Sable M.R., Wilkinson D.S.: Impact of perceived stress, major live events and pregnancy attitudes on low birth weight. *Perspectives on Sexual and Reproductive Health*, 2000, 32, 288-294.

[272] Cepicky P. Mandys F. Reproductive outcome in women who lost their husbands in the course of pregnancy. *Eur J Obstet Gynecol Reprod Biol* 1989,20,137-40

[273] Hedegaard M, Henriksen TB, Secher NJ, Hatch MC, Sabroe S. Do stressful life events affect duration of gestation and risk of preterm delivery? *Epidemiology* 1996, 7, 339-45

[274] Brooke Og, Anderson HR, Bland JM, Peacock JL, Stewart CM. Effects on birth weight of smoking, alcohol, caffeine, socioeconomic factors and psychosocial stress *BMJ* 1989, 298,795-801

[275] McCormick MC, Brooks Gunn J, Schoter T, Holmes JH, Wallace CY, Heagarty MC. Factors associated with smoking in low-income pregnant women: relationship to birth weight, stressful life events, social support, health behaviors, and mental distress. *J Clin Epidemiol* 1990, 43, 441-448

[276] Makowska Z, Makowiec-Dąbrowska T. Psycho-social work conditions as risk factors for preterm birth and newborn hypotrophy. *Medycyna Pracy* 1997, 48, 521-528.

[277] Tuntiseranee P, Geater A. et al. The effect of Heavy maternal workload on fetal growth retardation and preterm delivery. *JOEM American College of Occupational and Enviromental Medicine* 1998, 40, 1013-1021.

[278] Hobel C, Culhane J. Role of psychosocial and Nutritional Stress on Poor Pregnancy Outcome. *The Journal of Nutrition* 2003, 133, 5S, 1709-1717.

[279] Marcoux S, Berube S, Brisson H, Mondor M. Job Strain and Pregnancy-Induced Hypertension. *Epidemiology* 1999, 10, 376-82.

In: Textbook of Perinatal Epidemiology
Editor: Eyal Sheiner, pp. 237-250

ISBN: 978-1-60741-648-7
© 2010 Nova Science Publishers, Inc.

Chapter XIV

Fetal Risk Versus Safety of Medications in Pregnancy: Epidemiologic Considerations

Ilan Matok[*,1], *Amalia Levy*[1,6],
Rafael Gorodischer[2,3,4,6] *and Gideon Koren*[5,6]

[1]Epidemiology and [2]Pediatric Departments, Faculty of Health Sciences, Ben Gurion
University of the Negev
[3]Soroka Medical Center, [4]Clalit Health Services (Southern District), Beer-Sheva, Israel
[5]The Motherisk Program, Department of Clinical Pharmacology, Hospital for Sick
Children, The University of Toronto, Toronto, Canada
[6]BeMORE collaboration (Ben-Gurion Motherisk Obstetric Registry of Exposure
collaboration)

Introduction

Drugs are not tested in pregnant women before their introduction to the market [1]. Thus, their teratogenic effects are discovered only after they have been used during pregnancy. Animal studies may identify teratogenic drug effects, but they are not reliable in predicting drug effects in the human fetus, as demonstrated by the thalidomide tragedy [2-4]. Thalidomide did not cause congenital malformations in animal models, but its use by pregnant women resulted in an epidemic of phocomelia.

Medications are used widely in pregnancy. A large cohort study in the United Kingdom examined the use of medications in 11,545 pregnant women and found that 92.4% women had used at least one drug during their pregnancy (83% without including iron preparations and prenatal vitamins) [5]. Another study conducted in the United States found that out of

[*] For Correspondence: Ilan Matok; Department of Epidemiology and Health Services Evaluation, Faculty of Health Sciences, Ben Gurion University of the Negev, Beer-Sheva, Israel; E-mail: matoki@smile.net.il

578 pregnant women, 59.7% had used at least one prescription drug during their pregnancy (not including iron formulas and prenatal vitamins) and 92.6% of them used over-the-counter (OTC) drugs [6]. Another American study, conducted in two centers, found that the use of analgesic drugs was high (70.4% in one center and 76.1% in the other) [7]. Although medications are used extensively during pregnancy, for more than 90% of the drugs approved by the FDA in the past 20 years, there are insufficient human data to determine whether the benefits of therapy exceed the risk to the fetus [8].

For most medications available in the market, the package insert contains a statement such as "Use in pregnancy is not recommended unless the potential benefits justify the potential risk to the fetus". This is often interpreted as an indication that those medications may endanger the fetus, and due to this perceived risk pregnant mothers refrain from taking necessary medications (risking their own and also their fetus health). Conversely, as about 50% of pregnancies are unplanned, often the mother seeks termination of the pregnancy because of the perceived risk in view of the inadvertent fetal exposure. This issue is compounded because of the present trend of mothers to deliver at a more mature age, and larger numbers of women are diagnosed with chronic illnesses requiring long-term drug therapy before becoming pregnant.

Methods for Detection of Medication-Induced Teratogenic Effects

Medication-induced teratogenic effects could be detected in several ways after their introduction to the market [9]. Case reports are useful in situations wherein the drug causes a rare malformation or a characteristic pattern of malformations (for instance, thalidomide and isotretinoin) [4,10]. On the contrary, if the congenital malformation is common and the teratogen increases the background risk by a small percentage, the clinician may not recognize the deleterious effect of the drug on the fetus.

Cohort studies and case-control studies are also used to detect drug-induced congenital malformations, but each observational study method has its drawbacks.

Retrospective studies are affected by recall biases. In an effort to find an explanation of the unfavorable outcome, mothers of malformed infants are often more likely to remember unusual events in the course of their pregnancies than mothers who deliver normal infants. Cohort studies, and inclusion of data from available cohort investigations in meta-analysis, are other important sources of teratologic information; however publication bias is likely, as negative results are often not reported. Prospective observational studies are also subjected to bias, as patients are not randomly distributed between the different treatment groups, which may vary in the type and severity of the disease.

Another methodological problem concerning pharmacoepidemiological studies aimed to detect drug induced congenital malformations, is that data on over the counter drugs used during pregnancy are not documented. The same methodological problem occurs with herbal drugs and nutritional additives. There are also many confounding factors existing in the evaluation of drug- induced congenital malformations: for instance, fetal malformations may result from the maternal illness itself (e.g., diabetes mellitus, epilepsy) and from consanguineous marriage.

Computerized databases available today can be used to relate drug exposure of the fetus to the outcome of pregnancy. In the study of the adverse effect of drugs, it is crucial to validate the information as many of those databases are designed for administrative and/or clinical purposes rather than for epidemiological studies.

Computerized data bases have been used to detect drug- induced congenital malformations. Case reports and prospective cohorts are important as an immediate tool for signal generation in the first years of drug use. Case-control studies based on computerized databases can be conducted only later, when sufficient numbers of women have been exposed to the drug in the studied population.

One study that examined the risk for gastroschisis and small intestinal atresia in infants born to mothers who have used over the counter drugs against cough, cold and pain, found that aspirin increases the risk for gastroschisis; it also showed that pseaudoephedrine might increase the risk of gastroschisis and/or small intestinal atresia [11]. Drug status change from prescription drugs to OTC without consideration of their possibly teratogenic effects.

The value of the use of large computerized data bases in the investigation of adverse drug reactions is illustrated by a study by Cooper et al. who studied the safety of angiotensin-converting enzyme inhibitors (ACE inhibitors) after exposure during the first trimester [12]. They performed a linkage between maternal use of prescribed medications (determined from Medicaid pharmacy files) and a database containing information on pregnancy outcomes, including major congenital malformations. It was found that ACE inhibitors were significantly associated with an increased risk for congenital malformations. Another study found that exposure to paroxetine during the first trimester, if taken in dosage of more than 25 mg per day, is associated with an increased risk for congenital malformations [13]. That study linked between pharmacy records of medications dispensed to mothers during pregnancy and medical records including pregnancy outcome [13].

Adherence

Adherence to medication therapy should be addressed in any research involving consumption of medications. The use of databases raises the question of adherence to medication therapy. Usually, the databases contain information regarding medications dispensed to women, but we have no way of knowing whether they actually ingested them. Thus, there could be more doses prescribed and dispensed than actually ingested. Previous studies have shown that computerized pharmacy records provide accurate medication data and have high rates of concordance with self-reports of medications used by patients in general and specifically pregnant women [14-16,17]. A recent study found that the overall adherence to iron preparations dispensed for Israeli infants was high, as confirmed by laboratory tests [18].

To document some of the complexities of conducting epidemiological studies in pregnancy, we have selected several disease models which highlight different issues and how the scientific community has dealt with them.

The Use of Folic Acid during Pregnancy and Prevention of Birth Defects

It is widely accepted that the use of folic acid by pregnant women reduces the risk of neural tube defect in the fetus as long as other congenital malformations such as cardiovascular defects, orofacial clefts, urinary tract defects, limb reduction defects and omphalocele. In 1980, the results of a non-randomized clinical trial showed that the risk for neural tube defects was reduced in women who took multivitamins in the periconceptional period, as compared to women who did not [19]. Since then, observational studies have also demonstrated a reduced risk in women who took multivitamins supplements containing folic acid and to those who had higher dietary intake of folate during early pregnancy [20]. Mulinare et al. studied the data from the Atlanta Birth Defects Case-Control Study; in that observational case-controlled study there were 347 babies with neural tube defects live born or stillborn in the study period compared to 2,829 control babies born without a congenital malformation. The study showed that periconceptional use of multivitamins supplements reduced the incidence of neural tube defects in the fetus [20]. Another observational case-control study showed reduction in neural tube defects prevalence in infants born to women who took folic acid containing multivitamins supplements [21].

Later, two clinical studies demonstrated the effect of folic acid on the reduction of risk for neural tube defects [22,23]. In a very large interventional study, women in the intervention group were asked to take a pill containing 400 mcg of folic acid daily at the premarital exam until the end of the first trimester of pregnancy. There were significantly less infants identified with neural tube defects among more than 130 thousands fetuses or infants to women in the intervention group who took the pill than among 117 thousands of women in the controlled group (102 were with neural tube defects in the intervention, as compared to 173 in the control group). That study showed that taking folic acid in the periconceptional period reduces the risk for neural tube defects [23].

Pregnant women may be treated with medications which antagonize the action of folic acid. There are two groups of folic acid antagonists. One of them consists of dihydrofolate reductase inhibitors, such as trimetoprim and methotrexate, which block the conversion of folate to its more active metabolites [24]. The other group of folic acid antagonists affect folate metabolism in several ways, impair absorption of folate or increase its degradation. Medications in that group are primarily antiepileptic drugs such as phenytoin, carbamazepine, valproic acid and phenobarbital. One way to assess the role of folic acid in decreasing the prevalence of birth defects is to determine whether folic acid antagonists are associated with an increased risk for such defects. An observational retrospective case-control study found that folic acid antagonists increase the risk of birth defects in general [25]. The dihydrofolate reductase inhibitors group was shown to increase cardiovascular defects and oral clefts, while the antiepileptic group was shown to increase the risk for cardiovascular defects, oral clefts and urinary tract defects.

One cannot rule out the possibility of confounding in that study. Findings with regard to antiepileptic drugs may be confounded by the presence of the epilepsy itself. However, since other anti epileptic drugs, given for other indications, had the same effect on birth defects risk, it seems that epilepsy was not a confounder.

The teratogenic effect of antiepileptic medications has been reported in various studies and was summarized in several reviews [26].

The Centers for Disease Control and the U.S. Public Health Service as well as other health agencies around the world urge every woman who could become pregnant to receive 400 micrograms of synthetic folic acid every day [27]. In 1998 the FDA mandated the fortifications of grains because of the evidence that lack of folic acid may increase neural tube defects. An ecological study checked hospitalizations of newborns with folate sensitive birth defects such as neural tube defects; it compared the hospitalizations before and after the fortification of grains begun, between the years 2002 to 2007 and 1998 to 2002 and found a decline of hospitalizations because of neural tube defects [28].

Gestational Diabetes Mellitus

Gestational diabetes mellitus occurs in 2 to 9% in all pregnancies and it is associated with maternal and fetal complications [[29],[30]]. Macrosomia, shoulder dystocia, nerve palsies and hypoglycemia are among the perinatal risks that increase in gestational diabetes mellitus. Long-term risks for the infants born to mothers with gestational diabetes include sustained impairment of glucose tolerance and impaired intellectual achievements [31-34].

Studies have shown that timely and effective treatment of gestational diabetes reduces serious perinatal morbidity and may also improve the mother's health related quality of life [35, 36]. In a randomized clinical trial, Crowther et al. found that the rate of serious perinatal complications was significantly lower in the intervention group comparing the routine care group. The intervention included individualized dietary advice from dietitian, routine self monitoring of blood glucose levels and insulin therapy when diet was not sufficient. The rate of serious perinatal complications was 1% in the intervention group vs. 4% in the routine-care group (adjusted RR−0.33, 95% CI: 0.14-0.75) [35].

The current mainstream treatment for gestational diabetes is diet and insulin. Oral hypoglycemic medications are not used widely because of potential risk of fetal and neonatal hypoglycemia associated with their placental transfer to the fetus [29, 37].

Treatment of gestational diabetes by insulin has major challenges: affected women have been mostly healthy and the daily injection of insulin may be associated with poor adherence and subsequently poorer pregnancy outcomes [38]. Another significant challenge is the cost of insulin and associated devices for its injection which is financially prohibitive thus not affordable in many parts of the world [[39]]. An experimental study made by Elliott et al. has shown minimal placental transfer of glyburide across the perfused placental lobule [40]. Subsequent work has shown active transfer of glyburide from fetal to maternal circulation in the placenta, carried out by adenosine binding cassette placental transporters, including multidrug resistant-associated protein MDR-1 and MDR-3 and breast cancer-resistant protein [41]. Those findings represent advantages of glyburide in gestational diabetes mellitus. If indeed the placental transfer of glyburide is minimal and the risks to the fetus are not greater than those of insulin, then glyburide may be a safe alternative for insulin for the treatment of gestational diabetes.

Few studies investigated glyburide safety in gestational diabetes. Although their results supported its safety, their sample size was small and had no sufficient power to unequivocally state on the perinatal safety of glyburide.

Coetzee et al. performed a prospective cohort study with 23 pregnant women with gestational diabetes treated with glyburide and 39 with insulin. Glyburide was not significantly associated with large size for gestational age, but it was significantly associated with neonatal hypoglycemia [42].

Langer et al. compared between glyburide and insulin for the treatment of gestational diabetes in a prospective double blind randomized clinical trial [43]. There were 404 women participating, half in the glyburide treatment group, and the others at the insulin treatment group. They found similar glycemic control in both study groups. Amongst pregnancy outcomes that were investigated in that study were: large and small size for gestational age, macrosomia, hyperglycemia and hypoglycemia. The study did not find any significant association between glyburide and any of the pregnancy outcomes that were investigated. Yet, although not statistically significant, they reported 50% more instances of neonatal hypoglycemia in the neonates exposed to glyburide during pregnancy (18 out of 201 in the glyburide treatment group vs. 12 out of 203 in the insulin treatment group) [43].

In a retrospective cohort study, Jacobson et al. also investigated glyburide vs. insulin in gestational diabetes [44]. The study consisted of 236 women in the glyburide treatment group and 268 in the insulin treatment group. In this large study, no statistical significant difference was found between glyburide and insulin treatment groups in the following pregnancy outcomes: macrosomia, large or small for gestational age, hyperbilirubinemia, polycythemia, neonatal intensive care unit admission, ventilation and oxygen and neonatal hypoglycemia. However, they found that in the glyburide treatment group there were significantly more cases of preeclampsia and of infants requiring phototherapy [44]. A later retrospective cohort study done by Ramos et al. studied a subset of the cohort used by Jacobson et al. [45]. The subset chosen included pregnant women with 50 grams oral glucose challenge test equal or greater than 200 mg/dl and fasting plasma glucose of 105 mg/dl and above. This subset of the population is thought to represent a group of patients with increased insulin resistance and even pre-existing diabetes mellitus. In this retrospective study, there were 78 women in the insulin treatment group and 44 in the glyburide treatment group. No significant association between exposure to glyburide during pregnancy and the following pregnancy outcomes: preterm delivery, cesarean section, large or small for gestational age, macrosomia, birth injuries, preeclampsia and congenital anomalies. However, they found an increased association between exposure to glyburide and neonatal hypoglycemia (9 out of 12 in the glyburide treatment group vs. 5 out of 11 in the insulin treatment group). In this subset, more infants in the glyburide group required phototherapy although the difference did not reach statistical significance (3 out of 4 in the glyburide group compared to 6 out of 14 in the insulin treatment group, P=0.06) [45].

Recently, a meta-analysis was performed including studies published between 1985 and 2006 that compared glyburide use in gestational diabetes versus insulin [46]. They analyzed nine retrospective and prospective studies with a total of 801 women treated with glyburide for gestational diabetes and 637 with insulin [46]. Their conclusion was that the data regarding glyburide do not suggest that glyburide increased the overall perinatal risks. These studies and several other small cohort studies (retrospective and prospective) do not suggest overall increased perinatal risks with glyburide for gestational diabetes over insulin. However, most studies were not randomized; thus, selection bias could not be ruled out. Also, further investigation is needed to determine potential neonatal hypoglycemia caused by glyburide.

The Use of Metoclopramide for Nausea and Vomiting During Pregnancy

Nausea and vomiting of pregnancy are experienced by 50–80% of pregnant women during the first trimester. These symptoms may be severe and can continue beyond the first trimester [47-50]. Pregnant women and health professionals often refrain from pharmacological treatment of morning sickness due to perceived fears of teratogenic risks [47-50].

The first choice recommendation for the treatment of nausea and vomiting of pregnancy in the United States are pyridoxine and doxylamine, while metoclopramide is used only in the most severe cases [51].

There is extensive experience with metoclopramide use in non-pregnant patients, showing overall low rates of adverse events when used as recommended. Yet, only a few studies have assessed the safety of intrauterine exposure to metoclopramide during the first trimester, and their relatively small sizes had limited power to detect adverse effects of the drug if they exist [[52]-[56]].

A surveillance of Michigan Medicaid study investigated the exposure of 192 infants to metoclopramide during the first trimester [53]. The study was a retrospective cohort which used computer record linkage to connect between the mother and the infants. The study did not find any significant association between metoclopramide and the risk for congenital malformations. A prospective controlled cohort study by Berkovitch et al. that included five Teratogen Information Centers compared 126 infants exposed to metoclopramide during the first trimester for nausea and vomiting to 126 infants born to mothers who consulted at the same centers during the study period after taking nonteratogenic and nonembryotoxic drugs [54]. The following outcomes were studied: fetal malformations, spontaneous abortions, and decreased infant birth weight. The study found no significant association between exposure to metoclopramide and any of the investigated outcomes [54].

Another record linkage retrospective study done by Sørensen et al., linked databases from Jutland County in Denmark which contained information about medications dispensed to mothers during pregnancy and the Danish Medical Birth Registry [55]. The population studied comprised of 309 pregnancies exposed to metoclopramide during the first trimester, while 13,327 unexposed pregnancies served as the control group. The following pregnancy outcomes were investigated: congenital malformations, birth weight, preterm deliveries and stillbirths. The study did not find significant associations between metoclopramide and any of the pregnancy outcomes investigated [55]. Likewise, in another prospective controlled cohort study did not find any significant association between exposure to metoclopramide during the first trimester and congenital malformations as well as low birth weight [56]. The study consisted of 175 women in the exposure group; each one matched for age, maternal smoking and alcohol to women in the same center [56].

Despite the small number of studies on the safety of metoclopramide use during the first trimester and the relative small number of subjects, metoclopramide is widely used in many countries (particularly in Europe) and it is considered safe for usage in pregnancy. However, further larger studies are needed to confirm its safety during first trimester pregnancy.

Acid Reflux and Peptic Ulcer Treatment during Pregnancy

H_2-Blockers

Acid reflux affects 30–50% of pregnant women. H_2-blockers inhibit gastric secretion and are used for the treatment of peptic ulcer and gastroesophageal reflux during pregnancy [57,58].

H_2-blockers cross the human placenta by passive diffusion and accordingly millions of infants worldwide are exposed to H_2-blockers during embryogenesis [59]. Animal reproductive toxicology studies have failed to show teratogenicity of H_2-blockers [60]. Studies have reported on the safety of intrauterine exposure to H_2-blockers during the first trimester, however, the data are still scarce [61-69]. Cimetidine, ranitidine and famotidine have been the main drugs investigated. Controlled studies did not find any association between exposure to H_2-blockers and congenital malformations. Magee et al. studied the safety of H_2-blockers in a matched controlled cohort in which 178 women who were exposed to H_2-blockers during the first trimester were matched with 178 controls by maternal age, smoking and heavy alcohol drinking [61]. The following outcomes were investigated: congenital malformations, mode of delivery, gestational age, prematurity, birth weight, small for gestational age infants, neonatal health problems, and developmental milestones. No association was found between exposure to H_2-blockers and any of these pregnancy outcomes investigated [61]. In a prospective controlled study, Garbis et al. found that exposure to H_2-blockers during the first trimester of pregnancy was associated with increased risk for premature deliveries [65]. They also found a significant association between exposure to H_2-blockers during the first trimester and induced abortions. The study consisted of 553 women who were exposed to H_2-blockers during the first trimester and 1,390 women in the control group. That study did not find an association between exposure to H_2-blockers during the first trimester the risk for congenital malformation, spontaneous abortion and late fetal death [65].

Based on those studies with relatively small number of subjects, H_2-blockers appear to be safe for use during first trimester of pregnancy, but further larger studies are needed to confirm the safety of H_2-blockers during pregnancy.

Proton Pump Inhibitors (PPIs)

As with H_2-blockers, only a few studies are available to establish the safety of exposure to proton pump inhibitors (PPIs) during the first trimester of pregnancy [70-72]. The most studied drug has been omeprazole. Other proton pump inhibitors studied are pantoprazole and lansoprazole. Källén investigated 955 infants exposed to omeprazole during pregnancy, 863 of them during the first trimester [70]. That study did not find any association between exposure to omeprazole during pregnancy and any of the investigated pregnancy outcomes. Similar results were obtained in a multicenter controlled prospective cohort study, which included 295 pregnancies exposed to omeprazole (233 in the first trimester), 62 to lansoprazole (55 in the first trimester) 53 to pantoprazole (47 in the first trimester) and 868 infants in the control group [71]. That study did not find any significant association between exposure to PPIs and major congenital malformations or preterm delivery [71].

A meta-analysis study has analyzed all data regarding exposure to PPIs during the first trimester of pregnancy and the risk for congenital malformations [72]. The analysis, which included a total of 1,456 infants exposed to PPIs during the first trimester, did not find any significant association between exposure to PPIs and the risk for congenital malformations [72].

As with H_2-blockers, the limited available evidence indicates that PPIs appear to be safe for use during first trimester of pregnancy. Nevertheless, further larger studies are needed to confirm the safety of proton pump inhibitors for the unborn infant.

Synthesizing Existing Data

Over time, opposing studies on the same perinatal endpoint cause confusion among clinicians and parents. Over the last two decades, great progress has been made in synthesizing all existing studies into an overall estimate of fetal risk/safety. The method of meta-analysis of epidemiological studies has been developed in parallel to the development of meta-analysis of randomized studies. This method is especially appealing for pregnancy outcome studies, as the rates of malformations render most cohort studies insufficient to have sufficient statistical power. The combination of epidemiological studies and meta-analysis follows the method introduced by Einarson et al. in 1989 [73].

This method has been modified over the years to address bias against the null hypothesis (i.e., the fact that negative studies are more likely not to be published), as well as sample size, year of publication and study quality. It is imperative that studies in all languages are collected and analyzed. Moreover, there is increasing evidence that the quality of a study biases the results, with poor-quality studies tending more often to be positive.

With hundreds of new drugs introduced into the market every year, and with 50% of pregnancies unplanned, it is critical to employ all available epidemiological means to quantify, as soon as possible, the potential risks of drugs to the neonate and child.

References

[1]   Koren G, Pastuszak A, Ito, S. Drugs in pregnancy. *N Engl J Med*. 1998; 338:1128-
        1137.

[2]   Mitchell AA. Special considerations in studies of drug-induced birth defects. In: Strom
        BL ed., *Pharmacoepidemiology*. John Wiley & Sons; 2000:749-63.

[3]   Warkany J. Problems in applying teratogenic observations in animals to man.
        Pediatrics. 1974;53:820.

[4]   Lenz W. Thalidomide and congenital abnormalities. *Lancet*. 1962;4:45.

[5]   Headley J, Northstone K, Simmons H, Golding J; ALSPAC Study Team. Medication
        use during pregnancy: data from the Avon Longitudinal Study of Parents and Children.
        Eur J Clin Pharmacol. 2004;60:355-61.

[6]   Glover DD, Amonkar M, Rybeck BF, Tracy TS. Prescription, over-the-counter, and
        herbal medicine use in a rural, obstetric population. *Am J Obstet Gynecol*.
        2003;188:1039-45.

[7]   Werler MM, Mitchell AA, Hernandez-Diaz S, Honein MA. Use of over-the-counter
        medications during pregnancy. *Am J Obstet Gynecol*. 2005; 193:771-7.

[8]   Lo WY, Friedman JM. Teratogenicity of recently introduced medications in human
        pregnancy. *Obstet Gynecol*. 2002;100:465-73.

[9]   Mitchell AA. Systematic Identification of Drugs That Cause Birth Defects A New
        Opportunity. *N Engl J Med* 2003; 349: 2556-9.

[10]   Lammer EJ, Chen DT, Hoar RM, Agnish ND, Benke PJ, Braun JT, Curry CJ, Fernhoff
        PM, Grix AW Jr, Lott IT, et al. Retinoic acid embryopathy. *N Engl J Med*.
        1985;313:837-41.

[11]   Werler MM, Sheehan JE, Mitchell AA. Maternal medication use and risks of
        gastroschisis and small intestinal atresia. *Am J Epidemiol*. 2002;155:26-31.

[12]   Cooper WO, Hernandez-Diaz S, Arbogast PG, Dudley JA, Dyer S, Gideon PS, Hall K,
        Ray WA. Major congenital malformations after first-trimester exposure to ACE
        inhibitors. *N Engl J Med* 2006;354:2443-51.

[13]   Bérard A, Ramos E, Rey E, Blais L, St-André M, Oraichi D. First trimester exposure to
        paroxetine and risk of cardiac malformations in infants: the importance of dosage. *Birth
        Defects Res B Dev Reprod Toxicol* 2007;80:18-27.

[14]   Ray WA, Griffin MR. Use of Medicaid data for pharmacoepidemiology. *Am J
        Epidemiol* 1989;129:837-49.

[15]   West SL, Savitz DA, Koch G, Strom BL, Guess HA, Hartzema A. Recall accuracy for
        prescription medications: self-report compared with database information. *Am J
        Epidemiol* 1995;142:1103-12.

[16]   Johnson RE, Vollmer WM. Comparing sources of drug data about the elderly. *J Am
        Geriatr Soc* 1991;39:1079-84.

[17]   De Jong van den Berg LT, Feenstra N, Sorensen HT, Cornel MC. Improvement of drug
        exposure data in a registration of congenital anomalies. Pilot-study: pharmacist and
        mother as sources for drug exposure data during pregnancy. EuroMAP Group.
        European Medicine and Pregnancy Group. *Teratology*. 1999; 60: 33-6.

[18]   Meyerovitch J, Sherf M, Antebi F, Barhoum-Noufi M, Horev Z, Jaber L, Weiss D, Koren A. The incidence of anemia in an Israeli population: a population analysis for anemia in 34,512 Israeli infants aged 9 to 18 months. *Pediatrics*. 2006;118: 1055-60.

[19]   Smithells RW, Sheppard S, Schorah CJ, Seller MJ, Nevin NC, Harris R, Read AP, Fielding DW. Possible prevention of neural-tube defects by periconceptional vitamin supplementation. *Lancet*. 1980;1:339-40.

[20]   Mulinare J, Cordero JF, Erickson JD, Berry RJ. Periconceptional use of multivitamins and the occurrence of neural tube defects. *JAMA*. 1988;260:3141-5.

[21]   Milunsky A, Jick H, Jick SS, Bruell CL, MacLaughlin DS, Rothman KJ, Willett W. Multivitamin/folic acid supplementation in early pregnancy reduces the prevalence of neural tube defect. *JAMA*. 1989;262:2847-52.

[22]   MRC Vitamin Study Research Group. Prevention of neural tube defects: results of the Medical Research Council Vitamin Study. *Lancet*. 1991;338:131-7.

[23]   Berry RJ, Li Z, Erickson JD, Li S, Moore CA, Wang H, Mulinare J, Zhao P, Wong LY, Gindler J, Hong SX, Correa A. Prevention of neural-tube defects with folic acid in China. China-U.S. Collaborative Project for Neural Tube Defect Prevention. *N Engl J Med*. 1999;34:1485-90.

[24]   Lambie DG, Johnson RH. Drugs and folate metabolism. Drugs. 1985;30:145-55.

[25]   Hernández-Díaz S, Werler MM, Walker AM, Mitchell AA. Folic acid antagonists during pregnancy and the risk of birth defects. *N Engl J Med*. 2000;343:1608-14.

[26]   Tomson T, Battino D. Teratogenic effects of antiepileptic drugs. *Seizure*. 2008;17:166-71.

[27]   Centers for Disease Control and Prevention: Folic Acid. http://www.cdc.gov/ncbddd/folicacid/overview.htm, accessed on January 30 2009, at http://www.cdc.gov.

[28]   Robbins JM, Tilford JM, Bird TM, Cleves MA, Reading JA, Hobbs CA. Hospitalizations of newborns with folate-sensitive birth defects before and after fortification of foods with folic acid. *Pediatrics*. 2006;118:906-15.

[29]   Clinical management guidelines for obstetrician-gynecologists. ACOG practice bulletin no. 30. Washington, D.C.: American College of Obstetricians and Gynecologists, 2001.

[30]   Blank A, Grave G, Metzger BE. Effects of gestational diabetes on perinatal morbidity reassessed: report of the International Workshop on Adverse Perinatal Outcomes of Gestational Diabetes Mellitus, December 3-4, 1992. *Diabetes Care*. 1995;18:127-9.

[31]   Silverman B, Metzger BE, Cho NH, Loeb CA. Impaired glucose tolerance in adolescent offspring of diabetic mothers: relationship to fetal hyperinsulinism. *Diabetes Care*. 1995;18:611-7.

[32]   Petitt D, Bennett PH, Knowler WC, Baird HR, Aleck ICA. Gestational diabetes mellitus and impaired glucose tolerance during pregnancy: long-term effects on obesity and glucose intolerance in the offspring. *Diabetes Care*. 1985;34:Suppl 2:119-22.

[33]   Rizzo TA, Metzger BE, Dooley SL, Cho NH. Early malnutrition and child neurobehavioural development: insights from the study of children of diabetic mothers. *Child Dev*. 1997;68:26-38.

[34]   O'Sullivan J. The Boston Gestational Diabetes Studies. In: Sutherland HW, Stowers JM, Pearson DWM, eds. *Carbohydrate metabolism in pregnancy and the newborn*. London: Springer-Verlag; 1989:287-94.

[35] Crowther CA, Hiller JE, Moss JR, McPhee AJ, Jeffries WS, Robinson JS. Effect of Treatment of Gestational Diabetes Mellitus on Pregnancy Outcomes. *N Engl J Med.* 2005;352:2477-86.

[36] Langer O, Yogev Y, Most O, Xenakis EM. Gestational diabetes: the consequences of not treating. *Am J Obstet Gynecol.* 2005;192:989-97.

[37] Langer O. From educated guess to accepted practice: the use of oral antidiabetic agents in pregnancy. *Clin Obstet Gynecol.* 2007;50:959-71.

[38] Langer O. Management of gestational diabetes: pharmacologic treatment options and glycemic control. *Endocrinol Metab Clin North Am.* 2006;35:53-78.

[39] Moss JR, Crowther CA, Hiller JE, Willson KJ, Robinson JS. Costs and consequences of treatment for mild gestational diabetes mellitus - evaluation from the ACHOIS randomised trial. *BMC Pregnancy Childbirth.* 2007;7:27.

[40] Elliott BD, Langer O, Schenker S, Johnson RF. Insignificant transfer of glyburide occurs across the human placenta. *Am J Obstet Gynecol.* 1991;165:807-12.

[41] Kraemer J, Klein J, Lubetsky A, Koren G. Perfusion studies of glyburide transfer across the human placenta: implications for fetal safety. *Am J Obstet Gynecol.* 2006;195:270-4.

[42] Coetzee EJ, Jackson WP. The management of non-insulin-dependent diabetes during pregnancy. *Diabetes Res Clin Pract.* 1985-1986;1:281-7.

[43] Langer O, Conway DL, Berkus MD, Xenakis EM, Gonzales O. A comparison of glyburide and insulin in women with gestational diabetes mellitus. *N Engl J Med.* 2000;343:1134-8.

[44] Jacobson GF, Ramos GA, Ching JY, Kirby RS, Ferrara A, Field DR. Comparison of glyburide and insulin for the management of gestational diabetes in a large managed care organization. *Am J Obstet Gynecol.* 2005;193:118-24.

[45] Ramos GA, Jacobson GF, Kirby RS, Ching JY, Field DR. Comparison of glyburide and insulin for the management of gestational diabetics with markedly elevated oral glucose challenge test and fasting hyperglycemia. *J Perinatol.* 2007;27:262-7.

[46] Moretti ME, Rezvani M, Koren G. Safety of glyburide for gestational diabetes: a meta-analysis of pregnancy outcomes. *Ann Pharmacother.* 2008;42:483-90.

[47] Gadsby R, Barnie-Adshead AM, Jagger C. A prospective study of nausea and vomiting during pregnancy. *Br J Gen Prac.* 1993;43:245-8.

[48] Vellacott ID, Cooke EJA, James CE. Nausea and vomiting in early pregnancy. *Int J Gynaecol Obstet.* 1988;27:57-62.

[49] Weigel RM, Weigel MM. Nausea and vomiting of early pregnancy and pregnancy outcome: a meta-analytical review. *Br J Obstet Gynaecol.* 1989; 96: 1312-8.

[50] Deuchar N. Nausea and vomiting in pregnancy: a review of the problem with particular regard to psychological and social aspects. *Br J Obstet Gynaecol.* 1995;102:6-8.

[51] ACOG Practice Bulletin. Number 52, April 2004. *Obstet Gynecol.* 2004;103:803-15.

[52] Pradalier A, Chabriat H, Danchot J, Baudesson G, Joire JE. Safety and efficacy of combined lysine acetylsalicylate and metoclopramide repeated intake in migraine attacks. *Headache.* 1999;39:125-31.

[53] Rosa F. personal communication, FDA 1993, In: Briggs GG, Freeman RK, Yaffe SJ, eds. *Drugs in pregnancy and lactation*. 7th ed. Baltimore: Williams and Wilkins; 2005:1057-61.

[54] Berkovitch M, Elbirt D, Addis A, Schuler-Faccini L, Ornoy A. Fetal effects of metoclopramide therapy for nausea and vomiting of pregnancy. *N Engl J Med*. 2000; 343: 445-6.

[55] Sørensen HT, Nielsen GL, Christensen K, Tage-Jensen U, Ekbom A, Baron J. Birth outcome following maternal use of metoclopramide. The Euromap study group. *Br J Clin Pharmacol*. 2000; 49: 264-8.

[56] Berkovitch M, Mazzota P, Greenberg R, Elbirt D, Addis A, Schuler-Faccini L, Merlob P, Arnon J, Stahl B, Magee L, Moretti M, Ornoy A. Metoclopramide for nausea and vomiting of pregnancy: a prospective multicenter international study. *Am J Perinatol*. 2002;19: 311-6.

[57] Baron TH, Ramirez B, Richter JE. Gastrointestinal motility disorders during pregnancy. *Ann Intern Med*. 1993;118: 366-75.

[58] Better news on population. Lancet. 1992;339:1600.

[59] Howe JP, McGowan WA, Moore J, McCaughey W, Dundee JW. The placental transfer of cimetidine. *Anaesthesia*. 1981;36:371–75.

[60] Higasha N. Kamada S, Sakanova M, Takeuchi M, Simpo K, Tanable T. Teratogenicity studies in rats and rabbits. *J Toxol Sci*. 1984;9:53-72. As cited in Shepard TH. *Catalog of teratogenic Agents* 6th ed. Baltimore, MD. Johns Hopkins University Press; 1989:550.

[61] Magee LA, Inocencion G, Kamboj L, Rosetti F, Koren G. Safety of first trimester exposure to histamine H2-blockers. A prospective cohort study. *Dig Dis Sci*. 1996;41:1145–9.

[62] Källén B. Delivery outcome after the use of acid-suppressing drugs in early pregnancy with special reference to omeprazole. *Br J Obstet Gynaecol*. 1998;105: 877–81.

[63] Ruigómez A, Garcıa Rodrıguez LA, Cattaruzzi C, Troncon MG, Agostinis L, Wallander M-A, Johansson S. Use of cimetidine, omeprazole, and ranitidine in pregnant women and pregnancy outcomes. *Am J Epidemiol*. 1999;150:476–81.

[64] F. Rosa, personal communication, FDA 1993, In: Briggs GG, Freeman RK, Yaffe SJ, eds. *Drugs in pregnancy and lactation*. 7th ed. Baltimore: Williams and Wilkins; 2005: 627-8.

[65] Garbis H, Elefant E, Diav-Citrin O, Mastroiacovo P, Schaefer C, Vial T, Clementi M, Valti E, McElhatton P, Smorlesi C, Rodriguez EP, Robert-Gnansia E, Merlob P, Peiker G, Pexieder T, Schueler L, Ritvanen A, Mathieu-Nolf M. Pregnancy outcome after exposure to ranitidine and other H2 blockers. A collaborative study of the European Network of Teratology Information Services. *Reprod Toxicol*. 2005;19: 453-8.

[66] Schwethelm B, Margolis LH, Miller C, Smith S: Risk status and pregnancy outcome among Medicaid recipients. *Am J Prev Med*. 1989;5:157-63.

[67] Larson JD, Patatanian E, Miner PB, Rayburn WF, Robinson MG. Double-blind, placebo-controlled study of ranitidine for gastroesophageal reflux symptoms during pregnancy. *Obstet Gynecol*. 1997;90:83–7.

[68] Rayburn W, Liles E, Christensen H, Robinson M. Antacids vs antacids plus non-prescription ranitidine for heartburn during pregnancy. *Int J Gynecol Obstet*. 1999;66:35–7.

[69] Colin Jones DG, Langman MJ, Lawson DH, et al. Post-marketing surveillance of the safety of cimetidine: twelve-month morbidity report. *Q J Med*. 1985;54:253-68.

[70] Källén BA. Use of omeprazole during pregnancy--no hazard demonstrated in 955 infants exposed during pregnancy. *Eur J Obstet Gynecol Reprod Biol*. 2001;96:63-8.

[71] Diav-Citrin O, Arnon J, Shechtman S, Schaefer C, van Tonningen MR, Clementi M, De Santis M, Robert-Gnansia E, Valti E, Malm H, Ornoy A. The safety of proton pump inhibitors in pregnancy: a multicentre prospective controlled study. *Aliment Pharmacol Ther*. 2005;21:269-75.

[72] Nikfar S, Abdollahi M, Moretti ME, Magee LA, Koren G. Use of proton pump inhibitors during pregnancy and rates of major malformations: a meta-analysis. *Dig Dis Sci*. 2002;47:1526-9.

[73] Einarson TR, Leeder JS, Koren G: A method for meta analysis of epidemiological studies. *Drug Intell Clin Pharm*. 1988;22:813-24

In: Textbook of Perinatal Epidemiology
Editor: Eyal Sheiner, pp. 251-264

ISBN: 978-1-60741-648-7
© 2010 Nova Science Publishers, Inc.

Chapter XV

Bioeffects and Safety of Fetal Ultrasound Exposure: Why do we Need Epidemiology?

Jacques S. Abramowicz[*1], *J. Brian Fowlkes*[2],
Melvin E. Stratmeyer[3] *and Marvin C. Ziskin*[4],

Radiology and Biomedical Engineering, University of Michigan, Ann Arbor, MI[2]
Division of Biology, OSEL, Center for Devices and Radiological Health, Food and Drug
Administration, Silver Springs, MD[3]
Radiology and Medical Physics, Center for Biomedical Physics, Temple University
Medical School, Philadelphia, PA, 19140, USA[4]

Introduction

In 2005, the American Institute of Ultrasound in Medicine published the following Epidemiology Statement: "Based on the epidemiological data available and on current knowledge of interactive mechanisms, there is insufficient justification to warrant a conclusion of a causal relationship between diagnostic ultrasound and recognized adverse effects in humans. The epidemiological evidence is based on exposure conditions prior to 1992, the year in which acoustic limits of ultrasound machines were substantially increased for fetal/obstetrical applications" [1]. More recently, it published an In Vitro Biological Effects Statement. "It is often difficult to evaluate reports of ultrasonically induced in vitro biological effects with respect to their clinical significance. The predominant physical and biological interactions and mechanisms involved in an in vitro effect may not pertain to the in vivo situation..." [2] as well as a Prudent Use in Obstetrics statement: "The use of ultrasound

* For Correspondence: Jacques S. Abramowicz, MD; Frances T. and Lester B. Knight, Rush Fetal and Neonatal Medicine Program, Rush University Medical Center, Chicago, IL., USA; e-mail: Jacques_Abramowicz@rush.edu

without a medical indication to view the fetus, obtain a picture of the fetus or determine the fetal gender is inappropriate and contrary to responsible medical practice" [3]. These statements summarize the extent of the problem faced when discussing epidemiology of ultrasound bioeffects in humans: biological effects, some of them deleterious, have been demonstrated in laboratory animals at acoustic outputs identical to or close to those employed in obstetrics [4] but no population studies in humans have shown such harmful effects. It is critical to note that those epidemiological studies that exist were performed with machines manufactured prior to increases in the allowed outputs for OB ultrasound and "no demonstrated effects" does not necessarily equal "no effects" [5]. Given the quasi-universal use of diagnostic ultrasound in clinical obstetrics, it is appropriate to evaluate this issue in details. This is particularly relevant in today's clinical situations because of the use of modalities with potentially very high energy levels (such as spectral Doppler) and the expansion of diagnostic studies to the first trimester (e.g. nuchal translucency screening, ductus venosus waveform analysis or tricuspid valve function), which is known to be a period of high sensitivity of the fetus to teratological insults. Previously published analyses very rarely, if at all, involved scanning in the early first trimester [6]. A lack of uniformity in performing examinations and, more specifically, in reporting exposure conditions such as acoustic output and, particularly, duration of exposure, renders the task of delineating potential harmful effects extremely difficult. Only well performed epidemiological studies might shed some light on this concern. But these may be very complex to organize. Meanwhile prudence is recommended [3]. Of note: the mechanisms involved with the possible biological effects of ultrasound are extremely important but beyond the objectives of the present chapter. [7-12] Briefly, the two most likely effects are heating and cavitation. As the waveform travels through tissue, it loses amplitude by absorption and scatter. With absorption, energy is converted into heat. The latter can raise the temperature of the tissue being scanned. Cavitation is the oscillation of gas bubbles caused by ultrasound waves due to alternating pressures. These bubbles can implode resulting in mechanical effects, the release of extremely elevated heat (albeit for a fraction of time in a small area) and also, possibly, production of free radicals.

Why do we Need Epidemiological Studies in Ultrasound?

As extensively described in this book, epidemiology is the study of health and disease among groups or populations. It examines the distribution and determinants of disease frequency in human population. Included are analyses of causes, patterns and outcomes of diseases and effects thereof among many individuals. Applied to a medical procedure, such as diagnostic ultrasound, epidemiology is the study of effects of this procedure on human populations. In the case of obstetrical ultrasound, the population analyzed should include the pregnant patient as well as her infant, although most, if not all, studies deal exclusively with fetal effects and reports on safety and bioeffects in adults are exceedingly rare [13-15]. Effects have been shown under certain conditions in laboratory tissue and animal experiments under exposure levels similar to those used in diagnostic ultrasound [16-20]. Some effects have also been reported in humans but a definitive statement regarding risk should, ideally, include direct analysis of the effects in human populations. Several epidemiological studies have been published [5, 21]. For further discussion, including elements of statistics, in addition to that above, see Chapter 12 in NCRP Report number 140 [22], an extensive review by Newnham [23], a review by Ziskin [6] and AIUM document: Conclusions regarding Epidemiology for Obstetric Ultrasound [24].

Reports on the use of ultrasound in pregnancy to evaluate adverse outcomes of ultrasound over almost half a century include observational studies (case-control and cohort) and randomized controlled trials. There is a paucity of rigorously conducted epidemiological studies. Particular caution in interpreting case-control studies is necessary: the effect being studied (e.g. low estimated fetal weight) may be the clinical indication for performing the ultrasound exam (suspected growth delay) and may thus be found to be associated with it but not through a causal relationship.

Limitations of Epidemiology

Major limitations of published epidemiological studies are that (1) a testable hypothesis for causation of the studied effect is not always obvious and (2) information about ultrasound acoustic output and exposimetry (beam parameters, exposure duration and number of scanning episodes) is rarely presented or known, which makes comparisons between studies impossible. It has been recommended that these deficiencies be rectified in future research to arrive at truly valid and clinically meaningful results [25]. Furthermore, some of the studies have other serious limitations such as small samples and poorly matched controls [26]. While ultrasound may have bioeffects, based mainly on two mechanisms of action (thermal and mechanical), many uncertainties persist. These include, among others: existence of a threshold or lack thereof; importance of exposure duration which depends on the type of exam, the examiner's skills, and the presence of multiple examiners; influence of repeated scans (issue of cumulative doses), as well as biological response differences, secondary to tissue properties, susceptibility (fetus at different gestational ages, brain versus bones etc.) and environment (e.g. elevated temperature in the mother or medical conditions complicating the pregnancy). A further confounding factor is the fact that major congenital anomalies occur in 3-5% of the general human population. An increment of 1-2% over this "background" incidence would be a major clinical effect but might go undetected as an individual finding in routine clinical practice. In fact, the March of Dimes, until 2006, divided birth defects in 3 groups: defects observed at birth (3% of the general population), developmental issues, observed from 1-5 years of age (6-7%) and behavioral problems, observable only at school age (12-14%). This gave a total of 1 in 8 children with observable problems or 12.5% [27]. In 2006 [28], the March of Dimes somewhat altered its classification and divided known causes broadly into two groups: (1) genetic and partially genetic causes, originating mostly before conception (preconception) and (2) causes developing after conception, but before birth and at least 50% (birth, developmental, behavioral) have some genetic or partly genetic association. They described 8 million children born with anomalies. Those 8 million children represent about 6 percent of total births around the world, according to the report [28]. The birth prevalence of all genetic birth defects combined ranges worldwide from a high of 82 per 1,000 live births in low-income nations to a low of 39.7 per 1,000 live births in high-income countries [28]. It is therefore expected that some birth defects will be present in any study of ultrasound in relatively large (>1000) populations and yet, often, these studies describe no anomalies whatsoever, in the study group nor in the control population. An example of this is a survey of over 121,000 patients, among 68 examiners, combining 292 institute-years of experience where no anomalies are reported [29]. Finally, allowed acoustic outputs of instruments for obstetrical examinations has increased greatly since 1992 over the years and all available epidemiological data are from studies performed with lower outputs instruments [30]

End-Points for Ultrasound Bioeffects in Human Fetuses

Several biological endpoints have been analyzed in the human fetus/neonate to attempt to determine whether prenatal exposure to diagnostic ultrasound had observable effects [31-32]. Many studies are reported in Ziskin's 1999 review [6]. Among all endpoints, several are analyzed more in depth, including: intrauterine growth restriction (IUGR) and lower birth weight [33], delayed speech [34], lower intellectual performance [35], dyslexia [36], childhood malignancies [37], neurological and mental development or behavioral issues [38] and, more recently, non right-handedness [39-40]. With the exception of low birth weight, also demonstrated in monkeys [41], these findings have not been duplicated and the vast majority of studies have been negative for any association.

Low Birthweight

Several animal studies have described, albeit not always convincingly, that ultrasound may cause birth weight reduction. Decreased birth weight after prenatal exposure to ultrasound has been reported in the monkey [41] and the mouse [42] but not the rat [43]. In general, *in-situ* intensities were higher than what is considered routine in clinical obstetrical imaging in the human. High-level exposures were associated with decreased body weight *at birth* in exposed monkeys compared with controls but all showed catch-up growth when examined at 3 months of age [41]. Hence, the question of possible effects in humans has been raised. The mechanism whereby a fall in somatic growth could be induced by ultrasound is unclear. Tissue heating and effects on Insulin Growth Factors and heat shock proteins have been considered [44]. Moore et al.[45] examined over 2000 infants (half of them exposed to ultrasound) and found a small but statistically significant lower mean birth weight (116 grams at term) between exposed and non-exposed infants. While this is scientifically exact, the clinical importance, if any, is minimal at term. A serious concern is that no indications for the examination are known, no exposure information is available and information was collected several years after exposure. Furthermore, in a later study, the authors concluded that the relationship of ultrasound exposure and reduced birth weight may have been due to shared common risk factors, which lead to both exposure and a reduction in birth weight [46]. Another retrospective study, with Moore as a coauthor, reported a factor of 2 greater risk of low birth weight after 4 or more exposures to diagnostic ultrasound [47]. These results were not reproduced in other retrospective studies [48]. In fact, in a large study (originally 10,000 pregnancies exposed to ultrasound matched with 500 controls) with 6-year follow-up, Lyons et al.[48] did not find differences in birth weight (nor increased congenital malformations, chromosomal abnormalities, infant neoplasms, speech or hearing impairment or developmental problems). One oft-quoted study, which found significant birthweight reducing effects of prenatal ultrasound in humans involved over 2800 pregnancies [33]. In this randomized control trial, about half of the subjects received five ultrasound imaging and Doppler flow studies at 18, 24, 28, 34, and 38 weeks gestation and half received a single ultrasound imaging at 18 weeks. The authors found an increased risk of IUGR in fetuses exposed to frequent Doppler examinations. They speculate, with no clear scientific evidence, that this may be due to an effect on bone growth. However, when children from the study were examined at 1 year of age, there were no differences between the study and control groups. In addition, after examining their original subjects after 8 years, no evidence of long term adverse impact in neurological outcome was noted by the same group [49]. Similarly, no harmful effects of a single or two prenatal scans on growth were found in several randomized studies [50], [51]. In fact, in some studies, birth weight was slightly higher in the scanned group, but not significantly so, except in one where newborns who had been exposed to ultrasound *in utero* weighed on average 42g more than the control group [52]. Given the above and the fact that birth weight has been extensively analyzed in humans after diagnostic ultrasound exposure *in-utero,* it does not appear that such exposure is associated with reduced birth weight [53], except, possibly, for repeat Doppler exposure [54]. In a few studies that appear to favor such an effect of ultrasound on birth weight, a major problem is that there is an important confounding factor: many studies include pregnancies at risk for the primary outcome analyzed, i.e. IUGR, due to existing maternal or fetal conditions.

Delayed Speech

A second potential effect that has been extensively evaluated is delayed speech. In an attempt to determine if there is an association between prenatal ultrasound exposure and delayed speech in children, such children with delayed speech were compared to control subjects [34]. Among 72 children with delayed speech, a higher rate of ultrasound exposure in utero was found than in the 144 control subjects (Odds ratio = 2.8, 95% Confidence interval = 1.5 to 5.3, and p = 0.001). Certain concerns render these results less valid: There was neither a dose-response effect nor any relationship to time of exposure and many of the records were greater than five years old. Another large study of over 1100 children exposed in utero and over 1000 controls found no significant differences in delayed speech, limited vocabulary, or stuttering [55]. Interestingly, children exposed to ultrasound in utero were less likely to be referred to a speech therapist. Based on the above, there does not seem to be sufficient evidence to suspect an association of in utero ultrasound exposure and delayed speech.

Dyslexia

Dyslexia is another extensively studied subject. In one study over 400 children exposed to ultrasound *in utero* were used as a study group and compared to matched control to evaluate the appearance of adverse effects [36]. Numerous outcomes measures were examined, at birth (such as Apgar scores, gestational age, head circumference, birth weight, length, congenital abnormalities, neonatal infection, and congenital infection) or in early infancy, at 7 to 12 years of age (hearing, visual acuity and color vision, cognitive function, and behavior). No significant differences were found, except for a significantly greater proportion of dyslexia in those children exposed to ultrasound. However, the authors indicated that this could be an incidental finding, given the design of the study and the presence of several confounding factors that could have contributed to the possible dyslexia finding. On the other hand, it should be noted that exposure conditions were probably much lower than modern ultrasound systems given the fetal examinations were performed from 1968-1972. Subsequently, a long-term follow-up study was performed on over 2,100 children [50, 56]. Endpoints included evaluation for dyslexia along with additional hypotheses including an examination of non-right-handedness (see below) said to be associated with dyslexia. These studies [57-59] included the specific examination of more than 600 children with various tests for dyslexia such as spelling and reading. No statistically significant differences were found between ultrasound exposed children and controls for reading, spelling, arithmetic, or overall performance and intelligence scores, as reported by teachers or based on specific dyslexia tests. Since the original finding of dyslexia was not confirmed in subsequent randomized controlled trials, it is considered unlikely that routine ultrasound screening exams can cause dyslexia. These studies did, however, raise the issue of laterality (in terms of handedness; see below).

Neurological Development and Behavioral Issues

Neurons of the cerebral neocortex in mammals, including humans, are generated during fetal life in the brain proliferative zones and then migrate to their final destinations by following an inside-to outside sequence. This neuronal migration occurs, in the human fetal brain mainly from approximately 6-11 weeks gestation [60] but continuing until 32 weeks of gestation and it has long been thought that external factors, such as ultrasound, may, theoretically, affect this process [61]. Recently, Ang et al [62] evaluated the effect of ultrasound waves on neuronal position within the embryonic cerebral cortex of mice fetuses. Neurons generated at embryonic day 16 and known to normally migrate to the superficial cortical layers were chemically labeled. The pregnant mice were exposed to various ultrasound regimens. A small but statistically significant number of neurons remained scattered within inappropriate cortical layers and/or in the subjacent white matter and failed to acquire their proper position when exposed to ultrasound for a total of 30 min or longer during the period of their migration. While the authors appear to suggest their results imply that several neuropsychiatric disorders may result in humans, such as epilepsy, autism and schizophrenia, it is not clear whether a relatively small misplacement, in a relatively small number of cells that retain their origin cell class is of any clinical significance. Several major differences between the experimental setup of Ang et al, and the clinical use of ultrasound in humans, are noted [63]. The most notable difference was the length of exposure, of up to 7 hours in Ang's setup. No real mechanistic explanation was given for the findings and furthermore, there was no real dose-effect with high effects at the penultimate high dose but less so at the highest dose. Moreover, scans were performed over a small period of several days. The experimental setup was such that embryos received whole-brain exposure, which is rare in humans, although this is possible in very early pregnancy. In addition, brains of mice are much smaller than those in humans, and develop over days. Based on the above, the applicability to human embryology is questionable [63]. In another study, 2 out of 123 variables were found to be disturbed at birth but not at 1 year of age in children exposed *in utero*: grasp and tonic neck reflex [64]. Significance was not elaborated and some doubts exist regarding statistical validity. In a study mentioned above [36], vision and intelligence scores were identical among 425 exposed infants and 381 controls. Another large study found no association between routine exposure to prenatal ultrasound and school performance, deficits in attention, motor control, perception, vision and hearing [65]. In another large (>4900 children, aged 15-16), no differences were found in school performance between exposed and non-exposed children, except for a lower score for exposed boys in physical education [66]. Behavioral changes may be a more sensitive marker of subtle brain damage than obvious structural alterations [67]. Such changes have been described in animals [4, 68], albeit, often transient [41]. None have been reported in humans. In particular, schizophrenia and other psychoses have not been found to be associated with prenatal ultrasound exposure [69].

Childhood Malignancies

No association has been found between ultrasound exposure *in utero* and the later development of leukemia [70-71] or solid tumors in children [37, 72-76]. It should be noted that in a recent, prospective study, including first trimester scanning, no increased incidence of a particular brain tumor (primitive neuroectodermal tumor) was detected [76], as opposed to what was described for prenatal X-ray in a very similar population [77]. One must remember that although some of the above mentioned studies were published in 2007 or 2008, the populations studied were exposed to ultrasound *in utero* 20-30 years ago, i.e. with instruments generating lower outputs and with minmal or no information available on exposure conditions.

Non-Righthandedness

The issue of non-righthandedness as a result of prenatal exposure to ultrasound has been extensively debated. The first report of a possible link between prenatal exposure to ultrasound and subsequent non-right handedness at age 8-9 in the children who had been exposed to ultrasound *in utero*, was published in 1993 from Norway [59]. According to the authors the results were "only barely significant at the 5% level". In a later analysis of the data, the association was found to be restricted to males [78]. A second group of researchers (with Salvesen, a principal author of the first report, included, but with a new population of 3265 children, this time from Sweden) published similar findings of a statistically significant association between ultrasound exposure *in utero* and non-right handedness in males [39]. It should be noted that these studies by Kieler [39, 79] are population-based and observational rather than randomized and controlled as was Salvesen's. Furthermore the authors stretch their findings to suggest that non-right handedness is associated with brain damage. Salvesen then published a meta-analysis of these two studies and of previously unreported results [40]. No difference was found in general but, again, a small increase in non-right handedness was present when analyzing boys separately. Nowhere is a valid mechanistic explanation given in the studies to explain the findings. A word of caution is needed: the use of the term meta-analysis is somewhat of a misnomer. Only two studies were included. It is generally accepted that a meta-analysis should include at least six studies. A Cochrane review did not find any association between ultrasound exposure in early pregnancy and non-righthandedness, although they did not perform a gender analysis [53]. In conclusion, although there may be a small increase in the incidence of non-right handedness in male infants, there is not enough evidence to assume a direct effect on brain structure or function or even that non-right handedness is an adverse effect.

Congenital Malformations

Because hyperthermia is a known teratogen and ultrasound has the potential to elevate the temperature of insonated tissues [80] , the question has been asked whether ultrasound can induce fetal malformations [81-82]. Such malformations have been described in offsprings of pregnant animals whose temperature was raised not by ultrasound and examples of such congenital anomalies include anencephaly, microcephaly, other neural tube defects, ocular disorders and cleft lip and palate [83-87]. There is published scientific evidence to show that exposure to diagnostic ultrasound can produce significant temperature increases in the fetal guinea-pig brain near bone [88]. A detailed description of thermal effects of ultrasound and biological results is, however, beyond the scope of this chapter. In humans, prenatal ultrasound has not been shown to result in an increased incidence of congenital anomalies such as those mentioned in animals. Based on available data, it has been suggested that a diagnostic exposure producing a maximum temperature rise of 1.5°C above normal physiologic levels can be used without reservation in clinical examinations. However, if a diagnostic exposure produces an *in situ* temperature elevation to or above 41°C for 15 min, it should be considered potentially hazardous to embryonic or fetal development.[89]

Additional Caveats

It must once more be stressed that there has been *no* epidemiological study published on pregnant populations scanned after 1992, when regulations were altered and acoustic output of diagnostic instruments were permitted to reach levels many times higher than previously allowed (from 46 to 720 mW/cm^2 I$_{SPTA}$ for fetal applications). There are no epidemiological studies related to the output display standard (thermal and mechanical indices) and clinical outcomes [90]. There are no studies of effects related to first trimester exposure [91-92]. The safety of newer technologies (harmonic imaging, Doppler [spectral and color], 3D, the use of ultrasound contrast agents) as well as the issue of probe self-heating [93], have not been studied in terms of fetal exposure and need to be investigated particularly with the increased use of transvaginal scanning in early pregnancy [94].

Conclusions

Biological effects have been demonstrated using some forms of ultrasound in animal and *in vitro* models. However, epidemiological evidence is not sufficient to establish a causal association between fetal exposure to diagnostic ultrasound and adverse effects. Published human studies do not preclude the possibility that adverse effects may be found under certain conditions. Furthermore, present day instruments (as opposed to those used for all available epidemiological information) can deliver ultrasound energy (in particular thermal) at levels potentially hazardous with prolonged exposure [95] and epidemiological and statistical considerations show that minor chemical and behavioral changes could easily be beyond present detection techniques. Whether these might have long-term delayed or genetic effects is unclear. Hence the principle of prudent use seems advisable [96]. Although this may be financially, ethically and clinically extremely complex to organize, there is still a need for well-designed, randomized clinical studies addressing the risk for the fetus exposed *in utero*. Subtle or transient effects in humans are possible, but none proven so far, and, therefore, diagnostic ultrasound remains without any known risk. Moreover, while not always relevant in an analysis of epidemiological data, risk-benefit issues are extremely important in clinical practice. Since risks of adverse effects appear so low and clinical benefits so great, there is no justification based on epidemiological data to withhold the prudent use of diagnostic ultrasound in medically indicated conditions.

References

[1]   AIUM Official Statement: Conclusions Regarding Epidemiology for Obstetric Ultrasound. 2005; http://www.aium.org/publications /statements/_statementSelected. asp?statement=16. Accessed 9/30/2008.

[2]   AIUM Official Statement: In-Vitro Biological Effects 2007; http://www.aium.org/ publications/guidelinesStatementsX.aspx#statements. Accessed 11/20/08.

[3]   AIUM Official Statement:Prudent Use in Obstetrics. 2007; http://www.aium.org /publications/statements/_statementSelected.asp?statement=33. Accessed 9/20/2008.

[4]   Jensh RP, Brent RL. Intrauterine effects of ultrasound: animal studies. *Teratology.* Apr 1999;59(4):240-251.

[5]   Ziskin MC, Petitti DB. Epidemiology of human exposure to ultrasound: a critical review. *Ultrasound in medicine & biology.* 1988;14(2):91-96.

[6]   Ziskin MC. Intrauterine effects of ultrasound: human epidemiology. *Teratology.* Apr 1999;59(4):252-260.

[7]   Abramowicz JS. Ultrasound in obstetrics and gynecology: is this hot technology too hot? *J Ultrasound Med.* Dec 2002;21(12):1327-1333.

[8]   Barnett SB. Biophysical aspects of diagnostic ultrasound. *Ultrasound in medicine & biology.* May 2000;26 Suppl 1:S68-70.

[9]   Carstensen EL, Gates AH. The effects of pulsed ultrasound on the fetus. *J Ultrasound Med.* Apr 1984;3(4):145-147.

[10]   Merritt CR, Kremkau FW, Hobbins JC. Diagnostic ultrasound: bioeffects and safety. *Ultrasound Obstet Gynecol.* Sep 1 1992;2(5):366-374.

[11]   Nyborg WL. Biological effects of ultrasound: development of safety guidelines. Part II: general review. *Ultrasound in medicine & biology.* Mar 2001;27(3):301-333.

[12]   O'Brien WD, Jr. Ultrasound-biophysics mechanisms. *Progress in biophysics and molecular biology.* Jan-Apr 2007;93(1-3):212-255.

[13]   Church CC, Carstensen EL, Nyborg WL, Carson PL, Frizzell LA, Bailey MR. The risk of exposure to diagnostic ultrasound in postnatal subjects: nonthermal mechanisms. *J Ultrasound Med.* Apr 2008;27(4):565-592; quiz 593-566.

[14]   O'Brien WD, Jr., Deng CX, Harris GR, et al. The risk of exposure to diagnostic ultrasound in postnatal subjects: thermal effects. *J Ultrasound Med.* Apr 2008;27(4):517-535; quiz 537-540.

[15]   Brown BS. How safe is diagnostic ultrasonography? *Canadian Medical Association journal.* Aug 15 1984;131(4):307-311.

[16]   Dalecki D. Mechanical bioeffects of ultrasound. *Annual review of biomedical engineering.* 2004;6:229-248.

[17]   Rao S, Ovchinnikov N, McRae A. Gestational stage sensitivity to ultrasound effect on postnatal growth and development of mice. *Birth defects research.* Aug 2006;76(8):602-608.

[18]   Siddiqi TA, Meyer RA, Woods JR, Jr., Plessinger MA. Ultrasound effects on fetal auditory brain stem responses. *Obstetrics and gynecology.* Nov 1988;72(5):752-756.

[19]   Tarantal AF, Hendrickx AG. Evaluation of the bioeffects of prenatal ultrasound exposure in the cynomolgus macaque (Macaca fascicularis): I. Neonatal/infant observations. *Teratology.* Feb 1989;39(2):137-147.

[20]   Ziskin MC, Barnett SB. Ultrasound and the developing central nervous system. *Ultrasound in medicine & biology.* Jul 2001;27(7):875-876.

[21]   Salvesen KA, Eik-Nes SH. Is ultrasound unsound? A review of epidemiological studies of human exposure to ultrasound. *Ultrasound Obstet Gynecol.* Oct 1995;6(4):293-298.

[22]   *NCRP. (National Council on Radiation Protection and Measurements). Exposure Criteria for Medical Diagnostic Ultrasound: II. Criteria Based on All Known Mechanisms. Report No. 140.* Bethesda, MD2002.

[23]   Newnham JP. Studies of ultrasound safety in humans: clinical benefit vs. risk. In: Barnett SB, Kossoff G, eds. *Safety of Diagnostic Ultrasound* New York, London: The Parthenon Publishing Group; 1998:99-112.

[24]   Abramowicz JS, Fowlkes JB, Skelly AC, Stratmeyer ME, Ziskin MC. Conclusions regarding epidemiology for obstetric ultrasound. *J Ultrasound Med.* Apr 2008;27(4):637-644.

[25]   Edmonds PD, Abramowicz JS, Carson PL, Carstensen EL, Sandstrom KL. Guidelines for Journal of Ultrasound in Medicine Authors and Reviewers on Measurement and Reporting of Acoustic Output and Exposure. *J Ultrasound Med.* 2005;24:1171-1179.

[26] Kieler H. Epidemiological studies on adverse effects of prenatal ultrasound-which are the challenges? *Progress in biophysics and molecular biology.* 2007;93:301-308.

[27] Christianson A, Modell B. Medical genetics in developing countries. *Annual review of genomics and human genetics.* 2004;5:219-265.

[28] Christianson A, Howson CP, Modell B. *The March of Dimes Global Report on Birth Defects, The Hidden Toll of Dying and Disabled Children.* White Plains, NY2006.

[29] Ziskin MC. Survey of patients exposed to diagnostic ultrasound. In: Reid JM, Sikov MR, eds. *Interactions of ultrasound and biological tissues (Proceedings of a workshop held at Battelle Seattle Research Center, Seattle, Washington, November 8-11, 1971).* Rockville, Md: U.S. Dept. of Health, Education, and Welfare, Bureau of Radiological Health; 1973:203-206.

[30] Miller MW, Brayman AA, Abramowicz JS. Obstetric ultrasonography: a biophysical consideration of patient safety--the "rules" have changed. *American journal of obstetrics and gynecology.* Jul 1998;179(1):241-254.

[31] Brent RL, Jensh RP, Beckman DA. Medical sonography: reproductive effects and risks. *Teratology.* Aug 1991;44(2):123-146.

[32] Hellman LM, Duffus GM, Donald I, Sunden B. Safety of diagnostic ultrasound in obstetrics. *Lancet.* May 30 1970;1(7657):1133-1134.

[33] Newnham JP, Evans SF, Michael CA, Stanley FJ, Landau LI. Effects of frequent ultrasound during pregnancy: a randomised controlled trial. *Lancet.* Oct 9 1993;342(8876):887-891.

[34] Campbell JD, Elford RW, Brant RF. Case-control study of prenatal ultrasonography exposure in children with delayed speech. *Cmaj.* Nov 15 1993;149(10):1435-1440.

[35] Kieler H, Haglund B, Cnattingius S, Palmgren J, Axelsson O. Does prenatal sonography affect intellectual performance? *Epidemiology (Cambridge, Mass.* May 2005;16(3):304-310.

[36] Stark CR, Orleans M, Haverkamp AD, Murphy J. Short- and long-term risks after exposure to diagnostic ultrasound in utero. *Obstetrics and gynecology.* Feb 1984;63(2):194-200.

[37] 37. Cartwright RA, McKinney PA, Hopton PA, et al. Ultrasound examinations in pregnancy and childhood cancer. *Lancet.* Nov 3 1984;2(8410):999-1000.

[38] Bricker L, Neilson JP, Dowswell T. Routine ultrasound in late pregnancy (after 24 weeks' gestation). *Cochrane database of systematic reviews (Online).* 2008(4):CD001451.

[39] Kieler H, Axelsson O, Haglund B, Nilsson S, Salvesen KA. Routine ultrasound screening in pregnancy and the children's subsequent handedness. *Early human development.* Jan 9 1998;50(2):233-245.

[40] Salvesen KA, Eik-Nes SH. Ultrasound during pregnancy and subsequent childhood non-right handedness: a meta-analysis. *Ultrasound Obstet Gynecol.* Apr 1999;13(4):241-246.

[41] Tarantal AF, Hendrickx AG. Evaluation of the bioeffects of prenatal ultrasound exposure in the cynomolgus macaque (Macaca fascicularis): II. Growth and behavior during the first year. *Teratology.* Feb 1989;39(2):149-162.

[42] Hande MP, Devi PU. Effect of in utero exposure to diagnostic ultrasound on the postnatal survival and growth of mouse. *Teratology.* Nov 1993;48(5):405-411.

[43] Fisher JE, Jr., Acuff-Smith KD, Schilling MA, et al. Teratologic evaluation of rats prenatally exposed to pulsed-wave ultrasound. *Teratology.* Feb 1994;49(2):150-155.

[44] Kossoff G, Barnett SB. Take-home messages. In: Barnett SB, Kossoff G, eds. *Safety of diagnostic Ultrasound*. New York, London: Parthenon Publishing Group; 1998:133-139.

[45] Moore RM, Jr., Barrick MK, Hamilton TM. Effect of sonic radiation on growth and development. *Am J Epidemiol.* 1982;116:571.

[46] Moore RM, Jr., Diamond EL, Cavalieri RL. The relationship of birth weight and intrauterine diagnostic ultrasound exposure. *Obstetrics and gynecology.* Apr 1988;71(4):513-517.

[47] Marinac-Dabic D, Krulewitch CJ, Moore RM, Jr. The safety of prenatal ultrasound exposure in human studies. *Epidemiology (Cambridge, Mass.* May 2002;13(3 Suppl):S19-22.

[48] Lyons EA, Dyke C, Toms M, Cheang M. In utero exposure to diagnostic ultrasound: a 6-year follow-up. *Radiology.* 1988;166:687-690.

[49] Newnham JP, Doherty DA, Kendall GE, Zubrick SR, Landau LL, Stanley FJ. Effects of repeated prenatal ultrasound examinations on childhood outcome up to 8 years of age: follow-up of a randomised controlled trial. *Lancet.* Dec 4-10 2004;364(9450):2038-2044.

[50] Bakketeig LS, Eik-Nes SH, Jacobsen G, et al. Randomised controlled trial of ultrasonographic screening in pregnancy. *Lancet.* Jul 28 1984;2(8396):207-211.

[51] Saari-Kemppainen A, Karjalainen O, Ylostalo P, Heinonen OP. Ultrasound screening and perinatal mortality: controlled trial of systematic one-stage screening in pregnancy. The Helsinki Ultrasound Trial. *Lancet.* Aug 18 1990;336(8712):387-391.

[52] Waldenstrom U, Axelsson O, Nilsson S, et al. Effects of routine one-stage ultrasound screening in pregnancy: a randomised controlled trial. *Lancet.* Sep 10 1988;2(8611):585-588.

[53] Neilson JP. Ultrasound for fetal assessment in early pregnancy. *Cochrane database of systematic reviews (Online).* 2000(2):CD000182.

[54] Salvesen KA. Epidemiological prenatal ultrasound studies. *Progress in biophysics and molecular biology.* Jan-Apr 2007;93(1-3):295-300.

[55] Salvesen KA, Vatten LJ, Bakketeig LS, Eik-Nes SH. Routine ultrasonography in utero and speech development. *Ultrasound Obstet Gynecol.* Mar 1 1994;4(2):101-103.

[56] Eik-Nes SH, Okland O, Aure JC, Ulstein M. Ultrasound screening in pregnancy: a randomised controlled trial. *Lancet.* Jun 16 1984;1(8390):1347.

[57] Salvesen KA, Bakketeig LS, Eik-nes SH, Undheim JO, Okland O. Routine ultrasonography in utero and school performance at age 8-9 years. *Lancet.* Jan 11 1992;339(8785):85-89.

[58] Salvesen KA, Vatten LJ, Jacobsen G, et al. Routine ultrasonography in utero and subsequent vision and hearing at primary school age. *Ultrasound Obstet Gynecol.* Jul 1 1992;2(4):243-244, 245-247.

[59] Salvesen KA, Vatten LJ, Eik-Nes SH, Hugdahl K, Bakketeig LS. Routine ultrasonography in utero and subsequent handedness and neurological development. *BMJ.* Jul 17 1993;307(6897):159-164.

[60] Sidman RL, Rakic P. Neuronal migration, with special reference to developing human brain: a review. *Brain research.* Nov 9 1973;62(1):1-35.

[61] Mole R. Possible hazards of imaging and Doppler ultrasound in obstetrics. *Birth (Berkeley, Calif.* Dec 1986;13 Suppl:23-33 suppl.

[62] Ang ESBC, Gluncic V, Duque A, Schafer ME, Rakic P. Prenatal exposure to ultrasound waves impacts neuronal migration in mice. *Proc NY Acad Sci.* 2006;103:12903-12910.

[63] Abramowicz JS. Prenatal exposure to ultrasound waves: is there a risk? *Ultrasound Obstet Gynecol.* Apr 2007;29(4):363-367.

[64] Scheidt PC, Stanley F, Bryla DA. One-year follow-up of infants exposed to ultrasound in utero. *American journal of obstetrics and gynecology.* Aug 1 1978;131(7):743-748.

[65] Salvesen K. Routine ultrasonography in utero and development in childhood. In: Tejani N, ed. *Obstetrical events and developmental sequelae.* 2nd ed. Boca Raton: CRC Press, Inc; 1994.

[66] Stalberg K. *Prenatal ultrasound and X-ray-potentially adverse effects on the CNS.* Upsalla, Sweden: Women's and Children's Health, Obstetrics and Gynecology, Upsalla Universitet; 2008.

[67] Coyle I, Wayner MJ, Singer G. Behavioral teratogenesis: a critical evaluation. *Pharmacology, biochemistry, and behavior.* Feb 1976;4(2):191-200.

[68] Norton S, Kimler BF, Cytacki EP, Rosenthal SJ. Prenatal and postnatal consequences in the brain and behavior of rats exposed to ultrasound in utero. *J Ultrasound Med.* Feb 1991;10(2):69-75.

[69] Stalberg K, Haglund B, Axelsson O, Cnattingius S, Hultman CM, Kieler H. Prenatal ultrasound scanning and the risk of schizophrenia and other psychoses. *Epidemiology (Cambridge, Mass.* Sep 2007;18(5):577-582.

[70] Shu XO, Potter JD, Linet MS, et al. Diagnostic X-rays and ultrasound exposure and risk of childhood acute lymphoblastic leukemia by immunophenotype. *Cancer Epidemiol Biomarkers Prev.* Feb 2002;11(2):177-185.

[71] Naumburg E, Bellocco R, Cnattingius S, Hall P, Ekbom A. Prenatal ultrasound examinations and risk of childhood leukaemia: case-control study. *BMJ (Clinical research ed.* Jan 29 2000;320(7230):282-283.

[72] Kinnier Wilson LM, Waterhouse JA. Obstetric ultrasound and childhood malignancies. *Lancet.* Nov 3 1984;2(8410):997-999.

[73] Bunin GR, Buckley JD, Boesel CP, Rorke LB, Meadows AT. Risk factors for astrocytic glioma and primitive neuroectodermal tumor of the brain in young children: a report from the Children's Cancer Group. *Cancer Epidemiol Biomarkers Prev.* Apr-May 1994;3(3):197-204.

[74] Sorahan T, Lancashire R, Stewart A, Peck I. Pregnancy ultrasound and childhood cancer: a second report from the Oxford Survey of Childhood Cancers. *British journal of obstetrics and gynaecology.* Oct 1995;102(10):831-832.

[75] Salvesen KA, Eik-Nes SH. Ultrasound during pregnancy and birthweight, childhood malignancies and neurological development. *Ultrasound in medicine & biology.* Sep 1999;25(7):1025-1031.

[76] Stalberg K, Haglund B, Axelsson O, Cnattingius S, Pfeifer S, Kieler H. Prenatal ultrasound and the risk of childhood brain tumour and its subtypes. *British journal of cancer.* Apr 8 2008;98(7):1285-1287.

[77] Stalberg K, Haglund B, Axelsson O, Cnattingius S, Pfeifer S, Kieler H. Prenatal X-ray exposure and childhood brain tumours: a population-based case-control study on tumour subtypes. *British journal of cancer.* Dec 3 2007;97(11):1583-1587.

[78] Salvesen KA, Eik-Ness SH, Vatten LJ, Hugdahl K, Bakketeig LS. Routine ultrasound scanning in pregnancy. Authors' reply. *BMJ.* 1993;307:1562.

[79] Kieler H, Cnattingius S, Palmgren J, Haglund B, Axelsson O. First trimester ultrasound scans and left-handedness. *Epidemiology (Cambridge, Mass.* May 2002;13(3):370.

[80] Duck FA, Starritt HC. A study of the heating capabilities of diagnostic ultrasound beams. *Ultrasound in medicine & biology.* 1994;20(5):481-492.

[81] Abramowicz JS, Barnett SB, Duck FA, Edmonds PD, Hynynen KH, Ziskin MC. Fetal thermal effects of diagnostic ultrasound. *J Ultrasound Med.* Apr 2008;27(4):541-559; quiz 560-543.

[82] Miller MW, Ziskin MC. Biological consequences of hyperthermia. *Ultrasound in medicine & biology.* 1989;15(8):707-722.

[83] Chance PF, Smith DW. Hyperthermia and meningomyelocele and anencephaly. *Lancet.* Apr 8 1978;1(8067):769-770.

[84] Edwards MJ. Congenital defects in guinea pigs. Following induced hyperthermia during gestation. *Archives of pathology.* Jul 1967;84(1):42-48.

[85] Li Z, Ren A, Liu J, et al. Maternal flu or fever, medication use, and neural tube defects: a population-based case-control study in Northern China. *Birth defects research.* Apr 2007;79(4):295-300.

[86] Martinez-Frias ML, Garcia Mazario MJ, Caldas CF, Conejero Gallego MP, Bermejo E, Rodriguez-Pinilla E. High maternal fever during gestation and severe congenital limb disruptions. *American journal of medical genetics.* Jan 15 2001;98(2):201-203.

[87] Shiota K. Neural tube defects and maternal hyperthermia in early pregnancy: epidemiology in a human embryo population. *American journal of medical genetics.* Jul 1982;12(3):281-288.

[88] Horder MM, Barnett SB, Vella GJ, Edwards MJ, Wood AK. Ultrasound-induced temperature increase in guinea-pig fetal brain in utero: third-trimester gestation. *Ultrasound in medicine & biology.* Nov 1998;24(9):1501-1510.

[89] BMUS (British Medical Ultrasound Society) Guidelines for the Safe Use of Diagnostic Ultrasound Equipment. 2000; http://www.bmus.org/ultras-safety/us-safety03.asp. Accessed 11/8/2008.

[90] AIUM. How to interpret the ultrasound output display standard for higher acoustic output diagnostic ultrasound devices. *J Ultrasound Med.* 2004;23:723-726.

[91] Duck FA. Is it safe to use diagnostic ultrasound during the first trimester? *Ultrasound Obstet Gynecol.* Jun 1999;13(6):385-388.

[92] Sheiner E, Shoham-Vardi I, Hussey MJ, et al. First-trimester sonography: Is the fetus exposed to high levels of acoustic energy? *J Clin Ultrasound.* Jun 2007;35(5):245-249.

[93] Duck FA, Starritt HC, ter Haar GR, Lunt MJ. Surface heating of diagnostic ultrasound transducers. *The British journal of radiology.* Nov 1989;62(743):1005-1013.

[94] Calvert J, Duck F, Clift S, Azaime H. Surface heating by transvaginal transducers. *Ultrasound Obstet Gynecol.* Apr 2007;29(4):427-432.

[95] Church CC, Miller MW. Quantification of risk from fetal exposure to diagnostic ultrasound. *Progress in biophysics and molecular biology.* 2007;93:331-353.

[96] Miller DL. Safety assurance in obstetrical ultrasound. *Seminars in ultrasound, CT, and MR.* Apr 2008;29(2):156-164.

Maternal Morbidity

In: Textbook of Perinatal Epidemiology
Editor: Eyal Sheiner, pp. 267-297

Chapter XVI

Epidemiology of Obesity in Pregnancy

Adi Y. Weintraub[*] *and Eyal Sheiner*

Department of Obstetrics and Gynecology, Faculty of Health Sciences, Soroka
University Medical Center, Ben-Gurion University of the Negev, Beer-Sheva, Israel

Definitions

- BMI= body mass index, the weight in kilograms divided by the square of the height in meters (weight [kg]/height [m]).
- Obesity: BMI >30 kg/m^2

Introduction

When examining the history of obesity, it is evident that this health condition is seen throughout most of man's history. Ancient Egyptians considered obesity a disease and depicted it in drawings on a wall of illnesses. The most famous and earliest evidence of obesity is probably the Venus figures, statues of an obese female torso used in religious ceremonies and rituals. Mention of obesity appeared in the ancient Chinese and the ancient Aztec cultures. Hippocrates, the father of medicine, stated in his writings that sudden death was more common among obese men than lean ones.

[*] For Correspondence: Adi Y. Weintraub, Department of Obstetrics and Gynecology, Faculty of Health Sciences, Soroka University Medical Center, Ben-Gurion University of the Negev, Beer-Sheva, Israel, e-mail: adiyehud@bgu.ac.il

Throughout the history of obesity, the public's attitude towards obesity has been altered considerably, at times it was conceived as a symbol of wealth and social status and at times it was regarded as unfashionable, unhealthy and even sinful. Attitudes toward overweight people have varied in different times and places, depending on the availability of food. At times when food was scarce, fashion declared that overweight was a sign of prosperity and well-being; when food was plentiful, slender shapes were usually more fashionable. In the 20th century the incidence of obesity began to increase and become widespread.[1]

Early 20th century analysis of life insurance data demonstrates that obesity was associated with increased mortality rates. A familial basis (genetic or hormonal) for obesity was suggested in the 1920s; in the 1940s, psychological theories of obesity became popular; the marketing of diet food products began in the 1950s; and the use of behavior therapy to treat obesity began in the 1970s. Considerable advances have been made in diet, exercise and behavioral approaches to the treatment of obesity since their introduction. The World Health Organization (WHO) defined overweight and obesity as a global epidemic and convened in June, 1997 a consultation on obesity that reviewed epidemiological information, contributing factors and associated consequences of overweight and obesity. In particular, the Consultation considered the system for classifying overweight and obesity based on the body mass index (BMI), and concluded that a coherent system is available and should be adopted internationally.[2] The BMI was introduced as a statistical tool and index for diagnosis and follow-up of obesity. New drugs with better pharmacological profiles continue to regularly be introduced. Gastric surgery has had the most effective long-term success in treating the severely obese. However, despite this progress, obesity prevalence continues to increase sharply, and the challenge to clinicians and public health workers has never been greater.[2]

This chapter provides a review of the current literature regarding the prevalence of obesity in pregnancy, its short and long term health consequences for both the mother and neonate. The effects of prevention and management strategies for the treatment of obesity in reproductive aged women in general, and those of bariatric surgery in particular are discussed.

Definitions, Prevalence and Scope

Obesity is considered a chronic disease, prevalent in both developed and developing countries, and affecting all ages. Weight gain and obesity are posing a growing threat to health in countries all over the world. From a public health perspective, the well recognized worldwide public health concerns such as undernutrition and infectious disease have been replaced by overweight and obesity as a major contributor to poor health.[3-4] Overweight and obesity have been termed by the World Health Organization an epidemic and this term has been widely used in the literature. However, this is a misnomer. The word epidemic is defined as a temporary widespread outbreak of greatly increased frequency and severity. Unfortunately, the term endemic, defined as a condition that is consistently present, better defines the problem of overweight and obesity. Public health authorities began to address the problem of obesity in the late 1980s. Healthy People 2000 set as its goal reducing the prevalence of overweight people to less than 20% by the end of the 20th century.[5]

Unfortunately, this objective was not accomplished, and more than half the population was overweight at the beginning of 2000.

Overweight and obesity are defined as abnormal or excessive fat accumulation that may impair health.[6] Body mass index (BMI) is a simple index of weight-for-height that is commonly used in categorizing overweight and obesity in adult populations and individuals. It is defined as the weight in kilograms divided by the square of the height in meters (weight [kg]/height [m]^2). BMI provides the most useful measure of overweight and obesity as it is the same for both sexes and for all ages of adults.[6] Weight classification by BMI for pregnant adults is not valid; therefore, BMI and weight status should be assessed before and after pregnancy. Weight classification by BMI for adults is presented in table 1. The World Health Organization and the National Institutes of Health defined normal weight as a BMI of 18.5–24.9, overweight as a BMI of 25–29.9, and obesity as a BMI of 30 or greater. Obesity was further divided into classes: class I (30 –34.9), class II (35–39.9), and class III (greater than 40).[7]

Table 1. Weight classification by BMI for adults.

Classification		BMI
	Underweight	<18.50
	Normal range	18.50 - 24.99
	Overweight	25.00 - 29.99
	Obese	≥30.00
Obese class I		30.00 - 34-99
Obese class II		35.00 - 39.99
Obese class III		≥40.00

Excludes pregnant women

The prevalence of overweight and obesity in developed countries has increased dramatically over the past 20 years. In the United States, for example, approximately two thirds (65.1%) of Americans above the age of 20 have a body mass index (BMI) >25 kg/m^2 and are considered overweight. Nearly one third (30.5%) are considered obese (BMI >30 kg/m^2), and 4.9% are extremely obese (BMI >40 kg/m^2).[8-9] From 1999 to 2002, close to a third of childbearing age women (20–39 years) were classified as obese, and an additional quarter of this age cohort were overweight.[8,10-11] In Sweden the increase in overweight among women has been less prominent, but it is nevertheless indisputable.[9] In the UK up to 40% of women are overweight.[12] In Israel, obesity rates are high and are comparable to those in the United States.[13] In addition to the escalating prevalence of overweight and obesity among reproductive age women, the rates of adverse perinatal outcomes and co-morbidities are rising as well.

The worldwide increase in the prevalence of overweight and obesity has affected people of all ages including women of reproductive age. Close to a third of women of childbearing age (20–39 years) are classified as obese, and an additional quarter of women in this age group are overweight.[8,10-11] In the UK, overweight and obesity are common in antenatal clinics. Sebire et al.[12] examined a large unselected population from the North West Thames region and compared pregnancy outcomes based on maternal BMI measured at booking.[12] Of the entire cohort, 27.5% of women were overweight and 10.9% were obese, defined by BMI at booking. Kanagalingam et al.[14] examined booking BMI of women with singleton pregnancies in 1990 and 2002/2004. They reported a two-fold increase in women being recognized as obese at booking visits (from 9.4% to 18.9%). After adjusting for maternal age, parity, smoking status and deprivation status, the mean BMI elevated in 1.37 kg/m^2.[14] The scale of the obesity problem in different countries is presented in table 2. Maternal obesity represents an important modifiable risk factor for adverse pregnancy outcomes[15-19] with serious obstetric complications for both the mother and the fetus.[9,20–23]

Table 2. The scale of the obesity problem in different countries: estimates for 2005 and 2015.

Country	2005			2015	
	Mean BMI	Estimated BMI > 30	Estimated BMI > 25	Estimated BMI > 30	Estimated BMI > 25
Argentina	27.5	31	65.7	44.6	75.9
Australia	26.8	24.9	62.7	33.5	70
Bolivia	27.7	33.1	68.0	47.1	77.6
Brzil	25.6	18.3	53.5	31.3	66.5
Canada	26.1	23.2	57.1	28.2	61.9
China	22.8	1.9	24.7	6.3	39.8
Egypt	29.6	45.5	74.2	50.5	77.6
France	23.7	6.6	34.7	8.6	39.2
Germany	26	20.4	55.1	23.9	59
India	21.1	1.4	15.2	2.9	21.2
Israel	26.5	24.3	57.5	27.6	61.2
Japan	21.9	1.5	18.1	0.9	14.4
Kenya	22.2	1.9	21.7	2.6	24.9
Mexico	27.9	34.3	67.9	47.6	77.3
Nigeri	23.1	6.0	32.2	10.8	41.4
Sweden	24.6	10.9	44.9	13.9	49.5
Turkey	27.6	32.5	65.7	32.5	65.7
United kingdom	26.6	24.2	61.9	28.3	65.7
United states	28.8	41.8	72.6	54.3	80.2

The Viscous Cycle of Obesity and the Overnutrition Theory

A viscous cycle regarding obesity has been proposed.[24] During pregnancy, adult obesity causes an abnormal metabolic environment in utero. This in turn is associated with fetal-neonatal obesity even in the absence of frank gestational diabetes mellitus.[25] There is a large prevalence of overweight and obesity in those born large.[26] Increased prevalence of childhood obesity and probably a state of insulin resistance is related to an increased risk of the metabolic syndrome and accounts for the increase in type II diabetes particularly among the young. This increased prevalence in childhood obesity and insulin resistance is directly related to adolescent and adult obesity and the development of the metabolic syndrome.

Barker et al.[27] have been strong proponents of the fetal origin of adult disease hypothesis. Converging lines of evidence from epidemiological studies and animal models indicate that the origins of obesity and related metabolic disorders lie not only in the interaction between genes and traditional adult risk factors, such as unbalanced diet and physical inactivity, but also in the interplay between genes and the embryonic environment.[28] There is now convincing evidence that, in both human and animal models, the in utero environment may impact fetal developmental processes, altering offspring homeostatic regulatory mechanisms. "Gestational programming" may result in altered cell number, organ structure, hormonal set points or gene expression, with effects being permanent or expressed only at select offspring ages (e.g., newborn, childhood, adolescence, adulthood).[28]

It has been suggested that intrauterine overnutrition affects the lifelong risk of obesity. According to this hypothesis, high maternal plasma concentrations of glucose, free fatty acids, and amino acids result in permanent changes in appetite control, neuroendocrine functioning, or energy metabolism in the developing fetus and thus lead to obesity in later life. Since maternal BMI is positively associated with insulin resistance and glucose intolerance, and therefore higher plasma concentrations of glucose and free fatty acids, fetal overnutrition is more likely among mothers with greater BMI during pregnancy.[29] This hypothesis (if true) is important in explaining a pattern of anticipation in the prevalence of obesity and consequent decline in public health. This would mean that the obesity epidemic could accelerate through successive generations independent of further genetic or environmental factors.[30] In contrast, Lawler et al.[31] aimed to test this hypothesis by determining whether maternal BMI is more strongly related than paternal BMI to offspring fat mass, and by using genetic variants associated with maternal adiposity as instrumental variables for the causal association of maternal adiposity with offspring adiposity. They found that neither parental comparisons nor the use of genetic variants (fat mass and obesity associated (FTO) gene) as an instrumental variable, suggested that greater maternal BMI during offspring development had a marked effect on offspring fat mass at age 9-11 years. They concluded that developmental overnutrition related to greater maternal BMI was unlikely to have driven the recent obesity epidemic.[31]

Adverse Outcomes Associated with Maternal Overweight and Obesity

Overweight and obesity most likely contribute substantially to the burden of chronic health conditions. They are associated with a variety of adverse medical conditions such as cardiovascular disease, some types of cancer, diabetes mellitus, stroke, respiratory problems and arthritis.[32] Overweight and obesity have been associated with an increased risk of adverse pregnancy outcomes.[9,33-34] These complications could be divided into three groups:

1) Offspring complications from early pregnancy into adult life such as birth defects (including neural tube defects (NTD) and to a lesser degree some heart defect), miscarriages, perinatal mortality, impaired clinical and sonographic assessment of the fetus, macrosomia and long term complications into adult life.
2) Maternal complications such as infertility, preterm birth, hypertensive disorders (including preeclampsia/eclampsia), diabetes mellitus, thromboembolic disorders and postpregnancy weight retention.
3) Intrapartum and surgical complications including shoulder dystocia, inadequate labor progress, cesarean delivery, anesthetic complications and wound infections.

Offspring Complications from Early Pregnancy into Adult Life

Birth Defects and Congenital Malformations

An association between maternal obesity and congenital malformations (especially NTD) has been reported.[35-38] However, controversy exists regarding this association. While several studies suggested that obesity is indeed a risk factor for malformations, and mostly neural tube defects (NTD)[35-42], others did not find such an association[23,43]. Other reported anomalies include congenital heart defects,[44] multiple anomalies,[40] other defects of the central nervous system, great vessel defects, ventral wall defects and other intestinal defects.[36]

Recently, Rasmussen et al.[42] conducted a metaanalysis of published evidence on the relationship between maternal obesity and the risk of NTDs. Twelve studies met inclusion criteria. Unadjusted odds ratios for an NTD-affected pregnancy were 1.22 (95% CI, 0.99-1.49) among overweight women, 1.70 (95% CI, 1.34-2.15) among obese women, and 3.11 (95% CI, 1.75-5.46) among severely obese women, compared with normal-weight women. They concluded that maternal obesity is indeed associated with an increased risk of an NTD-affected pregnancy.[42]

Watkins et al.[40] explored the relation for several birth defects and obesity in a population-based case-control study, using data from the Atlanta Birth Defects Risk Factor Surveillance Study. Mothers who delivered an infant with and without selected birth defects in the five-county Atlanta metropolitan area between January 1993 and August 1997 were interviewed. The risks for obese women (BMI > or =30) and overweight women (BMI 25.0-29.9) were compared with those for average-weight women (BMI 18.5-24.9). Obese women were more likely than average-weight women to have an infant with spina bifida (unadjusted OR 3.5; 95% CI 1.2-10.3), omphalocele (OR: 3.3; 95% CI: 1.0-10.3), heart defects (OR: 2.0; 95% CI: 1.2-3.4), and multiple anomalies (OR: 2.0; 95% CI: 1.0-3.8). Overweight women were more likely than average-weight women to have infants with heart defects (OR: 2.0; 95% CI: 1.2-3.1) and multiple anomalies (OR: 1.9; 95% CI: 1.1-3.4). The authors concluded that obesity is significantly associated with spina bifida, omphalocele, heart defects, and multiple anomalies.[40]

Cedergren and Kallen[44] found a positive association between maternal obesity in early pregnancy and congenital heart defects in the offspring. They examined, in a prospective case-control study from the Swedish medical health registers, whether the offspring of obese women have an increased risk of cardiovascular defects compared with the offspring of average weight women. In the group of obese mothers, there was an increased risk for cardiovascular defects compared with average weight mothers [adjusted odds ratio (OR) = 1.18; 95% CI, 1.09 to 1.27], which was slightly more pronounced for the severe types of cardiovascular defects (adjusted OR = 1.23; 95% CI, 1.05 to 1.44). With morbid obesity, the OR for cardiovascular defects was 1.40 (95% CI, 1.22 to 1.64), and for severe cardiovascular defects, the OR was 1.69 (95% CI, 1.27 to 2.26). There was an increased risk for all specific defects studied among the obese women, but only ventricular septal defects and atrial septal defects reached statistical significance.[44]

The exact reasons for an association between congenital malformations and maternal obesity are poorly understood, although some explanations have been implicated such as: undetected pre-gestational diabetes mellitus, with an increase in serum insulin, triglycerides, uric acid and insulin resistance, technical problems with the ultrasound detection (reducing rates of early terminations) and lower folic acid levels. It is likely that yet unidentified explanations may exist.[45] Pre-gestational diabetes mellitus is a well-established risk factor for congenital anomalies[46-47] and the association with obesity is significant.[23,45,48] Sheiner et al.[23] investigated the association between obesity and congenital malformations after excluding patients with diabetes mellitus and did not find such an association.[23]

Lower circulating levels of folic acid has been suggested as an explanation for the increased prevalence of NTD's in the offspring of obese mothers.[45] However, the higher risk of NTD in obese patients remained even after universal folic acid flour fortification.[39] In Canada By late 1997, all refined wheat flour was fortified with folic acid. Because overweight women may consume greater quantities of refined wheat flour, Ray et al.[39] questioned whether their risk of NTD changed after flour fortification.[39] The presence of NTDs was systematically detected both antenatally and postnatally among Ontarian women who underwent antenatal maternal screening at 15 to 20 weeks of gestation. A total of 292 open NTDs were detected among 420,362 women. The adjusted OR for NTD was 1.2 (95% CI 1.1-1.3) per 10-kg incremental rise in maternal weight. The interaction between elevated maternal weight and the presence of folic acid flour fortification was of borderline significance (P = 0.09). Before fortification, greater maternal weight was associated with a modestly increased risk of NTD (adjusted OR 1.4, 95% CI 1.0-1.8); after flour fortification, this effect was more pronounced (adjusted OR 2.8, 95% CI 1.2-6.6). Thus, higher risk of

NTD is associated with increased maternal weight, even after universal folic acid flour fortification. It is noteworthy that maternal serum alpha-fetoprotein (AFP) levels between 15 and 20 weeks of pregnancy are significantly related to maternal weight (r = 0.24, p < 0.0001).[49] This is probably due to greater plasma volume in obese patients. It is possible that in obese women, the results of serum markers for NTD are harder to interpret.

Miscarriages

Obese women are at risk of various obstetrical problems at early pregnancy. Obesity is associated with an increased risk of early and recurrent miscarriages. In addition, Obesity has a negative impact on infertility treatment and if conception occurs, there is an increased risk of pregnancy loss.[50] Miscarriages in obese patients typically occur early in gestation, with the majority of studies describing pregnancy loss by 6-7 weeks gestation as detected by ultrasound.[51-53]

Lashen et al.[52] performed a nested case-control study, and compared a total of 1644 obese and 3288 age-matched normal weight controls (BMI 19-24.9 kg/m2). The risks of early miscarriage (OR 1.2, 95% CI 1.01-1.46; P = 0.04) and recurrent abortions (OR 3.5, 95% CI 1.03-12.01; P = 0.04) were significantly higher among the obese patients. The authors concluded that obesity is associated with an increased risk of first trimester and recurrent miscarriage.[52] Likewise, Sheiner et al.[23] conducted a large population-based study in the Negev, the southern part of Israel, and compared all pregnancies of obese (BMI >30 kg/m2) and non-obese patients. Recurrent abortions were significantly more common among the obese vs. the non-obese population (7.4% vs. 4.8%; OR 1.5; 95% CI 1.2-1.9; P<0.001). This association was significant for patients following fertility treatments as well as for those who conceived spontaneously.

Three cohort studies have suggested that obesity is an independent risk factor for spontaneous miscarriage in women who undergo fertility treatment[53-55]. In overweight women conceiving after IVF or intracytoplasmic sperm injection, an increased abortion rate over the first 6 weeks (22% versus 12%) was found, compared with lean or average weight women (RR 1.77; 95% CI 1.05–2.97).[53] Multivariate logistic regression analysis revealed that obesity and low oocyte count were independently associated with spontaneous abortion. Low oocyte count was associated with a higher increase in the risk of abortion in obese compared with lean patients. Interestingly, the effects of age, history of past pregnancies, or infertility diagnosis on the probability of miscarriage were not significant. The authors concluded that obesity is an independent risk factor for early pregnancy loss.[53] With ovulation induction using gonadotrophin-releasing hormone, there is a three-fold increase in the risk of pregnancy resulting in miscarriage,[54] and with egg donation in women with a BMI greater than 30 kg/m2, there is a four-fold increased risk of miscarriage.[53] Obesity is common among women with polycystic ovary syndrome (PCOS), occurring in 35–40% of patients.[50] The higher risk of spontaneous abortion observed in women with PCOS is most likely owed to their high prevalence of obesity.[55]

The preconception counseling of obese patients should point out the increased risk for sub-fertility as well as the risk for recurrent early abortions. Some authors suggest that obese patients should be denied treatment of any kind aimed to improve ovulation rates and achieve pregnancy until they have reduced their BMI.[56] It is recommended that weight loss be considered as a first option in women planning pregnancy, especially before undergoing infertility treatments.[56-58]

Perinatal and Neonatal Mortality

Maternal obesity has consistently been associated with increased rates of fetal and early neonatal death[10, 50, 59-60] .The mechanism of fetal compromise has not been fully determined and is likely to be multifactorial. The combination of rapid fetal growth induced by hyperinsulinemia that is noticed in obese women and the functional limitations of the placenta to transfer sufficient oxygen to the fetus leading to relative fetal hypoxia may be one explanation.[50,60]

In a prospective population-based cohort study (n = 3,480), a three-fold increase in antepartum stillbirth was found in morbidly obese women compared with women with a normal BMI.[33] In a large Swedish population-based cohort study (n = 167 750), the risk of late fetal death increased consistently with increasing prepregnancy BMI. Among nulliparous women, the risk of late fetal death was doubled among women with a normal BMI as compared with lean women, tripled among those who were overweight and quadrupled among those who were obese. Among the parous women, the risk of late fetal death was significantly increased only among obese women. For early neonatal death, the risk was doubled in nulliparous women with a higher BMI, but this was not true in parous women.[9]

Stephansson et al.[61] investigated The Swedish Medical Birth Register and also found that after controlling for multiple variables, overweight and obese women had a two-fold increase in the risk of term antepartum stillbirth. However, weight gain during pregnancy was not associated with an increased risk of antepartum stillbirth.[61]

In a study of 24,505 singleton pregnancies from Denmark, obesity was associated with a significantly greater risk of stillbirth (OR 2.8, 95% CI 1.5-5.3) and neonatal death (OR 2.6, 95% CI 1.2-5.8) compared with women of normal weight.[62] Another recent Danish study of 54,505 pregnant women, Nohr et al.[63] found that the risk for fetal death among obese women significantly increased with gestational age from a RR of 1.9 at 20-27 weeks gestation' to 2.1 at 28-36 weeks, and 4.6 beyond 40 weeks gestation. Overweight women were also at increased risk for fetal death beyond 28 weeks.[63]

Large population studies in the US and UK found that infants of obese women were nearly twice as likely to die in the first year of life, than those of normal weight women.[12,34] Chen et al [64] investigated the association of maternal obesity and infant death, neonatal and postneonatal death (infants who died with 28 days after birth and infants who died after 28 days but before one year, respectively) in the United States. They found that maternal obesity is associated with increased overall risk of infant death, mainly neonatal death.[64]

Suboptimal Clinical and Sonographic Assessment of the Fetus

Clinical guidelines for adequate fetal growth are unhelpful in morbidly obese women. Similarly, customized growth charts are not meaningful in this group. Fetal macrosomia on one hand and growth restriction on the other as well as malpresentation can all be easily missed.[60]

Ultrasound in obese women is often suboptimal.[50] Sonograms from 1622 consecutively scanned singleton pregnancies at a mean gestational age of 28.5 weeks were analyzed to determine whether maternal obesity affected visualization of fetal anatomy. Fetal head (cerebral ventricles), heart (four-chamber view), stomach, kidneys, bladder, diaphragm, intestines, spinal column, extremities, and umbilical cord were classified as visualized or suboptimally visualized. Maternal BMI was used as a measure of relative leanness. With a BMI beyond the 90th percentile, visualization fell by an average of 14.5%. Reduction in visualization was most marked for the fetal heart, umbilical cord, and spine. Among obese women, BMI was the best predictor of visualization.[65]

Likewise, Handler et al[66] examined the impact of maternal obesity on the rate of suboptimal ultrasound visualization of fetal anatomy in order to determine the optimal timing of prenatal ultrasound examination for the obese parturient. More than 11,000 pregnancies were studied, of which 38.6% of the patients were obese. The rate of suboptimal ultrasound visualization of the fetal structures was higher for obese compared to non-obese women. Increased severity of maternal obesity was associated with suboptimal ultrasound visualization rate for both the cardiac and the craniospinal structures.[67]

Macrosomia and Large for Gestational Age Neonates

Several studies have shown that maternal obesity and excessive weight gain during pregnancy are associated with macrosomic (> 4,000 g) or large for gestational age (LGA) neonates[23,34,63,68] (figure 1). Sukalich et al.[68] examined adverse obstetric outcomes in overweight adolescent parturients. They found a significantly increased incidence of macrosomia (OR 1.6; 95% CI 1.2-2.0) among overweight subjects as compared to appropriate-weight subjects.

The risk of macrosomia appears to be proportional to two independent risk factors, maternal prepregnancy weight and maternal weight gain during pregnancy.[60] A linear relationship between increasing maternal BMI and the incidence of macrosomia has been reported.[63,69] Ehrenberg et al.[70] studied the relative contribution of abnormal pregravid maternal body habitus and diabetes on the prevalence of LGA infants. They reviewed maternal and neonatal records for singleton term deliveries between January 1997 and June 2001. Subjects were characterized by pregravid BMI, divided into underweight (BMI <19.8 kg/m^2), normal (BMI 19.8-25 kg/m^2), overweight (BMI 25.1-30 kg/m^2), and obese (BMI >30 kg/m^2) subgroups. Diabetes was classified as gestational, treated with diet alone (A1GDM), or with insulin (A2GDM), and pregestaional diabetes (PDM). Newborns weighing more than the 90th percentile for gestational age were defined as LGA. The risk of LGA delivery for underweight, overweight, and obese women were compared with that of women with normal pregravid BMI. Multiple regression models were constructed to examine the relative effect of abnormal BMI and diabetes on the risk of the delivery of an LGA infant. Obesity and pregestational diabetes were independently associated an increased risk of LGA delivery.

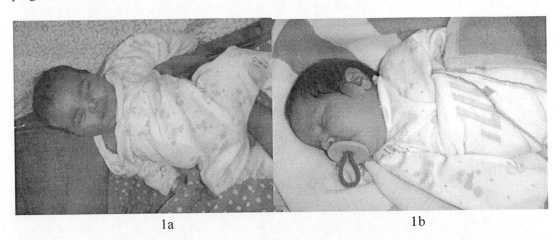

1a   1b

Figure 1. Two macrosomic babies delivered at the Soroka University Medical Center on July 4th , 2008: a) a female weighting 4510 grams, b) a male weighing 4700 grams.

Multiple factors have been associated with fetal overgrowth or macrosomia. Although maternal demographic factors such as age and weight gain play a significant role, they explain only a small fraction of the variance in fetal growth. In contrast, increased maternal pregravid weight and decreased pregravid insulin sensitivity are the strongest correlates with fetal growth, in particular fat mass at birth.[24] The mechanisms arc as yct not wcll dcfincd, but in early pregnancy increased maternal insulin resistance may be related to altered placental function as well as to increased fetoplacental availability of nutrients in late gestation, not only glucose but also free fatty acids and amino acids. Therefore, although women with GDM (even those who are treated and are under tight metabolic control) are at increased risk of having a macrosomic infant, women who are obese with normal glucose tolerance are potentially at a higher risk of having a macrosomic baby. Langer et al.[71] reported that, in obese women with GDM whose glucose was well controlled on diet alone, the odds of fetal macrosomia was significantly increased (OR=2.12) compared with women with well controlled (diet only) gestational diabetes mellitus (GDM) with normal BMI. Similar results were reported in women with GDM who were poorly controlled on diet or insulin.[71] The increase in birth weight or macrosomia may represent an increase in fat compared with fat free mass. Catalano et al.[72] reported that there is a significant increase in neonatal fat mass but not total body weight or fat free mass in appropriate birth weight infants of women with GDM as compared with a matched control group.[72]

Macrosomia raises the risk for additional labor and delivery complications such as shoulder dystocia, birth injury, and perinatal death. Furthermore, women with macrosomic neonates are more likely to undergo a cesarean delivery and suffer perineal trauma, chorioamnionitis or postpartum hemorrhage.[60]

Long Term Complications

Converging lines of evidence from epidemiological studies and animal models now indicate that the origins of obesity and related metabolic disorders lie not only in the interaction between genes and traditional adult risk factors, such as unbalanced diet and physical inactivity, but also in the interplay between genes and the embryonic, fetal and early postnatal environment [28].

Growth in utero is roughly summarized by birth weight, which if related to fatness later in life, might implicate the fetal environment in the development of obesity.[73] The relation between birth weight and fatness, measured in childhood or adulthood, is generally positive, although it is variable in magnitude.[74-75] A possible reason for this variability is that the strength of the relation may depend on the age at which fatness is measured. More importantly, several factors, such as gestational age, parental body size, and socioeconomic status, may confound the relation between birth weight and later fatness.[73] Parsons et al.[73] examined the influence of birth weight on BMI at different stages of later life and whether this relation persists after accounting for potential confounding factors. They found that in adulthood, BMI increased with increasing birth weight mainly at the heaviest birth weights. The relation between birth weight and BMI was influenced markedly by the mother's weight and BMI but was unaffected by the mother's height, age, or smoking habits, nor was it affected by the father's weight, or social class.[73]

Few studies were designed to investigate the direct association between maternal and offspring overweight or obesity, but several studies have indeed found a positive association. Laitinen et al.[76] reported that children of overweight or obese mothers had higher mean BMIs at each age point tested than did children born to underweight or normal weight mothers. At 31 years, overweight and obesity were more common in subjects whose mothers were overweight or obese before pregnancy (men: 43% overweight and 12% obese; women: 27% overweight and 14% obese) as compared to subjects whose mothers were underweight or of normal weight (men: 39% overweight and 7% obese; women: 18% overweight and 7% obese; P < 0.001). Circumferences of the waist and hip and waist-to-hip ratios of the offspring at 31 y increased as maternal BMI increased.[76]

Dabelea et al.[77] reported that the mean adolescent BMI was 2.6 kg/m2 greater in sibling offspring of diabetic pregnancies compared with the index siblings born when the mother previously had normal glucose tolerance. Since obesity and diabetes are closely associated, both maternal pregravid obesity and the presence of maternal diabetes may independently affect the risk of adolescent obesity in the offspring.

This risk of developing the metabolic syndrome (MS) in adolescents was recently addressed by Boney et al.[78] in a longitudinal cohort study of appropriate for gestational age (AGA) and large for gestational age (LGA) infants of women with normal glucose tolerance and GDM. The MS was defined as the presence of two or more of the following components: obesity, hypertension, glucose intolerance, and dyslipidemia. Maternal obesity was defined as a pregravid BMI greater than 27.3. Interestingly, they found that exposure of children to maternal obesity was as strong a predictor of risk for MS as LGA status (1.81, 95% CI 1.03–3.19, P<0.04 and 2.19, 95% CI 1.25–3.82, P<0.01 respectably). This suggests that, among obese mothers without clinical GDM, fetal hyperinsulinemia might develop because of mild maternal hyperglycemia that is below the threshold for a diagnosis of GDM or occurs later in the pregnancy, after screening. This is consistent with other studies showing that maternal obesity is a risk factor for LGA birth in the absence of evident GDM.[25]

Overweight and Obesity Associated Maternal Complications

Infertility

Fertility is extremely sensitive to bodyweight. In females a critical threshold of body fat is needed in order to enter puberty, ensuring she could bare a pregnancy to term. Obesity has a negative affect on fertility.[79] In women, early onset of obesity is responsible, at least in part, for the development of menses irregularities, chronic oligo/anovulation and infertility in the adult age.[80] Obesity may manifest several effects on female reproduction including altered levels of hypothalamic gonadotropins, anovulation, altered steroid production, reduced conception rates, and longer times to conception. Obesity also increases the risk of miscarriages and many pregnancy complications.[80] In women undergoing assisted reproductive technologies, obesity can impair the outcomes. These adverse effects of obesity are specifically evident in patients with polycystic ovary syndrome.[79]

Altered gonadotropin and steroid hormone levels initially contribute to anovulation.[80] Even in women who ovulate regularly, increased BMI correlates with reduced conception rates [81-82]. van der Steeg et al.[82] examined whether obesity affected the chance of a spontaneous pregnancy in a prospective cohort of 3029 consecutive subfertile couples. They found that the probability of a spontaneous pregnancy declined linearly with a BMI over 29 kg/m^2. When they corrected for possible confounders, they found that obese women had a 4% lower pregnancy rate per kg/m^2 increase [hazard ratio: 0.96 (95% CI 0.91-0.99)]. They concluded that obesity is associated with lower pregnancy rates in subfertile ovulatory women.[82]

Insulin excess and insulin resistance have been implicated as main factors responsible for the association of obesity and infertility.[79] These observations could also be explained by the affects of obesity on periconceptional oocyte and/or embryo quality. The decreased pregnancy rates seen with increasing BMI are primarily due to loss of the pre or peri implantation windows, which may indicate the presence of suboptimal embryos. Since the earliest stages of embryo growth are controlled by the oocyte developmental competence (quality of the oocyte), it is likely that alterations to the oocyte contribute to the reduced conception and pregnancy rates seen in obese women.[80]

It is almost impossible to evaluate oocyte quality in women attempting to conceive naturally. In vitro fertilization (IVF) enables close inspection of oocytes and their fertilization and subsequent development into blastocyst, before uterine transfer and implantation take place.[80] Clinical observations on the effect of BMI on IVF success are controversial.[51,83-89] While some authors have found no difference in IVF results between obese and normal weight women,[85-86] others have shown a decrease in pregnancy and live birth rates in overweight and obese women.[51,87-88] In a large Dutch study, BMI > 27 was associated with a lower birth rate per IVF cycle. However, no significant difference was found when live birth rate per oocyte retrieval was compared with the normal weight group.[89] Likewise, Dokras et al.[84] reported a significantly higher risk for IVF cycle cancellation in morbidly obese patients with no effect of BMI on clinical pregnancy or delivery rate.[84] Possible explanations for these differences include increased gonadotropin requirement during ovarian stimulation, fewer retrieved oocytes, decreased serum estradiol concentrations, increased cancellation rates and lower fertilization rates.[83]

In men, obesity is associated with low testosterone levels. In morbidly obese men, reduced spermatogenesis associated with severe hypotestosteronemia may cause infertility. Moreover, the frequency of erectile dysfunction increases with increasing BMI.[79]

Preterm Birth

Due to the increasing rate of obesity and of preterm births (PTB) investigations regarding an association between them have been published.[33-34] Cedergren[33] evaluated whether morbidly obese women have an increased risk of pregnancy complications and adverse perinatal outcomes. She conducted a prospective population-based cohort study, and compared 3,480 women with morbid obesity (BMI > 40), and 12,698 obese women (BMI 35.1-40) with normal-weight women (BMI 19.8-26). They found that for overweight women (BMI 29.1-35) the odds ratios (95% CI) for delivery before 37 and before 32 weeks of gestation were 1.22 (1.14-1.31) and 1.45 (1.32-1.59), respectively. For obese women (BMI 35.1-40) the odds ratios (95% CI) for delivery before 37 and before 32 weeks of gestation were 1.48 (1.37-1.59) and 1.95 (1.65-2.31), respectively. For morbidly obese women (BMI >40) the odds ratios (95% CI) for delivery before 37 and before 32 weeks of gestation were 1.85 (1.63-2.10) and 2.32 (1.73-3.12), respectively.[33]

Likewise, Baeten JM et al.[34] found that obese and overweight women were at elevated risk for delivering prematurely (<37 weeks' gestation) and very prematurely (≤32 weeks' gestation) compared with lean women, although only the risk for obese women of very premature delivery was more than marginal.[34]

Morbid obesity was associated with preterm birth. Even after excluding patients with preeclampsia, morbidly obese women were more likely to be induced.[33] Findings suggest that, while obesity may not be an independent risk factor for PTB, obesity does increase rates of medical complications (such as hypertension and diabetes) that have been shown to contribute to PTB. Hence, most of these preterm deliveries are probably elective due to maternal complications rather than being spontaneous preterm births. Indeed, while excluding cases of hypertensive disorders and diabetes mellitus, no significant differences in gestational age were noted between obese and non obese parturients (39.2 vs. 39.1 weeks; P=0.122).[23] Regardless of the etiology, these preterm infants have an increased risk of neonatal mortality and the surviving offspring is likely to have an increased risk of long term disability due to chronic respiratory problems and neurodevelopmental impairment.[90-91]

Hypertensive Disorders and Preeclampsia

Nonpregnant obese women have a significantly increased risk for what has been termed the metabolic syndrome, X syndrome or the insulin resistance syndrome. Central obesity defined by an elevated waist-to-hip ratio and insulin resistance lei at the core of this syndrome. Clinically, this syndrome is characterized by hypertension, glucose intolerance and dyslipidemia (hypercholesterolemia and hypertriglyceridemia).[48]

Chronic hypertension may be present prior to conception, or elevated blood pressure may appear initially in pregnancy (gestational hypertension), with or without other features of the preeclampsia syndrome (ie, proteinuria, elevated liver enzymes, and thrombocytopenia). The discriminations between pregnancy associated hypertension and essential hypertension is not clear and their diagnosis is not uniform throughout studies. This has led to a wide variation in the prevalence of hypertension in severely obese pregnant women from 5% to 66% in different studies.[50] Nevertheless, the overlapping spectrum of hypertensive disorders is definitely seen more commonly in obese women and its incidence is rising in the past two decades.[60]

In a large population-based cohort study using the Nova Scotia Atlee Perinatal Database, maternal outcomes in obese and nonobese women were compared. The study included 142,404 singleton pregnancies, 10,134 (7.2%) women were identified as obese (moderate obesity 92.3%, severe obesity 7.7%). Moderately obese women had an increased risk of pregnancy-induced hypertension (PIH) (adjusted OR 2.38, 95% CI 2.24-2.52) and severely obese women had an increased risk of PIH (adjusted OR 3.00, 95% CI 2.49-3.62).[92] In a prospective multicenter study of 16,102 women, 85% were controls (BMI less than 30), 9% were obese (BMI 30–34.9), and 6% were morbidly obese (BMI 35 or greater), Weiss et al., reported that obese women and morbidly obese women were 2.5 and 3.2 times respectively, more likely to develop gestational hypertension than the control group.[93] Similarly, in another recent prospective cohort study comparing consecutive deliveries of obese and nonobese patients from southern Israel, Burstein et al., found that obesity is a risk factor for developing gestational hypertension.[94]

The manifestations of the metabolic syndrome (obesity, insulin resistance and hypertriglyceridemia) are major contributors to the development of endothelial dysfunction, which in turn, is a central in the pathogenesis of preeclampsia. Endothelial dysfunction decreases prostacyclin secretion and enhances peroxydase production causing vasoconstriction and platelet aggregation.[60] Preeclampsia occurs in 5-7% of healthy nulliparous women and is a leading cause of maternal death and the most common cause of fetal death in the US.[95] Maternal obesity is a well established risk factor for the development of preeclampsia. Large population based studies have shown a two to threefold increased risk of developing preeclampsia in obese women compared with normal weight women.[96-97] A large Scandinavian study found that the incidence rose with maternal weight from 2.8% in lean women to 10.2% in obese women.[9] In the previously mentioned study by Weiss et al.[93], obese women and morbidly obese women were 1.6 and 3.3 times respectively, more likely to develop preeclampsia than the control group.

The association between obesity and hypertensive disorders may be confounded by the presence of chronic hypertension, diabetes mellitus and other elements of the metabolic syndrome. However, even in glucose-tolerant women, obesity is an independent predictor of preeclampsia.[98] A systematic overview of the literature conducted by O'brien et al.[96] included thirteen cohort studies, comprising nearly 1.4 million women. The risk of preeclampsia typically doubled with each 5-7 kg/m2 increase in prepregnancy body mass index. This relation persisted in studies that excluded women with chronic hypertension, diabetes mellitus or multiple gestations, or after adjustment for other confounders. Yogev et al.[99] showed that, in women with well-controlled GDM, there is a significant increased risk of preeclampsia in obese (10.8%) compared with average BMI women (8.2%). The risk of preeclampsia is also increased in obese women with GDM with poor glycemic control (14.9%).[99] Furthermore, Crowther et al.[100], in the Australian Carbohydrate Intolerance Study in Pregnant Women (ACHOIS), reported that the risk of preeclampsia in the intervention group for GDM was 12%, whereas in the routine care group the risk was 18% (P<0.02). Therefore, although currently proven therapies to prevent the development of preeclampsia in obese women are yet unknown, it has been suggested that tight glucose control in obese women with GDM may decrease the risk.[48]

Increase in oxidative stress generated from maternal adipose tissue has been suggested to play a role in the pathogenesis of preeclampsia in obese women. Therefore the use of antioxidants to prevent preeclampsia in obese women may have a theoretical benefit. However, two recent randomized controlled trials, have reported no benefit of antioxidants in the reduction of preeclampsia in treatment compared with placebo-controlled groups.[101-102] In the Vitamins in Preeclampsia trial, the investigators examined the risk of preeclampsia in primiparous women with a BMI greater than 30 at enrollment. In this subgroup, no benefit of antioxidants in decreasing the risk of preeclampsia was found.[102] To date, the results of clinical trials regarding the use of antioxidants to prevent preeclampsia are not definitive as to their efficacy and are currently still in progress.[48]

Diabetes Mellitus

Obesity is associated with tissue insulin resistance, decreased glucose uptake in skeletal muscle and adipose tissue, and enhancement of hepatic glucose production.[103] Obese pregnant women have higher fasting and postprandial insulin concentrations than non-obese women. Adipose tissue is a source of inflammatory cytokines and other metabolically active mediators. Obesity has been characterized as a state of low-grade chronic inflammation. Obese pregnant women have elevated concentrations of C-reactive protein and higher fasting and postprandial insulin concentrations than non-obese women.[104]

Gestational diabetes mellitus (GDM) is glucose intolerance first recognized during pregnancy and results in insufficient insulin secretion to compensate for the increase in insulin resistance during pregnancy. GDM may be the most significant obesity-related pregnancy complication, occurring in 3%-5% of all pregnancies and is a major cause of perinatal morbidity and mortality, as well as maternal morbidity.[105] Obesity has been repeatedly shown to be a risk factor for the development of GDM.[9,12,93-94,106] The risk of GDM increases with rising maternal BMI.

Weiss et al.[93] in the FASTER study reported that after adjusting for confounders, the odds ratio for the risk of GDM was 2.6 (95% CI 2.1-3.4, P<0.001) for obese and 4.0 (95% CI 3.1-5.2, P<0.01) for morbidly obese women. In a UK study, women with a BMI greater than 30 kg/m^2 were 3.6 times more likely to develop GDM compared with normal BMI women.[12] In a large study from Denmark that included 8092 women, the odds of developing GDM increased with increasing BMI (BMI < 25 kg/m^2, OR 1; BMI 25-29 kg/m^2, OR 3.4; BMI > 30 kg/m^2, OR 15.3).[106]

Weight change in obese women is another important factor in the development of GDM. In an observational study, after adjusting for maternal age, Glazer et al.[107], reported that women who lost 10 pounds between pregnancies were found to have a decreased risk of GDM with a relative risk (RR) of 0.63 (95% CI 0.38-1.02). However, a gain of 10 pounds between pregnancies was associated with an increased risk of GDM (RR = 1.47; 95% CI 1.05-2.04).[107]

Due to the increasing prevalence of obesity and advanced maternal age during pregnancy, a substantial increase in the prevalence of women entering pregnancy with type 2 diabetes mellitus (T2DM) has been noted.[60] T2DM is a condition that was previously considered to be a disease of old age and currently it is being encountered in younger women.[108]

Women with poorly controlled GDM at delivery are at increased risk of adverse outcomes such as respiratory distress, preeclampsia, preterm delivery, cesarean section as well as other complications.[103] A recent study of 4001 women with GDM treated either solely with a diet or with insulin found that obese women were at higher risk of adverse perinatal outcomes than normal weight women.[71]

T2DM, discovered in a pregnancy, is difficult to distinguish from GDM, until after delivery. The onset of hyperglycemia prior to 20 weeks gestation, development of fasting hyperglycemia or large insulin requirements are factors that may predict underlying T2DM. Screening for GDM is usually undertaken at 24-28 weeks gestation. In obese women with a family history of T2DM earlier screening tests may be justified due to an increased risk of T2DM with earlier onset of hyperglycemia.[60]

Thromboembolic Disorders

The risk of venous thromboembolism (VTE) in pregnancy is approximately six times greater than in non-pregnant women and is a major cause of death among women during pregnancy and the puerperium. Pulmonary embolism occurs in approximately 16% of patients with untreated deep vein thrombosis (DVT), and is the most common cause of maternal death. Maternal DVT is more common in the left leg (accounting for about 85% of leg thrombosis), occurs more commonly in iliofemoral veins than in calf veins (72% compared with 9%, respectively), and is more often associated with pulmonary embolism.[109]

Pregnancy is a hypercoagulable state, and obesity further increases the risk of thrombosis by promoting venous stasis, increasing blood viscosity and promoting activation of the coagulation cascade. The greatest risk is at term, and especially in association with caesarean delivery.[60]

In a retrospective study of 683 obese and 660 normal weight women, the incidence of thromboembolic disease was 2.3% in the obese group and 0.6% in the normal group.[110] In a recent study from Australia, it was noted that 75% of patients suffering thromboembolism during pregnancy were obese.[111]

Thromboembolism is the leading cause of maternal death in pregnancy and as a result of increasing rates of maternal obesity its incidence is likely to increase in the future. Based on safety data, a heparin-related compound (unfractionated heparin, and low molecular weight heparin) is the anticoagulant of choice during pregnancy for situations in which its efficacy is established.[112]

Postpregnancy Weight Retention

Women may experience significant weight retention after childbirth. Excess weight gain during pregnancy and a failure to lose weight thereafter are important predictors of long term weight change and higher BMI in later life.[10,60] Interpregnancy weight gain is strongly related with adverse maternal and perinatal outcomes. Gaining three or more BMI units during an average two year postpartum period, was related to an increased risk of adverse outcomes during the subsequent pregnancy, such as preeclampsia, gestational hypertension, gestational diabetes, caesarean delivery, stillbirth and deliveries of large-for-gestational-age neonates.[113] Over the decades of postreproductive life, the impact of pregnancy associated weight retention may increase the long term obesity-related-morbidity (ie. cardiovascular disease).[60]

A review of nine studies suggested that the average postpartum weight retention was 0.5-3 kg but could be as high as 17.7 kg.[114] These studies used varied methodologies to assess body weight, and different follow-up protocols. Therefore, drawing definite conclusions from these studies is limited.

Some studies have suggested that there is a direct association between weight increases during pregnancy and both the short term[115] and long term[116-117] postpartum weight retention. Rooney and Schauberger[116] followed 540 women for an average of 8.5 years after childbirth. Women, who gained less than the Institute Of Medicine (IOM)-recommended weight during pregnancy, increased their weight 4.1 kg from their prepregnancy weight. Those who gained the recommended amount of weight were 6.5 kg heavier than their prepregnancy weight, and those who gained more than recommended were 8.4 kg heavier (P =.01).[116] Similarly, Linne et al.[117], investigated women's weight in different time point (before, during, one year after and 15 years after pregnancy). Weight retention one year after pregnancy predicted 15 years later. In addition, normal weight women who gained weight excessively during pregnancy (average gain 18.8 kg) were more likely to become overweight. In should be noted that prepregnancy BMI was not found to be associated with long term weight retention.[117]

Intrapartum and Surgical Complications Associated with Maternal Obesity

Shoulder Dystocia

Shoulder dystocia (SD) occurs when delivery beyond the fetal head is obstructed by the encasement of the fetal shoulders and is considered an obstetric emergency. The consequences of SD include fetal fractures, neurological and hypoxic injury and in rare occasions death of the neonate.

Macrosomia is the single most important risk factor for SD and increasing fetal weight correlates directly with incidence of SD. Robinson et al.[118], found that obese women had a twofold increased risk of SD (OR: 2.1 95% CI 1.4-3.2), however, when controlled for confounders, obesity was no longer associated with SD[118]. Even more so, Mazouni et al.[119], found, in a univariate analysis, that SD was 3.6 times more likely in obese women (95% CI 2.1-6.3). In multiple regression analysis, obesity and multiparity were the most significant maternal risk factors for shoulder dystocia[119]. Likewise, in Sweden, Cedergren[33] found that the risk for SD increased with increased maternal BMI (adjusted OR 2.14, 95% CI 1.83-2.49 for women with BMI 29.1-35.0; adjusted OR 2.82, 95% CI 2.10-3.71 for women with BMI 35.1-40.0; and adjusted OR 3.14, 95% CI 1.86-5.31 for women with BMI >40.0).[33]

Inadequate Labor Progress

It has been suggested that initiation and progress of labor are more likely to be challenging in obese women. Induction and augmentation of labor in obese women, are more commonly employed (two to three times) than in lean women, with up to a quarter of obese women requiring intrapartum oxytocin treatment.[33,60,120-123] Among women undergoing induction of labor, those in the highest weight quartile, have slower progress of cervical dilation and longer labors.[123]

Cedergren[33] found that the risk for induction of labor increased with increased maternal BMI (adjusted OR 1.77, 95% CI 1.73-1.81 for women with BMI 29.1-35.0; adjusted OR 2.27, 95% CI 2.16-2.38 for women with BMI 35.1-40.0; and adjusted OR 2.53, 95% CI 2.32-2.75 for women with BMI >40.0).[33] Likewise, Nuthalapaty et al.[121] demonstrated that in nulliparous women, after adjusting for the confounders, the rate of cervical dilation was inversely associated with maternal weight. For each 10-kg increment in maternal weight, the rate of dilation was decreased by 0.04 cm/h (P =0.05). In addition, labor duration was positively associated with maternal weight. For each 10-kg increment in maternal weight, an increase in the oxytocin to delivery interval of 0.3 hours was observed (P =.02)[121]

Cesarean Delivery

In addition to increased risk for obstetric complications in obese women, several studies have reported that obese women are more likely to be delivered by caesarean delivery

(CD).[23,48,50,60,124] It is possible that CD in obese women are more often indicated for the management of pregnancy complications such as preeclampsia, GDM or suspected fetal macrosomia. Alternatively, it is possible that the soft tissue excess in the maternal pelvis complicates vaginal delivery and increases the necessity for CD in obese women.[60]

Some conditions that are independent risk factors for CD and constitute leading indications for surgery are more common among obese women. However, even in selected groups of patients without hypertension or diabetes mellitus, maternal obesity was found to be an independent risk factor for CD.[23] Among obese parturients higher rates of CD were found (27.8% vs. 10.8%; OR = 3.2; [95% CI 2.9, 3.5]; P < 0.001). After controlling for possible confounders, the association between maternal obesity and CD remained significant.

In an attempt to reduce morbidity associated with CD, vaginal birth after cesarean delivery (VBAC) is considered a reasonable and safe option. However, a decreased success rate has been reported in association with increased maternal BMI.[125] Durnwald et al.[125] investigated the impact of maternal obesity on the success of a trial of labor after a single low transverse cesarean delivery. In their study, 34% VBAC failure was noted. Decreased VBAC success was seen in obese women compared with women of normal BMI, (P = 0.003). When other factors were controlling for, the association between increasing pregravid BMI and BMI of 30 kg/m^2 or more, with decreased VBAC success, persisted (P = 0.03 and P = 0.006, respectively).[125]

Anesthetic Complications

The obese parturient poses a significant anesthetic risk. Women with a BMI of 35 kg/m^2 or greater are likely to have pre-existing medical conditions such as hypertension or diabetes, and this may further increase their anesthetic risks.[126-129]

Tracheal intubation is more difficult among obese parturients. Anatomical distortion and misidentification of anatomical landmarks have led to higher rates of epidural failure in obese mothers. Performing epidural anesthesia on morbidly obese patients may be extremely difficult.[126-129] Other intrapartum complications include increased risk of aspiration pneumonia due to an elevated gastric residual volume and lower gastric pH that is encountered in obese patients. In addition complications such as poor peripheral access, difficulty in monitoring maternal blood pressures, increased retention of lipid-soluble agents, increased drug distribution and more rapid desaturation have been reported.[60]

The significant difficulty in administering epidural analgesia should not prevent their use in labor. The prophylactic placement of an epidural catheter in laboring morbidly obese women, in order to potentially decrease anesthetic and perinatal complications associated with attempts at emergency provision of regional or general anesthesia, has been suggested.[126,128-130]

Wound Infections

Wound infections are a common surgical complication, often requiring a prolonged hospital stay and leading to increased costs. Multiple factors account for the increasing number of cesarean delivery wound complications, among these factors are the increase in the number of overweight and obese patients undergoing CD.[131-132]

In a prospective study from New Zealand, Beattie et al.[133] investigated factors involved in the development of post-CD wound infection. They found that maternal weight was a highly significant indicator of subsequent wound infection development (p = 0.0001), and that the relationship between increasing maternal weight and infection was a linear one.[133]

Overweight and obesity are independent risk factors for wound infection. Additionally, other factors associated with maternal obesity such as hypertensive disorders and diabetes mellitus have been recognized as independent risk factors for wound infection.[134] Schneid-Kofman et al. conducted a population-based study comparing women who have and have not developed a wound infection. During the study period, of 19,416 CD, 3.7% were complicated by wound infection. Obesity (OR 2.2; 95%CI 1.6-3.1) and diabetes mellitus (OR 1.4; 95%CI 1.1-1.7) were among the factors identified as associated with a wound infection in a multivariable logistic regression model. Furthermore, when obesity and diabetes (gestational and pregestational) were combined, the risk for wound infection was increased 9.3-fold (95%CI 4.5-19.2; P<0.001).[134] Information regarding higher rates of wound infection should be provided to obese women undergoing CD, especially when diabetes coexists.

The Treatment of Obesity

The goal of obesity treatment is to achieve and maintain a healthier weight. Both maternal and fetal complications are proportional to the degree of obesity and even moderate overweight amplifies the gestational risks. It has been shown that even small decreases in BMI, can improve women's health status and reduce the risk for some pregnancy complications as well as long-term consequences such as worsening of maternal obesity, maternal type 2 diabetes, and childhood obesity and metabolic disorders.

Achieving a healthy weight is usually done through dietary changes, increased activity and behavior modifications. In recent years prescription medication and weight-loss surgery (bariatric surgery) are becoming more popular. Optimal management includes preconception counseling, pregravid weight-loss programs, monitoring of gestational weight gain, repeated screening for pregnancy complications and long-term follow-up to minimize the social and economic consequences of pregnancy in overweight women.[135] Before conception, obese patients should receive tailored weight-loss counseling and be screened for obesity complications. Food intake during pregnancy should be tailored to achieve the minimum maternal weight gain required for normal fetal growth. Long-term follow-up is required to prevent worsening of maternal obesity after delivery, and the child's growth curve should be closely watched.

Bariatric Surgery for Obese Women

The best way to decrease the risk of medical and obstetric problems in obese women planning pregnancy is weight loss before conception. Given that lifestyle measures and medical treatments have had limited long-term success to date, more obese women of reproductive age are seeking bariatric surgery as an alternative.[48] Recently, it has been reported that pregnancies after bariatric surgery were uncomplicated and well tolerated by the mothers even in the presence of gestational diabetes mellitus.[43,136-137]

Although bariatric surgery appears to be the definitive answer for obesity-related gestational complications, pregnancy during the malnourished state following a successful weight loss procedure is not without potential risks.[138] Case reports and case series documenting poor perinatal outcomes and late surgical complications during pregnancies following bariatric surgery exist,[139–142] although systematic studies have generally failed to prove such associations.[43]

Available data suggests that risks for maternal complications, such as gestational diabetes and preeclampsia, may be lower following surgically induced weight loss than the risks in obese women and may approach rates of the general population. Similarly, neonatal complications, such as preterm delivery and macrosomia, may be lower in pregnancies following bariatric surgery. The effect of bariatric surgery on the need for CD is not entirely clear, since reported rates before and after surgery vary widely between studies.[143] A study from southern Israel, performed by our group, compared the perinatal outcomes of women who delivered before with women who delivered after bariatric surgery. A decrease in maternal complications, such as diabetes mellitus and hypertensive disorders, as well as a decrease in the rate of fetal macrosomia was found following bariatric surgery.[144]

Bariatric surgical procedures are categorized into two main types: malabsorptive procedures (jejunoileal bypass and biliopancreatic diversion) and restrictive procedures (gastric banding and vertical banded gastroplasty). Both types can result in deficiencies in iron, vitamin B_{12}, folate and calcium.[145] Nutritional problems during pregnancy following gastric banding or gastric bypass surgeries appear uncommon and many are attributed to supplement nonadherence. Reports of the relationship between bariatric surgery and fertility have shown normalization of sex hormones, menstrual irregularities, and improvement in polycystic ovarian syndrome following surgery. This suggested improved fertility is consistent with that observed in obese women after nonsurgically induced weight loss.[143]

Although rare, complications of bariatric surgery can manifest during pregnancy, internal hernia being the most common complication and may cause bowel compromise. There is no strong evidence to guide how long to delay pregnancy following bariatric surgery.[146] Typically, the recommended period is one year, coinciding with the cessation of the most rapid weight loss period. There is no convincing evidence to support or refute concerns about the use of oral contraceptive pills following bariatric surgery.[143]

Systematic studies have repeatedly failed to demonstrate elevated risk for adverse perinatal outcome in pregnancies following bariatric surgery. Although prevalence of certain complications (such as GDM and macrosomia) is higher in pregnancies following surgery compared with community controls,[43] rates are lower in comparison to obese cohorts,[144] suggesting bariatric surgery to be effective in preventing these obesity-related complications.[138]

Pregnancies following bariatric surgery appear to be safe but not all relevant concerns have been answered. Additional research is needed to clarify the optimal interval between the operation and subsequent pregnancy,[146] the effect that bariatric surgery might have on fertility, birth control, and risk for CD. Studies investigating differences in pregnancy outcomes between restrictive and malabsorptive procedures could better help clinicians in tailoring the appropriate bariatric procedure to the reproductive aged patient seeking pregnancy.

Summary

Obesity is a frequent condition with rising prevalence and it is recognized as a major worldwide health risk. One third of pregnant women are overweight and furthermore over one tenth are obese. Obesity in pregnancy is a predictor of obesity in later life and is associated with the development of the metabolic syndrome. A role for maternal obesity during pregnancy in the evolvement of the global obesity epidemic has been suggested. Several maternal, fetal and gestational complications have been recognized in association with obesity. Bariatric surgery seems to be safe and effective in preventing obesity-related complications. Obese reproductive aged patients seeking pregnancy should be counseled regarding pregnancy complications and adverse perinatal outcomes, and should be advised to lose weight prior to conception.

References

[1] Cassell JA. Anthropology and Nutrition: A Different Look at Obesity in America, Social, *J American Dietetic Assoc* 1995;95:424-427.

[2] World Health Organization. Obesity: preventing and managing the global epidemic. *Report of a WHO consultation presented at: the World Health Organization: June 3-5, 1997;* Geneva, Switzerland. Publication WHO/NUT/NCD/98.1.

[3] James PT, Leach R, Kalamara E, Shayeghi M. The worldwide obesity epidemic. *Obes Res.* 2001;9 Suppl 4:228S-233S.

[4] Chopra M, Galbraith S, Darnton-Hill I. A global response to a global problem: the epidemic of overnutrition. *Bull World Health Organ.* 2002;80:952-8.

[5] Public Health Service: Healthy People 2000: National Health Promotion And Disease Prevention Objectives. Washington, DC, US Department Of Health And Human Services, *Public Health Service*, DHHS Publication No. (PHS) 90-50212, 1990.

[6] Obesity and overweight. What are overweight and obesity? [Online]. 2006; Available from: *http://www.who.int/mediacentre/factsheets/fs311/en/index.html*

[7] World Health Organization. Obesity: preventing and managing a global epidemic. *World Health Organ Tech Rep Ser* 2000;894:1–4.

[8]   Hedley AA, Ogden CL, Johnson CL, Carroll MD, Curtin LR, Flegal KM. Prevalence of overweight and obesity among U.S. children, adolescents, and adults, 1999–2002. *JAMA* 2004;291:2847.

[9]   Cnattingius S, Bergstrom R, Lipworth L, Kramer MS. Prepregnancy weight and the risk of adverse pregnancy outcomes. *N Engl J Med* 1998;338:147–152.

[10] Sarwer DB, Allison KC, Gibbons LM, Markowitz JT, Nelson DB. Pregnancy and obesity: a review and agenda for future research. *J Womens Health (Larchmt).* 2006;15:720-33.

[11] O'Brien PE, Brown WA, Dixon JB. Obesity, weight loss and bariatric surgery. *Med J Aust.* 2005;183:310-4.

[12] Sebire NJ, Jolly M, Harris JP, Wadsworth J, Joffe M, Beard RW, Regan L, Robinson S. Maternal obesity and pregnancy outcome: a study of 287,213 pregnancies in London. *Int J Obes Relat Metab Disord.* 2001;25:1175-82.

[13] Keinan-Boker L, Noyman N, Chinich A, Green MS, Nitzan-Kaluski D. Overweight and obesity prevalence in Israel: findings of the first national health and nutrition survey (MABAT*). Isr Med Assoc J.* 2005;7:219-23.

[14] Kanagalingam MG, Forouhi NG, Greer IA, Sattar N. Changes in booking body mass index over a decade: retrospective analysis from a Glasgow Maternity Hospital. *BJOG.* 2005;112:1431-3.

[15] National Heart, Lung and Blood Institute. Clinical guidelines on the identification, evaluation and treatment of obesity in adults: The evidence report. Washington, D.C: *U.S. Department of Health and Human Services* 1998.

[16] Mokdad AH, Serdula MK, Dietz WH, Bowman BA, Marks JS, Koplan JP, The spread of the obesity epidemic in the United States, 1991–1998. *JAMA* 1999; 282: 1519–1522.

[17] Ehrenberg HM, Dierker L, Milluzzi C, Mercer BM. Prevalence of maternal obesity in an urban center. *Am J Obstet Gynecol* 2002;187:1189-93.

[18] Gross T, Sokol RJ, King KC. Obesity in pregnancy: risks and outcome. *Obstet Gynecol* 1980;56:446-50.

[19] Allison DB, Fonatine KR, Manson JE, Stevens J, Van Itallie TB. Annual deaths attributable to obesity in the United States. *JAMA* 1999;282:1530–1538.

[20] Isaacs JD, Magnon EF, Martin RW, Chauhan SP, Morrison JC. Obstetric challenges of massive obesity complicating pregnancy. *J Perinatol* 1994; 14: 10–14.

[21] Ratner RE, Hamner LH, Isada NB, Effects of gestational weight gain in morbidly obese women: Fetal morbidity. *Am J Perinatol* 1990;7:295–299.

[22] Kumari AS. Pregnancy outcome in women with morbid obesity. *Int J Gynaecol Obstet* 2001;73:101-7.

[23] Sheiner E, Levy A, Menes TS, Silverberg D, Katz M, Mazor M. Maternal obesity as an independent risk factor for caesarean delivery. *Paediatr Perinat Epidemiol.* 2004;18:196-201.

[24] Catalano PM. Obesity and pregnancy--the propagation of a viscous cycle? *J Clin Endocrinol Metab.* 2003;88:3505-6.

[25] Schäfer-Graf UM, Dupak J, Vogel M, Dudenhausen JW, Kjos SL, Buchanan TA, Vetter K. Hyperinsulinism, neonatal obesity and placental immaturity in infants born to women with one abnormal glucose tolerance test value. *J Perinat Med.* 1998;26:27-36.

[26] Curhan GC, Chertow GM, Willett WC, Spiegelman D, Colditz GA, Manson JE, Speizer FE, Stampfer MJ. Birth weight and adult hypertension and obesity in women. *Circulation.* 1996;94:1310-5.

[27] Barker DJ, Osmond C, Simmonds SJ, Wield GA. The relation of small head circumference and thinness at birth to death from cardiovascular disease in adult life. *BMJ.* 1993;306:422-6.

[28] Taylor PD, Poston L. Developmental programming of obesity in mammals. *Exp Physiol.* 2007;92:287-98.

[29] Lawlor DA, Smith GD, O'Callaghan M, Alati R, Mamun AA, Williams GM, Najman JM. Epidemiologic evidence for the fetal overnutrition hypothesis: findings from the mater-university study of pregnancy and its outcomes. *Am J Epidemiol.* 2007;165:418-24.

[30] Ebbeling CB, Pawlak DB, Ludwig DS. Childhood obesity: public-health crisis, common sense cure. *Lancet.* 2002;360:473-82.

[31] Lawlor DA, Timpson NJ, Harbord RM, Leary S, Ness A, McCarthy MI, Frayling TM, Hattersley AT, Smith GD. Exploring the developmental overnutrition hypothesis using parental-offspring associations and FTO as an instrumental variable. *PLoS Med.* 2008;5:e33.

[32] Must A, Spadano J, Coakley EH, Field AE, Colditz G, Dietz WH. The disease burden associated with overweight and obesity. *JAMA.* 1999;282:1523-9.

[33] Cedergren MI. Maternal morbid obesity and the risk of adverse pregnancy outcome. *Obstet Gynecol.* 2004;103:219-24.

[34] Baeten JM, Bukusi EA, Lambe M. Pregnancy complications and outcomes among overweight and obese nulliparous women. *Am J Public Health.* 2001;91:436-40.

[35] Källén K. Maternal smoking, body mass index, and neural tube defects. *Am J Epidemiol.* 1998;147:1103-11.

[36] Waller DK, Mills JL, Simpson JL, Cunningham GC, Conley MR, Lassman MR, Rhoads GG. Are obese women at higher risk for producing malformed offspring? *Am J Obstet Gynecol.* 1994;170:541-8.

[37] Shaw GM, Velie EM, Schaffer D. Risk of neural tube defect-affected pregnancies among obese women. *JAMA.* 1996;275:1093-6.

[38] Werler MM, Louik C, Shapiro S, Mitchell AA. Prepregnant weight in relation to risk of neural tube defects. *JAMA.* 1996;275:1089-92.

[39] Ray JG, Wyatt PR, Vermuelen MJ, Meier C, Cole DE. Greater maternal weight and the ongoing risk of neural tube defects after folic acid flour fortification. *Obstet Gynecol* 2005;105:261–5 .

[40] Watkins ML, Rasmussen SA, Honein MA, Botto LD, Moore CA. Maternal obesity and risk for birth defects. *Paediatrics* 2003;111:1152–8 .

[41] Watkins ML, Scanlon KS, Mulinare J, Khoury MJ. Is maternal obesity a risk factor for anencephaly and spina bifida? *Epidemiology* 1996;7: 507–12.

[42] Rasmussen SA, Chu SY, Kim SY, Schmid CH, Lau J. Maternal obesity and risk of neural tube defects: a metaanalysis. *Am J Obstet Gynecol.* 2008;198:611-9.

[43] Sheiner E, Levy A, Silverberg D, Menes TS, Levy I, Katz M, Mazor M. Pregnancy after bariatric surgery is not associated with adverse perinatal outcome. *Am J Obstet Gynecol* 2004;190: 1335-1340.

[44] Cedergren MI, Kallen BA. Maternal obesity and infant heart defects. *Obes Res.* 2003;11:1065-71.

[45] Krishnamoorthy U, Schram CM, Hill SR. Maternal obesity in pregnancy: Is it time for meaningful research to inform preventive and management strategies? *BJOG.* 2006;113:1134-40.

[46] Jenkins KJ, Correa A, Feinstein JA, Botto L, Britt AE, Daniels SR, Elixson M, Warnes CA, Webb CL; American Heart Association Council on Cardiovascular Disease in the Young. Noninherited risk factors and congenital cardiovascular defects: current knowledge: a scientific statement from the American Heart Association Council on Cardiovascular Disease in the Young: endorsed by the American Academy of Pediatrics. *Circulation.* 2007;115:2995-3014.

[47] Galindo A, Burguillo AG, Azriel S, Fuente Pde L. Outcome of fetuses in women with pregestational diabetes mellitus. *J Perinat Med.* 2006;34:323-31.

[48] Catalano PM. Management of obesity in pregnancy. *Obstet Gynecol.* 2007;109:419-33.

[49] Wald N, Cuckle H, Boreham J, Terzian E, Redman C. The effect of maternal weight on maternal serum alpha-fetoprotein levels. *Br J Obstet Gynaecol.* 1981 ;88:1094-6.

[50] Yu CK, Teoh TG, Robinson S. Obesity in pregnancy. *BJOG.* 2006 ;113:1117-25.

[51] Fedorcsak P, Dale PO, Storeng R, Ertzeid G, Bjercke S, Oldereid N, Omland AK, Abyholm T, Tanbo T. Impact of overweight and underweight on assisted reproduction treatment. *Hum Reprod.* 2004;19:2523-8.

[52] Lashen H, Fear K, Sturdee DW. Obesity is associated with increased risk of first trimester and recurrent miscarriage: matched case-control study. *Hum Reprod* 2004;19:1644-6.

[53]   Fedorcsak P, Storeng R, Dale PO, Tanbo T, Abyholm T. Obesity is a risk factor for early pregnancy loss after IVF or ICSI. *Acta Obstet Gynecol Scand.* 2000;79:43-8.

[54] Bellver J, Rossal LP, Bosch E, Zúñiga A, Corona JT, Meléndez F, Gómez E, Simón C, Remohí J, Pellicer A. Obesity and the risk of spontaneous abortion after oocyte donation. *Fertil Steril.* 2003;79:1136-40.

[55] Wang JX, Davies MJ, Norman RJ. Polycystic ovarian syndrome and the risk of spontaneous abortion following assisted reproductive technology treatment. *Hum Reprod.* 2001;16:2606-9.

[56] Nelson SM, Fleming RF. The preconceptual contraception paradigm: obesity and infertility. *Hum Reprod.* 2007;22:912-5.

[57] Nelson SM, Fleming R. Obesity and reproduction: impact and interventions. *Curr Opin Obstet Gynecol.* 2007;19:384-9.

[58] Clark AM, Thornley B, Tomlinson L, Galletley C, Norman RJ. Weight loss in obese infertile women results in improvement in reproductive outcome for all forms of fertility treatment. *Hum Reprod.* 1998;13:1502-5.

[59] Rosenn B. Obesity and diabetes: A recipe for obstetric complications. *J Matern Fetal Neonatal Med.* 2008;21:159-64.

[60] Ramachenderan J, Bradford J, McLean M. Maternal obesity and pregnancy complications: a review. *Aust N Z J Obstet Gynaecol.* 2008;48:228-35.

[61] Stephansson O, Dickman PW, Johansson A, Cnattingius S. Maternal weight, pregnancy weight gain, and the risk of antepartum stillbirth. *Am J Obstet Gynecol.* 2001;184:463-9.

[62] Kristensen J, Vestergaard M, Wisborg K, Kesmodel U, Secher NJ. Pre-pregnancy weight and the risk of stillbirth and neonatal death. *BJOG.* 2005;112:403-8.

[63] Nohr EA, Bech BH, Davies MJ, Frydenberg M, Henriksen TB, Olsen J. Prepregnancy obesity and fetal death: a study within the Danish National Birth Cohort. *Obstet Gynecol.* 2005;106:250-9.

[64] Chen A, Feresu SA, Fernandez C, Rogan WJ. Maternal Obesity and the Risk of Infant Death in the United States. *Epidemiology.* 2008 Sep 20. [Epub ahead of print].

[65] Wolfe HM, Sokol RJ, Martier SM, Zador IE. Maternal obesity: a potential source of error in sonographic prenatal diagnosis. *Obstet Gynecol.* 1990;76:339-42.

[66] Hendler I, Blackwell SC, Bujold E, Treadwell MC, Wolfe HM, Sokol RJ, Sorokin Y. The impact of maternal obesity on midtrimester sonographic visualization of fetal cardiac and craniospinal structures. *Int J Obes Relat Metab Disord.* 2004;28:1607-11.

[67] Hendler I, Blackwell SC, Bujold E, Treadwell MC, Mittal P, Sokol RJ, Sorokin Y. Suboptimal second-trimester ultrasonographic visualization of the fetal heart in obese women: should we repeat the examination? *J Ultrasound Med* 2005;24:1205-9.

[68] Sukalich S, Mingione MJ, Glantz JC. Obstetric outcomes in overweight and obese adolescents. *Am J Obstet Gynecol.* 2006;195:851-5.

[69] Johnson JW, Longmate JA, Frentzen B. Excessive maternal weight and pregnancy outcome. *Am J Obstet Gynecol.* 1992;167:353-70.

[70] Ehrenberg HM, Mercer BM, Catalano PM. The influence of obesity and diabetes on the prevalence of macrosomia. *Am J Obstet Gynecol.* 2004;191:964-8.

[71] Langer O, Yogev Y, Xenakis EM, Brustman L. Overweight and obese in gestational diabetes: the impact on pregnancy outcome. *Am J Obstet Gynecol.* 2005;192:1768-76.

[72] Catalano PM, Thomas A, Huston-Presley L, Amini SB. Increased fetal adiposity: a very sensitive marker of abnormal in utero development. *Am J Obstet Gynecol.* 2003;189:1698-704.

[73] Parsons TJ, Power C, Manor O. Fetal and early life growth and body mass index from birth to early adulthood in 1958 British cohort: longitudinal study. *BMJ.* 2001;323:1331-5.

[74] Parsons TJ, Power C, Logan S, Summerbell CD. Childhood predictors of adult obesity: a systematic review. *Int J Obes Relat Metab Disord.* 1999;23 Suppl 8:S1-107.

[75] Whitaker RC, Dietz WH. Role of the prenatal environment in the development of obesity. *J Pediatr.* 1998;132:768-76.

[76] Laitinen J, Power C, Järvelin MR. Family social class, maternal body mass index, childhood body mass index, and age at menarche as predictors of adult obesity. *Am J Clin Nutr.* 2001;74:287-94.

[77] Dabelea D, Hanson RL, Lindsay RS, Pettitt DJ, Imperatore G, Gabir MM, Roumain J, Bennett PH, Knowler WC. Intrauterine exposure to diabetes conveys risks for type 2 diabetes and obesity: a study of discordant sibships. *Diabetes.* 2000;49:2208-11.

[78] Boney CM, Verma A, Tucker R, Vohr BR. Metabolic syndrome in childhood: association with birth weight, maternal obesity and gestational diabetes mellitus. *Pediatrics* 2005;115:e290–6.

[79] Pasquali R, Patton L, Gambineri A. Obesity and infertility. *Curr Opin Endocrinol Diabetes Obes.* 2007;14:482-7.

[80] Robker RL. Evidence that obesity alters the quality of oocytes and embryos. *Pathophysiology.* 2008;15:115-21.

[81] Jensen TK, Scheike T, Keiding N, Schaumburg I, Grandjean P. Fecundability in relation to body mass and menstrual cycle patterns. *Epidemiology.* 1999;10:422-8.

[82] van der Steeg JW, Steures P, Eijkemans MJ, Habbema JD, Hompes PG, Burggraaff JM, Oosterhuis GJ, Bossuyt PM, van der Veen F, Mol BW. Obesity affects spontaneous pregnancy chances in subfertile, ovulatory women. *Hum Reprod.* 2008;23:324-8.

[83] Sneed ML, Uhler ML, Grotjan HE, Rapisarda JJ, Lederer KJ, Beltsos AN. Body mass index: impact on IVF success appears age-related. *Hum Reprod.* 2008;23:1835-9.

[84] Dokras A, Baredziak L, Blaine J, Syrop C, VanVoorhis BJ, Sparks A. Obstetric outcomes after in vitro fertilization in obese and morbidly obese women. *Obstet Gynecol.* 2006;108:61-9.

[85] Lashen H, Ledger W, Bernal AL, Barlow D. Extremes of body mass do not adversely affect the outcome of superovulation and in-vitro fertilization. *Hum Reprod.* 1999;14:712-5.

[86] Spandorfer SD, Kump L, Goldschlag D, Brodkin T, Davis OK, Rosenwaks Z. Obesity and in vitro fertilization: negative influences on outcome. *J Reprod Med.* 2004;49:973-7.

[87] Wang JX, Davies M, Norman RJ. Body mass and probability of pregnancy during assisted reproduction treatment: retrospective study. *BMJ.* 2000;321:1320-1.

[88] Nichols JE, Crane MM, Higdon HL, Miller PB, Boone WR. Extremes of body mass index reduce in vitro fertilization pregnancy rates. *Fertil Steril.* 2003;79:645-7.

[89] Lintsen AM, Pasker-de Jong PC, de Boer EJ, Burger CW, Jansen CA, Braat DD, van Leeuwen FE. Effects of subfertility cause, smoking and body weight on the success rate of IVF. *Hum Reprod.* 2005;20:1867-75.

[90] Allison KC, Sarwer DB, Paré E. Issues related to weight management during pregnancy among overweight and obese women. Expert Rev. Obstet. *Gynecol.*, 2007;2;249-254

[91] Smith GC, Shah I, Pell JP, Crossley JA, Dobbie R. Maternal obesity in early pregnancy and risk of spontaneous and elective preterm deliveries: a retrospective cohort study. *Am J Public Health.* 2007;97:157-62.

[92] Robinson HE, O'Connell CM, Joseph KS, McLeod NL. Maternal outcomes in pregnancies complicated by obesity. *Obstet Gynecol.* 2005;106:1357-64.

[93] Weiss JL, Malone FD, Emig D, Ball RH, Nyberg DA, Comstock CH, Saade G, Eddleman K, Carter SM, Craigo SD, Carr SR, D'Alton ME; FASTER Research Consortium. Obesity, obstetric complications and cesarean delivery rate--a population-based screening study. *Am J Obstet Gynecol.* 2004;190:1091-7.

[94] Burstein E, Levy A, Mazor M, Wiznitzer A, Sheiner E. Pregnancy outcome among obese women: a prospective study. *Am J Perinatol.* 2008;25:561-6.

[95] Sibai BM, Ewell M, Levine RJ, Klebanoff MA, Esterlitz J, Catalano PM, Goldenberg RL, Joffe G. Risk factors associated with preeclampsia in healthy nulliparous women. The Calcium for Preeclampsia Prevention (CPEP) Study Group. *Am J Obstet Gynecol.* 1997;177:1003-10.

[96] O'Brien TE, Ray JG, Chan WS. Maternal body mass index and the risk of preeclampsia: a systematic overview. *Epidemiology.* 2003;14:368-74.

[97] Eskenazi B, Fenster L, Sidney S. A multivariate analysis of risk factors for preeclampsia. *JAMA.* 1991;266:237-41.

[98] Jensen DM, Damm P, Sørensen B, Mølsted-Pedersen L, Westergaard JG, Ovesen P, Beck-Nielsen H. Pregnancy outcome and prepregnancy body mass index in 2459 glucose-tolerant Danish women. *Am J Obstet Gynecol.* 2003;189:239-44.

[99] Yogev Y, Xenakis EM, Langer O. The association between preeclampsia and the severity of gestational diabetes: the impact of glycemic control. *Am J Obstet Gynecol.* 2004;191:1655-60.

[100] Crowther CA, Hiller JE, Moss JR, McPhee AJ, Jeffries WS, Robinson JS; Australian Carbohydrate Intolerance Study in Pregnant Women (ACHOIS) Trial Group. Effect of treatment of gestational diabetes mellitus on pregnancy outcomes. *N Engl J Med.* 2005;352:2477-86.

[101] Rumbold AR, Crowther CA, Haslam RR, Dekker GA, Robinson JS; ACTS Study Group. Vitamins C and E and the risks of preeclampsia and perinatal complications. *N Engl J Med* 2006;354:1796–806.

[102] Poston L, Briley AL, Seed PT, Kelly FJ, Shennan AH; the Vitamins in Pre-eclampsia (VIP) trial consortium. Vitamin C and Vitamin E in pregnant women at risk for pre-eclampsia (VIP Trial): randomized placebo controlled trial. *Lancet* 2006; 367:1145–54.

[103] Catalano PM, Kirwan JP, Haugel-de Mouzon S, King J. Gestational diabetes and insulin resistance: role in short- and long-term implications for mother and fetus. *J Nutr.* 2003;133:1674S-1683S.

[104] Retnakaran R, Hanley AJ, Raif N, Connelly PW, Sermer M, Zinman B. C-reactive protein and gestational diabetes: the central role of maternal obesity. *J Clin Endocrinol Metab.* 2003;88:3507-12.

[105] Gabbe SG, Graves CR. Management of diabetes mellitus complicating pregnancy. *Obstet Gynecol.* 2003;102:857-68.

[106] Rode L, Nilas L, Wøjdemann K, Tabor A. Obesity-related complications in Danish single cephalic term pregnancies. *Obstet Gynecol.* 2005;105:537-42.

[107] Glazer NL, Hendrickson AF, Schellenbaum GD, Mueller BA. Weight change and the risk of gestational diabetes in obese women. *Epidemiology.* 2004;15:733-7.

[108] Hotu S, Carter B, Watson PD, Cutfield WS, Cundy T. Increasing prevalence of type 2 diabetes in adolescents. *J Paediatr Child Health.* 2004;40:201-4.

[109] Weintraub AY, Press F, Wiztitzer A, Sheiner E. Maternal Thrombophilia and Adverse Pregnancy Outcomes. *Expert Review Obstet Gynecol.* 2007;2:203-216.

[110] Edwards LE, Hellerstedt WL, Alton IR, Story M, Himes JH. Pregnancy complications and birth outcomes in obese and normal-weight women: effects of gestational weight change. *Obstet Gynecol.* 1996;87:389-94.

[111] Sharma S, Monga D. Venous thromboembolism during pregnancy and the post-partum period: incidence and risk factors in a large Victorian health service. *Aust N Z J Obstet Gynaecol.* 2008;48:44-9.

[112] Bates SM, Greer IA, Hirsh J, Ginsberg JS. Use of antithrombotic agents during pregnancy: the Seventh ACCP Conference on Antithrombotic and Thrombolytic Therapy. *Chest.* 2004;26, 627S-644S.

[113] Villamor E, Cnattingius S. Interpregnancy weight change and risk of adverse pregnancy outcomes: a population-based study. *Lancet.* 2006;368:1164-70.

[114] Gore SA, Brown DM, West DS. The role of postpartum weight retention in obesity among women: a review of the evidence. *Ann Behav Med.* 2003;26:149-59.

[115] Kac G, Benício MH, Velásquez-Meléndez G, Valente JG, Struchiner CJ. Gestational weight gain and prepregnancy weight influence postpartum weight retention in a cohort of brazilian women. *J Nutr.* 2004;134:661-6.

[116] Rooney BL, Schauberger CW. Excess pregnancy weight gain and long-term obesity: one decade later. *Obstet Gynecol.* 2002;100:245-52.

[117] Linné Y, Dye L, Barkeling B, Rössner S. Long-term weight development in women: a 15-year follow-up of the effects of pregnancy. *Obes Res.* 2004;12:1166-78.

[118] Robinson H, Tkatch S, Mayes DC, Bott N, Okun N. Is maternal obesity a predictor of shoulder dystocia? *Obstet Gynecol.* 2003;101:24-7.

[119] Mazouni C, Porcu G, Cohen-Solal E, Heckenroth H, Guidicelli B, Bonnier P, Gamerre M. Maternal and anthropomorphic risk factors for shoulder dystocia. *Acta Obstet Gynecol Scand.* 2006;85:567-70.

[120] Jensen H, Agger AO, Rasmussen KL. The influence of prepregnancy body mass index on labor complications. *Acta Obstet Gynecol Scand.* 1999;78:799-802.

[121] Nuthalapaty FS, Rouse DJ, Owen J. The association of maternal weight with cesarean risk, labor duration, and cervical dilation rate during labor induction. *Obstet Gynecol.* 2004;103:452-6.

[122] Usha Kiran TS, Hemmadi S, Bethel J, Evans J. Outcome of pregnancy in a woman with an increased body mass index. *BJOG.* 2005;112:768-72.

[123] Bhattacharya S, Campbell DM, Liston WA, Bhattacharya S. Effect of Body Mass Index on pregnancy outcomes in nulliparous women delivering singleton babies. *BMC Public Health.* 2007;7:168.

[124] Ehrenberg HM, Durnwald CP, Catalano P, Mercer BM. The influence of obesity and diabetes on the risk of cesarean delivery. *Am J Obstet Gynecol.* 2004;191:969-74.

[125] Durnwald CP, Ehrenberg HM, Mercer BM. The impact of maternal obesity and weight gain on vaginal birth after cesarean section success. *Am J Obstet Gynecol.* 2004;191:954-7.

[126] Hood DD, Dewan DM. Anesthetic and obstetric outcome in morbidly obese parturients. *Anesthesiology.* 1993;79:1210-8.

[127] Perlow JH, Morgan MA. Massive maternal obesity and perioperative cesarean morbidity. *Am J Obstet Gynecol.* 1994;170:560-5.

[128] Vallejo MC. Anesthetic management of the morbidly obese parturient. *Curr Opin Anaesthesiol.* 2007;20:175-80.

[129] Soens MA, Birnbach DJ, Ranasinghe JS, van Zundert A. Obstetric anesthesia for the obese and morbidly obese patient: an ounce of prevention is worth more than a pound of treatment. *Acta Anaesthesiol Scand*. 2008;52:6-19.

[130] Saravanakumar K, Rao SG, Cooper GM. Obesity and obstetric anaesthesia. *Anaesthesia*. 2006;61:36-48.

[131] Sarsam SE, Elliott JP, Lam GK. Management of wound complications from cesarean delivery. *Obstet Gynecol Surv*. 2005;60:462-73.

[132] Martens MG, Kolrud BL, Faro S, Maccato M, Hammill H. Development of wound infection or separation after cesarean delivery. Prospective evaluation of 2,431 cases. *J Reprod Med*. 1995;40:171-5.

[133] Beattie PG, Rings TR, Hunter MF, Lake Y. Risk factors for wound infection following caesarean section. *Aust N Z J Obstet Gynaecol*. 1994;34:398-402.

[134] Schneid-Kofman N, Sheiner E, Levy A, Holcberg G. Risk factors for wound infection following cesarean deliveries. *Int J Gynaecol Obstet*. 2005;90:10-5.

[135] Galtier F, Raingeard I, Renard E, Boulot P, Bringer J. Optimizing the outcome of pregnancy in obese women: from pregestational to long-term management. *Diabetes Metab*. 2008;34:19-25.

[136] Dixon JB, Dixon ME, O'Brien PE. Quality of life after lap-band placement: influence of time, weight loss, and comorbidities. *Obes Res* 2001; 9: 713-721.

[137] Sheiner E, Menes TS, Silverberg D, Abramowicz JS, Levy I, Katz M, Mazor M, Levy A. Pregnancy outcome of patients with gestational diabetes mellitus following bariatric surgery. *Am J Obstet Gynecol*. 2006;194:431-5.

[138] Karmon A, Sheiner E. Pregnancy after bariatric surgery: a comprehensive review. *Arch Gynecol Obstet*. 2008;277:381-8.

[139] Granström L, Granström L, Backman L. Fetal growth retardation after gastric banding. *Acta Obstet Gynecol Scand*. 1990;69:533-6.

[140] Haddow JE, Hill LE, Kloza EM, Thanhauser D. Neural tube defects after gastric bypass. *Lancet*. 1986;1:1330.

[141] Martin L, Chavez GF, Adams MJ Jr, Mason EE, Hanson JW, Haddow JE, Currier RW. Gastric bypass surgery as maternal risk factor for neural tube defects. *Lancet*. 1988;1:640-1.

[142] Huerta S, Rogers LM, Li Z, Heber D, Liu C, Livingston EH. Vitamin A deficiency in a newborn resulting from maternal hypovitaminosis A after biliopancreatic diversion for the treatment of morbid obesity. *Am J Clin Nutr*. 2002;76:426-9.

[143] Maggard MA, Yermilov I, Li Z, Maglione M, Newberry S, Suttorp M, Hilton L, Santry HP, Morton JM, Livingston EH, Shekelle PG. Pregnancy and fertility following bariatric surgery: a systematic review. *JAMA*. 2008;300:2286-96.

[144] Weintraub AY, Levy A, Levi I, Mazor M, Wiznitzer A, Sheiner E. Effect of bariatric surgery on pregnancy outcome. *Int J Gynaecol Obstet*. 2008;103:246-51.

[145] American College of Obstetricians and Gynecologists. Obesity in pregnancy. *ACOG Committee Opinion Number 315*, September 2005.

[146] Karmon A, Sheiner E. Timing of gestation after bariatric surgery: should women delay pregnancy for at least 1 postoperative year? *Am J Perinatol*. 2008;25:331-3.

In: Textbook of Perinatal Epidemiology
Editor: Eyal Sheiner, pp. 299-318

ISBN: 978-1-60741-648-7
© 2010 Nova Science Publishers, Inc.

Chapter XVII

Epidemiology of Asthma during Pregnancy

Ohad Katz [*] *and Eyal Sheiner*

Department of Obstetrics & Gynecology, Soroka University Medical Center, Faculty of
Health Sciences, Ben-Gurion University of the Negev, Beer-Sheva, Israel

Introduction

Chronic bronchial asthma is the most commonly encountered respiratory disorder complicating pregnancy and is a potentially serious medical condition that represents a significant public health issue [1–5]. The prevalence of asthma in pregnant women ranges between 0.4% and 12% [1–11] (with an average of 4–8%) and appears to have increased over recent decades. Kwon et al. [7] demonstrated a two-fold increase in the prevalence of asthma from 2.9% to 5.8% between 1976–1980 and 1988–1994. This diversity of statistics is presumably the result of differences in the definitions of asthma [5].

Diagnosis and Classification of Severity

Bronchial asthma is a chronic inflammatory airway disorder that is characterized by paroxysmal or persistent symptoms such as wheezing, coughing, sputum production, shortness of breath, or chest tightness. The diagnosis is based on a combination of a history of such symptoms, objective tests of lung function (i.e., an airflow obstruction that is at least partially reversible), and exclusion of alternative diagnoses [12–15].

---

[*] For Correspondence: Ohad Katz, M.D., Department of Obstetrics and Gynecology, Soroka University Medical Center, P.O. Box 151, Beer Sheva 84101, Israel. Tel: +972-8-640-3762; Fax: +972-8-640-3057; E-mail: katzoh@bgu.ac.il

During pregnancy, as well as in non-pregnant women with asthma, sequential measurement of forced expiratory volume in one second (FEV1) is the single best measure reflecting the severity of the disease. Peak expiratory flow rate (PEFR) is the largest expiratory flow achieved with a maximally forced effort from a position of maximal inspiration. It is usually attained within the initial 1 second of forced expiration. PEFR correlates well with FEV1 and can be measured reliably. Asthmatic patients will demonstrate an improvement in FEV1/PEFR values following administration of bronchodilators such as β2-agonists [12,13].

In 2004, the National Asthma Education and Prevention Program (NAEPP) Working Group on Asthma and Pregnancy classified asthma severity into four categories—mild intermittent, mild persistent, moderate persistent, and severe persistent. This classification was based on two criteria: clinical symptoms and objective pulmonary function tests (PEFR and FEV1). Regular medical treatment was not included as a criterion [12,15].

Physiologic Changes during Pregnancy

Pulmonary system—Throughout pregnancy, the enlarging uterus elevates the diaphragm about 4 cm and increases the transverse diameter of the thoracic cage about 2 cm [12,13]. The sub-costal angle widens appreciably and the thoracic circumference increases about 6 cm [13]. As a consequence, there is a reduction of the functional residual capacity (FRC) and residual volume (RV). Nevertheless, the vital capacity, PEFR, and FEV1 are not altered appreciably [12,13]. These changes result in hyperventilation in 60–70% of normal pregnancies and, occasionally, a sensation of dyspnea [13,14].

Brancazio et al. [16] measured PEFR in 57 women during each trimester and postpartum. PEFRs were normalized according to the accepted standard nomograms. No significant changes were demonstrated during the three trimesters and postpartum. Hassan et al. [17], however, studied the effect of gestational age on PEFR. They measured PEFRs in the standing, sitting, and supine positions in 38 healthy pregnant women at 4-week intervals starting at less than 10 weeks until delivery and again at 6 weeks postpartum. A small but significant decline in PEFR was demonstrated throughout pregnancy with a mean decline rate of 0.65 L/min per week (normal range of PEFR for reproductive women has been reported to be approximately 380–500 L/min). They concluded that PEFR measurements are affected by maternal position and advancing gestational age, especially in the supine position, and recommended an adjustment of patient's flow rate in relation to gestational age and maternal position, especially in pregnant women with asthma.

Gastrointestinal system—approximately one-third of the women have a gastroesophageal reflex disease (GERD) during pregnancy, especially during the second and third trimesters [13,14]. A reflux of gastric content can cause exacerbation of asthma.

Effects of Pregnancy on Asthma

The course of asthma during pregnancy is variable and may be influenced by the various physiologic changes during pregnancy as well as the severity of the pre-existing disease [14]. For many years, based on several historical cohort and prospective studies, the consensus has remained that about one-third of asthmatic women experience worsening of the disease during pregnancy, another third experience some kind of symptomatic improvement, and the rest have no change [3, 5,13,18,19]. Nevertheless, it is unclear whether this pattern is due to changes in asthma control, changes in asthma severity, or exacerbations related to pregnancy. Several studies have been done to answer these questions, but most are limited by their subjective nature. Only relatively few of these studies have examined objective measures such as spirometry [5].

The Course of Asthma during Pregnancy

In a multi-center, prospective, observational cohort study, Schatz et al. evaluated the relationship between asthma severity during pregnancy and gestational asthma exacerbations in 1734 asthmatic women. They found that about 30% of the women who were classified as having a mild disease at the beginning of their pregnancy became worse during pregnancy, and 23% of the women who were classified as having a moderate to severe disease improved [20]. In another prospective study, Schatz et al. followed the progression of asthma during pregnancy and puerperium in 330 women. The women were asked to subjectively rate their asthma symptoms during this period of time. Interestingly, 8% of the women who reported an improvement in their disease and 17% of the women who felt no change in their disease had an emergency department presentation for asthma during pregnancy, suggesting that even women who report an improvement in their asthma may require medical intervention during pregnancy [21]. Recently, Murphy et al. reviewed the literature for publications related to asthma exacerbations during pregnancy and found that exacerbations that required medical treatment occurred in about 20% of women [18]. In a prospective cohort study of 146 women, Murphy et al. [18] evaluated asthma exacerbations during pregnancy and observed that the exacerbation rate increased significantly with increasing asthma severity. Only 8% of women with mild asthma experienced an exacerbation compared with 47% of women with moderate asthma and 65% of women with severe asthma at a mean gestational age of 25 weeks. Respiratory viral infections were the most common precipitants of exacerbations (34%), followed by non-adherence to inhaled corticosteroid medication (29%). Exacerbation during labor and delivery were less common – ten to twenty percent [22]. Other Investigators reported similar results [23–25]. Stenius-Aarniala et al. investigated, prospectively, 198 asthmatic women during pregnancy; 42% of the women needed more medication, while 18% needed less medication and 40% were managed with the same anti-asthmatic medication as before pregnancy [23].

The findings of these studies challenge the concept mentioned above that only one-third of asthmatic women experience worsening of the disease during pregnancy, and suggest that the real risk of having an exacerbation during pregnancy is underestimated. These results also emphasize the importance of monitoring asthmatic women with pulmonary function testing during pregnancy, regardless of their asthma severity at the beginning of the pregnancy.

Fetal Sex

Several studies examined the possible influences of fetal sex on maternal asthma. In 1998, Beecroft et al. reported a possible association between asthma severity and fetal sex, based on the analysis of a questionnaire by 18 asthmatic women carrying a male fetus and 16 asthmatic women carrying a female fetus. They demonstrated that significantly more pregnant women carrying a female fetus experienced a worsening of symptoms, while pregnant women carrying a male fetus were more likely to report an improvement. The limitation of this study, however, is its small population [26]. One year later, Dodds et al. [27] reported a re-analysis of their population-based study from Canada that supported the association noted by Beecroft et al. Compared with women carrying a female fetus, fewer asthmatic women carrying a male fetus required steroid treatment (20% vs. 14%). Furthermore, more pregnant women carrying a male fetus used β2-agonists alone compared with women carrying a female fetus (40% vs. 35%), suggesting that asthma in pregnant women with a male fetus can be managed better than in pregnant women carrying a female fetus [27]. Between 1997 and 2000, Kwon et al. investigated prospectively the association between fetal sex and maternal airway lability among more than 700 pregnant asthmatic women. They significantly demonstrated a 10% improvement in airway lability among women carrying a male fetus compared with women carrying a female fetus. This difference persisted throughout pregnancy. In the authors' opinion, the assumption that sex hormones modulate asthma severity during pregnancy is reasonable [28]. Recently, Bakhireva et al. prospectively tested this hypothesis using a sample of 719 pregnant women with asthma. Pregnancy with a female fetus was associated with a higher incidence of asthma exacerbations (OR 1.84; 95% CI) independent of maternal age, BMI, ethnicity, smoking, and socioeconomic status [29]. Firoozi et al., however, failed to demonstrate such an association. In a large cohort study they compared 5529 pregnancies with a single female fetus and 5728 pregnancies with a single male fetus that gave birth between 1990 and 2002 in Quebec. No significant differences were found between mothers of a female or male fetus as to the occurrence of asthma exacerbations, the daily dose of inhaled corticosteroides (ICS), and the weekly dose of inhaled short-acting beta agonists (SABA) [30]. Other studies have failed to demonstrate such an association as well [31,32].

There is evidence that by potentiating the β-adrenergic-mediated relaxation of bronchial tissue and inhibiting the response to histamine, testosterone has a protective effect on asthmatic women, particularly from the second trimester onward. Another possible mechanism involves the activation of inflammatory pathways associated with asthma by sex-specific factors related to the female fetus [28]. Nevertheless, the fetal-sex related mechanisms responsible for the changes in the course of asthma during pregnancy are yet to be determined. The available literature has offered conflicting evidence and thus further research with large sample sizes is needed to clarify these potential effects.

Effects of Asthma on Pregnancy

A review of the studies investigating the association between maternal asthma and adverse pregnancy and perinatal outcomes reveals inconsistent data. While several studies have found an association between asthma and increased risk for adverse maternal and perinatal outcomes, other studies have failed to demonstrate such an association, especially among women with a better controlled disease (i.e., reduced number of exacerbations or higher maternal pulmonary function) [1,3,4]. The major retrospective and prospective studies investigating the association between maternal asthma and pregnancy/perinatal outcomes in the past two decades are summarized in Tables 1 and 2.

Retrospective Studies

Recently, Enriquez et al. reported the findings of one of the largest US cohort studies to date, regarding the relationship between maternal asthma, exacerbated asthma, and pregnancy outcomes. After controlling for confounding factors, there were dose-dependent relationships between asthma alone and exacerbated asthma with hypertensive disorders of pregnancy, membrane-related disorders, preterm labor, antepartum hemorrhage, and cesarean delivery. Maternal asthma was not associated with preterm birth or birth defects. They concluded that asthma is a risk factor for several common adverse outcomes of pregnancy, and poorly controlled asthma during pregnancy increases these risks [33].

The same year, Tata et al. [34] reported the results of a comprehensive analysis of adverse obstetric outcomes in women with and without asthma. All codes relating to stillbirth, miscarriage, therapeutic abortion, and obstetric complications were extracted from the Health Improvement Network database for (281,019) pregnancies between 1988 and 2004. Data regarding socioeconomic status and behavioral characteristics were extracted as well. Asthma severity was categorized into three levels according to the British Thoracic Society asthma guidelines for medication use. The unit of analysis was a pregnancy. Odds ratios of the outcomes comparing pregnancies in women with and without asthma were estimated using a logistic regression analysis. In 37,585 pregnancies of asthmatic women the risk of miscarriage was slightly higher (OR 1.10; 95% CI 1.06–1.13) than that of non-asthmatic women. The risks of stillbirth and therapeutic abortion, however, were similar. Risks of most obstetric complications (placental abruption, placenta previa, preeclampsia, hypertension, gestational diabetes, and assisted delivery) were not higher among asthmatic women, with the exception of increases in antepartum (OR 1.20; 95% CI 1.08–1.34) or postpartum (OR 1.38; 95% CI 1.21–1.57) hemorrhage, and caesarean section (OR 1.11; 95% CI 1.07–1.16). Risks of miscarriage and caesarean section increased moderately in women with more severe asthma and previous asthma exacerbations. According to the authors, these results indicate that asthmatic women have similar reproductive risks compared with women without asthma in the general population for most of the range of outcomes studied.

Table 1. Effects of maternal asthma on pregnancy outcomes—retrospective studies.

Author [Year]ref	Country	Control	Asthma	Significant association to asthma	No association to asthma
Lao and Huensgsburg (1990) [17]	Hong Kong	87	87	Low birth weight, Cesarean delivery	
Perlow et al. (1992) [38]	USA	130	81	Cesarean delivery, preterm labor, low birth weight	Pre-eclampsia, IUGR, congenital malformations
Lehrer et al. (1993) [39]	USA	22,680	1571	Pregnancy induced hypertension	
Demissie et al. (1998) [40]	USA	9156	2289	Low birth weight, preterm delivery, pre-eclampsia, congenital malformations, cesarean delivery	
Alexander et al. (1998) [6]	Canada	13709	817	Ante/postpartum hemorrhage, pregnancy induced hypertension (with steroid treatment)	Preterm delivery, pregnancy induced hypertension, Cesarean delivery
Kallen et al. (2000) [35]	Sweden	1.32M	36985	Preterm and postterm delivery, perinatal mortality, Low birth weight	Congenital malformations
Wen et al. (2001) [42]	Canada	34,668	8672	Pre-eclampsia, preterm delivery, low birth weight	
Liu et al. (2001) [41]	Canada	8772	2193	Pre-eclampsia, preterm delivery, small for gestational age, Cesarean delivery	Congenital malformations
Norjavaara and de Verdier (2003) [43]	Sweden	293,948	2968	Cesarean delivery	Still birth, Low birth weight, congenital malformations
Sheiner et al. (2005) [4]	Israel	137,205	1963	Cesarean delivery, IUGR	Perinatal mortality, low birth weight
Getahun et al. (2006) [37]	USA	36.9M	332,357	Placental abruption - modest (blacks)	
Enriquez et al. (2007) [37]	USA	131145	9154	Hypertensive disorders of pregnancy, membrane-related disorders, antepartum hemorrhage, cesarean delivery	Preterm birth, birth defects
Tata et al. (2007) [34]	GBR	24,3434	37,585	Miscarriage, antepartum and postpartum hemorrhage, cesarean delivery	Placental abruption, placenta previa, preeclampsia, hypertension, gestational diabetes, assisted delivery
Katz et al. (2007) [44]	Israel	196,707	2669	Preterm delivery (in winter season)	
Blais and Forget (2008) [36]	Canada		4344	Congenital malformations	
Tata et al. (2008) [45]	GBR			Congenital malformations (OR 1.1)	

Adapted from Katz and Sheiner, Asthma and pregnancy: A review of two decades. Expert Review Respiratory Medicine 2008;2:1-10; with permission of Expert Reviews Ltd.

Table 2. Effects of maternal asthma on pregnancy outcomes—prospective studies.

Author [Year]ref	Country	Control	Asthma	Significant association to asthma	No association to asthma
Stenius-Aarniala et al (1988) [23]	Finland	198	181	Pre-eclampsia (severe > mild), Cesarean delivery	Low birth weight, preterm delivery, perinatal mortality, congenital malformations
Doucette and Bracken (1993) [51]	USA	3859	32	Preterm delivery	Low birth weight
Jana et al. (1995) [25]	India	364	182	Low birth weight (in 15 women who had exacerbations)	Preterm delivery, low birth weight, perinatal mortality
Schatz et al. (1995) [8]	USA	486	486		Preterm delivery, perinatal mortality, low birth weight, pre-eclampsia, congenital malformations
Stenius-Aarniala et al. (1996) [49]	Finland	237	504	Cesarean delivery	Preterm delivery, perinatal mortality
Minerbi-Codish et al. (1998) [52]	Israel	77	101		Low birth weight, gestational hypertension, preterm delivery
Sobande et al. (2002) [54]	Saudi Arabia	10	88	Pre-eclampsia, Cesarean delivery, perinatal mortality, low birth weight	
Mihrshahi et al. (2003) [33]	Australia	271	340	hypertension	Cesarean delivery, pre-eclampsia, low birth weight
Bracken et al. (2003) [45]	USA	1333	872	Reduction of gestational age at delivery (with oral steroids or theophylline), intrauterine growth restriction	Preterm delivery
Triche et al. (2004) [47]	USA	1052	656	Pre-eclampsia (with moderate and severe asthma)	
Dombrowski et al. (2004) [48]	USA	881	1739	Cesarean delivery (with moderate or severe asthma), preterm delivery < 37 weeks (with severe asthma)	Preterm delivery < 32 or 37 weeks, pre-eclampsia
Murphy et al. (2005) [22]	Australia		146	Low birth weight in males (in 53 women who had exacerbations)	
Bakhireva et al. (2008) [50]	USA		716	Preterm delivery	IUGR

Adapted from Katz and Sheiner, Asthma and pregnancy: A review of two decades. Expert Review Respiratory Medicine 2008;2:1-10; with permission of Expert Reviews Ltd.

A few years earlier, Källén et al. [35] published the results of one of the largest retrospective studies on pregnancy outcomes in asthmatic women to date. They analyzed the pregnancy outcomes of nearly 37,000 asthmatic women who gave birth between 1984 and 1985. The analysis results were compared with the total births that occurred in Sweden during the same period of time (more than 1.3 million). Contrary to Tata et al., they found that the pregnancies of asthmatic women were significantly more likely to be complicated by preterm delivery, prolonged pregnancy (more than 41 weeks), low birth weight, pre-eclampsia, and perinatal mortality, with a correlation to asthma severity. No association to congenital malformations was noted.

Blais and Forget [36] conducted a large retrospective study of 4344 pregnancies of asthmatic women to investigate the association between first trimester exacerbations and increased risk for congenital malformations. The crude prevalence of malformations was 12.8% for women who had an exacerbation during the first trimester and 8.9% for women who did not. A 50% increased risk of congenital malformations was demonstrated for women who had an asthma exacerbation during the first trimester of pregnancy. Although it has limitations (residual confounding might be present and part of the observed association might be due to the use of oral corticosteroids), this study adds evidence to the necessity of keeping asthma under control during pregnancy to avoid exacerbations.

Getahun et al. [37] investigated the associations between maternal respiratory diseases and abruption in the United States. Data on women who delivered singleton births (n = 37,314,022) were derived from the National Hospital Discharge Survey for 1993 to 2003. ICD-9-CM codes were used to identify pregnant women hospitalized for respiratory disease and for placental abruption. RR and 95% CI were derived from multivariable logistic regression models to evaluate the associations after adjusting for maternal sociodemographic and behavioral characteristics. The association between asthma and abruption was modest (RR 1.1, 95% CI 1.0–1.2). Stratified analysis by maternal race showed that asthma was associated with abruption among black women but not white women.

The variable pregnancy outcomes were demonstrated by earlier studies as well. Lao and Huengsburg investigated pregnancy outcomes of 87 asthmatic women in Hong Kong between 1984 and 1987. Pregnancies of asthmatic women were significantly more likely to be complicated by preterm delivery (especially those who did not use medications) or cesarean delivery [19].

Perlow et al. [38] demonstrated an increased risk for preterm delivery and cesarean delivery, and low birth weight among women with severe asthma (oral steroid dependent). No association with pre-eclampsia or congenital malformations was noted. Nevertheless, this study included 187 asthmatic women and has a low power to detect such effects.

In a large study of about 24,000 women, of whom nearly 1,600 were asthmatic, Lehrer et al. [39] found a significant association between pregnancy-induced hypertension and asthma. This association persisted after adjustment for confounding factors. They also found a significant association between pregnancy-induced hypertension and a history of asthma. Nevertheless, after adjustment for potential confounders, this association failed to achieve statistical significance.

Demissie et al. [40] examined the association between asthma and maternal/perinatal outcomes, using a historical cohort analysis of singleton live deliveries in New Jersey hospitals between 1989 and 1992. A comparison of 2,289 women with an ICD-9-CM diagnosis code for asthma was conducted with a randomly-selected control sample of 9,156 women. After controlling for potential confounders, maternal asthma was significantly associated with preterm delivery, low birth weight, pre-eclampsia, and cesarean delivery. Unlike the previous studies, an increased risk for congenital malformations was noted.

Alexander et al. [6] conducted a similar study in Canada, but unlike the previous studies, during the examination of the medical records, the asthmatic women were classified into three groups of severity based on medication usage (no medication, beta agonist only, steroids). A total of 817 asthmatic women were compared with 13,709 non-asthmatic women for maternal complication and neonatal outcomes. Regardless of medication use, asthma was associated with ante-partum and post-partum hemorrhage. Asthmatic women using steroids were found to be at a slightly increased risk for gestational hypertension, possibly a complication of steroid use [6].

Using the Quebec hospital discharge records for 1991–1992 and 1995–1996, Liu et al. [41] investigated 2,193 asthmatic and 8,772 normal singleton pregnancies. After adjusting for potential confounders, maternal asthma was significantly associated with preterm birth, infants who are very small for gestational age, pre-eclampsia (and transient hypertension of pregnancy), and cesarean delivery. There was no association to congenital malformations. Wen et al. [42] demonstrated similar results.

Norjavaara et al. [43] investigated the influences of inhaled steroids on pregnancy outcomes during 1995 to 1998. Nearly 3,000 asthmatic women who used inhaled budesonide were compared to 7,700 women who used other asthma medications and to a control group of more than 293,000 healthy women. Other than cesarean delivery, the use of inhaled budesonide was not linked with any adverse pregnancy outcome.

Sheiner et al. [4] conducted a large retrospective population-based study, investigating pregnancy outcomes among asthmatic women. They compared all singleton pregnancies of asthmatic (1,963) and non-asthmatic (137,205) mothers who delivered between 1988 and 2002 in the Soroka University Medical Center (the sole hospital in the Negev, the southern part of Israel, which serves the entire obstetrical population in this region). After adjusting for potential confounders, the following adverse outcomes were associated with asthma: intrauterine growth restriction, hypertensive disorders, premature rapture of membranes, and cesarean delivery. Nevertheless, perinatal outcome was favorable.

Our group had investigated the seasonal effect on singleton deliveries, comparing all singleton pregnancies of asthmatic (n=2669) and non-asthmatic (n=196,707) women who gave birth between 1988 and 2006 [44]. A higher rate of preterm delivery was noted during the winter season among patients residing in semi-nomadic settlements compared to sedentary cities. Recently, Tata et al. [45] evaluated the association of maternal asthma and exposure to asthma medications during pregnancy with the risk of major congenital malformations. The unit of analysis was the child. A conditional logistic regression was used to assess the association of any major congenital malformation with maternal asthma and maternal asthma treatment. Live-born children with major congenital malformations numbering 5,124 cases were matched to 30,053 controls. Risk of any malformation in children born to asthmatic women was slightly higher (adjusted OR 1.10, 95% CI 1.01–1.20). No association, however, was demonstrated in children born to mothers receiving asthma treatment in the year before or during pregnancy. No increased risk of malformation was found with gestational exposures to short- or long-acting beta-agonists, inhaled corticosteroids, oral corticosteroids, or other bronchodilators. They concluded that commonly used asthma medications were found to be safe for use during pregnancy.

Prospective Studies

Large multi-center prospective cohort studies investigated pregnancy outcomes of asthmatic women [46–48]. These studies were unique in that they contained information regarding asthma severity and treatment. Bracken et al. [46] recruited 832 asthmatic women and 1,266 non-asthmatic women as a control group. Symptoms and treatment during pregnancy were closely monitored and recorded, and the women were classified according to the Global Initiative for Asthma guidelines as having mild intermittent, mild persistent, moderate persistent, or severe persistent asthma. Adjusted ORs for the associations between asthma status and pregnancy outcomes (preterm delivery and IUGR) were calculated from multiple logistic regression models. Preterm delivery was not associated with asthma diagnosis, regardless of severity classification. However, the need for treatment with daily oral steroid or theophylline was associated with reduction of gestational age at delivery by 2 weeks and 1 week, respectively. An increased risk IUGR was associated with severity of daily symptoms but not with medication type. In another analysis of the same prospective cohort study, Triche and Bracken [47] found that moderate to severe asthma symptoms are significantly associated with an increased risk for pre-eclampsia, regardless of asthma diagnosis or treatment before pregnancy. These results suggest that poor asthma control may affect maternal and fetal outcomes, possibly as a result of chronic maternal hypoxia and/or progressive inflammatory process.

Dombrowski et al. [48] conducted a multi-center prospective observational cohort study involving 16 university hospital centers. Preterm delivery of less than 32 weeks was the primary outcome; secondary outcome measures included pregnancy and neonatal outcomes. Asthma severity was defined according to the NAEPP classification and modified to include medication requirements. A total of 2,620 women were enrolled, of whom 873 had mild asthma, 814 had moderate asthma, and 52 had severe asthma; 881 non-asthmatic women served as a control group. In contrast to the study of Bracken et al., most of the asthmatic women were actively managed, including lung function testing. No significant differences in the rates of preterm delivery of less than 32 or 37 weeks of gestation were noted. Of all the other pregnancy outcomes explored, there were no significant differences for maternal complications except for an increase in overall cesarean delivery rate among the moderate/severe group compared with controls. After adjustment for confounding variables, however, preterm delivery less than 37 weeks and gestational diabetes were associated with severe asthma, most probably due to oral steroid use. These results, with regard to gestation age at delivery and oral steroid use, are similar to those of Bracken et al.

Over a decade earlier, Stenius-Aarniala et al. [49] prospectively followed 198 pregnancies of asthmatic women in Finland. Women were classified as having very mild, mild, moderately severe, or severe asthma. Information regarding the control group was collected retrospectively from labor records of women matched for age, parity, and gestational age. Asthma was significantly associated with mild pre-eclampsia compared with control subjects (15% vs. 5%) and occurred more often among women with severe asthma, compared to women with mild asthma (29% vs. 9%). The use of systemic corticosteroid was also associated with a higher rate of pre-eclampsia [23]. Several years later, the same group prospectively followed 504 pregnant women with asthma. As in their previous study, information regarding the control group was collected retrospectively from labor records of women matched for age, parity, and gestational age. Data on asthmatics with an acute exacerbation during pregnancy were compared with those with no recorded acute exacerbation and with the controls. Women who experienced an acute exacerbation were less likely to have used inhaled corticosteroids (ICS) prior to the exacerbation (17% vs. 4%). With regard to pregnancy outcomes, however, no significant differences were noted between the groups. The prompt use of ICS with these patients may have contributed to the reassuring outcomes [49].

Recently, Bakhireva et al. [50] evaluated the effect of maternal asthma on fetal growth and preterm delivery. A total of 719 pregnant asthmatic women were asked to evaluate their asthma control repeatedly during pregnancy and report hospitalizations and unscheduled clinic visits for asthma exacerbations. Independent of systemic corticosteroid treatment and other covariates, the incidence of preterm delivery was significantly higher among patients with inadequate asthma control during the first part of pregnancy (11.4%) compared with patients with adequate asthma control (6.3%). Similar results were demonstrated among patients who were hospitalized for asthma during pregnancy (16.4%) compared with patients without such history (7.6%). No such association was demonstrated with regard to IUGR. This study demonstrates a substantial risk for preterm delivery posed by poorly controlled maternal asthma and provides additional evidence regarding the importance of adequate treatment of asthma in pregnancy to maintain optimal asthma control.

Review of the recent prospective literature indicates that these results are consistent in the majority of the studies but not in all. Doucette and Bracken [51] compared pregnancy outcomes of 32 asthmatic women to 3,859 controls. Asthma was significantly associated with a two-fold risk for preterm delivery but not with low birth weight. Schatz et al. [8] examined pregnancy outcomes of 486 actively managed asthmatic women and the same number of controls. There were no significant differences between the groups with regard to pre-eclampsia, preterm delivery, IUGR, low birth weight, perinatal mortality, or congenital malformation. Jana et al. [25] reported similar findings in a study of 182 asthmatic and 364 non-asthmatic pregnant women that was conducted in India in 1983–1992. They found no significant increase in adverse pregnancy outcomes among asthmatic women. Nevertheless, in 15 asthmatic women who had a severe exacerbation during the pregnancy, a significant reduction in birth weight was noted. Minerbi-Codish et al. [52] compared 77 asthmatic mothers to 101 controls. Asthmatics were classified as mild, moderate, and severe according to their medical treatment. No significant association was found between maternal asthma or maternal use of corticosteroids and the following outcomes: gestational hypertension, low birth weight, preterm delivery, and Apgar scores. Mihrshahi et al. [53] examined pregnancy outcomes of 340 asthmatic and 271 non-asthmatic women. Asthma was not associated with increased risk for preterm delivery, low birth weight, pre-eclampsia cesarean delivery, and other outcomes. However, a limitation of this study is that women were recruited at 36 weeks' gestation, which may have led to an under-estimation of the adverse effects of asthma on pregnancy outcomes. By contrast, Sobande et al. [54] reported that compared to non-asthmatic women, pregnant asthmatic women are at increased risk for pre-eclampsia, perinatal mortality, low birth weight, and congenital malformations, but not for preterm delivery.

Summary: Effects of Asthma on Pregnancy

In contrast to the newer prospective studies, there is much less consensus among the retrospective studies with regard to pregnancy outcomes. Review of the retrospective literature reveals that asthma has been, but also has *not* been, associated with nearly every possible pregnancy complication. This inconsistency can be partially explained by the fact that the majority of these retrospective studies are limited by the little available information regarding asthma severity or treatment. Furthermore, many of the older studies have several methodologic inadequacies such as low power, lacking control for confounders, different inclusion/exclusion criteria.

The newer prospective studies have the advantage of being able to monitor clinical symptoms or effectiveness of treatment. However, the variation in population characteristics (general treatment, medication type, different criteria for severity classification) makes the comparison between the studies difficult.

Most of the prospective studies published in the past two decades indicate that adverse pregnancy outcomes are infrequent among asthmatic women with a well-controlled disease [8,23,25,52,53]. The two largest studies, by Dombrowski et al. [48] and Bracken et al. [46] (which contained information regarding asthma severity and treatment), indicate that therapy tailored to asthma severity can result in favorable pregnancy outcomes. Severe asthma, however, was found to be associated with an increased risk for preterm delivery, IUGR, and cesarean delivery.

An increased rate of cesarean delivery was also reported by other studies [23,48,50]. A recently published study provides a possible explanation for this finding. Linton and Peterson [55] reported that preexisting chronic conditions, including bronchial asthma, may increase the likelihood that a woman will deliver by cesarean section. It seems that uncertainly in guiding the delivery of asthmatic women, together with the misperception of increased risk of complications, account for the higher rate of cesarean deliveries among those women.

Contrary to previous retrospective publications [6,41,42], the majority of controlled prospective studies found no significant association between well-treated asthma and pre-eclampsia [8,46,48,52,53]. Triche et al. [47], however, found that moderate and severe asthma is significantly associated with an increased risk for pre-eclampsia, regardless of asthma diagnosis or treatment. Schatz [10] suggested that a release of local mediators during an asthma attack can be one of the mechanisms to explain this association. Other suggested mechanisms include hypoxia, inflammation, medication, and smoking [8,37,40-42].

In conclusion, there is extensive evidence that mild or moderate well-controlled asthma can result in excellent pregnancy and perinatal outcomes, whereas severe or poorly controlled asthma may result in adverse maternal and fetal outcomes such as preterm birth, pre-eclampsia, IUGR, and cesarean delivery.

Pharmacologic Therapy

According to the NAEPP Working Group Report on Managing Asthma During Pregnancy: Recommendations for Pharmacologic Treatment—Update 2004, it is safer for pregnant asthmatics to be medically treated than it is for them to have exacerbations. The stepwise approach, in which the dose, number of medications, and frequency of administration are changed in correlation to asthma severity, is used to achieve and maintain asthma control. For each step medications are defined as "preferred" or "alternative". Patients failing to respond are being stepped up. A step-down approach can be considered once control is sustained for several months [15].

Numerous studies examined the efficacy and safety of anti-asthma drug therapy during pregnancy. As a result, extensive evidence exists regarding the safety of the major drug classes.

Inhaled and Systemic Corticosteriods

Inhaled corticosteroids (ICS) are considered the therapy of choice for treating all levels of persistent asthma during pregnancy [3,12,15]. As mentioned earlier, Stenius-Aarniala et al. [49] demonstrated that women who experienced an acute exacerbation during pregnancy were less likely to have been using ICS prior to the exacerbation. ICS therapy was not associated with adverse pregnancy outcomes. Wendel et al. [56] prospectively studied 84 pregnant women with asthma exacerbations. The women were randomly assigned to receive either intravenous aminophylline and a beta-2 agonist or ICS (methylprednisolone) and a beta-2 agonist. Intravenous aminophylline offered no therapeutic advantages, while ICS reduced the need for subsequent admissions. .Using the Swedish Medical Birth Registry, Källén et al. [57] investigated the incidence of congenital malformations among over 2000 infants whose mothers had used inhaled budesonide for asthma in early pregnancy. No significant differences were demonstrated compared to the general population. Norjavaara and de Verdier [43] investigated, retrospectively, whether the reported use of ICS during pregnancy influenced birth outcomes. 2,968 mothers who reported use of ICS during early pregnancy gave birth to infants of normal gestational age, birth weight, with no increased rate of stillbirths. Schatz et al [58] evaluated the relationship between asthma medication therapy and adverse perinatal outcomes in 2,123 pregnancies. The use of inhaled beta-2 agonists, ICS, or theophylline was not significantly associated with adverse perinatal outcomes. After adjusting for potential confounders, oral corticosteroid use was significantly associated with both preterm delivery at less than 37 weeks' gestation and low birth weight. Dombrowski et al. [59] compared the efficacy of beclomethasone to oral theophylline for the prevention of asthma exacerbation in a prospective, double-blind, double placebo-controlled randomized clinical trial of pregnant women with moderate asthma. No significant differences were demonstrated between the groups with regard to treatment failure, proportion of peak expiratory flow rate less than 80% predicted, or maternal/perinatal outcomes. The theophylline cohort had a significantly higher incidence of treatment discontinuance caused by side effects. Rahimi et al. [60] reported the results of a meta-analysis of all clinical studies that evaluated the pregnancy and perinatal outcomes in women exposed to ICS. ICS therapy was not associated with increased risk for major malformations, preterm delivery, low birth weight, and pregnancy-induced hypertension. Silverman et al. [61] reported similar results.

In summary, the consistent findings provided by these studies indicate that ICS therapy is not associated with adverse pregnancy outcomes and is relatively safe for use during pregnancy. The safety of oral steroid treatment during pregnancy, however, is less clear. As mentioned earlier, an association between oral steroid treatment and an increased risk for preterm delivery was demonstrated by the two large prospective cohort studies of Dombrowski et al. [48] and Bracken et al. [46].

Beta-2 Agonists and Theophylline

Inhaled beta-2 agonists are recommended for all degrees of asthma during pregnancy [12] and, according to the NAEPP recommendations [15] (based on a review of six studies), inhaled beta-2 agonists are relatively safe to be used during pregnancy. As noted earlier, Schatz et al. [58] did not find an association between beta-2 agonist use and adverse pregnancy outcomes. Recently, Martel et al. [62] investigated, using a retrospective analysis, the effects of inhaled beta-2 agonists use on the risk of gestational hypertensive disorders (gestational hypertension, pre-eclampsia, eclampsia). Surprisingly, they found that use of inhaled beta-2 agonist during pregnancy was associated with reduced risk.

According to the NAEPP recommendations [15] (based upon a review of eight studies) theophylline is relatively safe for use during pregnancy at a serum concentration of 5–12 µg/mL. As noted earlier, the two large prospective studies of Dombrowski et al. and Schatz et al. confirmed these recommendations. Dombrowski's group [48] found that ICS and oral theophylline have the same efficacy in prevention of asthma exacerbation. Nevertheless, the theophylline cohort had a significantly higher incidence of treatment discontinuance caused by side effects. Schatz et al. [58] found that therapy with theophylline as well as with ICS or inhaled beta-2 agonists was not significantly associated with adverse perinatal outcomes.

Combined Therapy

Källén and Otterblad Olausson [63–65] conducted a large retrospective cohort study of over 24,000 pregnant asthmatics who reported the use of anti-asthmatic drugs in early pregnancy. They investigated the association between use of anti-asthmatic drugs during pregnancy and pregnancy complications, the risk for congenital malformations, and perinatal outcomes. The following complications occurred at an increased rate with the use of anti-asthmatic drugs, especially when three or more drugs had been used: preeclampsia, gestational diabetes, hemorrhage, premature rupture of membranes, labor induction, and cesarean delivery. Most of the increased risk for caesarean delivery (OR=1.79) could be explained by these pregnancy complications. Congenital malformations: After adjustment for confounding factors, a weak association between anti-asthmatic drug use and the risk for a congenital malformation was demonstrated (OR=1.09), specifically cardiac defects, orofacial clefts, and anal atresia. The use of inhaled corticosteroids showed a higher odds ratio for orofacial clefts and anal atresia, but the differences could be random. The authors concluded that "The use of anti-asthmatic drugs carry no major risk for congenital malformations, but a slight teratogenic effect cannot be excluded. It may be due to asthma, and arguments for a stronger effect of inhaled corticosteroids than of other anti-asthmatics are weak." Perinatal outcomes: An increased risk for preterm birth (OR=1.46), low birth weight (OR=1.67), small for gestational age (OR=1.70), hyperglycemia (OR=1.62), and mortality (OR=1.52) was found, with correlation to the number of drugs used by the mother during pregnancy, especially when three or more drugs had been used. An increased risk for neonatal icterus was mainly an effect of preterm birth. They concluded that "Infants whose mothers had asthma had a number of manifestations of poor outcome which appeared to be linked with the severity of the asthma."

Conclusions

Asthma is the most common respiratory disorder complicating pregnancy, with an increasing prevalence over recent years. The recent prospective studies investigating the influences of pregnancy on the course of asthma challenge the long-standing consensus that asthma will worsen in one-third, remain unchanged in one-third, and improve in one-third, and suggest that the real risk of having an exacerbation during pregnancy may be underestimated. Despite the controversy between retrospective and prospective cohort studies, it is clear that mild/moderate asthma, managed according to the NAEPP recommendations, is associated with favorable maternal and perinatal outcomes, while severe asthma or untreated asthma may be associated with increased risk for preterm birth, pre-eclampsia, IUGR, and cesarean delivery.

Management of asthma during pregnancy should include objective assessment of lung function, trigger avoidance, patient education, and stepwise therapy. ICS are the preferred treatment for all levels of persistent asthma, but other drug classes are efficient and relatively safe for use as well.

Since asthma is the most common respiratory disorder during pregnancy, further prospective studies should determine its clinical significance during pregnancy, in order to lead to a well-established protocol for surveillance in follow up during pregnancy.

References

[1]   Schatz M, Zeiger RS, Hoffman CP. Intrauterine growth is related to gestational pulmonary function in pregnant asthmatic women. Kaiser-Permanente Asthma and Pregnancy Study Group. *Chest* 1990;98:389-92.

[2]   Kwon HL, Belanger K, Bracken MB. Effect of pregnancy and stage of pregnancy on asthma severity: A systematic review. *Am J Obstet Gynecol*. 2004;190:1201-10.

[3]   Namazy JA, Schatz M. Treatment of asthma during pregnancy and perinatal outcomes. *Curr Opin Allergy Clin Immunol*. 2005;5:229-33.

[4]   Sheiner E, Mazor M, Levy A, Wiznitzer A, Bashiri A. Pregnancy outcome of asthmatic patients: a population-based study. *J Matern Fetal Neonatal Med*. 2005;18:237-40.

[5]   Murphy VE, Gibson PG, Smith R, Clifton VL. Asthma during pregnancy: mechanisms and treatment implications. *Eur Respir J*. 2005;25:731-50.

[6]   Alexander S, Dodds L, Armson BA. Perinatal outcomes in women with asthma during pregnancy. *Obstet Gynecol*. 1998;92:435-40.

[7]   Kwon HL, Belanger K, Bracken M. Asthma prevalence among pregnant and childbearing-aged women in the United States: estimates from national health surveys. *Ann Epidemiol* 2003;13:317-24.

[8]   Schatz M, Zeiger RS, Hoffman GP, Harden K, Forsythe A, Chilingar L, Saunders B, Porreco R, Sperling W, Kagnoff M, et al. Perinatal outcomes in the pregnancies of asthmatic women: A prospective controlled analysis. *Am J Respir Crit Care Med*. 1995;151:1170-4.

[9]   Clark SL. Asthma in pregnancy. National Asthma Education Program Working Group on Asthma and Pregnancy. National Institutes of Health, National Heart, Lung and Blood Institute. *Obstet Gynecol*. 1993;82:1036-40.

[10] Schatz M. Asthma during pregnancy: interrelationships and management. *Ann Allergy*. 1992;68:123-33.

[11] Katz O, Sheiner E. Asthma and pregnancy: A review of two decades. *Expert Rev. Resp. Med*. 2008;2:1-10.

[12] Dombrowski MP. Asthma and pregnancy. *Obstet Gynecol*. 2006;108:667-81.

[13] Cunningham FG, Leveno KJ, Bloom SL, Hauth JC, Gilstrap LC, Wenstrom KD, eds. *Williams Obstetrics*, 22nd ed. New York: McGraw-Hill Medical Publishing Division; 2006:136.

[14] Gluck JC. The change of asthma course during pregnancy. *Clin Rev Allergy Immunol*. 2004;26:171-80.

[15] NAEPP Expert Panel Report. Working Group Report on Managing Asthma During Pregnancy: Recommendations for Pharmacologic Treatment – update 2004. *Allergy Clin Immunol*. 2005;115:34-46.

[16] Brancazio LR, Laifer SA, Schwartz T. Peak expiratory flow rate in normal pregnancy. *Obstet Gynecol*. 1997;89:383-6.

[17] Hassan M, Donia SE, Nasrallah FK, Saade GR, Belfort MA. Effect of Gestational Age and Position on Peak Expiratory Flow Rate: A Longitudinal Study. *Obstet Gynecol*. 2005;105:372-5.

[18] Murphy VE, Clifton VL, Gibson PG. Asthma exacerbation during pregnancy: incidence and association with adverse pregnancy outcome. *Thorax* 2006;61:169-76.

[19] Lao TT, Huengsburg M. Labour and delivery in mothers with asthma. *Eur J Obstet Gynecol Reprod Biol*. 1990;35:183-90.

[20] Schatz M, Dombrowski MP, Wise R, Thom EA, Landon M, Mabie W, Newman RB, Hauth JC, Lindheimer M, Caritis SN, Leveno KJ, Meis P. Miodovnik M, Wapner RJ,

Paul RH, Varner MW, O'Sullivan MJ, Thurnau GR, Conway D, McNellis D. Asthma morbidity during pregnancy can be predicted by severity classification. *J Allergy Clin Immunol*. 2003;112:283-8.

[21] Schatz M, Harden K, Forsythe A, Chilingar L, Hoffman C, Sperling W, Zeiger RS. The course of asthma during pregnancy, post partum and with successive pregnancies: a prospective analysis. *J Allergy Clin Immunol*. 1988;81:509-17.

[22] Murphy VE, Gibson PG, Talbot PI, Clifton VL. Severe asthma exacerbations during pregnancy. *Obstet Gynecol*. 2005;106:1046-54.

[23] Stenius-Aarniala B, Piirilä P, Teramo K. Asthma and pregnancy: a prospective study of 198 pregnancies. *Thorax* 1988;43:12-8.

[24] Gluck JC, Gluck PA. The effect of pregnancy on the course of asthma. *Immunol Allergy Clin North Am*. 2006;26:63-80.

[25] Jana N, Vasishta K, Saha SC, Khunnu B. Effect of bronchial asthma on the course of pregnancy, labour and perinatal outcome. *J Obstet Gynaecol*. 1995;21:227-32.

[26] Beecroft N, Cochrane GM, Milburn HJ. Effect of sex of fetus on asthma during pregnancy: blind prospective study. *BMJ*. 1998;317:856-7.

[27] Dodds L, Armson BA, Alexander S. Use of asthma drugs is less among women pregnant with boys rather than girls. *BMJ*. 1999;318:1011.

[28] Kwon HL, Belanger K, Holford TR, Bracken MB. Effect of fetal sex on airway lability in pregnant women with asthma. *Am J Epidemiol*. 2006;163:217-21.

[29] Bakhireva LN, Schatz M, Jones KL, Tucker CM, Slymen DJ, Klonoff-Cohen HS, Gresham L, Johnson D, Chambers CD; OTIS Collaborative Research Group. Fetal sex and maternal asthma control in pregnancy. *J Asthma*. 2008;45:403-7.

[30] Firoozi F, Ducharme FM, Lemière C, Beauchesne MF, Perreault S, Forget A, Blais L. Effect of fetal gender on maternal asthma exacerbations in pregnant asthmatic women. *Respir Med*. 2009;103(1):144-51. Epub 2008 Aug 29.

[31] Kircher S, Schatz M, Long L. Variables affecting asthma course during pregnancy. *Ann Allergy Asthma Immunol*. 2002;89:463-6.

[32] Baibergenova A, Thabane L, Akhtar-Danesh N, Levine M, Gafni A. Is fetal gender associated with emergency department visits for asthma during pregnancy? *J Asthma*. 2006;43:293-9.

[33] Enriquez R, Griffin MR, Carroll KN, Wu P, Cooper WO, ebretsadik T, Dupont WD, Mitchel EF, Hartert TV. Effect of maternal asthma and asthma control on pregnancy and perinatal outcomes. *J Allergy Clin Immunol*. 2007;120:625-30.

[34] Tata LJ, Lewis SA, McKeever TM, Smith CJ, Doyle P, Smeeth L, West J, Hubbard RB. A Comprehensive Analysis of Adverse Obstetric and Pediatric Complications in Women with Asthma. *Am J Respir Crit Care Med*. 2007;175:991-7.

[35] Källén B, Rydhstroem H, Aberg A. Asthma during pregnancy-a population based study. *Eur J Epidemiol*. 2000;16:167-71.

[36] Blais L, Forget A. Asthma exacerbations during the first trimester of pregnancy and the risk of congenital malformations among asthmatic women. *J Allergy Clin Immunol*. 2008;121:1379-84.

[37] Getahun D, Ananth CV, Peltier MR, Smulian JC, Vintzileos AM. Acute and chronic respiratory diseases in pregnancy: Associations with placental abruption. *Am J Obstet Gynecol*. 2006;195:1180-4.

[38] Perlow JH, Montgomery D, Morgan MA, Towers CV, Porto M. Severity of asthma and perinatal outcome. Am J Obstet Gynecol. 1992;167:963-7.

[39] Lehrer S, Stone J, Lapinski R, Lockwood CJ, Schachter BS, Berkowitz R, Berkowitz GS. Association between pregnancy-induced hypertension and asthma during pregnancy. *Am J Obstet Gynecol*. 1993;168:1463-6.

[40] Demissie K, Breckenridge MB, Rhoads GG. Infant and maternal outcomes in the pregnancies of asthmatic women. Am J Respir Crit Care Med. 1998;158:1091-5.

[41] Liu S, Wen SW, Demissie K, Marcoux S, Kramer MS. Maternal asthma and pregnancy outcomes: a retrospective cohort study. *Am J Obstet Gynecol*. 2001;184:90-6.

[42] Wen SW, Demissie K, Liu S. Adverse outcomes in pregnancies of asthmatic women: results from a Canadian population. *Ann Epidemiol*. 2001;11:7-12.

[43] Norjavaara E, de Verdier MG. Normal pregnancy outcomes in a population-based study including 2,968 pregnant women exposed to budesonide. *J Allergy Clin Immunol*. 2003;111:736-42.

[44] Katz O, Mazor M, Wiznitzer A, Sheiner E. Seasonality in Deliveries of Asthmatic Patients. Presented at the World Asthma Meeting WAM, 22-25 June 2007, Istanbul, Turkey.

[45] Tata LJ, Lewis SA, McKeever TM, Smith CJ, Doyle P, Smeeth L, Gibson JE, Hubbard RB. Effect of maternal asthma, exacerbations and asthma medication use on congenital malformations in offspring: A UK population-based study. *Thorax* 2008;63(11):981-7. Epub 2008 Aug 4.

[46] Bracken MB, Triche EW, Belanger K, Saftlas A, Beckett WS, Leaderer BP. Asthma symptoms, severity, and drug therapy: a prospective study of effects on 2205 pregnancies. *Obstet Gynecol*. 2003;102:739-52.

[47] Triche EW, Saftlas AF, Belanger K, Leaderer BP, Bracken MB. Association of asthma diagnosis, severity, symptoms, and treatment with risk of preeclampsia. *Obstet Gynecol*. 2004;104:585-93.

[48] Dombrowski MP, Schatz M, Wise R, Momirova V, Landon M, Mabie W, Newman RB, McNellis D, Hauth JC, Lindheimer M, Caritis SN, Levenko KJ, Meis P, Miodovnik M, Wapner RJ, Paul RH, Varner MW, O'Sullivan MJ, Thurnau GR, Conway DL; National Institute of Child Health and Human Development Maternal-Fetal Medicine Units Network and the National Heart, Lung, and Blood Institute. Asthma during pregnancy. *Obstet Gynecol*. 2004;103:5-12.

[49] Stenius-Aarniala BS, Hedman J, Teramo KA. Acute asthma during pregnancy. *Thorax* 1996;51:411-4.

[50] Bakhireva LN, Schatz M, Jones KL, Chambers CD; Organization of Teratology Information Specialists Collaborative Research Group. Asthma control during pregnancy and the risk of preterm delivery or impaired fetal growth. *Ann Allergy Asthma Immunol*. 2008;101:137-43.

[51] Doucette JT, Bracken MB. Possible role of asthma in the risk of preterm labor and delivery. *J Obstet Gynaecol*. 1995;21:227-32.

[52] Minerbi-Codish I, Fraser D, Avnun L, Glezerman M, Heimer D. Influence of asthma in pregnancy on labor and the newborn. *Int J Gynaecol Obstet*. 2002;77:117-21.

[53] Mihrshahi S, Belousova E, Marks GB, Peat JK; Childhood Asthma Prevention Team. Pregnancy and birth outcomes in families with asthma. *J Asthma*. 2003;40:181-7.

[54] Sobande AA, Archibong EI, Akinola SE. Pregnancy outcome in asthmatic patients from high altitudes. *Int J Gynaecol Obstet*. 2002;77:117-21.

[55] Linton A, Peterson MR. Effect of preexisting chronic disease on primary cesarean delivery rates by race for births in U.S. military hospitals, 1999-2002. *Birth* 2004;31:165-75.

[56] Wendel PJ, Ramin SM, Barnett-Hamm C, Rowe TF, Cunningham FG. Asthma treatment in pregnancy: a randomized controlled study. *Am J Obstet Gynecol*. 1996;175:150-4.

[57] Källén B, Rydhstroem H, Aberg A. Congenital malformations after the use of inhaled budesonide in early pregnancy. *Obstet Gynecol* 1999;93:392-5.

[58] Schatz M, Dombrowski MP, Wise R, Momirova V, Landon M, Mabie W, Newman RB, Hauth JC, Lindheimer M, Caritis SN, Leveno KJ, Meis P, Miodovnik M, Wapner RJ, Paul RH, Varner MW, O'Sullivan MJ, Thurnau GR, Conway DL; Material-Fetal Medicine Units Network, The National Institute of Child Health and Development; The National Heart, Lung and Blood Institute. The relationship of asthma medication use to perinatal outcomes. *J Allergy Clin Immunol*. 2004;113:1040-5.

[59] Dombrowski MP, Schatz M, Wise R, Thom EA, Landon M, Mabie W, Newman RB, McNellis D, Hauth JC, Lindheimer M, Caritis SN, Leveno KJ, Meis P, Miodovnik M, Wapner RJ, Varner MW, O'Sullivan MJ, Conway DL; National Institute of Child Health and Human Development Maternal-Fetal Medicine Units Network; National Heart, Lung, and Blood Institute. Randomized trial of inhaled beclomethasone dipropionate versus theophylline for moderate asthma during pregnancy. *Am J Obstet Gynecol*. 2004;190:737-44.

[60] Rahimi R, Nikfar S, Abdollahi M. Meta-analysis finds use of inhaled corticosteroids during pregnancy safe: a systematic meta-analysis review. *Hum Exp Toxicol*. 2006;25:447-52.

[61] Silverman M, Sheffer A, Diaz PV, Lindmark B, Radner F, Broddene M, de Verdier MG, Pedersen S, Pauwels RA; START Investigators Group. Outcome of pregnancy in a randomized controlled study of patients with asthma exposed to budesonide. *Ann Allergy Asthma Immunol*. 2005;95:566-70.

[62] Martel MJ, Rey E, Beauchesne MF, Perreault S, Forget A, Maghni K, Lefebvre G, Blais L. Use of short-acting beta2-agonists during pregnancy and the risk of pregnancy-induced hypertension. *J Allergy Clin Immunol*. 2007;119:576-82.

[63] Källén B, Otterblad Olausson P. Use of anti-asthmatic drugs during pregnancy. 1. Maternal characteristics, pregnancy and delivery complications. *Eur J Clin Pharmacol*. 2007;63:363-73.

[64] Källén B, Otterblad Olausson P. Use of anti-asthmatic drugs during pregnancy. 2. Infant characteristics excluding congenital malformations. *Eur J Clin Pharmacol*. 2007;63:375-81.

[65] Källén B, Otterblad Olausson P. Use of anti-asthmatic drugs during pregnancy. 3. Congenital malformations in the infants. *Eur J Clin Pharmacol*. 2007;63:383-8.

In: Textbook of Perinatal Epidemiology
Editor: Eyal Sheiner, pp. 319-346

ISBN: 978-1-60741-648-7
© 2010 Nova Science Publishers, Inc.

Chapter XVIII

Epidemiology of Diabetes Mellitus during Pregnancy

Yariv Yogev[*] *and Avi Ben-Haroush*

Perinatal Division, Helen Schneider Hospital for Women, Rabin Medical Center, Petach Tikva and Sackler Faculty of Medicine, Tel Aviv University, Tel Aviv, Israel

Critical Points

- Differences in screening programs and diagnostic criteria make it difficult to compare frequencies of pregnancy complicated by diabetes among various populations.
- There are several predisposing risk factors for gestational diabetes mellitus (GDM) (see table).
- In the absence of risk factors, the incidence of GDM is low. Therefore, some authors suggest that selective screening may be cost effective, especially in view the forecasted rise in the burden of GDM.
- Polycystic ovary syndrome (PCOS) is an important risk factor for GDM, with special similarity in the existence of insulin resistance.
- The recurrence rate of GDM (35–80%) is influenced by parity, BMI, early diagnosis of GDM, insulin requirement, weight gain and by the interval between pregnancies.
- Pregnant women with impaired glucose tolerance (IGT) and an abnormal glucose challenge test (GCT) may be at increased risk of an adverse outcome relative to women with a normal glucose tolerance and a normal GCT.

---

[*] For Correspondence: Yariv Yogev, MD, Department of Obstetrics and Gynecology, Helen Schneider Hospital for Women, Rabin Medical Center, Petah Tiqwa 49100, Israel. Tel: +972-3-9377400; Fax: +972-3-9377409; E-mail: yarivyogev@hotmail.com

- GDM is characterized by an increased risk of a diabetic embryopathy, perhaps due to pre-existing but undetected type 2 DM. This should be considered in all patients with early diagnosis of GDM, accompanied by appropriate patient counseling.
- Hypertensive disorders in pregnancy and afterwards may be more prevalent in women with GDM. One possible mechanism is insulin resistance.
- Women with GDM are at increased risk of developing type 2 DM, especially obese patients, those who were diagnosed before 24 weeks' gestation and those who required insulin for glycemic control.

Introduction

There are three classifications of glucose intolerance in pregnancy: pre-existing type 1 diabetes, pre-existing type 2 diabetes and gestational diabetes mellitus (GDM) [1,2]. Type 1 diabetes is an autoimmune disease in which the pancreatic β-cells are destroyed. Type 2 diabetes is believed to be a combination of insulin resistance and relative insulin deficiency. Its etiology is traced to a strong genetic predisposition to insulin resistance further aggravated by obesity and diminished pancreatic β-cell function. Women with type 1 or type 2 are often grouped together for epidemiological purposes and classified as pre-existing or pre-gestational diabetes (PGDM). In contrast, women who develop glucose intolerance at any time during pregnancy are classified as GDM. However, some of these women are discovered to have type 1 or type 2 diabetes following pregnancy.

Although the aggregation of type 1 and type 2 diabetes into one classification and the need to confirm the diagnosis of GDM postpartum impedes our understanding of the epidemiology of diabetes during pregnancy, they do not lessen its significance. The need to measure the occurrence and consequence of diabetes in pregnancy is fundamental to an understanding of prevention, detection and treatment. Health systems rely on this information to identify individuals at risk and intervene with sufficient time to prevent adverse perinatal and neonatal outcomes. It is also essential to our understanding of whether interventions are effective.

Epidemiology requires that disease states be compared with non-disease states so that the relative risk of disease can be measured. Most epidemiologic information is expressed as a rate (number of events divided by the population at risk). The epidemiology of diabetes in pregnancy has two different denominators based on the events under investigation. One denominator is the number of pregnancies within a particular population during a specific year. For example, the number of women with GDM divided by the number of pregnancies provides the rate of GDM. A second denominator is live births within a single year.

The principal sources of epidemiological information are national and local statistics, hospital and ambulatory medical records, research studies and specialized registries. These epidemiological data vary as to their specificity, population size, criteria for ascertainment and definition of disease. Pregnancy-related statistics are generally based on state reports from birth certificates and hospital records. Whereas birth certificates tend to contain standardized data such as birth weight, hospital maternal and infant records vary in their completeness and comparability. Not all hospitals report maternal complications using the same terminology or criteria for identifying patients with disease. The balance among these various data sources and the conclusions that are drawn from them are, consequently, subject to wide interpretation.

Prevalence of Diabetes in Pregnancy

Estimates that diabetes (type 1, type 2 and GDM) occurs annually in 1% to 14% of all pregnancies in the United States are based on both national birth statistics and small community studies [1,2]. The data from these sources vary in their inclusion criteria. National data sources combine pre-gestational and gestational diabetes, reporting the total number of women with diabetes whose pregnancy resulted in a live birth [3]. The data are also reported by ethnicity (Asian, African-America, Hispanic, Native Americans, Pacific Islanders and Caucasian). Community studies tend to be more limited. They focus on one ethnic group with specific risk factors (e.g., family history (genetics), morphology (obesity), parity and previous GDM) [4]. In this section, national, regional and community reports of diabetes in pregnancy are combined to provide an estimate of the prevalence of maternal diabetes.

Pre-Gestational Diabetes

Based on the US Census Bureau report of the number of women between the ages of 15 and 44 (considered the principal period of fertility) adjusted for disease, there are an estimated 1.15 million women with type 1 or type 2 diabetes. Assuming that these women have a similar birth rate as the overall US birth rate (61/1000), it can be estimated that women with pre-gestational diabetes account for 71,000 births annually. However, published reports estimate that 10% of diabetes-related pregnancies are of women with pre-gestational diabetes. The United States Vital Statistics reported in 2002 that 132,000 women with diabetes had live births [3]. Consequently, pre-existing diabetes would account for 13,200 births (Caucasian, 7,100; African-American, 1,800; Hispanic, 2,800; with all other ethnic and racial groups accounting for the remainder). It is important to note that Native Americans and Hawaiian Natives, due to their especially high prevalence of type 2 diabetes, contribute disproportionately to the number of cases of pre-gestational diabetes. Both groups have rates of pre- gestational (type 2) diabetes that are higher than Caucasian, African-American and Hispanic women. Since the prevalence of type 1 and type 2 diabetes varies by both race and age, it is difficult to differentiate the number of births complicated by type 1 diabetes from those complicated by type 2 diabetes in the population as a whole or in any of its components.

The above data suggest that between 0.4% and 2% of US births are complicated by pre-gestational diabetes. Small population studies in the United States, as well as in other countries, indicate that the total number of women with pre-gestational diabetes is closer to 2% of US births [5-9]. This is based on several factors that were uncovered during the past decade: (1) increased incidence in type 2 diabetes among adolescents and women less than 25 years of age; (2) increased birth rate among adolescents; (3) population growth (due to immigration and higher birth rate) among groups with higher risk of diabetes (specifically Hispanic and Asian-American); (4) increased incidence of obesity in women of childbearing age; (5) increased incidence of impaired glucose homeostasis (elevated fasting blood glucose (100–125 mg/dl [5.6–6.9 mmo/l] and/or 2-hour post 75 gram glucose load (140–199 mg/dl [7.8–11.0 mmol/l). An examination of outcomes of pregnancy that are normally associated with hyperglycemia during pregnancy (such as macrosomia and neonatal hypoglycemia) may serve to improve the clarity of these estimates.

Gestational Diabetes Mellitus

The epidemiology of GDM is subject to substantial limitations due to disagreement over: (1) who should be screened; (2) when screening should occur; (3) screening test criteria; and, (4) diagnostic test criteria.

Screening recommendations range from the inclusion of all pregnant women (universal) to the exclusion of all women except those with very specific risk factors (selective): (e.g., age: >25; obesity: BMI >30; ethnicity: Hispanic, Native American, Asian American, African-American; family history: first degree relative; and, previous GDM or large for gestational age (LGA) infant). Screening by risk factor is estimated to omit more than 5% of the women with GDM [5]. With respect to the timing of the screening test, the controversy is whether to screen women with risk factors earlier (prior to the 13th gestational week) or waiting for the period between the 24th and 26th gestational week (when human placental lactogen is elevated). A second question is whether those women found negative during the early screening should be re-screened between the 24th–26th weeks when the highest yield of positive cases is likely to occur. A third question is whether women in very high risk populations, such as Native Americans and Hispanic Americans should be given a diagnostic test (such as the OGTT) in place of screening.

If universal screening is adopted, there is still disagreement as to the criteria for a positive screen. Current criteria, suggested by the American Diabetes Association and American College of Obstetrics and Gynecology, consider a positive screen as $\geq$ 140 mg/dl (8.3 mmol/l) one hour after a 50 gram glucose challenge. It has been reported that a decrease of 10 mg/dl in screening value will increase the positive predictive value of screening tests by 11% [2,6]. The consequences of inclusion policy and screening criteria can be significant. If selective screening and the 140mg/dl criteria continue to be employed, according to one report, it is likely that 16% of patients with GDM will go undetected [2,6].

Similar challenges are presented by variability in the diagnostic criteria for GDM. For example, there is a controversy as to whether the 75 gram 2-hour OGTT should be considered in place of the 100 gram 3-hour OGTT. The interpretation of OGTT criteria is also subject to debate. Some investigators have shown that women with high normal values or one abnormal value on the OGTT have the same risk of adverse perinatal outcome as do the women with two abnormal values [10,11]. Furthermore, a large number of pregnant women have poor or inadequate prenatal care and, therefore, are not included in the final statistics for diabetes in pregnancy.

In 2002, US data reported a total of 132,000 (3.3%) cases of diabetes among the approximately four million women with live births. If the prevalence rates of specific ethnic and racial groups were considered, this would significantly raise the number. Based on the US Vital Statistics database in 2002, GDM occurred in the pregnancies resulting in live births of 3.4% Hispanic women, 2.7% African-American women and 2.8% Caucasian women [3]. However, if small community studies are considered, the data suggest different estimates. Studies of Hispanic populations in the Southwestern region of the United States estimate the prevalence of GDM to be as high as 12% [8]. This is based on screening all women during their pregnancy and close surveillance throughout the gestational period. Studies of Native Americans also produce far higher rates than national data reflect. One study of Zuni tribal members uncovered a prevalence rate of 14%. Of course, these prevalence rates may not reflect the live birth rate. Even with adjustments for spontaneous abortions, the rate of pregnancies resulting in live births complicated by GDM is underestimated.

While the birth rate is stable for the Caucasian population, it is increasing for Hispanic, African-American and Asian populations. Taking into account the increase in birth rate (3%/year) combined with the increase in prevalence of GDM and type 2 diabetes (from 4 to 8% of women of childbearing age) in these populations, minority women would account for an additional 12,800 births affected by maternal diabetes. If universal screening were adopted with the criteria lowered to130 mg/dL, the net increase would be 24,000 cases. If women with impaired glucose were included, there would be an additional 60,000 cases of GDM. Thus, the overall increase in GDM might exceed 200,000 cases per year.

Racial Distribution of GDM

In a study of the prevalence of diabetes and Impaired Glucose tolerance (IGT) in diverse populations in women between the ages of 20 and 39, the World Health Organization (WHO) Ad Hoc Diabetes Reporting Group [12] noted lower rates of diabetes (< 1%) in Bantu (Tanzania), Chinese, rural Indian, Sri Lankan and some Pacific populations followed (1–3%) by Italian women, and white, black and Hispanic women in the US. Rural Fijian Indian and Aboriginal Australian women had 7% prevalence; the highest rate was found in Pima/Papago and Nauruan Indians (14–22%). The prevalence of IGT was low (< 3%) in Chinese and Malays, and was > 10% in black and Hispanic women in the US, urban Indian women in Tanzania, Pima and Nauruan Indians, and some other Pacific communities. The combined age-standardized prevalence of diabetes and IGT ranged from 0 to 36%, with >10% prevalence in one third of the populations, and > 30% prevalence in Pima and Nauruan Indians. Importantly, in some populations more than half of the cases of diabetes were undiagnosed prior to the survey. IGT was mostly overlooked in routine clinical practice. Thus, a substantial proportion of abnormal glucose tolerance in pregnancy will be undetected without screening.

It remains unclear, however, if this marked racial and geographic variation represents true differences in the prevalence of GDM, because of the remarkably variable approaches used across different studies, including different methods of screening, different oral and intravenous glucose loads, and different diagnostic criteria. For example, Dooley et al. [13]

demonstrated that race as well as maternal age and degree of obesity must be taken into account in comparing the prevalence of GDM in different populations. Their study included 3744 consecutive pregnant women who underwent universal screening. The population was 39.1% white, 37.7% black, 19.8% Hispanic and 3.4% Oriental/other. Black and Hispanic race, maternal age and percentage ideal body weight had a significant independent effect on the prevalence of GDM. The adjusted relative risk (RR) was higher in black (1.81, 95% [CI] 1.13–2.89) and Hispanic (2.45, 95% CI 1.48–4.04) women than in white women. The degree of carbohydrate intolerance was similar across racial groups; nevertheless, when the 92 GDM patients under dietary control were analyzed separately, mean birthweight was found to be highest in the Hispanic women, and was lowest in the blacks and Orientals. Hence, race had a significant independent effect on birthweight, with maternal percentage ideal body weight a significant covariate. These findings are supported by another study showing that Asian woman were more likely to have GDM than Caucasian woman (31.7 versus 14%, P = 0.02), despite their lower body mass index (BMI) [14].

Recently, Silva et al. [15] reported on ethnic differences in perinatal outcome of GDM; Neonates born to Native-Hawaiian/Pacific-Islander mothers and Filipino mothers had 4 and 2 times the prevalence of macrosomia, respectively, compared with neonates born to Japanese, Chinese, and Caucasian mothers. These differences persisted after adjustment for other statistically significant maternal and fetal characteristics. Ethnic differences were not observed for other neonatal or maternal complications associated with GDM, with the exception of neonatal hypoglycemia and hyperbilirubinemia. The authors concluded that this finding emphasizes the need to better understand ethnic-specific factors in GDM management and the importance of developing ethnic-tailored GDM interventions to address these disparities.

Risk Factors for GDM

The traditional and most often reported risk factors for GDM are high maternal age, weight and parity, previous delivery of a macrosomic infant and a family history of diabetes. These and other reported risk factors are summarized in Table-1. It is of great importance that the clinician understand and use these characteristics, along with others, such as the racial and geographic attributed risk, to improve screening programs and diagnostic accuracy, and perhaps to design better and more cost-effective selective screening and diagnostic tests. Jang et al. [16] examined 3581 consecutive Korean women and found a 2.2% prevalence of GDM. The affected women were older, had higher prepregnancy weights, higher BMI, higher parities and higher frequencies of known diabetes in the family. The risk of diabetes was closely associated with previous obstetric outcome, such as congenital malformation, stillbirth and macrosomia. The number of risk factors present in each individual increased the risk of diabetes, with the prevalence ranging from 0.6% in subjects without any risk factors to 33% in those with four or more. Thus, it is possible that selective screening may be cost-effective in situations where health resources are scarce and where total screening is impossible. Similar results were reported in a retrospective cohort study of 2574 pregnant women, which suggested that selective screening programs have a high true-positive yield

[17]. An age of ≥ 30, a family history of diabetes, obesity (BMI ≥ 27) and previous fetal macrosomia were the most frequent risk factors. Just over half (54.2%) of the population presented with one or more with the abovementioned risk factors. The positive predictive value (PPV) of screening increased with the number of risk factors, from 12% for the women with no risk factors to 40% for those with three or more risk factors. In another study, Jang et al. [18] demonstrated that in the racially homogeneous population of Seoul, Korea, besides prepregnancy BMI, age, weight gain and parental history of diabetes, short stature is an independent risk factor for GDM. Accordingly, Kousta et al. [17] reported that European and South Asian women with previous GDM were shorter than control women from the same ethnic groups, perhaps due to a common pathophysiological mechanism underlying GDM and the determination of final adult height. Others have reported similar results [19].

In a large retrospective cohort study in Canada, Xiong et al. [20] evaluated 111,563 pregnancies and detected a 2.5% prevalence of GDM. The risk factors identified were age > 35 years, obesity, history of prior neonatal death and a prior Cesarean section. Interestingly, teenage mothers and women who drank alcohol were less likely to have GDM. The risk factors mentioned above are mainly of maternal origin. However, cumulative knowledge about the long-term implications of exposure to the diabetic intrauterine environment has led to the addition of the mother's fetal history to the risk factor list. Egeland et al. [21] investigated whether the mother's own characteristics at birth could predict her subsequent risk of GDM. Using linked generation data from the Medical Birth Registry of Norway for all women born between 1967 and 1984, who gave birth between 1988 and 1998, the authors identified 498 women aged < 32 years with GDM in one or more singleton pregnancies. They found that the women whose mothers had had diabetes during pregnancy were at increased risk of GDM themselves. Significant inverse trends in diabetes were noted in relation to birthweight, with an increased risk of GDM of 80, 60 and 40% in women whose birthweights were ≤ 2500, 2500–2999 and 3000–3499 grams, respectively, compared with women in the 4000–4500 grams group. Similar findings were observed for categories of weight for gestational age.

Is GDM a cause or an effect? A retrospective study from Hong Kong [22] in 84 normotensive women showed that progressive glucose intolerance throughout pregnancy is associated with an upward shift in blood pressure in the third trimester. Hence, it is possible that blood pressure changes below the diagnostic threshold for hypertensive disorders of pregnancy may help to identify women at increased risk of GDM.

The relationship between dietary fat and glucose metabolism has been recognized for many years. Epidemiological data in humans suggest that subjects with a higher fat intake are more prone to disturbances in glucose metabolism [23]. Several researchers have hypothesized that polyunsaturated fatty acid plays an essential role in the maintenance of energy balance and, through regulation of gene transcription, may improve insulin resistance [24–26]. Accordingly, Bo et al. [27] investigated the relationship between lifestyle habits and glucose abnormalities in 504 Caucasian women with and without conventional risk factors for GDM. They identified 126 women with GDM and 84 with IGT. These patients were older and shorter than the women with normal pregnancies, and had significantly higher prepregnancy BMI, higher rates of diabetes in first-degree relatives and higher intakes of saturated fat.

Table 1. Summary of reported risk factors for GDM.

Risk Factor	Reference	Study and Population	Results
		Maternal factors	
	Jang et al., 1995 [16]	Universal screening with a 50-g glucose load at 24-28 weeks' gestation of 3581 consecutive Korean women. At 1-h plasma glucose ≥130 mg/dl, they underwent a 3-h 100-g OGTT. GDM prevalence was 2.2% (80 cases of GDM vs. 3432 normal controls).	Mean age of GDM and normal control groups, 31.7± 4.0 and 28.9±3.3 years, respectively (P<0.001).
	Jang et al., 1998 [18]	Same as above in 9005 pregnant women. GDM prevalence was 1.9% (173 GDM, 1735 IGT, and 6955 normal controls).	Mean age of GDM and IGT groups vs. normal controls, 31.1± 4.2, 29.4±3.5 and 28.5±3.4 years, respectively (P<0.001).
Older age	Xiong et al., 2001 [20]	Retrospective cohort study on 111563 deliveries from 1991 through 1997 in 39 hospitals in Canada. Average prevalence of GDM was 2.5% (2755 cases of GDM vs. 108,664 normal controls).	Age >35 years in 22.4% and 10.3% of GDM and normal patients, respectively (adjusted OR=2.34, 95% CI 2.13-2.58).
	Egeland et al., 2000 [21]	Medical Norwegian birth registry study of all women born in 1967-84 who gave birth in 1988-1998 (n=141,107), excluding 2393 non-singleton pregnancies.	GDM prevalence of 2.5%; age>35.
	Bo et al., 2001 [27]	126 pregnant women with GDM, 84 with IGT and 294 with normal glucose tolerance.	Prevalence of GDM increased with age, from 1.5 per 1000 deliveries for women aged ≤20 to 4.2 for women aged ≥30 (odds ratio 2.8; 95% confidence interval 1.9 to 4.3).

Table 1. (Continued)

	Jang et al., 1995 [16]	As described above.	Mean parity of GDM and normal control groups, 0.6±0.9 and 0.4± 0.5, respectively (P<0.05).
High parity	Jang et al., 1998 [18]	As described above.	Parity ≥2 in 9.8% of GDM and 4.7% of IGT groups and 2.6% of controls (P<0.001).
	Egeland et al., 2000 [21]	As described above.	Age-adjusted odds ratios (95%CI) for women with 2, 3, and 4 or more deliveries compared with 1delivery were 1.5 (1.2 to 1.9), 1.9 (1.4 to 2.5), and 3.3 (2.1 to 5.1), respectively.
Pre-pregnancy weight	Jang et al., 1995 [16]	As described above.	Mean weight of GDM and normal control groups, 56.4± 9.2 and 51.6±6.4 kg, respectively (P<0.001).
	Jang et al., 1998 [18]	As described above.	Mean weight of GDM and IGT groups vs. normal controls, 56.5± 9.5, 52.4±7.2 and 51.6±6.4 kg, respectively (P<0.001).
Pregnancy weight	Xiong et al., 2001 [20]	As described above.	Obesity ≥91 kg detected in 15.8% and 7.3% of GDM and normal groups, respectively (adjusted OR=2.40, 95% CI 2.06-2.98).
Pregnancy Weight gain	Jang et al., 1998 [18]	As described above.	Mean weight gain of GDM, IGT and normal control groups, of 8.4± 3.9, 8.3±3.3 and 8.1±8.1 kg, respectively (NS).

Table 1. (Continued)

BMI	Jang et al., 1995 [16]	As described above.	Only 1.3% of population was obese, but GDM prevalence increased significantly with increasing BMI. BMI≥27 in 8.8% of GDM and 1.1% of control group (P<0.001).
	Jang et al., 1998 [18]	As described above.	BMI≥27.3 in 9.8% of GDM, 2.4% of IGT, and 1.0% of controls (P<0.001).
	Bo et al., 2001 [27]	As described above.	Mean BMI in GDM, IGT, and normoglycemic group, 25.4± 5.3, 26.0±5.5 and 23.6±4.6, respectively (P=0.00002).
	Kousta et al., 2000 [17]	91 previous GDM and 73 normoglycemic control women, a median (interquartile range) of 20 (11-36) and 29 (17-49) months postpartum, respectively.	Women with previous GDM had higher BMI [26.4 (22.8-31.4) vs. 23.8 (21. 0-27.5) kg/m2, P = 0.002] and waist/hip ratio [0.82 (0.79-0.88) vs. 0. 77 (0.73-0.81), P<0.0001] than controls.
	Holte et al., 1998 [28]	34 women with GDM 3–5 years before the investigation and 36 controls with uncomplicated pregnancies, selected for similar age, parity, and date of delivery.	GDM patients had higher BMI than controls (25.2 vs. 22.2, P <0.001).

Table 1. (Continued)

Short stature	Jang et al., 1995 [16]	As described above.	Mean height of GDM and normal control groups, 158.1±4.8 and 159.7±4.2 cm, respectively (P<0.001).
	Jang et al., 1998 [18]	As described above.	≤157 cm, the odds ratio for GDM was two times greater compared the ≥163 cm group, even after controlling for age and BMI
	Kousta et al., 2000 [17]	346 women with previous GDM and 470 controls with no previous history of GDM.	European and South Asian women with previous GDM were shorter than control women from the same ethnic groups (European: 162.9 ± 6.1 vs. 165.3 ± 6.8 cm, P < 0.0001; South Asian: 155.2 ± 5.4 vs. 158.2 ± 6.3 cm, P = 0.003, adjusted for age).
	Bo et al., 2001 [27]	As described above.	GDM, IGT, and normoglycemic groups had a mean height of 1.62± 0.06, 1.61±0.006 and 1.63±0.07 cm, respectively (P=0.02).
	Branchtein et al., 2000 [19]	5564 Brazilian women	Height < 150 cm associated with a 60% increase in the odds of GDM, independently of age, obesity, skin color, parity, family history and previous GDM.
Low birth weight	Egeland et al., 2000 [21]	As described above.	Birth weight < 2500 a risk factor for GDM with OR=9.3 (CI 95% 4.1 to 21.1, P<0.001), as was weight for gestational age (centiles) < 10 with OR=1.7 (CI 95% 1.2 to 2.5).

Table 1. (Continued)

	Holte et al., 1998 [28]	As described above.	Compare with controls, GDM patients showed a higher prevalence of polycystic ovaries (14 of 34 [41%] *vs.* 1 of 36 [3%]); greater clinical and biochemical evidence of hyperandrogenism and insulin resistance; and a higher prevalence of pregnancy-induced hypertension (50% *vs.* 15%; P < 0.05) during the index pregnancy; 15% developed overt diabetes.
Polycystic ovary syndrome	Antilla et al., 1998 [30]	Retrospective comparative ultrasound study of ovaries in 31 women with GDM and 30 healthy controls matched for maternal age and BMI.	14 women with GDM (44%) and two controls exhibited PCO.
	Kousta et al., 2000 [29]	As described above.	Higher prevalence of PCO in previous-GDM group than controls (47/91 [52%] vs. 20/73 [27%]), P = 0. 002 overall, OR=2.7, P = 0.007 by logistic regression allowing for ethnicity].
	Mikola et al., 2001 [31]	Retrospective study of 99 pregnancies in women with PCOS compared with an unselected control population.	GDM developed in 20% of PCOS patients and 8.9% of controls (P < 0.001). BMI >25 important predictor of GDM (adjusted OR 5.1; CI 3.2-8.3), and PCOS an another, independent predictor (adjusted OR 1.9; CI 1.0-3.5).
	Koivunen et al., 2001 [32]	33 women with a history of GDM and 48 controls.	Higher prevalence of PCOS in GDM group (39.4% vs. 16.7%; P=0.03); also higher serum cortisol, androgens, and a greater area under the glucose curve.
High intake of saturated fat	Bo et al., 2001 [27]	As described above.	Only percentages of saturated fat (OR = 2.0; 95 %-CI = 1.2-3.2) and polyunsaturated fat (OR = 0.85; 95 %-CI = 0.77-0.92) were associated with gestational hyperglycemia, after adjustment for age, gestational age and BMI.

Table 1. (Continued)

Variable	Reference		Findings
Family history			
Familial history of diabetes	Jang et al., 1995 [16]	As described above.	35% of GDM vs. 15.4% of normal controls (P<0.001).
	Jang et al., 1998 [18]	As described above.	30.1% of GDM, 17.6% of IGT, and 13.2% of normal controls (P<0.001).
	Bo et al., 2001 [27]	As described above.	41% of GDM, 33% of IGT, and 28% of normal controls (P=0.04).
	Ho te al., 1998 [28]	As described above.	First-degree heredity of NIDDM more prevalent in previous-GDM than control group (24% vs. 6%; P < 0.05).
GDM in subject's mother	Egeland et al., 2000 [21]	As described above.	GDM rate 30.6 (per 1000 women) in women whose mother had GDM vs. 3.5 in controls (OR=9.3, CI 95% 4.1 to 21.1)
Previous obstetric outcome			
Congenital malformation	Jang et al., 1995 [16]	As described above.	GDM in 20.7% of patients who had previous malformation vs. 2.4% of patients who did not (OR=22.5; 95% CI, 7.15-70.96).
Still birth	Jang et al., 1995 [16]	As described above.	GDM in 14.3% of patients who had previous stillbirth vs. 2.6% of patients who did not (OR=8.5; 95% CI, 2.35-30.78).
	Xiong et al., 2001 [20]	As described above.	Previous neonatal death in 1.3% of GDM group vs. 0.6% of controls (adjusted OR=2.09; 95% CI 1.06-1.34).
Macrosomia	Jang et al., 1995 [16]	As described above.	GDM in 9.3% of patients who had previous macrosomia vs. 2.5% of patients who did not. (OR=5.8; 95% CI, 1.98-17.02).
Cesarean section	Xiong et al., 2001 [20]	As described above.	Previous CS in 14.8% of GDM group and 10.1% of controls (adjusted OR=1.55; 95% CI 1.11-1.25).

Table 1. (Continued)

	Study	Description	Findings
Previous GDM	MacNeill et al., 2001 [49]	A retrospective longitudinal study including 651 women.	Recurrence of GDM in 35.6% (95% CI = 31.9-39.3%). Infant birth weight in the index pregnancy and maternal pre-pregnancy weight were predictive of recurrent GDM.
	Major at al., 1998 [50]	78 patients with previous GDM.	Recurrence rate, 69%; more common with parity ≥1, BMI ≥ 30 kg/m2, GDM diagnosis at ≤ 24 gestational weeks, insulin requirement, weight gain of ≥ 15 pounds, and interval between pregnancies ≤ 24 months.
	Spong et al., 1998 [51]	164 Hispanic patients with previous GDM.	Recurrence rate 68%; more common with earlier diagnosis of GDM, requirement of insulin, and hospital admissions in index pregnancy.
	Foster-Powel and Cheung, 1998 [53]	Retrospective review of 540 women.	117 women had a subsequent pregnancy with recurrent GDM in 82 (70%). Risk factors were older age, race, BMI and weight gain.
Pregnancy factors			
High blood pressure in pregnancy	Yogev et al (66,67)	Retrospective study of 1813 GDM with and without preeclampsia	Increased rate of PET in GDM. Higher values of blood pressure in the first and second trimester on GDMs who developed PET.
Multiple pregnancy	Sivan et al., 2002 [34]	103 women with consecutive triplet pregnancies, compared to 85 women who elected to undergo fetal reduction to twins.	Higher GDM rate in the triplet than in reduction group (22.3% vs. 5.8%).
	Schwartz et al., 1999 [35]	Total 29,644 deliveries, 429 twins.	GDM increased in twin vs. singleton deliveries (7.7% vs. 4.1%; P < .05).
	Hoskins et al., 1995 [33]	3458 recorded twin live births. Calculated zygocity rate according to sex ratios.	Estimated risk for dizygotic twin pregnancies relative to monozygotic pregnancies of 8.6 (95% CI, 3.5-21.0).
	Wein et al., 1992 [36]	61,914 singleton and 798 twin pregnancies.	GDM prevalence of 7.4% in twins vs. 5.6% in singletons (P=0.025)

Table 1. (Continued)

		Protective factors
Young age	Xiong et al., 2001 [20]	As described above.	Age ≤19 years in 2.6% and 8.5% of GDM and normal patients, respectively (adjusted OR=0.35, 95% CI 0.27-0.44).
Alcohol use	Xiong et al., 2001 [20]	As described above.	Alcohol use in 0.7% and 2.0% of GDM and normal patients, respectively (adjusted OR=0.40, 95% CI 0.25-0.76).

In a multiple logistic regression model, all of these factors were associated with glucose abnormalities, after adjustment for gestational age. In the patients without conventional risk factors, only the percentages of saturated fats (odds ratio [OR] = 2.0, 95% CI 1.2–3.2) and polyunsaturated fats (OR = 0.85, 95% CI 0.77–0.92) were associated with gestational hyperglycemia, after adjustment for age, gestational age and BMI. Thus, the allegedly independent role of saturated fat in the development of gestational glucose abnormalities takes on greater importance in the absence of conventional risk factors. This suggests that glucose abnormalities may be prevented in some groups of women during pregnancy.

Polycystic Ovary Syndrome (PCOS) and GDM

PCOS is a heterogeneous disorder affecting 5–10% of women of reproductive age. It is characterized by chronic anovulation with oligo-/amenorrhea, infertility, typical sonographic appearance of the ovaries, and clinical or biochemical hyperandrogenism. Insulin resistance is present in 40–50% of patients, especially in obese women.

Holte et al. [28] reported a higher rate of ultrasonographic, clinical and endocrine signs of PCOS in 34 women who had had GDM 3–5 years before, compared to 36 matched controls with uncomplicated pregnancies. Five of the women (15%) with previous GDM had developed manifest diabetes. The authors concluded that women with previous GDM and PCOS may form a distinct subgroup from women with normal ovaries and previous GDM, who may be more prone to develop features of insulin-resistance syndrome. Other studies reported similar results. Kousta et al. [29] found a higher prevalence of PCOS in 91 women with previous GDM compared to 73 normoglycemic control women (52 versus 27%, P = 0.002), and Anttila et al. [30] reported a 44% prevalence of PCOS in women with GDM, with no differences in BMI before pregnancy or in weight gain during pregnancy compared to controls. They suggested a screening program for GDM for these patients. Mikola et al. [31] retrospectively evaluated 99 pregnancies in women with PCOS compared with an unselected control population. The average BMI and the nulliparity rate were higher in the PCOS group, as was the multiple pregnancy rate (9.1 versus 1.1%). GDM developed in 20% of the patients with PCOS but only in 8.9% of the controls (P < 0.001). A BMI > 25 was the best predictor of GDM (adjusted OR = 5.1, 95% CI 3.2–8.3), and PCOS was an additional independent predictor (adjusted OR = 1.9, 95% CI 1.0–3.5). Koivunen et al. [32] found that compared with 48 control women, 33 women with previous GDM more often had significantly abnormal oral glucose tolerance tests (OGTT), higher prevalences of polycystic ovaries (39.4 versus 16.7%, P = 0.03), higher serum concentrations of cortisol, dehydroepiandrosterone and dehydroepiandrosterone sulfate, and a greater area under the glucose curve.

Multiple Pregnancies and GDM

The number of fetuses in multifetal pregnancies is expected to influence the incidence of GDM owing to the increased placental mass and, thereby, the increase in diabetogenic hormones. However, the reports are somewhat conflicting, probably because of the heterogeneous populations studied. In an interesting study of the prevalence of GDM in dizygotic (DZ) twin pregnancies with two placentae compared to monozygotic (MZ) twin pregnancies with one placenta, Hoskins [33] evaluated 3458 recorded twin deliveries and found that a higher proportion of different-sex compared with same-sex twin pregnancies were complicated by GDM (3.5 versus 1.6%). The estimated risk for DZ twin pregnancies relative to MZ pregnancies was 8.6 (95% CI 3.5–21.0). The impact of fetal reduction on the incidence of GDM may support this theory. Sivan et al. [34] examined 188 consecutive triplet pregnancies of which 85 were reduced to twins. The rate of GDM was significantly higher in the triplet group than in the reduction group (22.3 versus 5.8%). Similar results were reported by Schwartz et al. [35] in a study of 29,644 deliveries. They found that GDM was significantly more frequent in the 429 twin deliveries (7.7 versus 4.1%, P < 0.05). However, insulin requirements were not different, suggesting a minor clinical impact. Wein et al. [36] compared the prevalence of GDM between 61,914 singleton and 798 twin deliveries performed between 1971 and 1991. The difference was significant only for the earlier decade (5.6 versus 7.4%, P = 0.025). Nevertheless, in a follow-up program there was a trend toward a higher prevalence of overt diabetes in the women who had had a diabetic twin pregnancy (18.5%) compared to those who had had a diabetic singleton pregnancy (7.4%). Whether this represents a true increased risk for diabetes is unknown.

By contrast, using data derived from the Medical Birth Registry of Norway, Egeland and Irgens [37] controlling for other risk factors such as advanced age, parity, maternal history of diabetes and the woman's own birthweight, found GDM in 6.6 per 1000 multiple pregnancies (n = 9271) and in 5.0 per 1000 singleton pregnancies (n = 640,700) (OR = 1.3, 95% CI 1.0–1.7, P = 0.03). However, analyses stratified by maternal age or parity yielded no elevated risk of GDM. Others have also failed to demonstrate a higher prevalence of GDM in multiple pregnancies [38,39].

Genetic Factors

Animal studies have shown that female fetuses exposed to a diabetic intrauterine milieu have an increased risk of subsequent GDM. In a family history study, Harder et al. [40] reported a significantly greater prevalence of diabetes (mainly type 2 DM) in the mothers of women with GDM than in their fathers. A significant aggregation of type 2 DM was also observed in the maternal-grandmaternal line compared to the paternal-grandpaternal line. However, in patients with type 1 diabetes there was no significant difference in the prevalence of any type of diabetes between mothers and fathers. Therefore, a history of type 2 DM on the mother's side might be considered as a particular risk factor for GDM via intergenerative transmission of type 2 DM, which might be prevented by strict avoidance of GDM. Dorner et al. [41] reported a significantly decreased familial diabetes aggregation on the maternal side in children with type 1 DM born between 1974 and 1984 compared to those born between 1960 and 1973. This finding was explained by the improved prevention of hyperglycemia during pregnancy since 1974, and particularly of GDM in women with familial diabetes aggregation. These authors also noted a highly significant predominance of type 2 DM in the great-grandmothers of individuals with infantile-onset diabetes compared to the paternal side. They suggested that GDM, which may represent a risk factor for diabetes transmission on the maternal side, is often followed by 'extra-gestational' type 2 DM at a later age. Like Harder et al. [40] these authors suggested that their findings were consistent with the suspected teratogenetic effect of GDM on diabetes susceptibility in the offspring, and that this was preventable by avoiding hyperglycemia in pregnant women and hyperinsulinism in fetuses.

Histocompatibility leukocytic antigen (HLA) studies are one way to establish a genetic linkage in certain diseases. In GDM, conflicting results have been reported. Kuhl [42] described similar frequencies of HLA DR2, DR3 and DR4 antigens in healthy pregnant women and women with GDM, and low prevalences of markers of autoimmune destruction of the beta cells in GDM pregnancies. Likewise, Vambergue et al. [43], in a study of 95 women with GDM, 95 with IGT and 95 control pregnant women, found no significant difference in the distribution of HLA class II polymorphism among the groups. However, the GDM and IGT groups presented some particular HLA patterns, pointing to a genetic heterogeneity of glucose intolerance during pregnancy. Lapolla et al. [44] evaluated 68 women with GDM and matched controls for the frequency of HLA A, B, C and DR antigens; the only significant differences were an increase in Cw7 and a decrease in A10 in the GDM group. Budowle et al. [45] reported that the Bf-F allele was found significantly less frequently in non-obese black women with GDM compared to controls, and suggested similar genetic associations in non-obese black women with GDM and with type 1 diabetes. Similarly, in another study, women with GDM who required insulin for glycemic control had a lower frequency of the Bf-F phenotype and a higher frequency of the Bf-f1 phenotype; they also had a lower frequency of the type 2 allele at the polymorphic locus adjacent to the insulin gene [46].

Freinkel et al. [47] evaluated 199 women with GDM and 148 patients with normal pregnancies, and found that the HLA DR3 and DR4 antigens occurred significantly more often in black women with GDM. Ferber et al. [48], in an analysis of 184 women with GDM, did not find an elevation in the frequency of any HLA class II alleles in GDM patients compared with non-diabetic unrelated subjects. However, the DR3 allele was noted significantly more frequently in 43 women with islet autoantibodies and in the 24 women who developed type 1 DM postpartum. The cumulative risk of developing type 1 DM within 2 years after pregnancy in the GDM women with DR3 or DR4 was 22%, and in the women without these alleles was 7% (P = 0.02). The risk rose to 50% in the DR3- and DR4-positive women who had required insulin during pregnancy (P = 0.006). These results indicate that women with GDM who have islet autoantibodies at delivery or develop type 1 DM postpartum have HLA alleles typical of late-onset type 1 diabetes, and that both HLA typing and islet antibodies can predict the development of type 1 DM postpartum.

Recurrence of GDM

MacNeill et al. [49] conducted a retrospective longitudinal study of 651 women who had had a diabetic pregnancy and at least one other thereafter. They found a 35.6% recurrence rate of GDM. Multivariate regression models showed that infant birthweight in the index pregnancy and maternal weight before the subsequent pregnancy was predictive of recurrent GDM.

Higher recurrence rates (69% of 78 patients) were reported by Major et al. [50]; recurrence was more common when the following variables were present in the index pregnancy: parity ≥ 1 (OR = 3.0), BMI ≥ 30 (OR = 3.6), GDM diagnosis ≤ 24 weeks gestation (OR = 20.4) and insulin requirement (OR = 2.3). A weight gain of ≥ 7kg (c. 15 pounds) (OR = 2.9) and an interval between pregnancies of ≤ 24 months (OR = 1.6) were also associated with a recurrence of GDM. Spong et al. [51] found a similarly high recurrence rate of 68% in 164 women with GDM. Risk factors for recurrence in this study were earlier diagnosis of GDM, insulin requirement and hospital admissions in the index pregnancy. Nohira et al. [52] evaluated the recurrence rate and risk factors of recurrent GDM in 32 patients with GDM and 37 with one abnormal OGTT value (OAV) in their index pregnancies. The recurrence rate from index GDM and OAV were 65.6% and 40.5%, respectively. Age, BMI prior to pregnancy, an increased weight gain between pregnancies and a short interval between pregnancies were risk factors for recurrence from the initial GDM. An increased weight gain between pregnancies and a short interval between pregnancies were risk factors of development to GDM from the initial OAV. They concluded that the control of weight gain and interval between pregnancies could be important to reduce GDM recurrence. Foster-Powel and Cheung [53] in a study of 117 women who had GDM, found that in a subsequent pregnancy the recurrence was 70%. Risk factors were older age, race, BMI and weight gain.

Abnormal Glucose Challenge Test (GCT) as a Risk Factor for Adverse Pregnancy Outcome

Is an abnormal GCT alone, without GDM, a risk factor for adverse pregnancy outcome? Using fetal weight and anthropometric characteristics as their parameters, Mello et al. [54] evaluated 1615 white women with singleton pregnancies who underwent universal screening for GDM in two periods of pregnancy. They divided the population into three groups according to the GCT results: (1) 172 patients with abnormal GCT in both periods; (2) 391 patients with a normal GCT in the early period and an abnormal GCT in the late period; (3) 1052 patients with a normal GCT in both periods (control group). The incidence of LGA infants was significantly higher in group 1 (40.7%) and group 2 (22.0%) than in the control group (8.3%), and significantly higher in group 1 than in group 2. The newborns of group 1 had higher birthweights than those of group 2 and the control group, and the newborns of the control group had significantly greater lengths and mean cranial circumferences. Group 1 babies had significantly lower ponderal indexes, thoracic circumferences and weight:length ratios than controls, and significantly larger cranial/thoracic circumferences. Additionally, Yogev et al. [55] studied the association between obesity, glucose challenge test (GCT) and pregnancy outcome in non diabetic gravid women. Overall, a positive GCT result (GCT > or = 130 mg/dl) was identified in 2541/6854 (37%) women. GDM was further diagnosed in 464/6854 (6.8%) of subjects. In both groups of screening results (> 130 mg/dl and < 130 mg/dl), the obese women were significantly older, gained more weight during pregnancy and had a lower rate of nulliparity in comparison to the non obese women. The obese women had higher rates of macrosomia, LGA and induction of labor. A gradual increase in the rate of macrosomia, LGA and cesarean section was identified in both obese and non-obese women in relation to increasing GCT severity categories. They concluded that both fetal size and cesarean section rate are associated with the degree of carbohydrate intolerance (screening results). Furthermore, obesity remains the main contributor impacting fetal size.

Weijers et al. [56] defined mild gestational hyperglycemia (MGH) as a positive GCT in the presence of a negative OGTT. Of the 1022 consecutive women evaluated, 813 (79.6%) were healthy, 138 (13.5%) had MGH and 71 (6.9%) had GDM. There was a stepwise significant increase in mean fasting glucose and C-peptide levels among the three diagnostic groups. Maternal age, non-Caucasian ethnicity and prepregnancy BMI were all associated with GDM, whereas only maternal age and prepregnancy BMI were associated with MGH. Therefore, it appears that additional factors promoting the loss of beta-cell function distinguish MGH from GDM. One of these factors is ethnicity.

Are women with one elevated 3-hour glucose tolerance test value at risk for adverse perinatal outcomes? Former studies have demonstrated higher perinatal morbidity if one abnormal value is not treated [10,11]. In a recent retrospective cohort study [57] perinatal outcomes in women with one elevated glucose tolerance test value were compared with the outcomes in women who screened negative by GCT. Of 14,036 women who met the study criteria, women with one elevated glucose tolerance test value exhibited higher rates of cesarean delivery (in nulliparous women only), preeclampsia, chorioamnionitis, birth weight > 4000 g and > 4500 g, and neonatal admission to the intensive care nursery as compared with women who screened negative (P < .05 for all).

Congenital Malformations

Schaefer-Graf et al. [58] in a review of 4180 pregnancies complicated by GDM (n = 3764) or type 2 DM (n = 416), reported that the congenital anomalies in the offspring affected the same organ systems described in pregnancies complicated by type 1 DM. The risk of anomalies rose with increasing hyperglycemia at diagnosis or presentation for care. However, most other reports had conflicting findings. Bartha et al. [59] failed to find an increase in major congenital malformations associated with GDM, as did Kalter [60] in a comprehensive review of the literature. An exception is the recent Swedish Health Registry study covering over 1.2 million births between 1987 and 1997 [61]. The authors identified 3864 infants born to women with pre-existing diabetes and 8688 infants born to women with GDM. The total malformation rate in the first group was 9.5% and in the second group 5.7%, similar to the rate in the general population. However, the GDM group was characterized by an excess of certain malformations, suggesting that a subgroup of GDM are at increased risk of diabetic embryopathy, perhaps due to pre-existing but undetected type 2 DM.

Martinez-Frias et al. [62] analyzed 19,577 consecutive infants with malformations of unknown cause and compared those born to mothers with GDM with those of non-diabetic mothers. Their findings indicated that GDM is a significant risk factor for holoprosencephaly, upper/lower spine/rib anomalies, and renal and urinary system anomalies. However, owing to the heterogeneous nature of GDM, which includes previously unrecognized and newly diagnosed type 2 DM, they could not rule out the possibility that the teratogenic effect is related to latent type 2 DM. Nevertheless, they concluded that pregnancies complicated by GDM should be considered at risk for congenital anomalies. Virtanen et al. [63] evaluated the prevalence of maternal glucose metabolism disorders during pregnancy in newborn boys having normal testicular descent or congenital cryptorchidism. After adjustment for possible confounding factors, abnormal maternal glucose metabolism was significantly more common in the group of cryptorchid boys [diet-treated gestational diabetes, P = 0.0001; OR, 3.98 (95% CI, 1.97–8.05); diet-treated gestational diabetes or only an abnormal result in oral glucose tolerance test, P = 0.0016; OR, 2.44 (95% CI, 1.40-4.25)] when compared with boys with normal testicular descent.

By contrast, the relationship between GDM and the development of congenital malformations was examined in another population-based retrospective study using birth certificate data for all live-born children delivered between 1984 and 1991 in Washington State [64]. The prevalence of congenital malformations was 7.2, 2.8 and 2.1% among the offspring of mothers with established diabetes (n = 8869), GDM (n = 1511) and no diabetes (n = 8934), respectively. That is, the rate of congenital malformations in the GDM group was only slightly higher than in the control group (OR = 1.3, 95% CI 1.0–1.6).

Hypertensive Disorders

Pre-eclampsia and gestational hypertension are apparently more frequent in women with GDM. A large study by Xiong et al. (20) detected pre-eclampsia in 2.7% of 2755 patients with GDM compared with only 1.1% of 108,664 patients with normal pregnancies (adjusted OR = 1.3, 95% CI 1.20–1.41). Similar results were observed for gestational hypertension. Likewise, Dukler et al. [65] studied 380 primiparous women with pre-eclampsia and 385 primiparous control women for a total of 1207 and 1293 deliveries, respectively. When adjusted for confounding variables, GDM was strongly associated with the recurrence of pre-eclampsia in the second pregnancy (OR = 3.72, 95% CI 1.45–9.53).

Yogev et al. [66] showed that GDM patients who developed pre-eclampsia were more obese, gained more weight during pregnancy and had more severe GDM in comparison to GDM patients who did not. Although all mean blood pressure measurements were within the normal range, significantly higher systolic and diastolic values were recorded in the GDM patients who developed pre-eclampsia throughout the first and the second trimesters of pregnancy. Logistic regression revealed that higher parity, maternal age and pre-pregnancy BMI were all contributing factors to pre-eclampsia. In contrast, weight gain during pregnancy and race were not related. In another study, Yogev et al. [67] demonstrated that the rate of preeclampsia is related to the severity GDM, and it can be decreased by optimizing glycemic control.

Conditions associated with increased insulin resistance, such as GDM, PCOS and obesity, may predispose patients to essential hypertension, hypertensive pregnancy, hyperinsulinemia, hyperlipidemia and high levels of plasminogen activator inhibitor-1, leptin and tumor necrosis factor-alpha. These findings may also be associated with a possible increased risk of cardiovascular complications in these women.

Risk for Future Type 2 Diabetes

Women with GDM have a 17–63% risk of type 2 DM within 5–16 years [68]. However, the risk varies according to different parameters. For example, Greenberg et al. [69], in a study of 94 patients with GDM, reported that the most significant predictor of 6-weeks postpartum diabetes was insulin requirement, with RR = 17.28 (95% CI 2.46–134.42), followed by poor glycemic control, IGT and a GCT $\geq$ 200mg/dl. All of these factors probably represent the magnitude of the insulin resistance, which is the hallmark of future diabetes and of other vascular complications. Similarly, Bian et al. [70] reported a diagnosis of diabetes 5–10 years postpartum in 33.3% of patients with previous GDM (n = 45), but only 9.7% (n = 31) of these with IGT and 2.6% (n = 39) of normal controls. Two or more abnormal OGTT values during pregnancy, a blood glucose level exceeding the maximal values at 1 and 2 hours after oral glucose loading, and high pregnancy BMI were all useful predictors of diabetes in later life. In a recent study of 227 women [71], in an average of 5.8 years after the diagnosis of GDM, the majority of women still had chronic insulin resistance. One third has IGT, IFG or type 2 DM. Nevertheless, only 37% of women with GDM were screened for postpartum type 2 DM according to guidelines published by the American Diabetes Association [72].

To determine if recurrent episodes of insulin resistance (i.e., another pregnancy) contribute to the decline in beta-cell function that leads to type 2 DM in high-risk individuals, Peters et al. [73] investigated 666 Latino women with a history of GDM. Among the 87 (13%) who completed an additional pregnancy, the rate ratio of type 2 DM increased to 3.34 (95% CI 1.80–6.19) compared with women without an additional pregnancy after adjustment for other potential diabetes risk factors during the index pregnancy (antepartum oral glucose tolerance, high fasting glucose, gestational age at diagnosis of GDM) and during follow-up (postpartum BMI, glucose tolerance, weight change, breastfeeding and months of contraceptive use). Weight gain was also independently associated with an increased risk of type 2 DM; the rate ratio was 1.95 (95% CI 1.63–2.33) for each 4.5kg gained during follow-up after adjustment for the additional pregnancy and the other potential risk factors. These data show that a single pregnancy, independent of the well-known effect of weight gain, accelerates the development of type 2 DM in women with a high prevalence of pancreatic beta-cell dysfunction.

What about milder, diet-controlled GDM? Damm [74] reported abnormal glucose tolerance in 34.4% of 241 women 2–11 years after a diabetic pregnancy (3.7% type 1 DM, 13.7% type 2 DM, 17% IGT) in contrast to a control group in which none of the women had diabetes and 5.3% had IGT. The independent risk factors for later development of diabetes were high fasting glucose levels at diagnosis of GDM, delivery > 3 weeks before term and abnormal OGTT 2 months postpartum. Low insulin secretion at diagnosis of GDM was also an independent risk factor. Even the non-obese glucose-tolerant women with previous GDM had a metabolic profile of type 2 DM, i.e., insulin resistance and impaired insulin secretion.

Thus, the first OGTT should probably be performed 2 months postpartum to identify women who are already diabetic and women at highest risk of later development of overt diabetes. Similarly, Lauenborg et al. [75] reported that the prevalence of metabolic syndrome was three times as high in women with prior diet-treated GDM compared with age-matched control subjects. Interestingly, according to a recent study, both women with a history of GDM as well as their children are at greater risk of progressing to type 2 DM [76]. Whether this effect is due to a genetic or an in utero influence has yet to be determined.

Summary

Diabetes is the second most common maternal/fetal complication of pregnancy. It effects between 3% and 15% of pregnancies depending upon race, ethnicity, weight, parity, pre-pregnancy glycemic status and a substantial number of other factors yet to be determined. There is neither a national registry nor a standard for reporting the myriad variables that are associated with maternal diabetes. There is variability in definitions, criteria and procedures for identifying women with pregnancies complicated by hyperglycemia. Differences in screening programs and diagnostic criteria make it difficult to compare frequencies of diabetes complicating pregnancy among various populations. Nevertheless, race has been proven to be an independent risk factor for GDM, which varies in prevalence in direct proportion to the prevalence of type 2 DM in a given population or ethnic group.

References

[1] *National Vital Statistics Reports, US Government.* 2003; 52(10).

[2] Ben-Haroush A, Yogev Y, Hod M. Epidemiology of gestational diabetes mellitus. In Hod M, Jovanovic L, Di Renzo GC, de Leiva A, Langer O. eds. *Textbook of Diabetes and Pregnancy*. London: Martin Dunitz, 2008; 15 :(118-129).

[3] Downs B. Fertility of American women in current population reports. *US Department of Commerce, US Census Bureau 2003.*

[4] American Diabetes Association, Clinical Practice Recommendations 2004. *Diabetes Care* 2004; 27(1):S88-S90.

[5] Brody SC, Harris R, Lohr K. Screening for gestational diabetes: A summary of the evidence of the US Preventive Services Task Force. *Obstet Gynecol* 2003;101(2): 380-92.

[6] Soonthornpun S, Soonthornpun K, Aksonteing J, Aksonteing J. A comparison between a 75-g and a 100-g oral glucose tolerance test in pregnant women. *Int J Gynecol Obstet* 2003; 81(2) 169-73.

[7] US Centers for Disease Control, Reproductive Health, Diabetes during pregnancy, United States 1993-95, (updated tables) 2004.

[8] American Diabetes Association: Type 2 diabetes in children and adolescents. *Diabetes Care* 2000; 23: 381-9.

[9] Benjamin E, Winters D, Mayfield J, Gohdes D. Diabetes in pregnancy in Zuni Indian women. *Diabetes Care* 1993; 16:1231-5.

[10] Langer O, Anyaegbunam A, Brustman L, Divon M. Management of women with one abnormal oral glucose tolerance test value reduces adverse outcome in pregnancy. *Am J Obstet Gynecol.* 1989; 161(3):593-9.

[11] Schäfer-Graf UM, Dupak J, Vogel M, Dudenhausen JW, Kjos SL, Buchanan TA, Vetter K. Hyperinsulinism, neonatal obesity and placental immaturity in infants born to women with one abnormal glucose tolerance test value. *J Perinat Med.* 1998; 26(1):27-36.

[12] WHO Ad Hoc Diabetes Reporting Group. Diabetes and impaired glucose tolerance in women aged 20–39 years. *World Health Stat* 1992; 45:321–7.

[13] Dooley SL, Metzger BE, Cho NH. Influence of race on disease prevalence and perinatal outcome in a US population. *Diabetes* 1991; 40:25–9.

[14] Gunton JE, Hitchman R, McElduff A. Effects of ethnicity on glucose tolerance, insulin resistance and beta cell function in 223 women with an abnormal glucose challenge test during pregnancy. *Aust N Z Obstet Gynaecol* 2001; 41:182–6.

[15] Silva JK, Kaholokula JK, Ratner R, Mau M. Ethnic differences in perinatal outcome of gestational diabetes mellitus. *Diabetes Care.* 2006; 29:2058-63.

[16] Jang HC, Cho NH, Jung KB, Oh KS, Dooley SL, Metzger BE. Screening for gestational diabetes mellitus in Korea. *Int J Gynecol Obstet* 1995; 51:115–22.

[17] Kousta E, Lawrence NJ, Penny A, Millauer BA, Robinson S, Johnston DG, McCarthy I. Women with a history of gestational diabetes of European and South Asian origin are shorter than women with normal glucose tolerance in pregnancy. *Diabet Med* 2000; 17:792–7.

[18] Jang HC, Min HK, Lee HK, Cho NH, Metzger BE. Short stature in Korean women: a contribution to the multifactorial predisposition to gestational diabetes mellitus. *Diabetologia* 1998; 41:778–3.

[19] Branchtein L, Schmidt MI, Matos MC, Yamashita T, Pousada JM, Duncan BB. Short stature and gestational diabetes in Brazil. Brazilian Gestational Diabetes Study Group. *Diabetologia* 2000; 43:848–51.

[20] Xiong X, Saunders LD, Wang FL, Demianczuk NN. Gestational diabetes mellitus: prevalence, risk factors, maternal and infant outcomes. *Int J Gynaecol Obstet* 2001; 75:221–8.

[21] Egeland GM, Skjærven R, Irgens LM. Birth characteristics of women who develop gestational diabetes: population based study. *Br Med* J 2000; 321:546–7.

[22] Ma RM, Lao TT. Maternal mean arterial pressure and oral glucose tolerance test results. Relationship in normotensive women. *J Reprod Med* 2001; 46:747–51.

[23] Lichtenstein AH, Schwab US. Relationship of diatary fat to glucose metabolism. *Atherosclerosis* 2000; 150:227–43.

[24] Clarke SD. Polyunsaturated fatty acid regulation of gene transcription: A mechanism to improve energy balance and insulin resistance. *Br J Nutr* 2000; 83(Suppl1):s59–s66.

[25] Clarke SD. Polyunsaturated fatty acid regulation of gene transcription: A molecular mechanism to improve the metabolic syndrome. *J Nutr* 2001; 131:1129–32.

[26] Rustan AC, Nenseter MS, Drevon CA. Omega-3 and omega-6 fatty acids in the insulin resistance syndrome. Lipid and lipoprotein metabolism and atherosclerosis. *Ann NY Acad Sci* 1997; 827:310–26.

[27] Bo S, Menato G, Lezo A, Signorile A, Bardelli C, De Michieli F et al. Dietary fat and gestational hyperglycaemia. *Diabetologia* 2001; 44:972–8.

[28] Holte J, Gennarelli G, Wide L, Lithell H, Berne C. High prevalence of polycystic ovaries and associated clinical, endocrine, and metabolic features in women with previous gestational diabetes mellitus. *J Clin Endocrinol Metab* 1998; 83:1143–50.

[29] Kousta E, Cela E, Lawrence N, Penny A, Millauer B, White D et al. The prevalence of polycystic ovaries in women with a history of gestational diabetes. *Clin Endocrinol* (Oxf) 2000; 53:501–7.

[30] Anttila L, Karjala K, Penttila RA, Ruutiainen K, Ekblad U. Polycystic ovaries in women with gestational diabetes. *Obstet Gynecol* 1998; 92:13–16.

[31] Mikola M, Hiilesmaa V, Halttunen M, Suhonen L, Tiitinen A. Obstetric outcome in women with polycystic ovarian syndrome. *Hum Reprod* 2001; 16:226–9.

[32] Koivunen RM, Juutinen J, Vauhkonen I, Morin-Papunen LC, Ruokonen A, Tapanainen JS. Metabolic and steroidogenic alterations related to increased frequency of polycystic ovaries in women with a history of gestational diabetes. *J Clin Endocrinol Metab* 2001; 86:2591–9.

[33] Hoskins RE. Zygosity as a risk factor for complications and outcomes of twin pregnancy. *Acta Genet Med Gemellol* 1995; 44:11–23.

[34] Sivan E, Maman E, Homko CJ, Lipitz S, Cohen S, Schiff E. Impact of fetal reduction on the incidence of gestational diabetes. *Obstet Gynecol* 2002; 99:91–4.

[35] Schwartz DB, Daoud Y, Zazula P, Goyert G, Bronsteen R, Wright D, Copes J. Gestational diabetes mellitus: metabolic and blood glucose parameters in singleton versus twin pregnancies. *Am J Obstet Gynecol* 1999; 181:912–14.

[36] Wein P, Warwick MM, Beischer NA. Gestational diabetes in twin pregnancy: prevalence and long-term implications. *Aust N Z J Obstet Gynaecol* 1992; 32:325–7.

[37] Egeland GM, Irgens LM. Is a multiple birth pregnancy a risk factor for gestational diabetes? *Am J Obstet Gynecol* 2001; 185:1275–6.

[38] Fitzsimmons BP, Bebbington MW, Fluker MR. Perinatal and neonatal outcomes in multiple gestations: assisted reproduction versus spontaneous conception. *Am J Obstet Gynecol* 1998; 179:1162–7.

[39] Henderson CE, Scarpelli S, Larosa D, Divon MY. Assessing the risk of gestational diabetes in twin pregnancies. *J Natl Med Assoc* 1995; 87:757–8.

[40] Harder T, Franke K, Kohlhoff R, Plagemann A. Maternal and paternal family history of diabetes in women with gestational diabetes or insulin-dependent diabetes mellitus type I. *Gynecol Obstet Invest* 2001; 51:160–4.

[41] Dorner G, Plagemann A, Reinagel H. Familial diabetes aggregation in type 2 diabetics: gestational diabetes an apparent risk factor for increased diabetes susceptibility in the offspring. *Exp Clin Endocrinol* 1987; 89:84–90.

[42] Kuhl C. Etiology and pathogenesis of gestational diabetes. *Diabetes Care* 1998; 21(Suppl2):B19–B26.

[43] Vambergue A, Fajardy I, Bianchi F et al. Gestational diabetes mellitus and HLA class II (-DQ, -DR) association: *The Digest Study. Eur J Immunogenet* 1997; 24:385–94.

[44] Lapolla A, Betterle C, Sanzari M et al. An immunological and genetic study of patients with gestational diabetes mellitus. *Acta Diabetol* 1996; 33:139–44.

[45] Budowle B, Huddleston JF, Go RC, Barger BO, Acton RT. Association of HLA-linked factor B with gestational diabetes mellitus in black women. *Am J Obstet Gynecol* 1988; 159:805–6.

[46] Bell DS, Barger BO, Go RC, Goldenberg RL, Perkins LL. Risk factors for gestational diabetes in black population. *Diabetes* 1990; 13:1196–201.

[47] Freinkel N, Metzger BE, Phelps RL, Simpson JL, Martin AO, Radvany R, et al. Gestational diabetes mellitus: a syndrome with phenotypic and genotypic heterogeneity. *Horm Metab Res* 1986; 18:427–30.

[48] Ferber KM, Keller E, Albert ED, Ziegler AG. Predictive value of human leukocyte antigen class II typing for the development of islet autoantibodies and insulin-dependent diabetes postpartum in women with gestational diabetes. *J Clin Endocrinol Metab* 1999; 84:2342–8.

[49] MacNeill S, Dodds L, Hamilton DC, Armson BA, Vanden Hof M. Rates and risk factors for recurrence of gestational diabetes. *Diabetes Care* 2001; 24:659–62.

[50] Major CA, deVeciana M, Weeks J, Morgan MA. Recurrence of gestational diabetes: Who is at risk? *Am J Obstet Gynecol* 1998; 179:1038–42.

[51] Spong CY, Guillermo L, Kuboshige J, Cabalum T. Recurrence of gestational diabetes mellitus: identification of risk factors. *Am J Perinatol* 1998; 15:29–33.

[52] Nohira T, Kim S, Nakai H, Okabe K, Nohira T, Yoneyama K. Recurrence of gestational diabetes mellitus: rates and risk factors from initial GDM and one abnormal GTT value. *Diabetes Res Clin Pract.* 2006; 71:75-81.

[53] Foster-Powel KA, Cheung NW. Recurrence of gestational diabetes. *Aust N Z J Obstet Gynaecol* 1998; 38:384–7.

[54] Mello G, Parretti E, Mecacci F et al. Anthropometric characteristics of full-term infants: effects of varying degrees of 'normal' glucose metabolism. *J Perinat Med* 1997; 25:197–204.

[55] Yogev Y, Langer O, Xenakis EM, Rosenn B. The association between glucose challenge test, obesity and pregnancy outcome in 6390 non-diabetic women. *J Matern Fetal Neonatal Med.* 2005; 17(1):29-34.

[56] Weijers RN, Bekedam DJ, Smulders YM. Determinants of mild gestational hyperglycemia and gestational diabetes mellitus in a large Dutch multiethnic cohort. *Diabetes Care* 2002; 25:72–7.

[57] McLaughlin GB, Cheng YW, Caughey AB. Women with one elevated 3-hour glucose tolerance test value: are they at risk for adverse perinatal outcomes? *Am J Obstet Gynecol.* 2006;194:e16-9.

[58] Schaefer-Graf UM, Buchanan TA, Songster G, Montoro M, Kjos SL. Patterns of congenital anomalies and relationship to initial maternal fasting glucose levels in pregnancies complicated by type 2 and gestational diabetes. *Am J Obstet Gynecol* 2000; 182:313–20.

[59] Kalter H. The non-teratogenicity of gestational diabetes. *Paediatr Perinat Epidemiol* 1998; 12:456–8.

[60] Bartha JL, Martinez-Del-Fresno P, Comino-Delgado R. Gestational diabetes mellitus diagnosed during early pregnancy. *Am J Obstet Gynecol* 2000; 182:346–50.

[61] Aberg A, Westbom L, Kallen B. Congenital malformations among infants whose mothers had gestational diabetes or preexisting diabetes. *Early Human Dev* 2001; 61:85–95.

[62] Martinez-Frias ML, Bermejo E, Rodriguez-Pinilla E, Prieto L, Frias JL. Epidemiological analysis of outcomes of pregnancy in gestational diabetic mothers. *Am J Med Genet* 1998; 78:140–5.

[63] Virtanen HE, Tapanainen AE, Kaleva MM, Suomi AM, Main KM, Skakkebaek NE, Toppari J. Mild gestational diabetes as a risk factor for congenital cryptorchidism. *J Clin Endocrinol Metab*. 2006;91:4862-5.

[64] Janssen PA, Rothman I, Schwartz SM. Congenital malformations in newborns of women with established and gestational diabetes in Washington State, 1984–91. *Paediatr Perinat Epidemiol* 1996; 10:52–63.

[65] Dukler D, Porath A, Bashiri A, Erez O, Mazor M. Remote prognosis of primiparous women with preeclampsia. *Eur J Obstet Gynecol Reprod Biol* 2001; 96:69–74.

[66] Yogev Y, Langer O, Brustman L, Rosenn B. Pre-eclampsia and gestational diabetes mellitus: does a correlation exist early in pregnancy? *J Matern Fetal Neonatal Med.* 2004;15(1):39-43.

[67] Yogev Y, Xenakis EM, Langer O. The association between preeclampsia and the severity of gestational diabetes: the impact of glycemic control. *Am J Obstet Gynecol.* 2004 ;191(5):1655-60.

[68] Kjos SL, Buchanan TA. Gestational diabetes mellitus. *N Engl J Med* 1999; 341:1749–56.

[69] Greenberg LR, Moore TR, Murphy H. Gestational diabetes mellitus: antenatal variables as predictors of postpartum glucose intolerance. *Obstet and Gynecol* 1995; 86:96–101.

[70] Bian X, Gao P, Xiong X, Xu H, Qian M, Liu S. Risk factors for development of diabetes mellitus in women with a history of gestational diabetes mellitus. *Chin Med J (Engl)* 2000; 113:759–62.

[71] Hunger-Dathe W, Mosebach N, Samann A, Wolf G, Muller UA. Prevalence of impaired glucose tolerance 6 years after gestational diabetes. *Exp Clin Endocrinol Diabetes*. 2006;114:11-7.

[72] Smirnakis KV, Chasan-Taber L, Wolf M, Markenson G, Ecker JL, Thadhani R. Postpartum diabetes screening in women with a history of gestational diabetes. *Obstet Gynecol.* 2005;106:1297-303.

[73] Peters RK, Kjos SL, Xiang A, Buchanan TA. Long-term diabetogenic effect of single pregnancy in women with previous gestational diabetes mellitus. *Lancet* 1996; 347:227–30.

[74] Damm P. Gestational diabetes mellitus and subsequent development of overt diabetes mellitus. *Dan Med Bull* 1998; 45:495–509.

[75] Lauenborg J, Mathiesen E, Hansen T, Glumer C, Jorgensen T, Borch-Johnsen K, Hornnes P, Pedersen O, Damm P. The prevalence of the metabolic syndrome in a

danish population of women with previous gestational diabetes mellitus is three-fold higher than in the general population. *J Clin Endocrinol Metab.* 2005;90:4004-10

[76] Fletcher B, Gulanick M, Lamendola C. Risk factors for type 2 diabetes mellitus. *J Cardiovasc Nurs* 2002; 16:17–23.

In: Textbook of Perinatal Epidemiology
Editor: Eyal Sheiner, pp. 347-385

ISBN: 978-1-60741-648-7
© 2010 Nova Science Publishers, Inc.

Chapter XIX

Epidemiology of Hypertensive Disorders during Pregnancy

Asnat Walfisch[*] *and Mordechai Hallak*

Department of Obstetrics and Gynecology, Hillel Yaffe Medical Center, Hadera, Israel

Introduction

Hypertensive disorders in pregnancy are a leading cause of maternal and perinatal morbidity and mortality. This chapter will focus on the four major disorders, their significance, related risks and the most widely accepted management options.

Definitions

The four major hypertensive disorders in pregnancy are:[1,2]

1) Preeclampsia – eclampsia
2) Gestational hypertension
3) Chronic hypertension
4) Preeclampsia superimposed on chronic hypertension

The diagnosis of a hypertensive disorder in a pregnant woman depends, in part, upon the gestational age at presentation:

Preeclampsia is defined as the new onset of hypertension and proteinuria after 20 weeks of gestation in a previously normotensive woman. It is classified as mild or severe (table 1

[*] For Correspondence: Asnat Walfisch MD, Department of Obstetrics and Gynecology, Hillel Yaffe Medical Center, Hadera, Israel. asnatwalfisch@yahoo.com

and 2). It may be associated with other symptoms and signs such as headache, edema, and visual disturbances. Rarely, preeclampsia may develop before 20 weeks of gestation in patients with antiphospholipid antibody (APLA) syndrome or in pregnancies with extensive hydatidiform changes.

Eclampsia is the development of a new onset generalized convulsions and/or coma in a woman whose condition also meets the criteria for gestational hypertension or preeclampsia. The seizures should not be attributable to another cause such as epilepsy.[3]

Gestational (transient) hypertension refers to elevated blood pressure first detected after 20 weeks of gestation without co-existing proteinuria.

Chronic hypertension is defined as systolic pressure $\geq$ 140 mmHg and/or diastolic pressure $\geq$ 90 mmHg that antedates pregnancy, is present before the 20th week of pregnancy, or persists longer than 12 weeks postpartum.[4]

Superimposed preeclampsia is worsening hypertension with new onset proteinuria in a woman with chronic hypertension. Women with both preexisting hypertension and proteinuria are considered preeclamptic if one of the following occurs:

An exacerbation of blood pressure to the severe range (systolic $\geq$160 mmHg or diastolic $\geq$110 mmHg) after 20 weeks of gestation, especially if accompanied by symptoms, increased liver enzymes, thrombocytopenia, or a sudden increase in the proteinuria.

Diagnoses may change over time: a patient with gestational hypertension may develop a new onset proteinuria and be considered preeclamptic, or have persistent blood pressure elevation postpartum and be considered as chronically hypertensive.

Incidence and Significance

Hypertensive disorders complicate 10 to 20 % of pregnancies, depending on the study population.

Chronic hypertension complicates about 3 % of pregnancies.[5]

Gestational hypertension occurs in about 6% of pregnancies.[5]

Preeclampsia occurs in up to 14% of all pregnancies worldwide, and about 5 - 8% in the United States.[1, 6-9] In high risk groups, the rates of preeclampsia may even be higher. Preeclampsia is mild in 75 percent of cases.[10] Ten percent of preeclampsia occur before 34 weeks of gestation. Preeclampsia-eclampsia is one of three most common causes of maternal mortality in the United States (thrombo-embolic disease and hemorrhage are the other two causes).[11] There is approximately one maternal death due to preeclampsia-eclampsia per 100,000 live births.[12, 13] Hypertensive disorders remain a leading cause of maternal death in developing countries as well, accounting for more than a quarter in Latin America and the Caribbean.[14]

Preeclampsia

Preeclampsia is defined as the new onset of hypertension and proteinuria after 20 weeks of gestation in a previously normotensive woman. It is classified as mild or severe (tables 1 and 2). It is a syndrome characterized by heterogeneous clinical and laboratory findings. The clinical findings of preeclampsia can manifest as either a maternal syndrome (hypertension, proteinuria, various symptoms), or a fetal syndrome (growth restriction), or both.[15]

Despite extensive research in this field, the cause of preeclampsia remains unknown. During the past decade, numerous pathophysiologic abnormalities have been suggested to explain the mechanisms leading to the development of preeclampsia. Some of these mechanisms have included impaired trophoblast differentiation and invasion, placental and endothelial dysfunction, immune mal-adaptation to paternal antigens, and exaggerated systemic inflammatory response. However, preeclampsia is a heterogeneous disorder, for which the mechanisms can differ in women with various risk factors. In addition, the diagnostic criteria for preeclampsia and its subtypes (mild, severe, superimposed on chronic hypertension) have not been consistent among published studies. As a result, research in this area has not resulted in significant improvement in methods of prediction, markers for confirming the diagnosis in various subtypes, prevention, or management of this disorder.[16]

Prediction

Many biomarkers and biophysical markers have been proposed to predict or confirm the development of preeclampsia. These markers have included serum placental growth factor (PLGF), soluble fms-like tyrosine kinase-1 receptor (sFLt-1), serum endoglin, placental protein-13, uterine artery Doppler measurements, and urinary podocyte excretion.

Widmer et al.[17] performed a systematic review evaluating the potential role of serum PLGF and sFLt-1 to be used for prediction of preeclampsia. The authors demonstrated that third trimester increases in sFLt-1 and decreases in PLGF levels are associated with preeclampsia, specifically in the severe disease. However, evidence is insufficient to recommend these markers for use as screening tests. This is due to the differences among the various studies regarding gestational age at the time of the measurements, methods used for analysis, population studies, and reporting of results. Another study[18] evaluated serum levels of various angiogenic factors at various gestational ages. This study demonstrated that circulating soluble endoglin levels increased significantly beginning 2–3 months before the onset of preeclampsia. The increased level of endoglin was usually accompanied by an increased ratio of sFLt-1:PLGF. Other studies have demonstrated similar findings.[19-21] However, despite the above literature on the association between abnormal angiogenic factors and subsequent preeclampsia, none of these studies provided adequate information that could be clinically useful for the prediction of preeclampsia. There is still a need for prospective studies with adequate sample sizes to address this question.

Placental protein-13 (PP-13) is produced in the placenta and is thought to be involved in implantation and maternal vascular remodeling. Several studies have shown that maternal screening with PP-13 levels in the first trimester may be useful for prediction of preeclampsia.[16,22]

An abnormal uterine artery Doppler velocimetry (high pulsatility index or the presence of a "notch") in the first and second trimester has been proposed as a good screening test to predict preeclampsia. This test has been studied alone and in combination with other prediction markers with good results.[23] An abnormal umbilical artery Doppler measurement is another common Doppler finding in women with established preeclampsia, particularly in those leading to delivery before 34 weeks' gestation.[24] Recent studies have shown that although abnormal umbilical artery Doppler measurements are very common in preeclampsia, such measurements had no prognostic value in the management of these patients.[25]

Risk Factors

The main risk factors for the development of preeclampsia include:

1) Past obstetrical history of preeclampsia. A systematic review of controlled studies reported that the relative risk of preeclampsia in women with a history of the disorder compared to women with no such history was 7.19 (95% CI 5.85-8.83).[26] In women who had mild preeclampsia during their first pregnancy, the recurrence incidence in a second pregnancy is up to 7 %, and women with early, severe preeclampsia are at the greatest risk of recurrence (25 -65% percent).[27-29]

2) Co-morbidity. Diabetes mellitus – pre-gestational, also increases the risk of preeclampsia (RR 3.56, 95% CI 2.54-4.99).[26] The reasons for this effect may be related to a variety of factors such as underlying vascular disease, renal disease, and abnormal lipid metabolism.[30] Preexisting hypertension, renal disease, obesity, and collagen vascular disorders are also well-described risk factors.

3) First pregnancy. This important predisposing factor increases the risk for developing preeclampsia with a relative risk of 2.91, (95% CI 1.28-6.61).[26] The reasons for this are unclear.

4) Positive family history and race. The relative risk is 2.9 (95% CI 1.70-4.93).[26] This finding suggests a possible heritable character to the disease, in some of the cases.[31-32] The paternal contribution to fetal genes may have a role in defective placentation and subsequent preeclampsia. Both men and women who were the product of a pregnancy complicated by preeclampsia are more likely to have a child who was the product of a pregnancy complicated by preeclampsia.[33] Of note, African American race is another independent risk factor.

5) Thrombophilia: The antiphospholipid antibody (APLA) syndrome has been associated with multiple pregnancy complications including preeclampsia as well as fetal loss, and maternal thrombosis.[34] Conflicting evidence exist in regards to association between preeclampsia and hereditary thrombophilias.

6) Multiple gestation increases the risk of preeclampsia. For twin pregnancies the relative risk is 2.93, 95% 2.04-4.21.[26] The risk rises with the number of fetuses.

7) Advanced maternal age is an independent risk factor for preeclampsia (maternal age > 40 RR 1.96, 95% CI 1.34-2.87).[26] This association may reflect undiagnosed underlying chronic hypertension with superimposed gestational hypertension. Very young women (adolescents) may also be at increased risk but this fact is more

controversial[6]; and a systematic review did not demonstrate a significant association.[26]

8) Laboratory markers: As mentioned above, a variety of laboratory tests have been investigated as possible markers for prediction of preeclampsia (eg, AFP, hCG, uE3, inhibin A). Most have not been shown to be sufficiently sensitive and specific to be clinically useful as a screening test. Measurement of angiogenic factors (eg, VEGF, sFlt-1, PlGF, sEng) in blood or urine is a promising although investigational approach for predicting preeclampsia.

9) Imaging markers: Uterine artery Doppler, although predictive, is not considered sufficiently sensitive and specific to be clinically useful as a screening test.

Other risk factors and their relationship to preeclampsia are unclear. An association between urinary tract infection during pregnancy and development of preeclampsia was shown (pooled odds ratio 1.57; 95% CI 1.45-1.70). [35] An association between periodontal disease and preeclampsia is also suspected (pooled odds ratio 1.76; 95% CI 1.43-2.18), but no association between preeclampsia and other common infections is known. These possible relationships require further investigation before drawing any conclusions regarding causality. However, women who smoke cigarettes have a lower risk of developing preeclampsia when compared with nonsmokers.[8]

Prevention

Many randomized trials and systematic reviews described the use of low dose aspirin, calcium, and vitamin C+E to prevent or reduce the incidence or severity of preeclampsia. Askie et al.[36] performed a meta-analysis of 31 randomized trials for prevention of preeclampsia using antiplatelet agents (mainly low dose aspirin). Antiplatelet agents were associated with a small reduction in the rate of preeclampsia, with a relative risk of 0.90 (95% CI, 0.85–0.97). The number of patients needed to be treated to prevent one case of preeclampsia depended on the baseline risk in the study population. Women with chronic hypertension had no reduction in the risk of preeclampsia, with RR 0.97 (95% CI, 0.84–1.12). Therefore, at present, the use of low dose aspirin to prevent preeclampsia should be individualized.

The benefits of calcium supplementation during pregnancy in reducing the incidence of hypertensive disorders were also extensively evaluated.

An evidence-based review by the United States Food and Drug Administration[37] concluded that the relationship between calcium and risk of hypertension in pregnancy is inconsistent and inconclusive, and the relationship between calcium and the risk of pregnancy-induced hypertension and preeclampsia is highly unlikely.

Unfortunately, the use of vitamin C (1000 mg/day) plus vitamin E (400 IU/day) supplementation during pregnancy for the prevention of preeclampsia did not prove beneficial as well. A systematic review[38] of four published trials that included 4680 randomized pregnant women concluded that combined vitamin C and E supplementation during pregnancy does not reduce the risk of preeclampsia.

Clinical Manifestations

Clinical manifestations of preeclampsia develop long after placental pathogenic changes. The gradual development of hypertension, proteinuria, and edema in pregnancy is usually due to preeclampsia, particularly in a primigravida. Typically, these findings appear after 20 weeks of gestation and progress until delivery.[1-2] Nevertheless, in few cases symptoms begin earlier, towards the end of the second trimester,[1] while others onset intra- or post-partum.[2]

The occurrence of signs and symptoms of preeclampsia before 20 weeks of gestation suggest an underlying molar pregnancy or the APLA syndrome. Other possibilities (chromosomal aneuploidy in the fetus, drug use) should also be considered.[39-40]

The clinical features of preeclampsia are attributable to different maternal responses to generalized endothelial dysfunction. Disturbed endothelial control of vascular tone causes hypertension, increased vascular permeability results in edema and proteinuria, and abnormal endothelial expression of pro-coagulants leads to coagulopathy. These changes may also cause ischemia of target organs (brain, liver, kidney, and placenta).

Furthermore, since poor perfusion is a major component of the disease process, attempts to lower blood pressure may exacerbate organ dysfunction even though the patient may become normotensive.

Hypertension - Hypertension in pregnancy is defined as the development of a systolic blood pressure ≥140 mmHg or a diastolic blood pressure ≥90 mmHg after 20 weeks of gestation in a previously normotensive woman.[4] The blood pressure must be measured with an appropriately sized cuff placed on the right arm at the same level as the heart with the woman sitting for at least 10 minutes. Disappearance of the fifth Korotkoff sound indicates the diastolic pressure. Two separate measures should be taken, six hours apart, for establishing the diagnosis. Hypertension is usually the earliest clinical finding of preeclampsia and is the most common clinical clue to the presence of preeclampsia. In the past, an increase from baseline of the systolic or the diastolic pressures was considered indicative of gestational hypertension, even in the absence of hypertension. These criteria have been rejected because of their low sensitivity (30%) and predictive values (30%), as well as lack of association with adverse pregnancy outcome.[41-42]

Importantly, before making a diagnosis of hypertension, the possibility of "white coat hypertension" should be considered. This phenomenon is not infrequent and if suspected may be diagnosed using a 24-hour ambulatory blood pressure monitoring. Pregnancy outcome in these cases is not different than normal pregnancies except for a higher cesarean section rates, perhaps due to a wrong decision-making processes based on the recorded high blood pressures.[43] Nevertheless, a Cochrane review concluded there is insufficient information on which to base a recommendation regarding the routine use of ambulatory blood pressure monitoring for new onset hypertension in pregnant women.[44]

Proteinuria - Proteinuria is defined as a total of ≥ 300 mg protein in a 24-hour urine specimen (or persistent 1+ on urine dipstick – at least twice, six hours apart). Proteinuria must be present, in addition to hypertension, to make a diagnosis of preeclampsia. Urinary protein excretion increases gradually, and is of variable magnitude in preeclampsia, occasionally reaching the nephrotic range (>5 g/day). This phenomenon is partially due to the impaired integrity of the glomerular barrier (both size and charge selectivity) and impaired tubular handling of filtered proteins (hypofiltration) leading to increased protein excretion.[45-46]

The protein-to-creatinine ratio may be calculated using a random urine sample with a threshold of 0.14 to 0.19.

Cardiovascular system - Increased afterload may lead to decrements in left ventricular performance although preeclampsia does not directly affect the myocardium.[47]After clinical manifestations become apparent, there is a marked reduction in cardiac output and increase in peripheral resistance.[47-49] Severe preeclampsia can be associated with a highly variable hemodynamic profile.[50-54]

Edema is a common finding in normal pregnancy. Thus, the presence of edema is no longer considered one of the diagnostic criteria for preeclampsia. Nevertheless, a sudden and rapid weight gain or the occurrence of facial edema warrants evaluation for other clinical manifestations of preeclampsia.

The intravascular volume is lower in preeclamptic pregnancies. The reduced volume may be a consequence of vasoconstriction and not under-filling of the arterial circulation. Thus, diuretics should be avoided in the absence of pulmonary edema. The etiology of pulmonary edema in preeclampsia, which occurs particularly in the postpartum period, is multifactorial. Excessive elevations in pulmonary vascular hydrostatic pressure (PCWP) compared to plasma oncotic pressure, capillary leak, left heart failure, and iatrogenic volume overload may be the explanations for this phenomenon in some cases.[55]

Renal findings - The kidney is the organ most likely to manifest endothelial injury related to preeclampsia. Glomerular filtration rate (GFR) decreases by 30 - 40% and renal plasma flow decreases (to a lesser extent) when compared to pregnant controls. GFR can be estimated using serum and urine creatinine together with age and weight of the patient. The plasma creatinine concentration is generally normal or only slightly elevated and renal failure is an unusual complication that can occur in patients who develop severe disease. Hyperuricemia and hypocalciuria also occur resulting from unclear mechanisms.[45, 56-57] The rise in serum uric acid concentration is thought to reflect renal ischemia which induces increased proximal sodium and urate reabsorption. Other explanations for hyperuricemia in preeclampsia include underlying metabolic syndrome, tissue damage, oxidative stress, and inflammation.[58] The underlying renal lesion of preeclampsia is a variant of thrombotic microangiopathy (TMA) called Glomerular Endotheliosis. The histologic features of Glomerular Endotheliosis include endothelial cell swelling and loss of fenestrations with resulting occlusion of capillary lumens.[59] Fibrin deposition may also be observed.

Liver - Vasospasm and precipitation of fibrin are typical of liver as well as kidney involvement.[60] Other histologic findings observed in the liver of a preeclamptic woman include: Periportal hemorrhage, ischemic lesions, and microvesicular fat deposition.[61]

The clinical manifestations of liver involvement include right upper quadrant or epigastric pain, elevated transaminases and, in the most severe cases, subcapsular hemorrhage or hepatic rupture, which may be a part of HELLP syndrome (Hemolysis, Elevated Liver function tests, Low Platelets – see below).

Hematologic system - Thrombocytopenia (due to formation of microthrombi) is the most common coagulation abnormality observed in preeclampsia.[62] Unless there are additional complications (abruption of the placenta or severe liver involvement) the prothrombin time, partial thromboplastin time, and fibrinogen concentration are not affected. Examination of a blood smear may reveal schistocytes and helmet cells as evidence of microangiopathic hemolysis. Hemolysis is associated with a low hematocrit, and elevation in the serum lactate dehydrogenase concentration. The presence of both hemolysis and hemoconcentration in preeclampsia may negate each other, resulting in a normal hematocrit value.

Central nervous system - Headache, blurred vision, scotomata, and, rarely, transient cortical blindness may be signs of central nervous system involvement. Seizures in a preeclamptic woman signify a change in diagnosis to eclampsia. Two percent of severely preeclamptic women and 0.25%-0.5% of mildly preeclamptic women will develop eclampsia.[10]Luckily stroke, which is the most serious complication of severe preeclampsia/eclampsia, is rare.

Histopathologic and imaging findings include: hemorrhage, petechiae, vasculopathy, ischemic brain damage, microinfarcts, fibrinoid necrosis, cerebral edema and ischemic/hemorrhagic changes in the posterior hemispheres. [63-66]

Blindness related to retinal pathology (retinal artery or venous thrombosis, retinal detachment, optic nerve damage, retinal artery spasm, and retinal ischemia) may be permanent.[67]

Fetus and uteroplacental circulation - Chronic placental hypo-perfusion results in fetal growth restriction and oligohydramnion. Severe preeclampsia results in 12% fetal growth restriction and early onset preeclampsia in 23%.[68] Abruption of the placenta occurs in less than 1 percent in women with mild preeclampsia, but has been reported in 3 percent of those with severe disease.[69] Fetal or maternal complications may lead to iatrogenic preterm delivery, while preeclampsia does not appear to accelerate fetal maturation, as once believed.[70]

Diagnosis and Evaluation

Characteristic clinical features developing after 20 weeks of gestation in a woman who was previously normotensive are the basis for diagnosis of preeclampsia (Table 1).

Table 1. Criteria for the diagnosis of preeclampsia.

	Criteria
1.	Systolic blood pressure ≥140 mmHg or diastolic blood pressure≥ 90 mmHg*§
2.	Proteinuria ≥ 300mg in a 24-hour urine specimen**

* In two measurements at least six hours apart, but no more than seven days.
§ Diastolic blood pressure is determined with patient sitting and based upon the fifth Korotkoff sound.
**A random +1 on urine dipstick is suggestive, but not diagnostic, of the presence of this criterion.

Screening urine for proteinuria is an integral part of antepartum care strategy to detect preeclampsia. Women with proteinuria on a dipstick should undergo quantitative measurement of protein excretion (urine protein to creatinine ratio or 24-hour urine protein excretion) as urinary protein dipstick values do not correlate well with 24-hour urinary protein excretion values. Severe disease is defined by the criteria in the table 2.

Table 2. Criteria for the diagnosis of severe preeclampsia.

The presence of preeclampsia together with at least one of the following:	Criteria
Severe hypertension:	Systolic blood pressure ≥ 160 mm Hg or diastolic ≥110 mm Hg on two occasions at least six hours apart.
Severe proteinuria:	≥ 5 grams in a 24 hours urine collection.
Symptoms of the central nervous system:	Severe headache, blurred vision, scotomata, altered mental status.
Symptoms of liver capsule distention:	Right upper quadrant or epigastric pain.
Signs of hepatocellular injury:	Serum transaminase concentration at least twice the upper normal limit.
Thrombocytopenia:	< 100,000 platelets per mm^3
Severe fetal growth restriction	EFW ≤ 5th percentile
Oliguria	< 0.5cc/Kg/hr or < 500 cc/24hr
Pulmonary edema	Demonstrated by chest X ray or by a clinical evaluation
Cerebrovascular accident	Demonstrated using an imaging study or a clinical evaluation

Preeclampsia should be suspected in any pregnant woman with new onset hypertension even if proteinuria is absent. In order to distinguish preeclampsia from other hypertensive disorders of pregnancy, such as gestational hypertension and chronic hypertension, clinical and laboratory findings are used. Nevertheless, frequently, signs and symptoms of these disorders overlap (Table 3).

A variety of other disorders can present with symptoms or signs similar to preeclampsia, eclampsia, and HELLP syndrome. Although preeclampsia is the most common cause of hypertension, coagulation abnormalities, liver abnormalities, and renal abnormalities in pregnant women, the following conditions must be considered: Acute fatty liver, thrombotic thrombocytopenic purpura / hemolytic uremic syndrome (TTP/HUS), migraine, cerebral hemorrhage, gestational thrombocytopenia and autoimmune thrombocytopenia, exacerbation of systemic lupus erythematosus, cholestasis, hepatitis and pancreatitis.

The main goal is to support the diagnosis by excluding other disorders characterized by hypertension and proteinuria. Following the diagnosis of preeclampsia, the severity of the disease is assessed. Mild preeclampsia includes those women who satisfy the criteria for preeclampsia but do not have any features of a severe disease. Laboratory evaluation helps to determine disease severity by characterizing end organ involvement (Table 4).[4]

Table 3. Differential diagnosis (DD) of common causes of hypertension during pregnancy.

	Mild preeclampsia	Severe preeclampsia	Chronic hypertension	Gestational hypertension
Onset	After 20 weeks of gestation	After 20 weeks of gestation	Before 20 weeks of gestation	After 20 weeks of gestation
Proteinuria	Present, increases with time.	Present, increases with time, occasionally reaching the nephrotic range	Usually absent or less than 1 g/day in hypertensive nephrosclerosis	Absent
Parity	More common in primiparas	More common in primiparas	Not more common in primiparas	Mildly more common in primiparas
Age	More common in older (>40 years) primigravidas	More common in older (>40 years) primigravidas	Older primi-and multigravidas	More common in older (>40 years) primigravidas
Plasma uric acid concentration	Level rises to above 5.5 mg/dL (327 mmol/L)	Level rises to above 5.5 mg/dL (327 mmol/L)	Usually remains below 5.5 mg/dL (327 mmol/L)	Level rises to above 5.5 mg/dL (327 mmol/L)
Hematologic changes	Usually normal	Often accompanied by thrombocytopenia, and signs of hemoconcentration or hemolysis	Usually normal	Usually normal
Liver function tests	Usually normal	Often abnormal	Usually normal	Usually normal
Resolution	Usually within two to six weeks postpartum (may last 12 weeks)	Usually within two to six weeks postpartum (may last 12 weeks)	Does not resolve postpartum	Usually within one week postpartum (may last 12 weeks)

Table 4. Initial laboratory evaluation of preeclampsia.

Test	Purpose
Hematocrit / Hemoglobin	Hemoconcentration, Hemolysis
Platelet count	Thrombocytopenia
Quantification of protein excretion	≥300 mg in 24 hours - mild disease ≥5gr in 24 hours – severe disease
Serum creatinine concentration	Elevation (≥1.2mg/dl) suggests severe disease
Serum ALT and AST	Elevation suggests hepatic dysfunction indicative of severe disease
Serum lactate dehydrogenase (LDH) concentration	Hemolysis
Peripheral blood smear	Red cell fragmentation (schistocytes or helmet cells)
Serum uric acid concentration	Elevation suggests the diagnosis
Coagulation function tests	Usually normal in the absence of thrombocytopenia or liver dysfunction, and do not need to be monitored routinely

There are no data from randomized trials on which to base recommendations for the optimal type and frequency of fetal monitoring. It should however include serial assessments of: fetal movement counts, fetal nonstress testing and assessment of amniotic fluid volume (biophysical profile). Early fetal growth restriction may be the first manifestation of preeclampsia or a sign of severe preeclampsia. Therefore, a sonographic estimation of fetal weight should be performed at the time of diagnosis of preeclampsia and then repeated periodically. Doppler velocimetry is useful for assessing fetal status if fetal growth restriction is present.

Management

Delivery is the definitive treatment of preeclampsia which in itself is a completely reversible disease. As long as the patient remains undelivered, there are increased risks of complications such as seizures, placental abruption, HELLP syndrome, renal failure and cerebral hemorrhage. Although the fetus is at increased risk of stillbirth and intrauterine growth restriction, delivery may not always be beneficial. Conservative management may be pursued in well selected cases.

Once the diagnosis of preeclampsia is well established, subsequent management will depend on the results of initial maternal and fetal assessment. Safety of the mother and fetus is the main objective of management. Specifically, the main goals of therapy are prevention of convulsions and other complications as well as delivery of a surviving child. The decision between delivery and continued pregnancy depends on gestational age, fetal status, and severity of maternal condition at the time of the initial assessment. Fetal survival in preeclamptic pregnancies has improved during the last 2 decades because of more aggressive clinical management (early detection, fetal monitoring, use of steroids, and timely delivery).[18]

Women with mild preeclampsia at term are induced if there are no contraindications to vaginal birth. Delivery minimizes the risk of progression to severe disease and its complications. Most experts advise delivery by no later than 40 weeks of gestation for all preeclamptic women.[4,71-72] Women with mild disease remote from term can be managed expectantly to enable further fetal growth and maturation.

Preeclamptic women are at risk of preterm delivery. Although it was once thought that preeclampsia accelerated fetal lung maturation, respiratory distress syndrome is not less common in preterm infants of preeclamptic women[73] and antenatal corticosteroids to promote fetal lung maturity are recommended before 34 weeks of gestation.

The indications for delivery for women with preeclampsia are the following:

- Fetal indications - Severe fetal growth restriction, oligohydramnios and non-reassuring fetal status.
- Maternal indications – Term pregnancy ($\geq$37w), HELLP syndrome, deterioration in renal function, abruption of the placenta, persistent severe headaches or visual changes, persistent severe epigastric pain, nausea, or vomiting.

Severe preeclampsia (Table 2) is usually regarded as an indication for delivery in order to minimize the risk of development of maternal and fetal complications.

Women who develop severe preeclampsia at or beyond 32- 34 weeks of gestation should be delivered. Delivery should be planned at an institution with appropriate facilities for care of the preterm neonate.

Management of early onset (before 32-34 weeks of gestation) severe preeclampsia is a challenge. Immediate delivery leads to high neonatal mortality and morbidity rates, whereas, expectant management to increased maternal mortality and morbidities and possible fetal death or asphyxial damage. Sibai and Barton[74] conducted a review of published studies from 1990 to 2006 evaluating the risks and benefits of expectant management in severe preeclamptic pregnancies. It included two randomized trials and 11 observational studies. The authors showed that expectant management is safe and improves neonatal outcome in a selected group of patients with severe preeclampsia between 24 and 33 weeks of gestation. With close monitoring, expectantly managed pregnancies complicated by severe preeclampsia can be extended by 5 to 19 days, on average, with good maternal and neonatal outcomes.[75]

For gestational age below 24 weeks, expectant management is associated with high maternal morbidity and limited perinatal benefit. In cases of severe preeclampsia and severe fetal growth restriction data to support this management is limited and expectant management may increase stillbirth.[76]

Bed Rest

Although widely recommended, there are no large randomized trials evaluating the risks and benefits of bed rest. A Cochrane review analyzed four trials including 449 women.[77] Although one small trial suggested that bed rest may be associated with reduced risk of severe hypertension and preterm birth, at present, there is insufficient evidence to provide clear guidance. Restrictive activity may be associated with an increased risk of thrombo-embolic events and therefore, bed rest should not be recommended routinely for hypertension in pregnancy. Nevertheless, bed-rest in the lateral decubitus position augments utero-placental blood flow, which can be of value if there is utero-placental insufficiency. Thus, some rest in this position remains part of the routine management of women with suspected utero-placental insufficiency (such as those with fetal growth restriction).

Control of Hypertension

Although guidelines derived from systematic reviews are limited due to lack of standardized clinical trials, many physicians withhold treatment unless the systolic pressure is ≥ 160 mmHg or the diastolic pressure is ≥ 110 mmHg. The higher the blood pressure, the higher the risk of cerebral hemorrhage.[1,4,78-80] There is, however, concern that lowering maternal blood pressure may compromise placental perfusion and fetal well-being.[81-84] There is no consensus as to the optimal blood pressure threshold for initiating therapy. The only benefit of antihypertensive therapy in women with mild hypertension is a reduced risk of developing severe hypertension. This is considered insufficient to warrant exposing the fetus to the potential adverse effects on its placental perfusion. The target blood pressures are usually around 140 mm Hg systolic and 90 mm Hg diastolic.

Two clinical settings require consideration of antihypertensive therapy:

1) Acute management of severe hypertension, which may require parenteral therapy.
2) Chronic blood pressure control in the selected cases of expectant management of severe preeclampsia.[4,85]

Acute Setting Parenteral Therapy

Labetalol - Labetalol has been shown to be effective and safe in pregnancy, although data are limited.[85] Initialy, 20 mg are administered intravenously followed by 20 to 80 mg at 10 minute intervals and up to a maximum cumulative dose of 300 mg. The fall in blood pressure begins within 5 to 10 minutes and lasts up to six hours. Constant infusion of 1 to 2 mg/min can be used instead of intermittent therapy.

Hydralazine - Although used extensively in the setting of preeclampsia, intravenous hydralazine is associated with significant maternal hypotension when compared with other antihypertensive drugs.[83] Thus, hydralazine is not recommended as a first-line drug for treatment of severe hypertension in pregnant women, although evidence is not sufficient for making a definitive conclusion. Initially, IV 5 mg is administered over two minutes; and, depending upon the initial response, a 5 to 10 mg bolus is given after 20 minutes. The maximum bolus dose is 20 mg. The fall in blood pressure begins within 10 to 30 minutes and lasts up to four hours.

Calcium channel blockers - Experience with nifedipine (30 mg) and nicardipine in pregnancy is more limited than for labetalol and hydralazine.[86-88] Administration of IV calcium channel blockers together with Mg So4 may lead to serious side effects such as pulmonary edema. Use of immediate release sublingual nifedipine (10 mg) has been associated with an excessive reduction in blood pressure leading to serious cardiovascular morbidity and is discouraged.[89-91]

Diazoxide - Although rarely necessary, this drug can be used when adequate blood pressure control cannot be achieved with labetalol or hydralazine.[1] There is potential value to small doses of diazoxide (15 mg every three minutes to a maximum dose of 300 mg) when compared to hydralazine in terms of safety and effectiveness.[92]

Nitroprusside is contraindicated in late pregnancy due to possible fetal cyanide poisoning. However, the drug may be considered as a last resort for emergency control of refractory severe hypertension (0.5 to 10 mcg/kg/min)

Chronic Setting Oral Therapy

Occasionally, severe preeclamptic women are not delivered immediately. Oral antihypertensive therapy is often indicated for these patients. Options for oral antihypertensive therapy are the same as for women with chronic hypertension (see below) and the blood pressure targets usually are 140 to 150 mm Hg systolic and 90 to 100 mm Hg diastolic.

Outcome

The major adverse outcomes associated with preeclampsia are:

- Maternal: Central nervous system, hepatic, and renal dysfunction (eg, cerebral hemorrhage, hepatic rupture, renal failure), and bleeding (related to thrombocytopenia, placental abruption).
- Fetal: Preterm delivery, fetal growth restriction, and perinatal death.

Factors that influence outcome include: Severity of the disease, gestational age at onset and presence of coexisting conditions (eg, multiple gestation, diabetes mellitus, renal disease, thrombophilia, or preexisting hypertension).[93]

With mild preeclampsia neonatal outcomes are generally good except for a higher frequency of labor induction.[94] On the other hand, severe preeclampsia is associated with increased rates of maternal liver and kidney dysfunction, induced labor, cesarean delivery, preterm birth, fetal growth restriction, and neonatal respiration difficulties.[94] The highest risk of maternal and neonatal morbidity is in pregnancies complicated by early onset severe preeclampsia.

Postpartum Course

Preeclampsia related hypertension usually resolves within a few weeks and is almost always gone by 12 weeks postpartum.[95-96]

If hypertension persists beyond this period it should be evaluated and treated as in any non-pregnant woman. If the hypertension is severe, antihypertensive agents may be required temporarily postpartum. Oral antihypertensive medications similar to those used in the non-pregnant population may be appropriate. Beta-adrenergic blockers, calcium channel blockers, diuretics, and even angiotensin converting enzyme (ACE) inhibitors are suitable choices for non-breastfeeding mothers. The blood pressure should be monitored regularly to avoid hypotension. Usually within 3 weeks the blood pressure returns to its baseline values and therapy is stopped. In breastfeeding mothers calcium channel blockers and beta-adrenergic blockers appear to be safe although both enter breast milk. Labetalol and propranolol are preferred because these drugs are not concentrated in breast milk.[4] ACE inhibitors and angiotensin receptor antagonists should be avoided during lactation, and may be considered again after lactation cessation. Diuretics may reduce the milk volume, but this does not occur at doses ≤ 50 mg daily.[97]

Long Term Course

Women with early onset severe preeclampsia are at greatest risk of recurrence (25-65%) while in women who had mild preeclampsia during the first pregnancy the incidence is much lower (5-7%).[27, 29, 98-100] Patients with severe preeclampsia, particularly if occurring in the second trimester, have a high risk for recurrent preeclampsia in subsequent pregnancies and for chronic hypertension, perhaps due to irreversible vascular injury.[27, 29,100]
Observational studies have shown that preeclampsia is a risk factor for future development of cardiovascular disease. A systematic review evaluating this risk has shown that compared with women with no history of the disease, women with preeclampsia were at increased risk of the following: hypertension (RR 3.70, 95% CI 2.70-5.05 at mean follow-up of 14 years),ischemic heart disease (RR 2.16, 95% CI 1.86-2.52 at mean follow-up of 11.7 years), stroke (RR 1.81, 95% CI 1.45-2.27 at mean follow-up of 10.4 years), and venous thrombo-embolism (RR 1.79, 95% CI 1.37-2.33 at mean follow-up of 4.7 years).[101]
The reason for this observation may be the presence of unrecognized latent hypertension, an inherited thrombophilia, or other genetic or environmental factors predisposing to hypertension.

In contrast to high risk women (early onset preeclampsia, recurrent preeclampsia, severe preeclampsia, or preeclampsia with onset as a multipara), preeclampsia/eclampsia occurring late in gestation in primigravid women and followed by a second normotensive pregnancy does not appear to be associated with increased remote cardiovascular risk.[102]
A study from Israel reported an increased risk of cancer in women with a history of preeclampsia (hazard ratio 1.27, 95% CI 1.03-1.57) with a median follow-up of 29 years.[103] Site-specific increases were noted for cancer of the stomach, lung or larynx, breast, and ovary. However, a systematic review did not find any such association.[101]The discordant results may be explained by several factors including differences in patient populations, insufficient adjustment for confounders, differences in length of follow-up and more.

HELLP Syndrome

HELLP syndrome (Hemolysis, Elevated Liver enzymes, Low Platelets) probably represents a severe form of preeclampsia but this relationship remains controversial. Both these entities are probably part of a disease spectrum. Up to 20% of patients with HELLP syndrome do not have hypertension or proteinuria.[104-106] Both severe preeclampsia and HELLP syndrome may be associated with hepatic involvement including infarction, hemorrhage, and rupture.

Most cases are diagnosed between 28 and 36 weeks of gestation with an incidence of 1-2 per 1000 pregnancies overall and 10 -20% of women with severe preeclampsia/eclampsia. The disease may less often present postpartum (about a third of the cases)[107] usually within 48 hours of delivery, but occasionally as long as seven days postpartum. In these cases of postpartum HELLP syndrome, most patients are not diagnosed with preeclampsia antepartum.

Abdominal mid-epigastric or right upper quadrant pain and tenderness is the most common clinical presentation although some patients are asymptomatic.[107] The signs and symptoms by incidence according to Weinstein and Sibai are as follows:[104,108] Right upper quadrant or epigastric pain (86-90%), nausea and/or vomiting (45-84%), headache (50%), right upper quadrant tenderness on palpation (86%), diastolic blood pressure above 110 mm Hg (67%), proteinuria - above 2+ on dipstick (85-96%), and demonstrable edema (55-67%). Only in approximately 85 percent of cases hypertensive proteinuria is present.[109]Serious maternal morbidity includes disseminated intravascular coagulation (DIC), sub-capsular liver hematoma, abruption of the placenta, acute renal failure, and pulmonary edema.[107]

The diagnosis of HELLP syndrome is based on the presence of specific laboratory abnormalities in the blood count, smear, liver enzymes and LDH.[109] No consensus exists regarding the degree of laboratory abnormality diagnostic of HELLP syndrome. Nevertheless, the following criteria are usually met: [107]Platelet count $\leq$ 100,000 cells / microL, serum AST $\geq$ 70 IU/L, serum LDH $\geq$ 600 IU/L or total bilirubin $\geq$1.2 mg/dL as well as blood smear with signs of microangiopathic hemolytic anemia. If not all criteria are met the diagnosis is referred to as "partial HELLP". The diagnosis of HELLP syndrome may sometimes be hard to differentiate from other diseases complicating pregnancy such as: thrombotic thrombocytopenic purpura, hemolytic-uremic syndrome, acute fatty liver of pregnancy, lupus flare, idiopathic thrombocytopenic purpura, antiphospholipid syndrome, gastroenteritis, hepatitis, appendicitis or gallbladder disease.[109]

The principal elements of management include stabilization of the patient, assessment of the fetus and consideration of delivery. Delivery is the definitive treatment for HELLP syndrome and indications for immediate delivery include: [109]
Near term pregnancy ($\geq$34w), abruption of the placenta, non-reassuring fetal status or maternal multi-organ dysfunction including active deterioration of the laboratory parameters.
If gestational age is less than 34 weeks, glucocorticoid course may be administered assuming maternal and fetal status are reassuring. However, attempts to delay delivery beyond 48 hours are not recommended. Few data[110-111] on expectant management of HELLP syndrome have shown the following: Although maternal complications were uncommon with careful maternal monitoring and laboratory abnormalities reversed in a subgroup of patients, perinatal outcome was not improved. Thus, expectant management is not recommended.[109]

As in preeclampsia, severe hypertension can usually be controlled using labetalol, hydralazine, nifedipine or, in severe cases, with sodium nitroprusside.[112] For convulsion prevention and treatment, IV magnesium sulfate is administered.

Platelet transfusion is indicated only in the presence of significant maternal bleeding or if the platelet count drops to < 20,000 cells/microL.

Dexamethazone was suggested by some to be associated with a more rapid improvement in laboratory and clinical parameters.[113-116] However, well designed clinical trials did not support these findings.[117-118]

The mode of delivery, as in severe preeclampsia, depends on gestational age, cervical score, and maternal and fetal status. Following delivery, laboratory values may initially worsen. Platelet count reaches its nadir usually around 24-48 hours postpartum. LDH concentration peak earlier.[119-120] Maternal outcome following HELLP syndrome is generally good; however, serious complications may occur. The complications are interdependent:

placental abruption may lead to DIC which may cause renal failure and pulmonary edema. As for the fetus, 70% of cases lead to preterm delivery, and rates of intra uterine growth retardation are high.[121] Perinatal mortality may reach 20% and is closely related to gestational age, growth restriction and the presence of placental abruption.[109] Women with a history of HELLP syndrome are at a high risk of developing preeclampsia in subsequent pregnancies. However, recurrent HELLP or hepatic rupture is rare.[122-124]

Eclampsia

Eclampsia is defined as the development of generalized convulsions and/or coma in a woman with gestational hypertension or preeclampsia. These seizures should not be attributable to another coincidental neurologic disease.[3]

In general, eclampsia may develop anytime from 20th week of gestation to the puerperium. Eclampsia prior to 20 weeks of gestation should raise the possibility of an alternative diagnosis (see differential diagnosis below) or of an underlying APLA (antiphospholipid antibody) syndrome or molar pregnancy. APLA syndrome and molar pregnancies may lead to eclamptic seizures before 20 weeks of gestation.

The seizures are one of several clinical manifestations of severe preeclampsia and not the end result of preeclampsia. Thus, risk factors for eclampsia are similar to those for preeclampsia. Approximately a half of the cases develop before term pregnancy and a third at term, intra-partum or within 48 hours of delivery.[125] Eclampsia occurring beyond 48 hours postpartum is rare (see table 5).[126-128] The exact cause of eclamptic seizures is not known. It may be related to cerebral overregulation and vasospasm of cerebral arteries or to the loss of auto-regulation resulting in hyper-perfusion, or to both. Both processes may be a result of high systemic blood pressure.[129]

Table 5. Timing of eclampsia relative to gestational age[130, 195].

Gestational age	Frequency (%)
Antepartum	38-55
Intrapartum	13-36
≤48 hours postpartum	5-39
>48 hours postpartum	5-17

Incidence

Approximately 2% of severely preeclamptic women and 0.5% of mildly preeclamptic women develop eclampsia.[10] The incidence of eclampsia varies around the world with 5 cases per 10,000 live births in developed countries versus 6 -100 cases per 10,000 live births in developing countries.[125,130-131]

Clinical Manifestations

Eclampsia is a clinical diagnosis. The generalized, tonic-clonic seizures usually last 3-4 minutes and are self-limiting. Persistent headache, blurred vision, photophobia, right upper quadrant or epigastric pain, and altered mental status may occur before the seizure. If the seizure is typical electroencephalographic or cerebral imaging studies are not required.[132] Prolonged fetal bradycardia is common during an eclamptic seizure, and does not necessarily require emergent cesarean delivery. Fetal bradycardia is a result of maternal hypoxia and uterine hyper-stimulation. Stabilizing the mother by administration of oxygen, anticonvulsant and antihypertensive drugs can help the fetus recover in-utero. However, the possibility of placental abruption should be kept in mind mainly if the fetal heart rate remains non-reassuring for more than 10 minutes despite resuscitative efforts.[129]

Differential Diagnosis

Eclamptic seizures are indistinguishable from other generalized tonic-clonic seizures. When convulsions occur during pregnancy, delivery, or the preuperium, eclampsia is diagnosed until proven otherwise. Other etiologies should be considered if seizures occur before 20 weeks of gestation or in cases of focal neurologic deficits, prolonged coma, or atypical eclampsia.

These include: epilepsy, intracranial hemorrhage or CVA (cerebrovascular accident), space-occupying lesions of the CNS (central nervous system), hypertensive encephalopathy, metabolic disorders, CNS infection (meningitis or encephalitis) or vasculitis, thrombotic thrombocytopenic purpura (TTP) or thrombophilia, drug abuse, post-dural puncture syndrome and finally hyperventilation syndrome.[133]

Management

The definitive treatment of eclampsia is delivery to reduce the risk of maternal morbidity and mortality. Immediate management issues include prevention of hypoxia and acidosis, management of hypertension, control of convulsion, prevention of recurrence, and delivery of the fetus and the placenta.

During a seizure, airway maintenance and aspiration prevention are the first step. The bed side rails should be raised to prevent fall and trauma. Supplemental oxygen should be provided. Since 20% of deaths in eclampsia are due to hypertensive CVAs, emergent antihypertensive therapy should be instituted in hypertensive women.[134]

Options for treatment include labetalol or hydralazine. Pharmacologic treatment of mild hypertension is not recommended, as neither maternal nor fetal benefits have been demonstrated.[135] The initial convulsion is usually short and treatment is primarily directed at prevention of recurrent convulsions rather than control of the initial seizure. As many as ten percent of women will experience another seizure if not treated.[136]

Anticonvulsant Therapy for Prevention and Treatment of Eclampsia

Magnesium sulfate is the drug of choice for prevention of eclampsia and of recurrent seizures.[137] Anticonvulsant therapy should be administered to prevent seizures in women with severe preeclampsia or recurrent seizures in eclamptic women.[9,138] Anticonvulsant therapy may also be used for prevention of seizures in women with mild preeclampsia, but its role in this setting is controversial.[12,139-142] The largest study performed on preeclamptic women, enrolled over 10,000 women with preeclampsia. The patients were randomly assigned to receive magnesium sulfate or placebo. Therapy significantly reduced the risk of eclamptic convulsions (0.8 versus 1.9 percent, RR 0.42, 95% CI 0.29-0.60). However, to prevent one convulsion, 63 women with severe preeclampsia or 109 women with mild preeclampsia would need to be treated.[140]

Magnesium's mechanism of action as an anticonvulsant in preeclampsia is not clearly understood. Some investigators attribute the anticonvulsant effect of magnesium to blocked neuronal calcium influx through the glutamate channel. [143] Magnesium is believed to block the N-methyl-D-aspartate (NMDA) receptors in the central nervous system as implicated from rat models.[144] Other mechanisms may be related to vasodilatation of the cerebral vessels, inhibition of platelet aggregation, protection of endothelial cells from damage by free radicals and more.[145]

Therapy is generally initiated during labor, induction of labor, or prior to planned delivery while administering corticosteroids. If the patient is improving, therapy is discontinued 24 hours postpartum since the risk of developing seizures drops.

The superiority of magnesium sulfate over phenytoin for prevention of eclamptic seizures was illustrated in a randomized, controlled trial comparing these two drugs.[137] Eclamptic seizures developed in 10 of 1089 women assigned to phenytoin compared to none of 1049 women assigned to magnesium sulfate. Maternal and neonatal outcomes were similar in both groups. When compared to a lytic cocktail (a mixture of chlorpromazine , promethazine and pethidine), a Cochrane review concluded that magnesium sulfate is more effective and safe.[146]

An overview of randomized, controlled trials of magnesium sulfate therapy compared to placebo or other anticonvulsants in severe preeclampsia included 6343 patients.[139] Seizures rate was significantly lower with magnesium sulfate therapy (RR 0.39, 95% CI 0.28-0.55).

Magnesium sulfate's effectiveness for prevention of recurrent seizures in women with eclampsia was clearly demonstrated in randomized controlled trials. Its use can reduce the rate of recurrent seizures by one-half to two-thirds (RR 0.44, 95% CI 0.32-0.51) and the rate of maternal death by one-third (RR 0.62, 95% CI 0.39-0.99).[10] Moreover it is cheaper, relatively easily administered and less sedative than other anticonvulsant therapies.

The initial dose varies from 4 to 6 g intravenously over 15 minutes.[9] This dose is safe even in the presence of renal insufficiency. The maintenance dose is 2gper hour administered as a continuous intravenous infusion. In women with myasthenia gravis, magnesium sulfate is contraindicated since it can lead to a severe myasthenic crisis. Concurrence with calcium channel blockers may produce hypotension. During the maintenance phase monitoring of patellar reflex, respirations and urine output is imperative. A serum concentration range of

4.8 to 8.4 mg/dL is recommended.[147] Calcium gluconate (1 g intravenously) may be administered in cases of magnesium toxicity.

As mentioned above, the definitive treatment for eclampsia is delivery. After maternal stabilization, the mode of delivery is considered. The gestational age, cervical score and fetal condition and position are taken into account. Cesarean delivery is a reasonable option, for women remote from term with an unfavorable cervix, since less than one third will successfully deliver vaginally.[136, 148-149]

Outcome

Maternal mortality rates of 0 to 14 percent have been reported depending on prenatal care, resource availability and gestational age.[125,150-151] Perinatal mortality ranges from 9-23%.[125,151] Complications occur in up to 70 percent of women with eclampsia. These include: Premature delivery, abruption of the placenta, perinatal death, acute renal failure, hepato-cellular injury, intra-cerebral hemorrhage, cardio-respiratory arrest, postpartum hemorrhage, coagulopathy and more.[139] Although most of these complications resolve postpartum, cerebro-vascular damage may result in permanent neurologic damage and is the most common cause of death.[152-153] HELLP syndrome develops in up to 20 percent of eclamptic women.

Gestational Hypertension

Gestational hypertension is defined as systolic blood pressure $\geq$ 140 mmHg and/or a diastolic blood pressure $\geq$ 90 mmHg, in the absence of proteinuria, in a previously normotensive pregnant woman at or after 20 weeks of gestation.[72, 154] The onset of mild hypertension without proteinuria is occasionally seen late in the third trimester. Gestational hypertension is a diagnosis which may enclose three types of patients: Transient hypertension of pregnancy- without progression to preeclampsia, progression to preeclampsia and lastly women with previously unrecognized chronic hypertension. Therefore, the diagnosis of gestational hypertension should be used during pregnancy only in women who do not meet criteria for preeclampsia or chronic hypertension. The final diagnosis is verified only twelve weeks postpartum after chronic hypertension has been ruled out.

Some evidence suggests that gestational hypertension and preeclampsia are actually the same entities which only vary in the disease stage. Others argue that these are two different entities which carry different risk factors. For example, first pregnancy is a strong risk factor for preeclampsia, but not for gestational hypertension.[155] However, as many as 50 percent of women with gestational hypertension go on to develop preeclampsia and the risk correlates inversely with gestational age.[156-157] The highest risk of progression to preeclampsia is in women who develop gestational hypertension before 30 weeks of gestation.[156-158]

Gestational hypertension has little adverse effect on the mother or fetus, [1] unless hypertension is severe ($\geq$ 160/110 mmHg).[94, 158] Pregnancy outcome in mild gestational hypertension are generally favorable.[72, 94,157-159] However, in cases of severe gestational hypertension the risk of maternal and perinatal morbidity rises and is comparable to severe preeclampsia rates.[72, 94,155,157-160] Morbidity includes: preterm delivery, small for gestational age infants, and abruption of the placenta.

The hypertension typically resolves shortly postpartum,[4] but may recur in subsequent pregnancies.

As mentioned above, gestational hypertension may not be benign in the following two situations:

1) Remote from term — May be related to the development of preeclampsia and adverse neonatal outcome.[157]

2) Clinical features of severe disease — Symptoms and signs of severe disease (severe hypertension, persistent headache, visual changes, growth restriction, oligohydramnios, epigastric or right upper abdominal pain, thrombocytopenia, or liver function abnormalities).

In these two situations, women are at high risk of maternal and/or fetal morbidity and should be managed as if they have preeclampsia.[94, 158,160]

Maternal Evaluation

Primarily gestational hypertension should be distinguished from preeclampsia (Table 3) and its severity must be determined. White coat hypertension should also be excluded.

The presence or absence of proteinuria will determine whether the patient is diagnosed with gestational hypertension or preeclampsia. Urine protein can be quantified using a 24-hour urine collection or a urine protein-to-creatinine ratio on a random urine sample. These methods are preferred over a simple urine dipstick which carries higher false negative and false positive rates. Signs and symptoms of end organ damage should be ruled out by questioning, physical examination and laboratory evaluation.

Twenty percent of women who develop eclampsia have no proteinuria,[161] and 10 percent of women with other clinical or histological manifestations of preeclampsia have no proteinuria.[162] Therefore close follow-up of women with gestational hypertension is prudent.

Fetal well-being should be assessed with a biophysical profile including a nonstress test. A sonographic estimation of fetal weight is obtained to exclude growth restriction. Umbilical artery Doppler velocimetry is performed in cases of growth restriction.[72]

Management and Prognosis

Due to the increased risk of developing preeclampsia and other complications, patient counseling is important. Any symptoms suggestive of severe disease should be reported. As in preeclampsia, antihypertensive agents are not given unless hypertension is severe. Medical therapy of mild hypertension does not improve neonatal outcome[15, 163] and may mask severe disease.[72] There is no evidence from large randomized trials that any maternal and fetal routine surveillance method decreases perinatal morbidity or mortality. Mild gestational hypertension is usually diagnosed at or beyond 37 weeks of gestation and hence antenatal corticosteroids are rarely indicated.[72] Delivery before 34 weeks occurres in as little as 1-5% of cases.[72] Since some studies have reported that pregnancies complicated by gestational hypertension are at increased risk of perinatal mortality and pregnancy complications, [155,164-165] patients with mild gestational hypertension are usually delivered no later than 40 weeks of gestation.

The indications and choice of antihypertensive therapy in gestational hypertension are the same as for women with preeclampsia. Severe hypertension is treated medically to reduce the risk of stroke although there are no data showing that these women are at increased risk of stroke. Women with severe gestational hypertension are managed differently due to comparable rates of pregnancy complications as with severe preeclampsia. In these cases, maternal and fetal surveillance are more extensive and similar to that for women with severe preeclampsia. Hypertension is treated with antihypertensive agents and delivery is considered.

During labor, the woman is monitored for development of proteinuria, worsening hypertension, and symptoms of severe disease since preeclampsia may develop intra-partum. Magnesium sulfate seizure prophylaxis is administered if severe gestational hypertension or severe preeclampsia develop.

Most women with gestational hypertension become normotensive soon postpartum.[95] If the woman is still hypertensive by the 12th postpartum week, she is diagnosed as chronically hypertensive (about 15% of cases).[166] Gestational hypertension does not affect the endothelium, hence the prompt resolution of the hypertension postpartum when compared with preeclampsia (one week versus two weeks).[167] Gestational hypertension tends to recur with subsequent pregnancies[165] and is associated with hypertension later in life.[166,169] A retrospective cohort study[169] of over 3500 women who had gestational hypertension demonstrated a significant association to hypertension later in life (adjusted odds ratio 2.47, 95% CI 1.74-3.51).

Chronic Hypertension

In pregnant women, chronic hypertension is defined as abnormally elevated blood pressure (140/90 mmHg or greater) that is documented before pregnancy.[170] Because of the physiologic decrease in blood pressure seen in mid-pregnancy, chronic hypertensive patients may actually have pressures in the normotensive range for a good portion of their pregnancy. This will make the diagnosis difficult in those with scant prenatal care. When pre-pregnancy blood pressure is unknown, the diagnosis is based on the presence of hypertension before 20 weeks of gestation. Patients with mild chronic hypertension are those with systolic blood pressures between 140-159 mmHg and diastolic pressures between 90-109 while those with a systolic blood pressure ≥160 mmHg or a diastolic ≥ 110 mmHg are classified as severe. This is a relatively common disorder occurring in 1-5% of pregnant women.[170] There are at least 120,000 pregnant women with chronic hypertension per year in the United States, a rate expected to increase.[171] Essential hypertension is responsible for 90% of chronic hypertension associated with pregnancy. Causes of secondary hypertension include renal disease, endocrinologic disorders, or collagen vascular disease. In chronic hypertension elevated blood pressure is the cardinal pathophysiologic feature, whereas in preeclampsia increased blood pressure is only a sign of the underlying disorder. Thus, the impact of the two conditions on mother and fetus are different, as is the management. The cost of managing chronic hypertension in pregnancy is high, maternal and fetal related.

Adverse Pregnancy Outcome

Women with chronic hypertension are at increased risk of adverse pregnancy outcome. The most common complication is superimposed preeclampsia, where the incidence is up to four-fold higher when compared to the general obstetric population.[170,172] In addition, when evaluating the magnitude of fetal and maternal risk, in this setting, a five-fold increase in low birth weight (RR 5.5, 95% CI 2.6-11.9), a three-fold increase in perinatal mortality (OR 3.4, 95% CI 3.0-3.7), a two-fold increase in abruption of the placenta (OR 2.1, 95% CI 1.1-3.9), and an increased frequency of impaired fetal growth even in the absence of superimposed preeclampsia have all been shown.[173-174]

The absolute ranges of risk for adverse pregnancy outcome reported in observational studies of women with mild and severe chronic hypertension are high and include preterm birth, superimposed preeclampsia, fetal growth restriction and abruption of the placenta (Table 6).[170]

Table 6. Chronic hypertension – Main adverse pregnancy outcome.

Adverse Outcome	Severe chronic HTN	Mild chronic HTN
Preterm birth <37 weeks	62-70%	12-34%
Superimposed preeclampsia	50%	10-25%
Fetal growth restriction	31-40%	8-16%
Abruption of the placenta	5-10%	0.7-1.5%

Other potential problems are the known long term risks of any hypertensive disease and include: retinopathy, renal failure, heart failure, hypertensive encephalopathy and cerebral hemorrhage.[175]

Women with severe chronic hypertension and those with adverse outcomes in previous pregnancies are at a higher risk of superimposed preeclampsia, fetal growth restriction and abruption of the placenta.[171] These women should therefore undergo thorough counseling about these risks before conception and should be advised about the importance of adequate blood pressure control before conception and early in pregnancy.

The treatment of chronic hypertension during pregnancy, despite these risks, is controversial. Treatment holds limited beneficial effects; mainly partial prevention of maternal morbidity which largely depend upon the severity of the hypertensive disease.

Maternal Evaluation and Approach

The primary objective in the management of pregnancies complicated by chronic hypertension is to reduce maternal risks and achieve optimal perinatal survival. This objective can be achieved using an approach that includes pre-conceptional evaluation and counseling, early antenatal care, frequent antepartum visits to monitor both maternal and fetal well-being, timely delivery with intensive intra-partum monitoring, and proper postpartum management.

For management and counseling purposes, women with chronic hypertension should be categorized as having either low-risk or high-risk hypertension in pregnancy.[170] Women are considered at low risk when they have mild essential hypertension without any target organ involvement. All other women should be considered to have high risk chronic hypertension. The initial evaluation of the hypertensive patient is beyond the scope of this chapter. However secondary hypertension must always be considered in young women, especially if white, non-obese and under 30 years of age with a confirmed negative family history of hypertension. Women with chronic hypertension who desire pregnancy should be encouraged to receive pre-pregnancy care. The cause and severity of the hypertension should be established. The patient should cautiously and gradually be taken off anti-hypertensive drugs with potential adverse effects on the fetus. Renal function and proteinuria should be assessed. Once conception has occurred, early prenatal care within an appropriate setting is important. Frequent care is essential to optimize perinatal outcome in these patients. During the initial visits, if not determined earlier, a detailed evaluation of the etiology and severity of the chronic hypertension should be made and careful attention given to co-morbidities and to the outcome of previous pregnancies. Baseline laboratory tests recommended in pregnancy include, at least, serum creatinine, blood urea nitrogen, glucose, and electrolytes as well as urinalysis and urine culture.[79,170] These tests will effectively rule out many causes of previously unrecognized secondary hypertension and will identify important co- morbidities. Women who develop evidence of proteinuria on a urine dipstick should have a quantitative test for urine protein. Patients with severe hypertension or proteinuria should also have a retinal evaluation, chest x-ray, EKG, antinuclear antibody testing, and, when indicated, serum complement studies. An echocardiogram should be performed to evaluate cardiac function in cases of long standing hypertension. Patients with recurrent pregnancy loss or a history of thrombo-embolic disease should be evaluated for APLA syndrome. Pregnancies in high risk hypertensive women with additional risk factors are associated with increased maternal and perinatal complications. These pregnancies should be managed in consultation with appropriate specialists. Close monitoring and multiple hospitalizations may be necessary to control hypertension and associated complications.

Indications for Treatment

There is no consensus on the best treatment approach for women with mild chronic hypertension. Women with uncomplicated chronic hypertension who are stable on medication may continue their therapy or have it tapered or stopped during pregnancy as long as their blood pressure is monitored closely.[4, 170] Many times, acceptable blood pressures will be achieved during the second trimester in the absence of the usual antihypertensive therapy due to the physiological decrease in blood pressure at this time.

Mild Chronic Hypertension

Although a large number of trials were conducted focusing on the potential benefits of antihypertensive therapy in pregnancy, these trials, even with meta-analysis, lack sufficient power to detect modest treatment effects. Mild essential hypertension is defined as systolic pressure of 140-159 or diastolic pressure of 90- 109 mmHg.

Neither the fetus nor the patient appears to be at risk from mild hypertensive disease.

Furthermore, controlled trials have not demonstrated any reduced risk of preeclampsia or abruption, or any improvement in fetal or maternal outcome when antihypertensive medications were given in this setting.[78,83-84,174,176-177] The only demonstrated benefit, as concluded in two systematic reviews, is the decreased incidence of severe hypertension.[84,178] Up to 13 women would need to be treated to prevent one episode of severe hypertension.[84] Based on the available data, treatment is usually not initiated in pregnant women with uncomplicated mild essential hypertension, especially in the first trimester. If the patient is already on antihypertensive therapy and measured blood pressures during early pregnancy are less than 120/80 mmHg, discontinuation of therapy should strongly be considered. Nevertheless, signs of hypertensive end-organ damage or persistent high blood pressures (systolic pressures greater than 150 mmHg or diastolic pressures of over 100 mmHg) should promote initiation of therapy. These thresholds, although not necessarily in the severe range, allow a non-emergent approach with oral drugs.

Specific subgroups of women with mild hypertension appear to be at greater risk of fetal and maternal complications and may benefit from antihypertensive therapy (Table 7).[170] Target blood pressures of around 140 / 90 mmHg are desirable.

Table 7. Suggested indications for therapy in mild chronic hypertension.

	Secondary hypertension (eg, renal disease, collagen vascular disease, coarctation of the aorta)
	End-organ damage (eg, retinopathy, ventricular dysfunction)
	Maternal age over 40 years old
	Microvascular disease
	History of stroke
	Previous perinatal loss
	Diabetes
	Dyslipidemia
	Persistent high blood pressures of mild hypertensive disease (systolic pressures ≥150 mmHg or diastolic pressures ≥95 mmHg)

Severe Chronic Hypertension

Severe hypertension is defined as blood pressure ≥ 160/100 mmHg. Even in the absence of associated signs of early hypertensive encephalopathy, severe hypertension should be treated to protect the mother from serious co -morbidity, such as heart failure, renal failure or stroke.

Drug Therapy

All antihypertensive drugs cross the placenta. There are no data from large well-designed randomized trials on which to base a recommendation for use of one drug over another. The pharmacologic approach to blood pressure control should be individualized depending on the presence of other conditions, such as renal disease, diabetes, and left ventricular dysfunction. Usually, if maternal blood pressure is controlled with her own medications prior to conception, it may be continued throughout the pregnancy and after delivery, except for angiotensin-converting enzyme inhibitors, angiotensin receptor blockers and atenolol.[170, 179]
If however the patient is not treated and an indication exists, treatment is usually started with either labetalol or methyldopa. Calcium channel blockers (long acting) may be added. These drugs have been extensively used during pregnancy and are reasonably safe and effective.[1]

Methyldopa - This mild antihypertensive drug is one of the most widely used drugs in pregnant women and is considered safe for the fetus.[1,176,180-183] However, blood pressure goals may not be achieved, and the drug may have a sedative effect.

Labetalol - Labetolol is the most widely used beta-adrenergic blocker in pregnancy. Beta-adrenergic blockers are not associated with an increased risk of congenital anomalies however their safety is somewhat controversial due to few reports of preterm delivery, fetal growth restriction, and hypoglycemia.[182]Labetalol has both alpha- and beta-adrenergic blocking activity, and may preserve utero-placental blood flow better than other drugs in this class. Beta blockers are more effective in avoiding episodes of severe hypertension and are better tolerated than methyldopa.[84, 183]

Calcium channel blockers - These agents appear to be safe for use in pregnancy according to accumulating experience.[178] Long-acting nifedipine (30 to 90 mg once daily as sustained release tablet, increase at 7 to 14 day intervals, maximum dose 120 mg/day) has been used without major problems.[81, 184-185]

Thiazide diuretics - Although previously controversial, current recommendations suggest that these agents can be continued as long as volume depletion is avoided.[1,4,181,186] Volume depletion is unlikely with chronic therapy, assuming that drug dose and dietary sodium intake are constant, since fluid loss occurs during the first two weeks of use.

Angiotensin converting enzyme (ACE) inhibitors and angiotensin II receptor blockers (ARBs) are fetopathic and are contraindicated during pregnancy.

Antepartum Assessment

This assessment is directed toward early diagnosis of superimposed preeclampsia and signs of placental insufficiency. Frequent prenatal visits are recommended for monitoring maternal blood pressure, proteinuria, renal function and fundal growth as well as periodic sonographic estimation of fetal size and growth.[4,170] Nevertheless, an uncomplicated pregnancy is expected in over 85 % of hypertensive women.[1]

There is no consensus regarding the role of antepartum fetal assessment in pregnancies complicated by mild maternal hypertension. Gestational age should be determined to avoid uncertainty when fetal growth delay is suspected.[170] In the absence of superimposed preeclampsia or fetal growth restriction, the frequency of antepartum fetal assessment is controversial. Nevertheless, many clinicians perform a nonstress test with amniotic fluid index or biophysical profile weekly or twice per week in the later third trimester.

In cases of utero-placental vasculopathy or intrauterine growth restriction, close fetal surveillance is warranted.[79] In these cases, serial sonographic assessments of fetal growth are indicated as well as frequent nonstress testing and/or biophysical profile examination.[4,79]

Delivery

Women with mild, uncomplicated chronic hypertension can be allowed to go into spontaneous labor and deliver at term[79] although the practice of inducing labor at 39-40 weeks of gestation is common. Earlier delivery should be considered for women with the following: severe hypertension, superimposed preeclampsia, fetal growth restriction or other signs of placental insufficiency, and in any other cases of suspected pregnancy complications.

Intrapartum management is directed at the avoidance of acute maternal and fetal complications. Maternal blood pressure can be controlled with oral or intravenous hydralazine or labetalol. Close attention must be given to the use of intravenous fluids and to the noninvasive hemodynamic parameters. Fetuses may be compromised by long-standing growth restriction and hypoxemia prior to the onset of labor. Therefore, continuous fetal monitoring and fetal scalp pH sampling, as needed, are important to assess the ability of the fetus to tolerate labor.

Postpartum, high risk patients should be monitored closely for at least 48 hours due to the risk of developing hypertensive encephalopathy, pulmonary edema and renal failure. Either oral or intravenous antihypertensive drugs can be used to control severe hypertension. In some women, it is often necessary to switch to a new agent such as an angiotensin-converting enzyme inhibitor, particularly in those with pre-gestational diabetes mellitus and those with cardiomyopathy.

In patients with evidence of circulatory congestion or pulmonary edema, diuretic therapy should be used. High risk patients should be evaluated after the postpartum period for cardiac or renal function change and for adjustment of antihypertensive medication as stated above. Some patients may wish to breast-feed their infants. As discussed previously, all antihypertensive drugs are found in the breast milk, although drugs differ in the amount transferred to the milk.[187] Long-term effect of maternal antihypertensive drugs on breastfeeding infants is not known. Methyldopa appears to be safe since milk concentrations are low. The use of methyldopa as a first-line oral therapy appears to be a reasonable choice. Labetalol or propanolol are a better choice than atenolol and metoprolol due to lower concentrations in breast milk.[187-188] There is little information about the transfer of calcium channel blockers to breast milk, but there are no apparent side effects. Diuretic agents may induce a decrease in milk production.[187] Angiotensin-converting enzyme inhibitors and angiotensin II receptor antagonists should be avoided because of their effects on neonatal renal function.

Preeclampsia Superimposed on Chronic Hypertension

Women with chronic hypertension should be monitored closely for early detection of superimposed preeclampsia, the most frequent complication associated with hypertension during pregnancy. Superimposed preeclampsia is defined as worsening hypertension with new onset proteinuria in a woman with chronic hypertension. Women with both preexisting hypertension and proteinuria are considered preeclamptic if one of the following occurs:

An exacerbation of blood pressure to the severe range (systolic $\geq$ 160 mmHg or diastolic $\geq$110 mmHg) after 20 weeks of gestation, especially if accompanied by symptoms or increased liver enzymes or thrombocytopenia, or a sudden increase in the proteinuria.

However, current diagnostic criteria for hypertensive disorders of pregnancy are not adequate in women who have preexisting hypertension or proteinuria or both. In these women, the definitions for superimposed preeclampsia are arbitrary and lack reliable data to support their validity.[16] Many clinical, biophysical, and biochemical markers have been proposed to either predict or detect the development of superimposed preeclampsia.[17,189-192] These have included markers related to impaired trophoblast differentiation and invasion, placental and endothelial dysfunction, coagulation and complement activation, immune mal-adaptation to paternal antigens, and exaggerated systemic inflammatory response. Some authors have suggested the diagnostic usefulness of serum sFLt-1, soluble endoglin, and uric acid values in differentiating women with preeclampsia from those with various other hypertensive disorders of pregnancy.[16] However, major limitations regarding the diagnostic criteria of preeclampsia used as well as sample size make these studies insufficient.

Superimposed preeclampsia complicates approximately 5-50% of the chronic hypertensive pregnancies, depending on whether the diagnosis of preeclampsia was made simply on the basis of exacerbation of the hypertension or if significant proteinuria was part of the definition. In patients with risk factors, the incidence of superimposed preeclampsia is 25-50%. Importantly, the incidence of superimposed preeclampsia (or placental abruption) is not influenced by the use of antihypertensive medications.[193] Decreased utero-placental perfusion can lead to worsening of the fetal growth restriction. Spontaneous or intentional interruption of the pregnancy adds the compounding complications of prematurity. Severe superimposed preeclampsia developing after 28 weeks is an indication for delivery; prior to 28 weeks the pregnancy may be followed conservatively in a tertiary center with daily evaluation of maternal and fetal condition, although this latter approach remains controversial.[194]

References

[1]   Cunningham FG, Lindheimer MD. Hypertension in pregnancy. *N Engl J Med* 1992; 326:927.

[2]   Sibai BM. Pitfalls in diagnosis and management of preeclampsia. *Am J Obstet Gynecol* 1988; 159:1.

[3]   American College of Obstetricians and Gynecologists. Hypertension in Pregnancy. ACOG. Technical Bulletin #219. *American College of obstetricians and Gynecologists*, Washington, DC, 1996.

[4]   Working group report on high blood pressure in pregnancy. *National Institutes of Health*, Washington, DC 2000.

[5]   Lain KY, Roberts JM. Contemporary concepts of the pathogenesis and management of preeclampsia. *JAMA* 2002; 287:3183.

[6]   Saftlas AF, Olson DR, Franks AL, et al. Epidemiology of preeclampsia and eclampsia in the United States, 1979-1986. *Am J Obstet Gynecol* 1990; 163:460.

[7]   Maternal mortality--United States, 1982-1996. MMWR *Morb Mortal Wkly Rep* 1998; 47:705.

[8]   Sibai BM, Gordon T, Thom E, et al. Risk factors for preeclampsia in healthy nulliparous women: a prospective multicenter study. The National Institute of Child Health and Human Development Network of Maternal-Fetal Medicine Units. *Am J Obstet Gynecol* 1995; 172:642.

[9]   ACOG practice bulletin. Diagnosis and management of preeclampsia and eclampsia. Number 33, January 2002. *Obstet Gynecol* 2002; 99:159.

[10]   Sibai BM. Magnesium sulfate prophylaxis in preeclampsia: Lessons learned from recent trials. *Am J Obstet Gynecol* 2004; 190:1520.

[11]   www.cdc.gov. (accessed October 18, 2006).

[12]   Livingston JC, Livingston LW, Ramsey R, et al. Magnesium sulfate in women with mild preeclampsia: a randomized controlled trial. *Obstet Gynecol* 2003; 101:217.

[13]   MacKay AP, Berg CJ, Atrash HK. Pregnancy-related mortality from preeclampsia and eclampsia. *Obstet Gynecol* 2001; 97:533.

[14]   Khan KS, Wojdyla D, Say L, et al. WHO analysis of causes of maternal death: a systematic review. *Lancet* 2006; 367:1066–1074.

[15]   Sibai B, Dekker G, Kupfermic M. Preeclampsia. *Lancet* 2005; 365:785–799.

[16]   Sibai B. Hypertensive disorders of pregnancy: the United States perspective *Curr Opin Ob Gyn* 2008, 20:102–106.

[17]   Widmer M, Villar J, Benigni A, et al. Mapping the theory of preeclampsia and the role of angiogenic factors: A systemic review. *Obstet Gynecol* 2007;109:168–180.

[18]   Levine RJ, Lam C, Qian C, et al. Soluble endoglin and other circulating angiogenic factors in preeclampsia. *N Engl J Med* 2006; 355:992–1005.

[19] Vatlen LJ, Eskild A, Nilsen TIL, et al. Changes in circulating level of angiogenic factors from the first to second trimester as predictors of preeclampsia. *Am J Obstet Gynecol* 2007; 196:239.e1–239.e6.

[20] Smith GCS, Crossley JA, Aitken DA, et al. Circulating angiogenic factors in early pregnancy and the risk of preeclampsia, intrauterine growth restriction, spontaneous preterm birth, and stillbirth. *Obstet Gynecol* 2007; 109:1316–1324.

[21] Rana S, Karumanchi A, Levine RJ, et al. Sequential changes in antiangiogenic factors in early pregnancy and risk of developing preeclampsia. *Hypertension* 2007; 50:137–142.

[22] Chafetz I, Kuhnreich I, Sanner M, et al. First-trimester placental protein 13 screening for preeclampsia and intrauterine growth restriction. *Am J Obstet Gynecol* 2007; 197:35.e1–35.e7.

[23] Papageorghiou AT, Leslie K. Uterine artery Doppler in the prediction of adverse pregnancy outcome. *Curr OpinObstet Gynecol* 2007; 19:103–109.

[24] Li H, Gudnason H, Olofsson P, et al. Increased uterine artery vascular impedance is related to adverse outcome of pregnancy but is present in only one-third of late third-trimester preeclamptic women. *Ultrasound Obstet Gynecol* 2005; 25:459–463.

[25] Geerts I, Odendaal HJ. Severe early onset preeclampsia: prognostic value of ultrasound and Doppler assessment. *J Perinatol* 2007; 27:335–342.

[26] Duckitt K, Harrington D. Risk factors for pre-eclampsia at antenatal booking: systematic review of controlled studies. *BMJ* 2005; 330:565.

[27] Sibai BM, El-Nazer A, Gonzalez-Ruiz A. Severe preeclampsia-eclampsia in young primigravid women: Subsequent pregnancy outcome and remote prognosis. *Am J Obstet Gynecol* 1986; 155:1011.

[28] van Rijn BB, Hoeks LB, Bots ML, et al. Outcomes of subsequent pregnancy after first pregnancy with early-onset preeclampsia. *Am J Obstet Gynecol* 2006; 195:723.

[29] Sibai BM, Mercer B, Sarinoglu C. Severe preeclampsia in the second trimester: Recurrence risk and long-term prognosis. *Am J Obstet Gynecol* 1991; 165:1408.

[30] Dekker GA, Sibai BM. Etiology and pathogenesis of preeclampsia: current concepts. *Am J Obstet Gynecol* 1998; 179:1359.

[31] Dawson LM, Parfrey PS, Hefferton D, et al. Familial risk of preeclampsia in newfoundland: a population-based study. *J Am Soc Nephrol* 2002; 13:1901.

[32] Nilsson E, Salonen Ros H, Cnattingius S, Lichtenstein P. The importance of genetic and environmental effects for pre-eclampsia and gestational hypertension: a family study. *BJOG* 2004; 111:200.

[33] Esplin MS, Fausett MB, Fraser A, Kerber R, Mineau G, Carrillo J, Varner MW. Paternal and maternal components of the predisposition to preeclampsia. *N Engl J Med* 2001 22; 344(12):867-72.

[34] Stella CL, How HY, Sibai BM. Thrombophilia and adverse maternal-perinatal outcome: controversies in screening and management. *Am J Perinatol* 2006; 23:499.

[35] Conde-Agudelo A, Villar J, Lindheimer M. Maternal infection and risk of preeclampsia: systematic review and metaanalysis. *Am J Obstet Gynecol* 2008; 198:7.

[36] Askie LM, Duley L, Henderson-Smart DJ, Stewart LA, On behalf of the PARIS Collaborative Group. Antiplatelet agents for prevention of preeclampsia: a meta-analysis of individual patient data. *Lancet* 2007; 369:1791–1798.

[37] Trumbo PR, Ellwood KC. Supplemental calcium and risk reduction of hypertension, pregnancy-induced hypertension, and preeclampsia: An evidence-based review by the US Food and Drug Administration. *Nutr Rev* 2007; 65:78–87.

[38] Polyzos NP, Mauri D, Tsappi M, et al. Combined Vitamin C and E supplementation during pregnancy for preeclampsia prevention: A systematic review. *Obstet Gynecol Survey* 2007; 62:202–206.

[39] Towers CV, Pircon RA, Nageotte MP, et al. Cocaine intoxication presenting as preeclampsia and eclampsia. *Obstet Gynecol* 1993; 81:545.

[40] Broekhuizen FF, Elejalde R, Hamilton PR. Early-onset preeclampsia, triploidy and fetal hydrops. *J Reprod Med* 1983; 28:223.

[41] Villar MA, Sibai BM. Clinical significance of elevated mean arterial blood pressure in second trimester and threshold increase in systolic or diastolic blood pressure during third trimester [see comments]. *Am J Obstet Gynecol* 1989; 160:419.

[42] Levine RJ, Ewell MG, Hauth JC, et al. Should the definition of preeclampsia include a rise in diastolic blood pressure of < 15 mm Hg to a level <90 mm Hg in association with proteinuria? *Am J Obstet Gynecol* 2000; 183:787.

[43] Bellomo G, Narducci PL, Rondoni F, et al. Prognostic value of 24-hour blood pressure in pregnancy. *JAMA* 1999; 282:1447.

[44] Bergel E, Carroli G, Althabe F. Ambulatory versus conventional methods for monitoring blood pressure during pregnancy (Cochrane Review). *Cochrane Database Syst Rev* 2002;CD001231.

[45] Moran P, Lindheimer MD, Davison JM. The renal response to preeclampsia. *Semin Nephrol* 2004; 24:588.

[46] Moran P, Baylis PH, Lindheimer MD, Davison JM. Glomerular ultrafiltration in normal and preeclamptic pregnancy. *J Am Soc Nephrol* 2003; 14:648.

[47] Lang RM, Pridjian G, Feldman T, et al. Left ventricular mechanics in preeclampsia. *Am Heart J* 1991; 121:1768.

[48] Bosio PM, McKenna PJ, Conroy R, O'Herlihy C. Maternal central hemodynamics in hypertensive disorders of pregnancy. *Obstet Gynecol* 1999; 94:978.

[49] Visser W, Wallenburg HC. Central hemodynamic observations in untreated preeclamptic patients. *Hypertension* 1991; 17:1072.

[50] Hankins GD, Wendel GD Jr, Cunningham FG, Leveno KJ. Longitudinal evaluation of hemodynamic changes in eclampsia. *Am J Obstet Gynecol* 1984; 150:506.

[51] Cotton DB, Lee W, Huhta JC, Dorman KF. Hemodynamic profile of severe pregnancy-induced hypertension. *Am J Obstet Gynecol* 1988; 158:523.

[52] Phelan JP, Yurth DA. Severe preeclampsia. I. Peripartum hemodynamic observations. *Am J Obstet Gynecol* 1982; 144:17.

[53] Clark SL, Greenspoon JS, Aldahl D, Phelan JP. Severe preeclampsia with persistent oliguria: management of hemodynamic subsets. *Am J Obstet Gynecol* 1986; 154:490.

[54] Mabie WC, Ratts TE, Sibai BM. The central hemodynamics of severe preeclampsia. *Am J Obstet Gynecol* 1989; 161:1443.

[55] Benedetti TJ, Kates R, Williams V. Hemodynamic observations in severe preeclampsia complicated by pulmonary edema. *Am J Obstet Gynecol* 1985; 152:330.

[56] Taufield PA, Ales KL, Resnick LM, et al. Hypocalciuria in preeclampsia. *N Engl J Med* 1987; 316:715.

[57] August P, Marcaccio B, Gertner JM, et al. Abnormal 1,25 dihydroxyvitamin D metabolism in preeclampsia. *Am J Obstet Gynecol* 1992; 166:1295.

[58] Powers RW, Bodnar LM, Ness RB, et al. Uric acid concentrations in early pregnancy among preeclamptic women with gestational hyperuricemia at delivery. *Am J Obstet Gynecol* 2006; 194:160.

[59] Stillman IE, Karumanchi SA. The glomerular injury of preeclampsia. *J Am Soc Nephrol* 2007; 18:2281.

[60] Arias F, Mancilla-Jimenez R. Hepatic fibrinogen deposits in pre-eclampsia. Immunofluorescent evidence. *N Engl J Med* 1976; 295:578.

[61] Minakami H, Oka N, Sato T, et al. Preeclampsia: a microvesicular fat disease of the liver?. *Am J Obstet Gynecol* 1988; 159:1043.

[62] Stubbs TM, Lazarchick J, Van Dorsten JP, et al. Evidence of accelerated platelet production and consumption in nonthrombocytopenic preeclampsia. *Am J Obstet Gynecol* 1986; 155:263.

[63] Sheehan HL, Lynch JB. Pathology of toxaemia of pregnancy. *Churchill and Livingstone,* London 1973.

[64] Richards A, Graham D, Bullock R. Clinicopathological study of neurological complications due to hypertensive disorders of pregnancy. *J Neurol Neurosurg Psychiatry* 1988; 51:416.

[65] Drislane FW, Wang AM. Multifocal cerebral hemorrhage in eclampsia and severe pre-eclampsia. *J Neurol* 1997; 244:194.

[66] Morriss MC, Twickler DM, Hatab MR, et al. Cerebral blood flow and cranial magnetic resonance imaging in eclampsia and severe preeclampsia. *Obstet Gynecol* 1997; 89:561.

[67] Carpenter F, Kava HL, Plotkin D. The development of total blindness as a complication of pregnancy. *Am J Obstet Gynecol* 1953; 66:641.

[68] Odegard RA, Vatten LJ, Nilsen ST, et al. Preeclampsia and fetal growth. *Obstet Gynecol* 2000; 96:950.

[69] Sibai BM, Mercer BM, Schiff E, Friedman SA. Aggressive versus expectant management of severe preeclampsia at 28-32 weeks' gestation: A randomized controlled trial. *Am J Obstet Gynecol* 1994; 171:818.

[70] Friedman SA, Schiff E, Kao L, Sibai BM. Neonatal outcome after preterm delivery for preeclampsia. *Am J Obstet Gynecol* 1995;172:1785.

[71] Nicholson JM, Kellar LC, Kellar GM. The impact of the interaction between increasing gestational age and obstetrical risk on birth outcomes: evidence of a varying optimal time of delivery. *J Perinatol* 2006; 26:392.

[72] Sibai BM. Diagnosis and management of gestational hypertension and preeclampsia. *Obstet Gynecol* 2003; 102:181.

[73] Chang EY, Menard MK, Vermillion ST, et al. The association between hyaline membrane disease and preeclampsia. *Am J Obstet Gynecol* 2004; 191:1414.

[74] Sibai BM, Barton JR. Expectant management of severe preeclampsia remote from term: patient selection, treatment, and delivery indications. *Am J Obstet Gynecol* 2007; 196:514.e1–514.e9.

[75] Norwitz ER, Edmund F, Funai EF. Expectant management of severe preeclampsia. *UPTODATE* January 3, 2008.

[76] Haddad B, Kayem G, Deis S, Sibai BM. Are perinatal and maternal outcomes different during expectant management of severe preeclampsia in the presence of intrauterine growth restriction? *Am J Obstet Gynecol* 2007; 196:237.e1–237.e5.

[77] Meher S, Abalos E, Carroli G, Meher S. Bed rest with or without hospitalisation for hypertension during pregnancy. *Cochrane Database Syst Rev* 2005; :CD003514.

[78] Remuzzi G, Ruggenenti P. Prevention and treatment of pregnancy-associated hypertension: What have we learned in the last 10 years? *Am J Kidney Dis* 1991; 18:285.

[79] American College of Obstetricians and Gynecologists. Chronic hypertension in pregnancy. ACOG practice bulletin #29. *American College of Obstetricians and Gynecologists,* Washington, DC 2001.

[80] Martin JN Jr, Thigpen BD, Moore RC, et al. Stroke and severe preeclampsia and eclampsia: a paradigm shift focusing on systolic blood pressure. *Obstet Gynecol* 2005; 105:246.

[81] Sibai BM, Barton JR, Akl S, et al. A randomized prospective comparison of nifedipine and bed rest versus bed rest alone in the management of preeclampsia remote from term. *Am J Obstet Gynecol* 1992; 167:879.

[82] von Dadelszen P, Magee LA. Fall in mean arterial pressure and fetal growth restriction in pregnancy hypertension: an updated metaregression analysis. *J Obstet Gynaecol Can* 2002; 24:941.

[83] Magee LA, Ornstein MP, von Dadelszen P. Fortnightly review: management of hypertension in pregnancy. *BMJ* 1999; 318:1332.

[84] Abalos E, Duley L, Steyn DW, Henderson-Smart DJ. Antihypertensive drug therapy for mild to moderate hypertension during pregnancy (Cochrane Review). *Cochrane Database Syst Rev* 2007; :CD002252.

[85] Duley L, Henderson-Smart DJ, Meher S. Drugs for treatment of very high blood pressure during pregnancy. *Cochrane Database Syst Rev* 2006;3:CD001449.

[86] Hanff LM, Vulto AG, Bartels PA, et al. Intravenous use of the calcium-channel blocker nicardipine as second-line treatment in severe, early-onset pre-eclamptic patients. *J Hypertens* 2005; 23:2319.

[87] Elatrous S, Nouira S, Ouanes Besbes L, et al. Short-term treatment of severe hypertension of pregnancy: prospective comparison of nicardipine and labetalol. *Intensive Care Med* 2002; 28:1281.

[88] Jannet D, Carbonne B, Sebban E, Milliez J. Nicardipine versus metoprolol in the treatment of hypertension during pregnancy: a randomized comparative trial. *Obstet Gynecol* 1994; 84:354.

[89] O'Mailia JJ, Sander GE, Giles TD. Nifedipine-associated myocardial ischemia or infarction in the treatment of hypertensive urgencies. *Ann Intern Med* 1987; 107:185.

[90] Grossman E, Messerli FH, Grodzicki T, Kowey P. Should a moratorium be placed on sublingual nifedipine capsules given for hypertensive emergencies and pseudoemergencies?. *JAMA* 1996; 276:1328.

[91] Impey L. Severe hypotension and fetal distress following sublingual administration of nifedipine to a patient with severe pregnancy induced hypertension at 33 weeks. *Br J Obstet Gynaecol* 1993; 100:959.

[92] Hennessy A, Thornton CE, Makris A, et al. A randomised comparison of hydralazine and mini-bolus diazoxide for hypertensive emergencies in pregnancy: *The PIVOT trial. Aust N Z J Obstet Gynaecol* 2007; 47:279.

[93] Heard AR, Dekker GA, Chan A, et al. Hypertension during pregnancy in South Australia, Part 1: Pregnancy outcomes. *Aust N Z J Obstet Gynaecol* 2004; 44:404.

[94] Hauth JC, Ewell MG, Levine RJ, et al. Pregnancy outcomes in healthy nulliparas who developed hypertension. Calcium for Preeclampsia Prevention Study Group. *Obstet Gynecol* 2000; 95:24.

[95] Ferrazzani S, De Carolis S, Pomini F, et al. The duration of hypertension in the puerperium of preeclamptic women: relationship with renal impairment and week of delivery. *Am J Obstet Gynecol* 1994; 171:506.

[96] Podymow T, August P. Postpartum course of gestational hypertension and preeclampsia. *Hypertension in pregnancy* 20006; 25:210.

[97] *http://toxnet.nlm.nih.gov/cgi-bin/sis/search/f?./temp/~0BtRSx:1 (accessed November 2, 2007).*

[98] Campbell DM, MacGillivray I. Preeclampsia in second pregnancy. *Br J Obstet Gynaecol* 1985; 92:131.

[99] Xiong X, Fraser WD, Demianczuk NN. History of abortion, preterm, term birth, and risk of preeclampsia: A population-based study. *Am J Obstet Gynecol* 2002; 187:1013.

[100] Sibai BM, Sarinoglu C, Mercer BM. Eclampsia. VII. Pregnancy outcome after eclampsia and long-term prognosis. *Am J Obstet Gynecol* 1992; 166:1757.

[101] Bellamy L, Casas JP, Hingorani AD, Williams DJ. Pre-eclampsia and risk of cardiovascular disease and cancer in later life: systematic review and meta-analysis. *BMJ* 2007; 335:974.

[102] Chesley LC, Annitto JE, Cosgrove RA. The remote prognosis of eclamptic women: Sixth periodic report. *Am J Obstet Gynecol* 1976; 124:446.

[103] Paltiel O, Friedlander Y, Tiram E, et al. Cancer after pre-eclampsia: follow up of the Jerusalem perinatal study cohort. *BMJ* 2004; 328:919.

[104] Sibai BM, Taslimi MM, el-Nazer A, et al. Maternal-perinatal outcome associated with the syndrome of hemolysis, elevated liver enzymes, and low platelets in severe preeclampsia-eclampsia. *Am J Obstet Gynecol* 1986; 155:501.

[105] Reubinoff BE, Schenker JG. HELLP syndrome — a syndrome of hemolysis, elevated liver enzymes, and low platelet count — complicating pre-eclampsia-eclampsia. *Int J Gynaecol Obstet* 1991; 36:95.

[106] Sibai BM. The HELLP syndrome (hemolysis, elevated liver enzymes, and low platelets): Much ado about nothing? *Am J Obstet Gynecol* 1990; 162:311.

[107] Sibai BM, Ramadan MK, Usta I, et al. Maternal morbidity and mortality in 442 pregnancies with hemolysis, elevated liver enzymes, and low platelets (HELLP syndrome). *Am J Obstet Gynecol* 1993; 169:1000.

[108] Weinstein L. Preeclampsia/Eclampsia with hemolysis, elevated liver enzymes, and thrombocytopenia. *Obstet Gynecol* 1985;66:657-60.

[109] Sibai BM. Diagnosis, controversies, and management of the syndrome of hemolysis, elevated liver enzymes, and low platelet count. *Obstet Gynecol* 2004; 103:981.

[110] Visser W, Wallenburg HC. Temporising management of severe pre-eclampsia with and without the HELLP syndrome. *Br J Obstet Gynaecol* 1995; 102:111.

[111] van Pampus MG, Wolf H, Westenberg SM, et al. Maternal and perinatal outcome after expectant management of the HELLP syndrome compared with pre-eclampsia without HELLP syndrome. *Eur J Obstet Gynecol Reprod Biol* 1998; 76:31.

[112] Stone JH. HELLP syndrome: Hemolysis, elevated liver enzymes, and low platelets. *JAMA* 1998; 280:559.

[113] O'Brien JM, Shumate SA, Satchwell SL, et al. Maternal benefit of corticosteroid therapy in patients with HELLP (hemolysis, elevated liver enzymes, and low platelet count) syndrome: impact on the rate of regional anesthesia. *Am J Obstet Gynecol* 2002; 186:475.

[114] Matchaba P, Moodley J. Corticosteroids for HELLP syndrome in pregnancy. *Cochrane Database Syst Rev* 2004; :CD002076.

[115] Isler CM, Barrilleaux PS, Magann EF, et al. A prospective, randomized trial comparing the efficacy of dexamethasone and betamethasone for the treatment of antepartum HELLP (hemolysis, elevated liver enzymes, and low platelet count) syndrome. *Am J Obstet Gynecol* 2001; 184:1332.

[116] Martin JN Jr, Thigpen BD, Rose CH, Cushman J. Maternal benefit of high-dose intravenous corticosteroid therapy for HELLP syndrome. *Am J Obstet Gynecol* 2003; 189:830.

[117] Fonseca JE, Mendez F, Catano C, Arias F. Dexamethasone treatment does not improve the outcome of women with HELLP syndrome: a double-blind, placebo-controlled, randomized clinical trial. *Am J Obstet Gynecol* 2005; 193:1591.

[118] Katz L, de Amorim MM, Figueiroa JN, Pinto e, Silva JL. Postpartum dexamethasone for women with hemolysis, elevated liver enzymes, and low platelets (HELLP) syndrome: a double-blind, placebo-controlled, randomized clinical trial. *Am J Obstet Gynecol* 2008; 198:283.

[119] Martin JN Jr, Blake PG, Perry KG Jr, et al. The natural history of HELLP syndrome: Patterns of disease progression and regression. *Am J Obstet Gynecol* 1991; 164:1500.

[120] Hupuczi P, Nagy B, Sziller I, et al. Characteristic laboratory changes in pregnancies complicated by HELLP syndrome. *Hypertens Pregnancy* 2007; 26:389.

[121] Sibai BM, Spinnato JA, Watson DL, et al. Pregnancy outcome in 303 cases with severe preeclampsia. *Obstet Gynecol* 1984; 64:319.

[122] Greenstein D, Henderson J, Boyer T. Liver hemorrhage: Recurrent episodes during pregnancy complicated by preeclampsia. *Gastroenterology* 1994; 106:1668.

[123] Sibai BM, Ramadan MK, Chari RS, Friedman SA. Pregnancies complicated by HELLP syndrome (hemolysis, elevated liver enzymes, and low platelets): Subsequent pregnancy outcome and long-term prognosis. *Am J Obstet Gynecol* 1995; 172:125.

[124] Wust MD, Bolte AC, de Vries JI, et al. Pregnancy outcome after previous pregnancy complicated by hepatic rupture. *Hypertens Pregnancy* 2004; 23:29.

[125] Douglas KA, Redman CW. Eclampsia in the United Kingdom. BMJ 1994; 309:1395.

[126] Lubarsky SL, Barton JR, Friedman SA, et al. Late postpartum eclampsia revisited. *Obstet Gynecol* 1994; 83:502.

[127] Miles JF Jr, Martin JN Jr, Blake PG, et al. Postpartum eclampsia: a recurring perinatal dilemma. *Obstet Gynecol* 1990; 76:328.

[128] Chames MC, Livingston JC, Ivester TS, Barton JR. Late postpartum eclampsia: A preventable disease? *Am J Obstet Gynecol* 2002; 186:1174.

[129] Morriss MC, Twickler DM, Hatab MR, et al. Cerebral blood flow and cranial magnetic resonance imaging in eclampsia and severe preeclampsia. *Obstet Gynecol* 1997; 89:561.

[130] Tuffnell DJ, Jankowicz D, Lindow SW, et al. *Outcomes of severe pre-eclampsia/eclampsia in Yorkshire* 1999/2003. BJOG 2005; 112:875.

[131] Geographic variation in the incidence of hypertension in pregnancy. World Health Organization International Collaborative Study of Hypertensive Disorders of Pregnancy. *Am J Obstet Gynecol* 1988; 158:80.

[132] Dahmus MA, Barton JR, Sibai BM. Cerebral imaging in eclampsia: Magnetic resonance imaging versus computed tomography. *Am J Obstet Gynecol* 1992; 167:935.

[133] Cunningham FG, Grant NF, Leveno KJ, et al (eds): Hypertensive disorders in pregnancy. *In Williams Obstetrics, 21st ed.*New York, McGraw-Hill, 2001, pp 567-618.

[134] Lindenstrom E, Boysen G, Nyboe J. Influence of systolic and diastolic blood pressure on stroke risk: a prospective observational study. *Am J Epidemiol* 1995; 142:1279.

[135] Norwitz ER. Eclampsia. *UPTODATE* May 2008.

[136] Pritchard JA, Cunningham FG, Pritchard SA. The Parkland Memorial Hospital protocol for treatment of eclampsia: evaluation of 245 cases. *Am J Obstet Gynecol* 1984; 148:951.

[137] Lucas MJ, Leveno KJ, Cunningham FG. A comparison of magnesium sulfate with phenytoin for the prevention of eclamspia. *N Engl J Med* 1995; 333:201.

[138] Roberts JM, Villar J, Arulkumaran S. Preventing and treating eclamptic seizures. *BMJ* 2002; 325:609.

[139] Hall DR, Odendaal HJ, Smith M. Is the prophylactic administration of magnesium sulphate in women with pre-eclampsia indicated prior to labour?. *BJOG* 2000; 107:903.

[140] Altman D, Carroli G, Duley L, Farrell B, Moodley J, Neilson J, Smith D; Magpie Trial Collaboration Group. Do women with pre-eclampsia, and their babies, benefit from magnesium sulphate? The Magpie Trial: a randomized placebo-controlled trial. *Lancet* 2002; 359:1877.

[141] Alexander JM, McIntire DD, Leveno KJ, Cunningham FG. Selective magnesium sulfate prophylaxis for the prevention of eclampsia in women with gestational hypertension. *Obstet Gynecol* 2006; 108:826.

[142] Witlin AG, Friedman SA, Sibai BM. The effect of magnesium sulfate therapy on the duration of labor in women with mild preeclampsia at term: a randomized, double-blind, placebo-controlled trial. *Am J Obstet Gynecol* 1997; 176:623.

[143] Lipton SA, Rosenberg PA: Excitatory amino acids as a final common pathway for neurologic disorders. *N Engl J Med* 1994; 330:613.

[144] Hallak M, Hotca JW, Evans JB. Magnesium sulfate affects the N-methyl-D-aspartate receptor binding in maternal rat brain. *Am J Obstet Gynecol* 1998;178:S112.

[145] Roberts JM. Magnesium for preeclampsia and eclampsia. N Engl J Med 1995; 333:250.

[146] Duley L, Gulmezoglu AM. Magnesium sulphate versus lytic cocktail for eclampsia. *Cochrane Database Syst Rev* 2001; :CD002960.

[147] Sibai BM, Lipshitz J, Anderson GD, Dilts PV Jr. Reassessment of intravenous MgSO4 therapy in preeclampsia-eclampsia. *Obstet Gynecol* 1981; 57:199.

[148] Alexander JM, Bloom SL, McIntire DD, Leveno KJ. Severe preeclampsia and the very low birth weight infant: is induction of labor harmful? *Obstet Gynecol* 1999; 93:485.

[149] Nassar AH, Adra AM, Chakhtoura N, et al. Severe preeclampsia remote from term: labor induction or elective cesarean delivery? *Am J Obstet Gynecol* 1998; 179:1210.

[150] Sibai BM, McCubbin JH, Anderson GD, et al. Eclampsia. I. Observations from 67 recent cases. *Obstet Gynecol* 1981; 58:609.

[151] López-Llera M. Main clinical types and subtypes of eclampsia. *Am J Obstet Gynecol* 1992; 166:4.

[152] Sibai BM, Spinnato JA, Watson DL, et al. Eclampsia. IV. Neurological findings and future outcome. *Am J Obstet Gynecol* 1985; 152:184.

[153] Okanloma KA, Moodley J. Neurological complications associated with the pre-eclampsia/eclampsia syndrome. *Int J Gynaecol Obstet* 2000; 71:223.

[154] Report of the National High Blood Pressure Education Program Working Group on High Blood Pressure in Pregnancy. *Am J Obstet Gynecol* 2000;183:S1.

[155] Villar J, Carroli G, Wojdyla D, et al. Preeclampsia, gestational hypertension and intrauterine growth restriction, related or independent conditions?. *Am J Obstet Gynecol* 2006; 194:921.

[156] Saudan P, Brown MA, Buddle ML, Jones M. Does gestational hypertension become pre-eclampsia? *Br J Obstet Gynaecol* 1998; 105:1177.

[157] Barton JR, O'brien JM, Bergauer NK, Jacques DL, et al. Mild gestational hypertension remote from term: progression and outcome. *Am J Obstet Gynecol* 2001; 184:979.

[158] Buchbinder A, Sibai BM, Caritis S, et al. Adverse perinatal outcomes are significantly higher in severe gestational hypertension than in mild preeclampsia. *Am J Obstet Gynecol* 2002; 186:66.

[159] Hnat MD, Sibai BM, Caritis S, et al. Perinatal outcome in women with recurrent preeclampsia compared with women who develop preeclampsia as nulliparas. *Am J Obstet Gynecol* 2002; 186:422.

[160] Knuist M, Bonsel GJ, Zondervan HA, Treffers PE. Intensification of fetal and maternal surveillance in pregnant women with hypertensive disorders. *Int J Gynaecol Obstet* 1998; 61:127.

[161] Chesley LC: Hypertensive Disorders in Pregnancy, *AppletonCenturyCrofts,* New York 1978.

[162] Fisher KA, Luger A, Spargo BH, Lindheimer MD. Hypertension in pregnancy: Clinical-pathological correlations and late prognosis. *Medicine* (Baltimore) 1981; 60:267.

[163] Sibai BM, Eclampsia, VI. Maternal-perinatal outcome in 254 consecutive cases. *Am J Obstet Gynecol* 1990; 163:1049.

[164] Magee LA, von Dadelszen P, Bohun CM, et al. Serious perinatal complications of non-proteinuric hypertension: an international, multicentre, retrospective cohort study. *J Obstet Gynaecol* Can 2003; 25:372.

[165] Steer PJ, Little MP, Kold-Jensen T, et al. Maternal blood pressure in pregnancy, birth weight, and perinatal mortality in first births: prospective study. *BMJ* 2004; 329:1312.

[166] Reiter L, Brown MA, Whitworth JA. Hypertension in pregnancy: The incidence of underlying renal disease and essential hypertension. *Am J Kidney Dis* 1994; 24:883.

[167] Magloire L, Funai EF. Gestational hypertension. *UPTODATE* June 2007.

[168] Hjartardottir S, Leifsson BG, Geirsson RT, Steinthorsdottir V. Recurrence of hypertensive disorder in second pregnancy. *Am J Obstet Gynecol* 2006; 194:916.

[169] Wilson BJ, Watson MS, Prescott GJ, Sunderland S, et al. Hypertensive diseases of pregnancy and risk of hypertension and stroke in later life: results from cohort study. *BMJ* 2003; 326:845.

[170] Sibai BM. Chronic hypertension in pregnancy. *Obstet Gynecol*. 2002;100:369-377.

[171] Sibai BM. Caring for women with hypertension in pregnancy. *JAMA* 2007;298:1566.

[172] Powrie RO. A 30-year-old woman with chronic hypertension trying to conceive. *JAMA* 2007; 298:1548.

[173] Ferrer RL, Sibai BM, Mulrow CD, et al. Management of mild chronic hypertension during pregnancy: a review. *Obstet Gynecol* 2000; 96:849.

[174] Mulrow CD, et al. Management of chronic hypertension in pregnancy. Agency for Healthcare Research and Quality, August 2000. *Evidence report/Technology assessment 14. AHRQ publication 00-E011.*

[175] Gilbert WM, Young AL, Danielsen B. Pregnancy outcomes in women with chronic hypertension. *J Reprod Med* 2007; 52:1046.

[176] Redman CW. Controlled trials of antihypertensive drugs in pregnancy. *Am J Kidney Dis* 1991; 17:149.

[177] Sibai BM, Mabie WC, Shamsa F, et al. A comparison of no medication versus methyldopa or labetalol in chronic hypertension during pregnancy. *Am J Obstet Gynecol* 1990; 162:960.

[178] Magee LA, Duley L. Oral beta-blockers for mild to moderate hypertension during pregnancy. *Cochrane Database Syst Rev* 2003; :CD002863.

[179] Umans JG, Lindheimer MD. Antihypertensive treatment. *In: Lindheimer MD, Roberts JM, Cunningham FG, eds. Chesley's Hypertensive Disorders in Pregnancy*. 2nd ed. Norwalk, CT: Appleton & Lange; 1998:581-604.

[180] Cockburn J, Moar VA, Ounsted M, Redman CW. Final report of study on hypertension during pregnancy: the effects of specific treatment on the growth and development of the children. *Lancet* 1982; 1:647.

[181] Ferris TF. Hypertension in pregnancy. *The Kidney* 1990; 23: Number 1.

[182] Montan S, Ingemarsson I, Marsal K, Sjöberg NO. Randomised controlled trial of atenolol and pindolol in human pregnancy: Effects on fetal hemodynamics. *BMJ* 1992; 304:946.

[183] Lydakis C, Lip GY, Beevers M, Beevers DG. Atenolol and fetal growth in pregnancies complicated by hypertension. *Am J Hypertens* 1999; 12:541.

[184] Fenakel K, Fenakel G, Appelman Z, et al. Nifedipine in the treatment of severe preeclampsia. *Obstet Gynecol* 1991; 77:331.

[185] Smith P, Anthony J, Johanson R. Nifedipine in pregnancy. *BJOG* 2000; 107:299.

[186] Collins R, Yusuf S, Peto R. Overview of randomised trials of diuretics in pregnancy. *Br Med J* (Clin Res Ed) 1985; 290:17.

[187] Briggs GG, Freeman RK, Yaffee SJ. Drugs in pregnancy and lactation: *A reference guide to fetal and neonatal risk. 5th ed.* Baltimore:Williams & Wilkins, 1998.

[188] White WB. Management of hypertension during lactation. *Hypertension* 1984;6: 297–300.

[189] Sibai BM. Biomarker for hypertension-preeclampsia: are we close yet? *Am J Obstet Gynecol.* 2007;197(1):1-2.

[190] Conde-Agudelo A, Villar J, Linheimer M. World Health Organization systemic review of screening tests for preeclampsia. *Obstet Gynecol.* 2004;104(6): 1367-1391.

[191] Nicolaides KH, Bindra R, Twian OM, et al. A novel approach to first-trimester screening for early preeclampsia combining serum PP-13 and Doppler ultrasound. *Ultrasound Obstet Gynecol.* 2006;27(1):13-17.

[192] Espinoza J, Romero R, Nien JK, et al. Identification of patients at risk for early onset and/or severe preeclampsia with the use of uterine artery Doppler velocimetry and placental growth factor. *Am J Obstet Gynecol.* 2007;196:326.e1- 326.e13.

[193] Sibai BM. Chronic hypertension in pregnancy. *Clin Perinatol* 1991;18:833-44.

[194] Sibai BM, Akl S, Fairlie F, Moretti M. A protocol for managing severe preeclampsia in the second trimester. *Am J Obstet Gynecol* 1990;163:733-8.

[195] Sibai BM. Diagnosis, prevention, and management of eclampsia. *Obstet Gynecol* 2005; 105:402.

In: Textbook of Perinatal Epidemiology
Editor: Eyal Sheiner, pp. 387-408

ISBN: 978-1-60741-648-7
© 2010 Nova Science Publishers, Inc.

Chapter XX

Thrombophilia and Adverse Pregnancy Outcomes

Adi Y. Weintraub[*], Gali Pariente and Eyal Sheiner

Department of Obstetrics and Gynecology, Soroka University Medical Center, Faculty of Health Science, Ben Gurion University of the Negev, Beer-Sheva, Israel

Definitions

- Early abortion: fetal loss that occurs during the first trimester
- Late abortion: fetal loss that occurs during the second trimester
- Stillbirth: pregnancy loss beyond 24 weeks of gestation
- Antiphospholipid syndrome (APLA syndrome): the presence of lupus anticoagulant or anticardiolipin antibodies of medium to high titer found in association with a history of thrombosis (arterial or venous) or adverse pregnancy outcomes

Introduction

Thrombophilias are inherited or acquired conditions, which predispose an individual to thromboembolism. During pregnancy, maternal thrombophilia has been identified as a major risk factor for adverse pregnancy outcomes (APO) including venous and arterial thrombosis, preeclampsia, placental abruption, intrauterine growth restriction (IUGR), intrauterine fetal losses, and recurrent miscarriages [1-15]. However, great controversy exists regarding the association between inherited and acquired thrombophilia and their associated APO since

[*] For Correspondence: Adi Y. Weintraub M.D, Department of Obstetrics and Gynecology, Soroka University Medical Center, P.O Box 151, Beer-Sheva, Israel. Tel 972-8-6400774, Fax 972-8-6275338, E-mail adiyehud@bgu.ac.il

such an association was not found by other investigators [16-18]. In a recent systematic review, Rasmussen and Ravn [19] concluded that the association between congenital thrombophilia and preeclampsia, IUGR, placental abruption and fetal losses relies on poor evidence; thus, any recommendations and clinical guidelines are based on weak scientific proof.

Sufficient development of a functioning placenta is paramount for a successful pregnancy. The perfusion to the placenta might be impaired due to thrombosis resulting from microthrombi in the placental vascular bed. These microthrombi can cause multiple infarcts that could eventually lead to placental insufficiency and associated pregnancy complications [12,20-22].

The known thrombotic nature of the placental vascular lesions and the increased thrombotic risk associated with the existence of thrombophilias strongly suggest a causative relationship between inherited thrombophilias and these adverse pregnancy complications and outcomes [3, 5, 23]. As adequate placental circulation is dependant on the normal balance of procoagulant and anticoagulant mechanisms, inherited thrombophilia may be associated with placental insufficiency [5].

The common inherited disorders are deficiencies in antithrombin III, protein C, and protein S, activated protein C resistance (APCR) due to the factor V Leiden (FVL) mutation, a function-enhancing mutation in the prothrombin (PT) gene (G20210A), and thermo labile mutation for methylenetetrahydrofolate reductase (C677T) (MTHFR) [3,24-25]. The most common acquired thrombophilia is the APLA syndrome. It is an autoimmune condition that is characterized by the presence of circulating antibodies such as the lupus anticoagulant (LAC) and anticardiolipin (ACL).

In this chapter, aspects of certain APO and thrombophilia are discussed, as well as prophylactic and therapeutic implications.

Adverse Pregnancy Outcomes

A causative relationship between thrombophilia and APO has been a subject of great controversy. An association between thrombophilia and pregnancy complications has been widely reported in the literature. In contrast, other studies report different results [16, 17, 26, 27]. Our group [23] found a statistically significant increase in the frequency of obstetrical risk factors and pregnancy complications (i.e., recurrent abortions, perinatal mortality, severe preeclampsia and IUGR) among women diagnosed with inherited thrombophilia as compared to those without known thrombophilia. Previous fetal losses, recurrent abortions, fertility treatments and IUGR were found to be independently associated with thrombophilia, using a multivariable analysis.

Recently, the Thrombosis: Risk and Economic Assessment of Thrombophilia Screening (TREATS) study published their findings. Meta-analysis was used to calculate pooled odds ratios (OR) associated with individual clinical outcomes, stratified by thrombophilia type. The authors concluded that thrombophilia is associated with increased risks of venous thromboembolism (VTE) and APO [28]. The association between selected thrombophilias and APO are presented in Table 1.

Table 1. The association between selected thrombophilias and APO.

	Preeclampsia	IUGR	Placental Abruption	Early Pregnancy Loss	Late Pregnancy Loss
PT homozygote	0	0	0	√√	0
PT heterozygote	√√	√√	√√√	0	√√
FVL homozygote	√√	√√ √	√	√√√	0
FVL heterozygote	√√	√	√√√	√√*	√√
MTHFR homozygote	√√	√	√	√	√
AT deficiency	√	0	-	-	0
Protein C deficiency	√	√	√	√	√
Protein S deficiency	√	√	√	√	√√√
ACL Ab	√√	√	√	√√√	√√√
LAC	√	√√√*	0	√√	√
Acquired APCR	√	0	-	√√√	0
Hyperhomocysteinemia	√√√	√	√√√	√√√	0
Total	√√	√√	√√√	√√	√√

APO: Adverse pregnancy outcome; IUGR: intrauterine growth restriction; FVL: factor V leiden; PT: prothrombin; MTHFR: methylenetetrahydrofolate reductase; AT: antithrombin; ACL Ab: anticardiolipin antibodies; LAC: lupus anticoagulant; APCR: activated protein C resistance.

√√√ statistically significant highly increased risk (>threefold) for APO

√√ statistically significant increased risk for APO

√ increased risk for APO that did not reach statistical significance increased risk for APO has not been established data not sufficient

* borderline significance

Adapted from Expert Review Obstet Gynecol. 2, 203-216 (2007) with permission of Expert Reviews Ltd.

Several studies have shown that multiparous women with thrombophilias and severe pregnancy complications suffer from a high recurrence rate in subsequent pregnancies (66–83%) [2, 7, 21, 29]. Nevertheless, the type of complication may differ from one pregnancy to another, e.g., severe preeclampsia to IUGR or recurrent fetal loss to preeclampsia [2, 7, 21, 29].

Preeclampsia

There is a growing body of evidence that associates gestational hypertensive disorders and the presence of inherited or acquired thrombophilias [30]. Severe early onset preeclampsia was initially reported in women with thrombotic disorders such as APCR, hyperhomocysteinemia, protein S, protein C and antithrombin deficiencies and anticardiolipin antibodies by Dekker et al. [31].

When compared with controls, women with preeclampsia were more likely to be heterozygous FVL mutation carriers (OR 1.6, 95% CI, 1.2–2.1), carriers of the PT gene G20210A mutation (OR 2.4, 95% CI, 1.2–4.7) and homozygous for the MTHFR C677T gene mutation (OR 1.7, 95% CI, 1.2–2.3). Protein C and protein S deficiencies and APCR were also found more prevalent among women with preeclampsia (OR 21.5, 95% CI, 1.1–414.4; OR 12.7, 95% CI, 4.0–39.7; and OR 4.6, 95% CI, 2.8–7.6; respectively) [25].

Lin et al. [32] conducted a meta-analysis of 31 case-control studies from 13 countries. FVL was found to be associated with a twofold increased risk for preeclampsia (cases with mild preeclampsia OR 1.81, 95% CI, 1.14–2.87 and for cases with severe preeclampsia, OR 2.24, 95% CI, 1.28–3.94). In the same meta-analysis, a slightly elevated, though not statistically significant, pooled OR (1.38) was demonstrated between the MTHFR C667T polymorphism and severe preeclampsia. A non-significant twofold increased risk for severe preeclampsia was suggested in this meta-analysis, in association with the PT 20210 polymorphism [32].

In his review of 190 articles, Kupferminc [33] found no association between the MTHFR C677T mutation and severe preeclampsia, a possible association between the PT G20210A gene mutation and preeclampsia and an established association between preeclampsia and the antithrombin, protein C and protein S deficiencies as well as with APCR, FVL, hyperhomocysteinemia, APLA syndrome and combined defects.

A large-scale case-control study published by Mello et al. [34] included 808 caucasion patients who developed preeclampsia (cases) and 808 women with previous uneventful pregnancies (controls). Matched for age and parity they were evaluated for inherited and acquired thrombophilia in order to determine whether thrombophilia increases the risk of preeclampsia or interferes with its clinical course. FVL, PT G20210A, MTHFR C677T, anticardiolipin antibodies, lupus anticoagulant, and hyperhomocysteinemia were found to be significantly associated with severe preeclampsia. Moreover, thrombophilic patients with severe preeclampsia were found to be at an increased risk for acute renal failure, disseminated intravascular coagulation, placental abruption and perinatal mortality as compared with non-thrombophilic preeclamptic patients. In women with mild preeclampsia (402 cases), only PT and homozygous MTHFR gene mutations were significantly more prevalent as compared to the controls [34].

Conversely, in a case-control study that investigated the association between single thrombophilic patterns and different pregnancy complications, no association was found between preeclampsia and the FVL or PT gene mutations. Deficiency in AT III was significantly linked with preeclampsia (RR 0.88, 95% CI, 0.83–0.94) [35].

Recently Muetze et al. [36] assessed the prevalence of the FVL, the PT G20210A mutation and the MTHFR C677T polymorphism in 71 women with HELLP syndrome and in their fetuses from the same index pregnancy. The study was performed retrospectively in a case-control design. Maternal heterozygosity for FVL was significantly more prevalent in the HELLP group than in controls (OR 4.45, 95% CI, 1.31–15.31). No significant association was observed for maternal PT mutation (p=0.89) or MTHFR polymorphism (p=0.19). The fetal genotype was not associated with HELLP syndrome in these mutations. Analysis of gene-gene interactions and genotype-phenotype correlation with respect to clinical parameters and perinatal outcomes revealed no further differences.

Facchinetti et al. [37] investigated recurrence of preeclampsia in women with thrombophilias. In a multicenter, observational, cohort design, 172 caucasion patients with a previous pregnancy complicated by preeclampsia were observed in the following pregnancy. They were evaluated for heritable (FVL and PT G20210A mutations, protein S, protein C, and antithrombin deficiencies) and acquired (hyperhomocystinemia, lupus anticoagulant, and anticardiolipin antibodies) thrombophilias. In 60 women (34.9%), the presence of a thrombophilic defect was demonstrated. They had a higher risk for recurrent preeclampsia (OR 2.5, 95% CI, 1.2–5.1) compared to patients without thrombophilia. Similar findings were found when only heritable thrombophilias were considered. Thrombophilic patients were at increased risk for the occurrence of very early preterm delivery (< 32 weeks; OR 11.6, 95% CI, 3.4–43.2) [37]. The association between selected thrombophilias and preeclampsia is presented in Table 1.

Intrauterine Growth Restriction

Few reports have examined the association and suggest a possible correlation between IUGR and thrombophilia, but data are not homogeneous. Kupferminc et al. [21] found a genetic thrombophilic mutation in 50% of women with severe IUGR, and a total prevalence of thrombophilia in women with IUGR of 61.4% [21]. A higher prevalence of thrombophilias was found by the same group in another study that examined the association between unknown mid-trimester severe IUGR and thrombophilia. The frequency of thrombophilias in the study group was 69% compared with 14% in the control group (OR 4.5, 95% CI, 2.3–9, P < 0.001) [38]. The FVL [39,40], PT [2,39,40] and MTHFR [39] gene mutations, as well as hyperhomocysteinemia [41] were significantly more prevalent in women with IUGR compared with controls. These thrombophilias were found to be independently associated with IUGR in a regression analysis model performed by Martinelli et al. [39]. Mello et al. [34] investigated thrombophilias in women with pregnancy complications. Thirteen of them were complicated by IUGR. A thrombophilic abnormality was found in 85% of these patients. The most prominent thrombophilias in women with IUGR were hyperhomocysteinemia, protein S deficiency and FVL [34].

Conversely, other studies failed to find an association between thrombophilia and IUGR [26,42]. These observations may be attributed to variations in birth weight and gestational age between the different groups; mean birth weight of 2393 ± 606 grams in the study by Infante-Rivard et al. [26] with 83% of the patients delivered at 36–40 weeks gestation versus mean birth weight of 1387 ± 616 grams and a mean gestational age of 33.2 ± 4 weeks in the study by Kupferminc et al. [21]. Similarly, Martinelli et al. [39] reported a mean gestational age at delivery of 34.6 ± 3 weeks with a mean birth weight of 1584 ± 586 grams. A later study by this group reported that neonates from thrombophilic mothers formed 30% of those weighting < 1000 grams [40]. The use of the 10th percentile in the former study may include many constitutionally small fetuses, which do not carry the clinical risks of growth-restricted fetuses. Conversely, the combination of prematurity and IUGR reported in other studies carries a high risk of serious long-term outcomes. It is evident from these differences in birth weight and gestational age that the different studies differ in fetal and neonatal populations and these have diverse clinical relevance.

Two systematic reviews and meta-analyses examined the association between thrombophilia and IUGR [43,44]. Howley et al. [44], in his systematic review of the association between thrombophilia and IUGR, found a significantly increased risk for IUGR in women with FVL (OR 2.7, 95% CI, 1.3–5.5) and the PT gene mutation (OR 2.5, 95% CI, 1.3–5.0) [44].

In a previously-mentioned review of 190 studies, Kupferminc [33] did not find an association between the MTHFR C677T and FVL mutations and IUGR, but did find an association between preeclampsia and the antithrombin, protein C and protein S deficiencies as well as with APCR, hyperhomocysteinemia, PT G20210A gene mutation, APLA syndrome and combined defects.

Recently, Kocher et al. [45], in a large cohort of 5000 patients, investigated the correlation between the presence of the FVL and PT G20210A mutations with a history of adverse pregnancy events including IUGR. Patients carrying the FVL or PT G20210A mutations were compared with three times as many matched controls for the occurrence of obstetric complications. The patients were matched according to pregnancy order and maternal age. The association of IUGR with FVL (OR 1.92, 95% CI, 0.77–4.77; $P = 0.16$) was not significant. However, a non-significant positive trend towards an association between PT G20210A and IUGR was found [45]. The association between selected thrombophilias and IUGR is presented in Table 1.

Placental Abruption

There is a growing body of evidence that connects between different thrombophilic abnormalities and placental abruption [2,4,43,46-49]. Thrombophilic abnormalities were found in 65%–70% of patients with placental abruption in different studies. It is worth noting that thrombophilia poses a risk for placental abruption that is independent from the development of preeclampsia [48,49].

Kupferminc [33] did not find an association between protein C deficiency and placental abruption. However, a possible association was noted between antithrombin deficiency and MTHFR gene mutation and placental abruption. Larciprete et al. [35] in their case-control study have shown APCR to be significantly related to placental abruption (RR 0.71, 95% CI, 0.61–0.82) [35]. Likewise, a significant association was documented by Kupferminc [33] between placental abruption and the APCR, as well as with APLA syndrome, hyperhomocysteinemia, FVL, PT G20210A gene mutation, protein S deficiency and combined defects [33]. Recently, Karakantza et al. [50] investigated the impact of inherited thrombophilic factors on the gestational outcome of unselected pregnant women. Thrombophilic genotypes were significantly higher in women with placental abruption. Heterozygocity for FVL increased the risk for placental abruption 9.1 times. The MTHFR mutation genotype increased the risk for placental abruption 4.8 times despite folate supplements, and normal serum folate and B12 levels [50]. The association between selected thrombophilias and placental abruption is presented in Table 1.

Fetal Loss

Early and late abortions are defined on the basis of the trimester (first and second) in which they occur. Stillbirth is defined when pregnancy loss occurs beyond 24 weeks of gestation [51]. Miscarriage is common (around 25% of conceptions) and an identifiable cause is found in only a few of these cases. Therefore, greater attention focuses on women with recurrent miscarriages (RM). Recurrent miscarriages, three or more successive pregnancy losses affect 1%–2% of pregnancies. Two or more successive losses affect 5% of pregnancies, causing much grief and distress. Unfortunately, a definite cause has been established in less than 50% of the cases, leading to the frustration of both patient and caregiver [29,52]. It has been suggested that maternal thrombophilia might be a risk factor for fetal loss. Many studies have been conducted in order to examine this possible association. Controversial results have been reported depending on timing and definition of fetal loss. Some indirect and direct evidence support the role of thrombophilia in fetal loss.

Indirect evidence: Many women, who suffered a pregnancy loss, are at an increased risk of developing APO of preeclampsia, IUGR, placental abruption and stillbirth. It has been postulated that these pregnancy outcomes represent a spectrum of disorders that share a common origin [29,53]. Women with previous RM are in a prothrombotic state even while not pregnant [53]. Women with RM have been reported to be at a chronic state of endothelial stimulation that is associated with activation of the coagulation system [53]. Women with RM have excess thromboxane production and a shift in the thromboxane/prostacyclin ratio in favor of the procoagulant agent thromboxane when compared with women with no history of RM [54]. This could lead to vasospasm and platelet aggregation, causing the development of microthrombi and placental necrotic lesions [53]. The preliminary data that are accumulating and reports of improved pregnancy outcomes after anticoagulant prophylaxis and treatment, can also serve as an indirect evidence for the association between thrombophilia and fetal loss. The association between selected thrombophilias and early and late fetal loss is presented in Table 1. Anticoagulant prophylaxis and treatment will be later addressed.

Direct evidence: Studies finding a higher prevalence of thrombophilias in women with RM serve as a direct evidence for a causative relationship between thrombophilia and pregnancy loss [10,24,27,55-58]. Although there are inconsistencies between studies that may reflect problems such as a small sample size, inconsistent case definitions, a potential selective bias and retrospective designs, these studies suggest an overall association between thrombophilia and fetal loss.

The most compelling evidence relates to APLA syndrome [59,60]. Antiphospholipid antibodies and in turn increased thrombin generation and thrombotic placental infarction [61] are found in 15% of women with RM [60] that may manifest as either early miscarriage, late miscarriage or both. Recently, Ruffatti et al. [62] investigated the relationship between antibody profile and pregnancy outcome in patients with a previous diagnosis of primary APLA syndrome. A total of 97 pregnancies occurring in 79 primary APLA syndrome patients were evaluated for the presence of: Lupus Anticoagulant (LA), IgG/IgM anticardiolipin (aCL), IgG/IgM anti-human beta-2-glycoprotein-I antibodies. Twelve of 97 pregnancies were unsuccessful, of which 11 had more than one positive laboratory test and one had a single positive test. The rate of pregnancy loss was more frequent in pregnancies that had three positive tests than in pregnancies that had two positive tests (adjusted HR 23, 95% CI, 1.3–408, p=0.03) [62].

In a meta-analysis [24], 31 studies on thrombophilic disorders and fetal loss were analyzed. FVL was associated with early and late recurrent fetal loss, and late non-recurrent fetal loss. APCR was associated with early recurrent fetal loss, and PT G20210A mutation with early recurrent and late non-recurrent fetal loss. Protein S deficiency was associated with recurrent fetal loss and late non-recurrent fetal loss. MTHFR mutation, protein C, and antithrombin deficiencies were not found to be significantly associated with fetal loss [24]. Recently, in their large cohort study Kocher et al. [45] found a statistically significant association between FVL and stillbirth [45].

In a systematic review, Robertson et al. [43] evaluated the correlation between miscarriage and thrombophilia (a total of 50 studies were selected, 35 studies with 7167 patients with early miscarriage and 15 studies with 4038 patients with late miscarriage). Both adverse outcomes revealed the existence of a statistically significant association with some hereditary and acquired thrombophilias. Early abortions were found to be associated with the FVL both heterozygote (OR 2.71, 95% CI, 1.32–5.58) and homozygote (OR 1.68, 95% CI, 1.09–2.58), PT heterozygosity (OR 2.49, 95% CI, 1.24–5.0) and ACL antibodies (OR 3.40, 95% CI, 1.33–8.68). Late abortions were found to be associated with FVL heterozygosity (OR 2.06, 95% CI, 1.10–3.86), PT heterozygosity (OR 2.66, 95% CI, 1.28–5.53) and ACL antibodies (OR 3.30, 95% CI, 1.62–6.70) [43].

Venous Thromboembolism

Venous thromboembolism (VTE) is a common and important cause of maternal morbidity and mortality. The estimated incidence of pregnancy associated venous thrombosis is approximately 1 in 1000 deliveries, and the estimated age-adjusted incidence of venous thrombosis ranges from 6 to 10 times higher in pregnant than nonpregnant women [63].

VTE is a leading cause of death among women in the United States during pregnancy and the puerperium. Pulmonary embolism (PE) occurs in approximately 16% of patients with untreated deep vein thrombosis (DVT), and is one of the most common causes of maternal death [33,64-65]. The overall risk of DVT in pregnancy is high and even higher in women with a previous history of VTE, with a recurrence rate of close to 11% [66]. The incidence of recurrent VTE during subsequent pregnancies among women with pregnancy-associated VTE is higher compared to women with unprovoked VTE [67]. Maternal DVT is often associated with PE [68]. In pooled data from the Centers for Disease Control and Prevention National Pregnancy Mortality Surveillance system from 1991 to 1999, PE was the second most common cause of pregnancy-related death when the fetus was undelivered and accounted for 20% of all pregnancy-related deaths [69]. It occurs more commonly in iliofemoral veins than in calf veins (72% compared with 9%, respectively), and is more common in the left leg (accounting for about 85% of leg thrombosis).

The risk of venous thrombosis in women with an inherited or acquired thrombophilia is increased during pregnancy. However, not all women with thrombophilia will develop VTE during pregnancy. The risk of VTE depends on the type of thrombophilia and the existence of additional risk factors [64-66].

Recently, 52 double heterozygous carriers of FVL and PT G20210A mutation who had remained pregnant at least once before knowledge of thrombophilia were retrospectively investigated with respect to the occurrence of first VTE during pregnancy and puerperium. They were compared with 104 heterozygous carriers of FVL, 104 heterozygous carriers of PT G20210A and 104 women without thrombophilia. No VTE during pregnancy was observed in all four groups of women. However, in the puerperium VTE occurred in two double carriers (1.8% of pregnancies, 95% CI, 0.5–6.3), three single FVL carriers (1.5% of pregnancies, 95% CI, 0.5–4.3), two single PT carriers (1% of pregnancies, 95% CI, 0.2–3.6) and one non-carrier (0.4%, 0–2.5) [70].

The MEGA study [71] evaluated pregnancy and the postpartum period as risk factors for VTE in 285 patients and 857 non-pregnant control subjects. The risk of VTE was increased 5-fold (OR 4.6, 95% CI, 2.7–7.8) during pregnancy and increased 60-fold (OR 60.1, 95% CI, 26.5–135.9) during the first 3 months after delivery compared with non-pregnant women. A 14-fold increased risk of DVT was found compared with a 6-fold increased risk of PE. The risk was highest in the third trimester of pregnancy (OR 8.8, 95% CI, 4.5–17.3) and during the first 6 weeks after delivery (OR 84.0, 95% CI, 31.7–222.6). The risk of pregnancy-associated VTE was increased by 52-fold in FVL carriers (OR 52.2, 95% CI, 12.4–219.5) and increased by 31-fold in PT G20210A mutation carriers (OR 30.7, 95% CI, 4.6–203.6) compared with non-pregnant women without the mutation. Risk factors for VTE in pregnancy and the puerperium are listed in Table 2.

The utility of thrombophilia testing in pregnant women with thrombosis is questionable. Some studies state that because of the increased risk of VTE during pregnancy and the puerperium, thrombophilia screening is indicated only in selected patients with a previous history of VTE or a positive family history [72]. Others claim that screening for thrombophilias in obstetrics has become too widely spread, despite data that are lacking or inconclusive and despite the fact that it does not necessarily alter management and use of anticoagulation in present of future pregnancies [63].

Table 2. Risk factors for VTE in pregnancy and the puerperium.

Primary risk factors	Potentially reversible risk factors
Inherited and acquired thrombophilia	Surgical procedure in pregnancy or puerperium
Age over 35 years	Hyperemesis and dehydration
Obesity (BMI > 30)	Severe infection (e.g., pyelonephritis)
Multiparity (> 4)	Immobility after delivery(>4 days)
Gross varicose veins	Ovarian hyperstimulation syndrome
Paraplegia	Preeclampsia
Sickle cell disease	Excessive blood loss and blood transfusions
Some medical disorders (e.g., nephritic syndrome, certain cardiac diseases)	Instrumental delivery
Inflammatory disorders (e.g., inflammatory bowel disease)	Prolonged labor
Myeloproliferative disorders (e.g., essential thrombocytopenia, polycythemia vera)	

Adapted from Expert Review Obstet Gynecol. 2, 203-216 (2007) with permission of Expert Reviews Ltd.

Anticoagulant Therapy and Thromboprophylaxis

The identification of a link between thrombophilic factors and APO opens up treatment possibilities. Until recently, it has not been clear whether antithrombotic therapy is useful in women with previous placental dysfunction and inherited thrombophilia. Many physicians have been treating such women with antithrombotic therapy on the basis of logic and anecdotal evidence [73].

Anticoagulant therapy is indicated during pregnancy for the prevention and treatment of VTE, for the prevention and treatment of systemic embolism in patients with mechanical heart valves and, often in combination with aspirin, for the prevention of pregnancy complications in women with APLA syndrome or other thrombophilias and previous pregnancy complications [51,74].

At present, there are limited data regarding the efficacy of anticoagulants during pregnancy, recommendations about their use during pregnancy are based largely on data extrapolated from nonpregnant patients, from case reports, and from case series of pregnant patients [74-75]. The antithrombotics currently available for the prevention and treatment of VTE and arterial thromboembolism include heparin and heparin-like compounds (unfractionated heparin (UFH), low molecular weight heparin (LMWH), and heparinoids), coumarin derivatives, and aspirin. Based on safety data, a heparin-related compound (LMWH or UFH) is the anticoagulant of choice during pregnancy for situations in which its efficacy is established [74-75]. There is accumulating experience with the use of LMWHs, both in pregnant and nonpregnant patients, for the prevention and treatment of VTE [76-78] and the prevention of APO [79-81]. Although a variety of antithrombotics exist we will hereby address only the three most common agents: UFH, LMWH and warfarin.

Antithrombotic Agents

Unfractionated heparin: UFH is the drug of choice for the prophylaxis and treatment of thromboembolic manifestations in pregnancy [51]. Because of its molecular weight, it does not cross the placenta and therefore does not cause hemorrhagic complications and is not considered teratogenic [74]. The most common maternal side effects are osteoporosis, thrombocytopenia (heparin induced thrombocytopenia [HIT]), allergy and hemorrhage with an overall 3% incidence rate [74]. The half-life of UFH is short, with an anticoagulant effect of approximately 8–12 hours. Heparin is partially reversible with protamin sulfate. Recent administration is not a contraindication for regional analgesia if partial thromboplastin time (PTT) is not prolonged [82].

Recently it has been suggested that heparin may act by mechanisms other than anticoagulation. Heparin has been shown to have the potential to reduce trophoblast invasion in cell lines and first trimester extra villous trophoblast cells [83].

Low molecular weight heparin: LMWH is comparable to UFH with regard to effectiveness and safety in the prophylaxis and treatment of VTE. It too does not cross the placenta as well and can be considered safe during pregnancy. When compared with UFH, LMWH demonstrates a better bioavailability, a longer half-life and a predictable anticoagulant activity, allowing fixed dosing based on body weight without the need to monitor the PTT [51,74].

In the nonpregnant patient with VTE, LMWH is usually administered once daily with the use of a weight-adjusted dose regimen. Opinion is divided as to the optimal regimen for LMWH in pregnant women. Because of increased renal excretion, the half-life of LMWH decreases in pregnancy [84]. Consequently, a twice-daily weight-based regimen has been recommended [85]; however, many clinicians use once-daily dosing to simplify administration.

The half-life of LMWH is longer than that of UFH and cannot be reversed with protamin sulfate. Regional analgesia within 18–24 hours of LMWH administration may be associated with epidural hematomas [82]. Because the evaluation of LMWH in pregnancy has been limited to case series, there is uncertainty about their value in pregnant women requiring antithrombotic therapy. However, given their advantages over UFH, the clear-cut evidence of their efficacy in nonpregnant patients, and the fact that they are safe for the fetus, their use during pregnancy is a reasonable clinical practice [74,86]. Le Templier and Rodger [87] have recently assessed the effect of LMWH on bone mineral density in an ongoing multicenter multinational randomized trial designed to compare the effect of LMWH prophylaxis on pregnancy outcomes in thrombophilic pregnant women. The results revealed that there was no significant difference in mean bone mineral density between a LMWH prophylaxis group and the non prophylaxis group. It should be noted that the study was not adequately powered to detect differences in absolute fracture risk [87].

Warfarin: Warfarin is the most commonly used oral anticoagulant. In pregnancy it is typically used on patients with prosthetic heart valves [82]. It readily crosses the placenta and has been associated with adverse events in the fetus, including teratogenicity and bleeding. Warfarin embryopathy is characterized by nasal hypoplasia, telecanthus as well as displasia of the epiphyses of the long bones and cervical and lumbar vertebrae. It is associated with exposure between 6 and 9 weeks of gestation and has an incidence of 10%–15%. The rates of spontaneous abortions and stillbirths are also elevated with warfarin use during pregnancy, partly on the basis of placental hemorrhage. The use of warfarin in the second trimester and early in the third trimester is associated with fetal intra-cranial hemorrhage and schizencephaly. Warfarin appears to be safe during breastfeeding [51,74].

The half-life of warfarin is long. The production of vitamin K dependent clotting factors is inhibited for 36–48 hours. Warfarin should be discontinued near term and replaced with UFH. If delivery is anticipated shortly after warfarin administration, vitamin K can hasten the production of the vitamin K dependent clotting factors. If the patient is in labor or requires a cesarean section and the prothrombin time is prolonged, fresh frozen plasma administration is warranted for clotting factor replacement [82].

Management of Thrombophilia during Pregnancy

The management of thrombophilia during pregnancy includes primary thromboprophylaxis for VTE in asymptomatic women, secondary prophylaxis of recurrences in women who have previously developed thrombosis, and the treatment of acute thrombotic episodes. Recently, the American College of Chest Physicians published their Evidence-Based Clinical Practice Guidelines for the management of VTE and thrombophilia, as well as the use of antithrombotic agents, during pregnancy [85]. For patients with a higher risk thrombophilia (antithrombin deficiency) antepartum prophylactic of intermediate-dose LMWH or UFH should be given, in addition to postpartum prophylaxis. For all other pregnant women with thrombophilia but no prior VTE, they suggest antepartum clinical surveillance or prophylactic dose LMWH or UFH, plus postpartum anticoagulants as routine care [85].

It is rather difficult to establish guidelines for antithrombotic therapy due to the lack of relevant and well-controlled trials. Thus, the recommendations regarding prophylactic and therapeutic strategies in pregnancy are largely based on clinical trials in non-pregnant populations [33]. The limitations upon which these recommendations are based are examplified in the study by Brill-Edwards et al. [88]. Among 44 patients with a history of VTE following a reversible risk factor (Table 2) who had a negative thrombophilia screening no recurrences of VTE were noted. One might interpret the risk of thrombosis in this group to be nonexistent. However, the upper limit of the 95% confidence interval is 8%, meaning that a potential risk of recurrence as high as 8% exists. In addition, although it does appear that homozygosity for FVL or the PT mutation, heterozygosity for both of the above, or antithrombin III deficiency may be associated with a higher risk for recurrence, there are no prospective data to adequately evaluate the risks and benefits of therapeutic anticoagulation with regard to prevention of recurrent clot vs. the risk of hemorrhagic complications [63].

Fox et al. [89] evaluated anti-factor Xa activity in pregnant patients receiving LMWH for VTE prophylaxis. Only 59% of anti-Xa concentrations were in the prophylactic range, whereas 26% were subprophylactic, and 15% were supraprophylactic. Anti-Xa values were not more likely to be prophylactic in early compared with late pregnancy, obese compared with nonobese patients, or in patients receiving a weight-based minimal dose compared with patients receiving less than a weight-based minimal dose. Anti-factor Xa levels did not correlate with maternal age, weight, body mass index, or gestational age, but there was a positive correlation with the percent of the minimal weight-based dose [89].

The risk for VTE in a pregnant patient with thrombophilia should be stratified based on the type of thrombophilia and VTE status. The thrombophylaxis and treatment based on thrombophilia type and previous VTE status is presented in Table 3. Patients at the highest risk group should be treated with antenatal high prophylactic or therapeutic dose LMWH and at least 6 weeks postnatal warfarin. Patients with moderate risk should receive prophylactic dose LMWH both antenatally and 6 weeks postnatally. Patients with relatively low risk should receive prophylactic LMWH 6 weeks postnatally.

Attempts have been made to create risk prediction scores with some success although they are not yet widely implemented. Dargaud et al. [90] evaluated the usefulness of score based management of pregnancies with high risk of VTE. They studied 116 consecutive pregnancies in 109 women with confirmed thrombophilia and/or a history of VTE. A VTE risk prediction score was established. All patients with a positive score (n=57, 49.1%) have been treated with an antenatal thrombophylaxis. Negative score patients (n=55 cases), did not receive antenatal prophylaxis. During the study period, there was only one episode of VTE. The authors concluded that implementing this scoring system has resulted in favorable outcomes and a low risk of recurrent thrombosis in a limited series of women with increased risk of VTE. Further prospective multicenter clinical trials with larger populations of pregnant women with high risk of VTE are required to test the applicability of this scoring system.

Table 3. Thrombophylaxis and treatment in pregnancy based on thrombophilia type and previous VTE status.

Risk	Previous VTE and thrombophilia status	Prophylaxis and treatment
High risk	VTE in current pregnancy Previous VTE on long term anticoagulants Previous recurrent VTE Previous VTE in patients with highly thrombogenic thrombophilias (AT deficiency, combined defects, homozygotes or compound heterozygotes for th FVL or PT mutations) APLA syndrome and previous thrombosis (arterial or venous) or RPL	Antenatal high prophylactic or therapeutic dose LMWH and at least 6 weeks postnatal warfarin.
Moderate risk	Previous VTE in patients with lesser thrombogenic thrombophilias VTE with family history of VTE Asymptomatic highly thrombogenic thrombophilias	Antenatal and 6 weeks postnatal prophylactic LMWH.
Relatively low risk	Single previous VTE with reversible risk factor Asymptomatic lesser thrombogenic thrombophilias	6 weeks postnatal prophylactic LMWH.

VTE: venous thromboembolism; LMWH: low molecular weight heparin; AT: antithrombin; FVL: factor V Leiden; PT: prothrombin; RPL: recurrent pregnancy loss. Adapted from *Expert Review Obstet Gynecol.* 2, 203-216 (2007) with permission of Expert Reviews Ltd.

There is now compelling evidence that inherited and acquired thrombophilias are associated with a proportion of cases of VTE and placental dysfunction in the second and third trimester (e.g. stillbirth, IUGR, preeclampsia and placental abruption) [73]. Anecdotally, antithrombotic therapy has been shown to be of benefit in improving fetal outcome in women with thrombophilia and previous second and third trimester placental dysfunction [79,81], although a randomized double blind trial has never been conducted. Until recently, it has not been clear whether antithrombotic therapy is useful in women with previous placental dysfunction and inherited thrombophilia. Many physicians have been treating such women with antithrombotic therapy on the basis of logic and anecdotal evidence [73].

Antiphospholipid Syndrome

Antiphospholipid syndrome is defined as the presence of lupus anticoagulant or anticardiolipin antibodies of medium to high titer on two occasions eight weeks apart, found in association with a history of thrombosis (arterial or venous) or APO (three or more unexplained miscarriages before ten weeks of gestation, a fetal death after ten weeks of gestation or a premature (less than 35 weeks) birth due to severe preeclampsia or IUGR [91].

The risk of recurrent thrombosis in women with APLA syndrome is up to 70% and may even be higher during pregnancy [92]. Pregnant women with APLA syndrome and previous thrombosis should receive antenatal and postnatal thrombophylaxis with LMWH [93]. As previously mentioned, pregnancy complications associated with APLA syndrome include recurrent pregnancy loss, preeclampsia, IUGR and thrombosis. The mechanisms of APO in women who have APLA syndrome are not clearly understood [94].

Evidence based recommendations for the treatment of pregnancy complications in APLA syndrome patients are difficult to provide, due to the lack of large randomized clinical trials [94]. Heparin may improve pregnancy outcome in women who have APLA syndrome. Randomized trials have found the combination of aspirin and UFH to be associated with improved outcomes when compared with aspirin alone in women who had RM [95-96]. In contrast, another trial compared the efficacy of LMWH as adjunctive therapy to low dose aspirin and did not find that the addition of LMWH significantly improved pregnancy outcomes [97]. In other settings, LMWH has been compared with UFH and was found to be as good as or better than UFH for the prevention or treatment of thromboembolism. Resent data from observational studies and systematic reviews support the use of LMWH as a safer alternative than UFH in pregnancy [76,86]. LMWH has a lower incidence of heparin-induced thrombocytopenia and osteoporosis [98] and does not require laboratory monitoring or dose adjustments [94]. Compared with recurrent thrombosis, the management of women with obstetric manifestations of APLA syndrome is controversial. Low dose aspirin has been shown to improve pregnancy outcome, and is recommended for all women with APLA syndrome [93]. For patients diagnosed with APLA syndrome that suffered no previous pregnancy loss, treatment with LMWH is not mandatory [99].

Goldman et al. [100] examined how practicing obstetricians evaluate and manage thrombophilias in selected clinical situations. They mailed a questionnaire investigating knowledge and practice patterns pertaining to thrombophilia to 300 randomly selected American College of Obstetricians and Gynecologists Fellows and Junior Fellows. More than 50% reported sending an inherited thrombophilia panel and antiphospholipid antibodies screen for patients with a history of fetal demise, intrauterine growth restriction (less than 5th percentile), placental abruption, and severe preeclampsia. Ninety-two percent reported testing patients with RM for antiphospholipid antibodies. Despite no clear evidence, 80% also reported testing these patients for inherited thrombophilias. The majority intervene with either thromboprophylaxis or low-dose aspirin when managing patients at risk for thromboembolism. Seventy percent use LMWH (fractionated) for patients requiring therapeutic anticoagulation, while 62% also use it for prophylactic anticoagulation. Thirty eight percent of physicians using LMWH monitor anti-factor Xa levels. It is clear by the results that most responding obstetricians do not manage thrombophilia patients according to expert opinion. Despite the fact that often there is no clear evidence for treatment, many physicians are inclined to intervene in patients at risk for thromboembolism. Educational endeavors are needed to guide obstetricians caring for patients at risk for thromboembolism.

Statistical Pitfalls in the Association between Thrombophilias and APO

The question of whether the relationship between acquired and inherited thrombophilias and APO can be considered causal is rather philosophical. Middeldorp [30] reviewed the consistency and strengths of associations, potential mechanisms and the possibility to intervene with anticoagulants and found that relevant methodological issues in the case of thrombophilia and pregnancy complications consist of differences between observational and experimental research and quality issues in randomized controlled trials. Observational research is hampered by severe methodological flaws or inconsistent results. For example, two randomized control trials have not used an adequate comparator (i.e., no treatment or placebo) [81,101].

Kist et al. [102] investigated the relationship of thrombophilias with APO. They analyzed the influence of confounders such as ethnicity, severity of illness and method of testing in case-control studies conducted between 1966 and 2006. They concluded that reports on the prevalence of maternal thrombophilias and APO are influenced by various confounders, which are not always appropriately analysed. They identified differences that reflect the differential impact of the confounders [102]. The importance of more uniform research data should be emphasized.

Summary

Thrombophilias are inherited or acquired conditions, which predispose an individual to thromboembolism. The most common inherited disorders are deficiencies in antithrombin III, protein C, and protein S, APCR due to FVL mutation, a function-enhancing mutation in the prothrombin (PT) gene (G20210A), and thermo labile mutation for methylenetetrahydrofolate reductase (C677T) (MTHFR). During pregnancy, thrombophilia has been identified as a major risk factor for APO, including venous and arterial thrombosis, preeclampsia, placental abruption, IUGR, intrauterine fetal losses and recurrent miscarriages. The risk of VTE in pregnancy is approximately six times greater than in non-pregnant women and is a major cause of death among women during pregnancy and the puerperium. Pulmonary embolism occurs in approximately 16% of patients with untreated DVT and is the most common cause of maternal mortality. The risk of venous thrombosis in women with inherited or acquired thrombophilia is increased during pregnancy. Women with previous VTE should be screened for inherited and acquired thrombophilia, preferably before pregnancy. LMWH has become the treatment of choice for thrombophilia; it does not cross the placenta and can be considered safe during pregnancy.

References

[1]   Romero R, Dekker G, Kupferminc M, Saade G, Livingston J, Peaceman A, Mazor M, Yoon BH, Espinoza J, Chaiworapongsa T, Gomez R, Arias F, Sibai B. Can heparin prevent adverse pregnancy outcome? *J Matern Fetal Neonatal Med.* 2002;12:1-8.

[2]   Kupferminc MJ, Fait G, Many A, Gordon D, Eldor A, Lessing JB. Severe preeclampsia and high frequency of genetic thrombophilic mutations. *Obstet Gynecol.* 2000;96:45-49.

[3]   Kupferminc MJ. Thrombophilia and preeclampsia: the evidence so far. *Clin Obstet Gynecol.* 2005;48:406-415.

[4]   Wiener-Megnagi Z, Ben-Shlomo I, Goldberg Y, Shalev E. Resistance to activated protein C and the leiden mutation: high prevalence in patients with abruptio placentae. *Am J Obstet Gynecol*. 1998;179:1565-1567.

[5]   Vossen CY, Preston FE, Conard J, Fontcuberta J, Makris M, van der Meer FJ, Pabinger I, Palareti G, Scharrer I, Souto JC, Svensson P, Walker ID, Rosendaal FR. Hereditary thrombophilia and fetal loss: a prospective follow-up study. *J Thromb Haemost*. 2004;2:592-596.

[6]   Verspyck E, Borg JY, Le Cam-Duchez V, Goffinet F, Degré S, Fournet P, Marpeau L. Thrombophilia and fetal growth restriction. *Eur J Obstet Gynecol Reprod Biol*. 2004;113:36-40.

[7]   Sheiner E, Levy A, Katz M, Mazor M. Pregnancy outcome following recurrent spontaneous abortions. *Eur J Obstet Gynecol Reprod Biol*. 2005;118:61-65.

[8]   Raziel A, Kornberg Y, Friedler S, Schachter M, Sela BA, Ron-El R. Hypercoagulable thrombophilic defects and hyperhomocysteinemia in patients with recurrent pregnancy loss. *Am J Reprod Immunol*. 2001;45:65-71.

[9]   Rai R, Shlebak A, Cohen H, Backos M, Holmes Z, Marriott K, Regan L. Factor V Leiden and acquired activated protein C resistance among 1000 women with recurrent miscarriage. *Hum Reprod*. 2001;16:961-965.

[10]   Preston FE, Rosendaal FR, Walker ID, Briët E, Berntorp E, Conard J, Fontcuberta J, Makris M, Mariani G, Noteboom W, Pabinger I, Legnani C, Scharrer I, Schulman S, van der Meer FJ. Increased fetal loss in women with heritable thrombophilia. *Lancet*. 1996;348:913-916.

[11]   Peeters LL. Thrombophilia and fetal growth restriction. *Eur J Obstet Gynecol Reprod Biol*. 2001;95:202-205.

[12]   Dudding TE, Attia J. The association between adverse pregnancy outcomes and maternal factor V Leiden genotype: a meta-analysis. *Thromb Haemost*. 2004;91:700-711.

[13]   Dizon-Townson DS, Nelson LM, Easton K, Ward K. The factor V Leiden mutation may predispose women to severe preeclampsia. *Am J Obstet Gynecol*. 1996;175:902-905.

[14]   Weintraub AY, Sheiner E. Anticoagulant therapy and thromboprophylaxis in patients with thrombophilia. *Arch Gynecol Obstet*. 2007;276:567-571.

[15]   Weintraub AY, Wiznitzer A, Sheiner E. Maternal thrombophilia and adverse pregnancy outcomes. *Expert Review Obstet Gynecol*. 2007;2:203-216.

[16]   McCowan LM, Craigie S, Taylor RS, Ward C, McLintock C, North RA. Inherited thrombophilias are not increased in "idiopathic" small-for-gestational-age pregnancies. *Am J Obstet Gynecol*. 2003;188:981-985.

[17]   Livingston JC, Barton JR, Park V, Haddad B, Phillips O, Sibai BM. Maternal and fetal inherited thrombophilias are not related to the development of severe preeclampsia. *Am J Obstet Gynecol*. 2001;185:153-157.

[18]   Alfirevic Z, Mousa HA, Martlew V, Briscoe L, Perez-Casal M, Toh CH. Postnatal screening for thrombophilia in women with severe pregnancy complications. *Obstet Gynecol*. 2001;97:753-759.

[19] Rasmussen A, Ravn P. High frequency of congenital thrombophilia in women with pathological pregnancies? *Acta Obstet Gynecol Scand*. 2004;83:808-817.

[20] Many A, Schreiber L, Rosner S, Lessing JB, Eldor A, Kupferminc MJ. Pathologic features of the placenta in women with severe pregnancy complications and thrombophilia. *Obstet Gynecol*. 2001;98:1041-1044.

[21] Kupferminc MJ, Eldor A, Steinman N, Many A, Bar-Am A, Jaffa A, Fait G, Lessing JB. Increased frequency of genetic thrombophilia in women with complications of pregnancy. *N Engl J Med*. 1999;340:9-13.

[22] Eldor A. Thrombophilia, thrombosis and pregnancy. *Thromb Haemost*. 2001;86:104-111.

[23] Weintraub AY, Sheiner E, Levy A, Yerushalmi R, Mazor M. Pregnancy complications in women with inherited thrombophilia. *Arch Gynecol Obstet*. 2006;274:125-129.

[24] Rey E, Kahn SR, David M, Shrier I. Thrombophilic disorders and fetal loss: a meta-analysis. *Lancet*. 2003;361:901-908.

[25] Alfirevic Z, Roberts D, Martlew V. How strong is the association between maternal thrombophilia and adverse pregnancy outcome? A systematic review. *Eur J Obstet Gynecol Reprod Biol*. 2002;101:6-14.

[26] Infante-Rivard C, Rivard GE, Yotov WV, Génin E, Guiguet M, Weinberg C, Gauthier R, Feoli-Fonseca JC. Absence of association of thrombophilia polymorphisms with intrauterine growth restriction. *N Engl J Med*. 2002;347:19-25.

[27] Alonso A, Soto I, Urgelles MF, Corte JR, Rodriguez MJ, Pinto CR. Acquired and inherited thrombophilia in women with unexplained fetal losses. *Am J Obstet Gynecol*. 2002;187:1337-1342.

[28] Wu O, Robertson L, Twaddle S, Lowe GD, Clark P, Greaves M, Walker ID, Langhorne P, Brenkel I, Regan L, Greer I. Screening for thrombophilia in high-risk situations: systematic review and cost-effectiveness analysis. The Thrombosis: Risk and Economic Assessment of Thrombophilia Screening (TREATS) study. *Health Technol Assess*. 2006;10:1-110.

[29] Weintraub AY, Sheiner E, Bashiri A, Shoham-Vardi I, Mazor M. Is there a higher prevalence of pregnancy complications in a live-birth preceding the appearance of recurrent abortions? *Arch Gynecol Obstet*. 2005;271:350-354.

[30] Middeldorp S. Thrombophilia and pregnancy complications: cause or association? *J Thromb Haemost*. 2007;5:276-282.

[31] Dekker GA, de Vries JI, Doelitzsch PM, Huijgens PC, von Blomberg BM, Jakobs C, van Geijn HP. Underlying disorders associated with severe early-onset preeclampsia. *Am J Obstet Gynecol*. 1995;173:1042-1048.

[32] Lin J, August P. Genetic thrombophilias and preeclampsia: a meta-analysis. *Obstet Gynecol*. 2005;105:182-192.

[33] Kupferminc MJ. Thrombophilia and pregnancy. *Reprod Biol Endocrinol*. 2003;1:111.

[34] Mello G, Parretti E, Marozio L, Pizzi C, Lojacono A, Frusca T, Facchinetti F, Benedetto C. Thrombophilia is significantly associated with severe preeclampsia: results of a large-scale, case-controlled study. *Hypertension*. 2005;46:1270-1274.

[35]   Larciprete G, Gioia S, Angelucci PA, Brosio F, Barbati G, Angelucci GP, Frigo MG, Baiocco F, Romanini ME, Arduini D, Cirese E. Single inherited thrombophilias and adverse pregnancy outcomes. *J Obstet Gynaecol Res*. 2007;33:423-430.

[36]   Muetze S, Leeners B, Ortlepp JR, Kuse S, Tag CG, Weiskirchen R, Gressner AM, Rudnik-Schoeneborn S, Zerres K, Rath W. Maternal factor V Leiden mutation is associated with HELLP syndrome in Caucasian women. *Acta Obstet Gynecol Scand*. 2008;87:635-642.

[37]   Facchinetti F, Marozio L, Frusca T, Grandone E, Venturini P, Tiscia GL, Zatti S, Benedetto C. Maternal thrombophilia and the risk of recurrence of preeclampsia. *Am J Obstet Gynecol*. 2009;200:46.e1-5.

[38]   Kupferminc MJ, Many A, Bar-Am A, Lessing JB, Ascher-Landsberg J. Mid-trimester severe intrauterine growth restriction is associated with a high prevalence of thrombophilia. *BJOG*. 2002;109:1373-1376.

[39]   Martinelli P, Grandone E, Colaizzo D, Paladini D, Sciannamé N, Margaglione M, Di Minno G. Familial thrombophilia and the occurrence of fetal growth restriction. *Haematologica*. 2001;86:428-431.

[40]   Grandone E, Margaglione M, Colaizzo D, Pavone G, Paladini D, Martinelli P, Di Minno G. Lower birth-weight in neonates of mothers carrying factor V G1691A and factor II A(20210) mutations. *Haematologica*. 2002;87:177-188.

[41]   Vollset SE, Refsum H, Irgens LM, Emblem BM, Tverdal A, Gjessing HK, Monsen AL, Ueland PM. Plasma total homocysteine, pregnancy complications, and adverse pregnancy outcomes: the Hordaland Homocysteine study. *Am J Clin Nutr*. 2000;71:962-968.

[42]   Franchi F, Cetin I, Todros T, Antonazzo P, Nobile de Santis MS, Cardaropoli S, Bucciarelli P, Biguzzi E. Intrauterine growth restriction and genetic predisposition to thrombophilia. *Haematologica*. 2004;89:444-449.

[43]   Robertson L, Wu O, Langhorne P, Twaddle S, Clark P, Lowe GD, Walker ID, Greaves M, Brenkel I, Regan L, Greer IA; The Thrombosis: Risk and Economic Assessment of Thrombophilia Screening (TREATS) Study. Thrombophilia in pregnancy: a systematic review. *Br J Haematol*. 2006;132:171-196.

[44]   Howley HE, Walker M, Rodger MA. A systematic review of the association between factor V Leiden or prothrombin gene variant and intrauterine growth restriction. *Am J Obstet Gynecol*. 2005;192:694-708.

[45]   Kocher O, Cirovic C, Malynn E, Rowland CM, Bare LA, Young BA, Henslee JG, Laffler TG, Huff JB, Kruskall MS, Wong G, Bauer KA. Obstetric complications in patients with hereditary thrombophilia identified using the LCx microparticle enzyme immunoassay: a controlled study of 5,000 patients. *Am J Clin Pathol*. 2007;127:68-75.

[46]   van der Molen EF, Verbruggen B, Novakova I, Eskes TK, Monnens LA, Blom HJ. Hyperhomocysteinemia and other thrombotic risk factors in women with placental vasculopathy. *BJOG*. 2000;107:785-791.

[47]   Goddijn-Wessel TA, Wouters MG, van de Molen EF, Spuijbroek MD, Steegers-Theunissen RP, Blom HJ, Boers GH, Eskes TK. Hyperhomocysteinemia: a risk factor for placental abruption or infarction. *Eur J Obstet Gynecol Reprod Biol*. 1996;66:23-29.

[48] Facchinetti F, Marozio L, Grandone E, Pizzi C, Volpe A, Benedetto C. Thrombophilic mutations are a main risk factor for placental abruption. *Haematologica*. 2003;88:785-788.

[49] de Vries JI, Dekker GA, Huijgens PC, Jakobs C, Blomberg BM, van Geijn HP. Hyperhomocysteinaemia and protein S deficiency in complicated pregnancies. *BJOG*. 1997;104:1248-1254.

[50] Karakantza M, Androutsopoulos G, Mougiou A ,Sakellaropoulos G, Kourounis G, Decavalas G. Inheritance and perinatal consequences of inherited thrombophilia in Greece. *Int J Gynaecol Obstet*. 2008;100:124-129.

[51] De Santis M, Cavaliere AF, Straface G, Di Gianantonio E, Caruso A. Inherited and acquired thrombophilia: pregnancy outcome and treatment. *Reprod Toxicol*. 2006;22:227-233.

[52] Greer IA. Thrombophilia: implications for pregnancy outcome. *Thromb Res*. 2003;109:73-81.

[53] Regan L, Rai R. Thrombophilia and pregnancy loss. *J Reprod Immunol*. 2002;55:163-180.

[54] Tulppala M, Viinikka L, Ylikorkala O. Thromboxane dominance and prostacyclin deficiency in habitual abortion. *Lancet*. 1991;337:879-881.

[55] Sottilotta G, Oriana V, Latella C, Luise F, Piromalli A, Ramirez F, Mammì C, Santoro R, Iannaccaro P, Muleo G, Lombardo VT. Genetic prothrombotic risk factors in women with unexplained pregnancy loss. *Thromb Res*. 2006;117:681-684.

[56] Onderoglu L, Baykal C, Al RA, Demirtas E, Deren O, Gurgey A. High frequency of thrombophilic disorders in women with recurrent fetal miscarriage .*Clin Exp Obstet Gynecol*. 2006;33:50-54.

[57] Many A, Elad R, Yaron Y, Eldor A, Lessing JB, Kupferminc MJ. Third-trimester unexplained intrauterine fetal death is associated with inherited thrombophilia. *Obstet Gynecol*. 2002;99:684-687.

[58] Kujovich JL. Thrombophilia and pregnancy complications. *Am J Obstet Gynecol*. 2004;191:412-424.

[59] Triplett DA, Harris EN. Antiphospholipid antibodies and reproduction. *Am J Reprod Immunol*. 1989;21:123-131.

[60] Rai RS, Clifford K, Cohen H, Regan L. High prospective fetal loss rate in untreated pregnancies of women with recurrent miscarriage and antiphospholipid antibodies. *Hum Reprod*. 1995;10:3301-3304.

[61] Vincent T, Rai R, Regan L, Cohen H. Increased thrombin generation in women with recurrent miscarriage. *Lancet*. 1998;352:116.

[62] Ruffatti A, Tonello M, Cavazzana A, Bagatella P, Pengo V. Laboratory classification categories and pregnancy outcome in patients with primary antiphospholipid syndrome prescribed antithrombotic therapy. *Thromb Res*. 2009;123:482-487.

[63] Scifres CM, Macones GA. The utility of thrombophilia testing in pregnant women with thrombosis: fact or fiction? *Am J Obstet Gynecol* Oct. 2008;199:344e341-347.

[64] Martinelli I, De Stefano V, Taioli E, Paciaroni K, Rossi E, Mannucci PM. Inherited thrombophilia and first venous thromboembolism during pregnancy and puerperium. *Thromb Haemost*. 2002;87:791-795.

[65] Gerhardt A, Scharf RE, Beckmann MW, Struve S, Bender HG, Pillny M, Sandmann W, Zotz RB. Prothrombin and factor V mutations in women with a history of thrombosis during pregnancy and the puerperium. *N Engl J Med*. 2000;342:374-380.

[66] Pabinger I, Grafenhofer H, Kyrle PA, Quehenberger P, Mannhalter C, Lechner K, Kaider A. Temporary increase in the risk for recurrence during pregnancy in women with a history of venous thromboembolism. *Blood*. 2002;100:1060-1062.

[67] White RH, Chan WS, Zhou H, Ginsberg JS. Recurrent venous thromboembolism after pregnancy-associated versus unprovoked thromboembolism. *Thromb Haemost*. 2008;100:246-252.

[68] Ginsberg JS ,Brill-Edwards P, Burrows RF, Bona R, Prandoni P, Büller HR, Lensing A. Venous thrombosis during pregnancy: leg and trimester of presentation. *Thromb Haemost*. 1992;67:519-520.

[69] Chang J, Elam-Evans LD, Berg CJ, Herndon J, Flowers L, Seed KA, Syverson CJ. Pregnancy-related mortality surveillance—United States, 1991–. 1999MMWR Surveill Summ. 2003;52:1-8.

[70] Martinelli I, Battaglioli T, De Stefano V, Tormene D, Valdrè L, Grandone E, Tosetto A, Mannucci PM; GIT (Gruppo Italiano Trombofilia). The risk of first venous thromboembolism during pregnancy and puerperium in double heterozygotes for factor V Leiden and prothrombin G20210A. *J Thromb Haemost*. 2008;6:494-498.

[71] Pomp ER, Lenselink AM, Rosendaal FR, Doggen CJ. Pregnancy, the postpartum period and prothrombotic defects: risk of venous thrombosis in the MEGA study. *J Thromb Haemost*. 2008;6:632-637.

[72] Lindhoff-Last E, Luxembourg B. Evidence-based indications for thrombophilia screening. *Vasa*. 2008;37:19-30.

[73] Greer I, Hunt BJ. Low molecular weight heparin in pregnancy: current issues. *Br J Haematol*. 2005;128:593-601.

[74] Bates SM. Treatment and prophylaxis of venous thromboembolism during pregnancy. *Thromb Res*. 2002;108:97-106.

[75] Bates SM, Greer IA, Hirsh J, Ginsberg JS. Use of antithrombotic agents during pregnancy: the Seventh ACCP Conference on Antithrombotic and Thrombolytic Therapy. *Chest*. 2004;126:627S-644S.

[76] Lepercq J, Conard J, Borel-Derlon A, Darmon JY, Boudignat O, Francoual C, Priollet P, Cohen C, Yvelin N, Schved JF, Tournaire M, Borg JY. Venous thromboembolism during pregnancy: a retrospective study of enoxaparin safety in 624 pregnancies. *BJOG*. 2001;108:1134-1140.

[77] Gould MK, Dembitzer AD, Sanders GD, Garber AM. Low-molecular-weight heparins compared with unfractionated heparin for treatment of acute deep venous thrombosis. A cost-effectiveness analysis. *Ann Intern Med*. 1999;130:789-799.

[78] Dolovich LR, Ginsberg JS, Douketis JD, Holbrook AM, Cheah G. A meta-analysis comparing low-molecular-weight heparins with unfractionated heparin in the treatment of venous thromboembolism: examining some unanswered questions regarding location of treatment, product type, and dosing frequency. *Arch Intern Med*. 2000;160:181-188.

[79]   Kupferminc MJ, Fait G, Many A, Lessing JB, Yair D, Bar-Am A, Eldor A. Low-molecular-weight heparin for the prevention of obstetric complications in women with thrombophilias. *Hypertens Pregnancy*. 2001;20:35-44.

[80]   De Carolis S, Ferrazzani S ,De Stefano V, Garofalo S, Fatigante G, Rossi E, Leone G, Caruso A. Inherited thrombophilia: treatment during pregnancy. *Fetal Diagn Ther*. 2006;21:281-286.

[81]   Brenner B, Bar J, Ellis M, Yarom I, Yohai D, Samueloff A. Effects of enoxaparin on late pregnancy complications and neonatal outcome in women with recurrent pregnancy loss and thrombophilia: results from the Live-Enox study. *Fertil Steril*. 2005;84:770-773.

[82]   Chasen ST. Peripartum and perioperative management of the anticoagulated patient. *Obstet Gynecol Clin North Am*. 2006;33:493-497.

[83]   Ganapathy R, Whitley GS, Cartwright JE, Dash PR, Thilaganathan B. Effect of heparin and fractionated heparin on trophoblast invasion. *Hum Reprod*. 2007;22:2523-2527.

[84]   Sephton V, Farquharson RG, Topping J, Quenby SM, Cowan C, Back DJ, Toh CH. A longitudinal study of maternal dose response to low molecular weight heparin in pregnancy. *Obstet Gynecol*. 2003;101:1307-1311.

[85]   Bates SM, Greer IA, Pabinger I, Sofaer S, Hirsh J. Venous thromboembolism, thrombophilia, antithrombotic therapy, and pregnancy :American College of Chest Physicians Evidence-Based Clinical Practice Guidelines (8th Edition). *Chest*. 2008;133:844S-886S.

[86]   Sanson BJ, Lensing AW, Prins MH, Ginsberg JS, Barkagan ZS, Lavenne-Pardonge E, Brenner B, Dulitzky M, Nielsen JD, Boda Z, Turi S, Mac Gillavry MR, Hamulyák K, Theunissen IM, Hunt BJ, Büller HR. Safety of low-molecular-weight heparin in pregnancy: a systematic review. *Thromb Haemost*. 1999;81:668-672.

[87]   Le Templier G, Rodger MA. Heparin-induced osteoporosis and pregnancy. *Curr Opin Pulm Med*. 2008;14:403-407.

[88]   Brill-Edwards P, Ginsberg JS, Gent M, Hirsh J, Burrows R, Kearon C, Geerts W, Kovacs M, Weitz JI, Robinson KS, Whittom R, Couture G; Recurrence of Clot in This Pregnancy Study Group. Safety of withholding heparin in pregnant women with a history of venous thromboembolism. Recurrence of Clot in This Pregnancy Study Group. *N Engl J Med*. 2000;343:1439-1444.

[89]   Fox NS, Laughon SK, Bender SD, Saltzman DH, Rebarber A. Anti-factor Xa plasma levels in pregnant women receiving low molecular weight heparin thromboprophylaxis. *Obstet Gynecol*. 2008;112:884-889.

[90]   Dargaud Y, Rugeri L, Ninet J, Negrier C, Trzeciak MC. Management of pregnant women with increased risk of venous thrombosis. *Int J Gynaecol Obstet*. 2005;90:203-207.

[91]   Wilson WA, Gharavi AE, Koike T, Lockshin MD, Branch DW, Piette JC, Brey R, Derksen R, Harris EN, Hughes GR, Triplett DA, Khamashta MA. International consensus statement on preliminary classification criteria for definite antiphospholipid syndrome: report of an international workshop. *Arthritis Rheum*. 1999;42:1309-1311.

[92] Khamashta MA, Cuadrado MJ, Mujic F, Taub NA, Hunt BJ, Hughes GR. The management of thrombosis in the antiphospholipid-antibody syndrome. *N Engl J Med.* 1995;332:993-997.

[93] Shehata HA, Nelson-Piercy C, Khamashta MA. Management of pregnancy in antiphospholipid syndrome. *Rheum Dis Clin North Am.* 2001;27:643-659.

[94] Dentali F, Crowther M. Acquired thrombophilia during pregnancy. *Obstet Gynecol Clin North Am.* 2006;33:375-388.

[95] Rai R, Cohen H, Dave M, Regan L. Randomised controlled trial of aspirin and aspirin plus heparin in pregnant women with recurrent miscarriage associated with phospholipid antibodies (or antiphospholipid antibodies). *BMJ.* 1997;314:253-257.

[96] Kutteh WH. Antiphospholipid antibody-associated recurrent pregnancy loss: treatment with heparin and low-dose aspirin is superior to low-dose aspirin alone. *Am J Obstet Gynecol.* 1996;174:1584-1589.

[97] Farquharson RG, Quenby S, Greaves M. Antiphospholipid syndrome in pregnancy: a randomized, controlled trial of treatment. *Obstet Gynecol.* 2002;100:408-413.

[98] Wawrzynska L, Tomkowski WZ, Przedlacki J, Hajduk B, Torbicki A. Changes in bone density during long-term administration of low-molecular-weight heparins or acenocoumarol for secondary prophylaxis of venous thromboembolism. *Pathophysiol Haemost Thromb.* 2003;33:64-67.

[99] Pattison NS, Chamley LW, Birdsall M, Zanderigo AM, Liddell HS, McDougall J. Does aspirin have a role in improving pregnancy outcome for women with the antiphospholipid syndrome? A randomized controlled trial. *Am J Obstet Gynecol.* 2000;183:1008-1012.

[100] Cleary-Goldman J, Bettes B, Robinson JN, Norwitz E, Schulkin J. Thrombophilia and the obstetric patient. *Obstet Gynecol.* 2007;110:669-674.

[101] Gris JC, Mercier E, Quere I, Lavigne-Lissalde G, Cochery-Nouvellon E, Hoffet M, Ripart-Neveu S, Tailland ML, Dauzat M, Marès P. Low-molecular-weight heparin versus low-dose aspirin in women with one fetal loss and a constitutional thrombophilic disorder. *Blood.* 2004;103:3695-3699.

[102] Kist WJ, Janssen NG, Kalk JJ, Hague WM, Dekker GA, de Vries JI. Thrombophilias and adverse pregnancy outcome—A confounded problem! *Thromb Haemost.* 2008;99:77-85.

Fetal Morbidity
and Neonatal Complications

In: Textbook of Perinatal Epidemiology
Editor: Eyal Sheiner, pp. 411-438

ISBN: 978-1-60741-648-7
© 2010 Nova Science Publishers, Inc.

Chapter XXI

Epidemiology of Neural Tube Defects

PJ Lupo, AJ Etheredge, A. Agopian and LE Mitchell[*]

Institute of Biosciences and Technology, Texas A&M University System Health Science
Center, Houston, TX., USA

Definitions

- Anencephaly: Lethal malformation caused by failure of fusion in the cranial region of the neural tube during neurulation.
- Malformation: Structural birth defect resulting from an intrinsically abnormal developmental process. Malformations may occur in isolation, in association with other malformations, or as part of a syndrome.
- Maternal genetic effect: Effect of the maternal genotype on the phenotype of offspring that is not attributable to the Mendelian transmission of genes.
- Myelomeningocele: Severe malformation caused by failure of fusion in the caudal region of the neural tube during neurulation; commonly referred to as spina bifida.
- Neural tube: Embryonic precursor of the brain and spinal cord.
- Neural tube defects (NTDs): Structural malformations resulting from a failure in the process of neural tube development (e.g. anencephaly and myelomingocele).
- Neurulation: Embryological processes that result in the formation of the neural tube.
- Population stratification: Differences in the frequencies of genetic variants (i.e. alleles) between cases and controls, due to systematic differences in ancestry rather than association of genes with disease. Failure to adequately account for

[*] For Correspondence: Laura E. Mitchell, Ph.D., University of Texas School of Public Health, 1200 Herman Pressler Dr., E547, Houston, TX 77030, laura.e.mitchell@uth.tmc.edu, 713-500-9954 (T), 713-500-9958 (F)

population stratification can lead to false positive genetic associations or population stratification bias.

Introduction

Birth defects have a considerable global health impact, as they are both common and associated with significant morbidity and mortality. Worldwide, it is estimated that 6% of infants (~8 million/year) are born with a serious birth defect, at least 3.3 million children under age 5 die each year from birth defects, and approximately 3.2 million children born with a birth defect each year survive with lifelong, birth defect-related disabilities.[1] In the United States (U.S.), birth defects represent the principal cause of pediatric hospitalizations[2] and death in the first year of life,[3] and are a major source of medical expenditures; the national lifetime costs for infants born with one or more of 17 common birth defects in a single year has been estimated to exceed 5 billion dollars.[4]

Some of the most common birth defects involve malformations of the spinal cord and brain (i.e. neural tube defects). Such birth defects represent a vastly heterogeneous set of conditions with diverse etiologies. Despite this diversity, epidemiological strategies have been successfully used to characterize and identify risk factors for many of these malformations.

Embryology

Neural tube defects (NTDs) are a group of structural malformations that result from abnormal development of the neural tube, the embryonic structure that develops into the brain and spinal cord. During the third week post-conception, the embryonic precursor of the neural tube, known as the neural plate, develops from ectoderm cells.[5] This plate is transformed into the neural tube by a process referred to as primary neurulation. During primary neurulation, the neural plate undergoes a series of shaping and folding events followed by midline fusion, which results in the formation of the cylindrical neural tube. In humans, primary neurulation forms the region of the neural tube that will develop into the brain and the majority of the spinal cord, and is completed by about 25 days post-conception.[6, 7] Upon completion of primary neurulation, the neural tube is extended caudally by a process known as secondary neurulation. During secondary neurulation, a solid rod of mesenchymal cells is transformed into an epithelial tube.[8]

Classification and Clinical Impact

NTDs are often classified as being "open" or "closed". Open NTDs result from defects in primary neurulation and are characterized by exposure of the affected region of the neural tube to the body surface. Annually, the most common open NTDs, myelomeningocele and anencephaly, occur in 3,000 pregnancies in the U.S. and 324,000 births worldwide.[1, 9] Closed NTDs include a range of conditions that result from defects in secondary neurulation. The closed NTDs are entirely covered by skin and are generally less severe than open NTDs (Table 1).[10]

Table 1. Types of open and closed neural tube defects (NTDs).

Defect	Description
Open NTDs	
Myelomingocele (spina bifida)	Meninges and neural tissue protrude through spinal defect
Anencephaly	Absence of cranial skull and forebrain (lethal)
Craniorachischisis	Severe spinal and cranial skull defects expose brain and spinal cord (lethal)
Closed NTDs	
Occult spinal dysraphism (spina bifida occult)	Spinal defect without protrusion of tissue
Meningocele	Meninges protrude through spinal defect
Lipomeningocele	Lipomatous mass protrudes through spinal defect
Encephalocele	Brain tissue protrudes through skull defect
Iniencephaly	Severe spinal defects with cranial retroflexion (lethal)
Sacral agenesis	Complete or partial absence of sacrum

Open NTDs

Myelomeningocele: Myelomeningocele, also referred to as spina bifida cystica, or often simply spina bifida, results from failure of fusion in the caudal region of the neural tube during primary neurulation. This condition is characterized by an open lesion on the spine, through which an abnormally formed spinal cord and damaged membranes and nerves are exposed to the body surface. Although the open lesions can be surgically closed, the underlying neurological damage is permanent.

Spina bifida related morbidity and mortality are associated with both the size and location of the neural tube defect, with the worst outcomes generally occurring among infants with the largest and highest lesions. However, with appropriate medical care, most infants with spina bifida will survive the neonatal period (e.g. one-year survival of infants with spina bifida born in the U.S. between 1995 and 2001 was 92%[11]) and into adulthood.[12-14] Morbidity among affected individuals is related to secondary nervous system malformations (e.g. Arnold-Chiari II malformation, hydrocephalus)[15] and disabilities including lower extremity weakness and paralysis, sensory loss, bowel and bladder dysfunction, orthopedic abnormalities, and specific learning disabilities.[15]

Healthcare management for individuals with spina bifida often involves an array of approaches, including surgical interventions (e.g. shunting for hydrocephalus), ambulation-assistive devices and therapies, orthopedic treatments, urologic management, and psychosocial care, and is extremely costly. Average medical expenditures for children with spina bifida in the U.S. are estimated to be 13 times greater than that for children without spina bifida,[16] with estimated national lifetime medical costs for children born with spina bifida in a given year of over $200,000,000.[4]

Anencephaly: Anencephaly results from failure of fusion in the cranial region of the neural tube during primary neurulation. This condition is characterized by incomplete formation of the forebrain and skull, resulting in exposure of the brain to the body surface.[10] Anencephaly is a lethal condition for which there is no treatment. Many fetuses affected with anencephaly die *in utero*, and those that survive to term are either stillborn or die in early infancy.[17]

Craniorachischisis: Craniorachischisis is an open NTD that is generally quite rare. This condition results from failure of neural tube fusion along the entire body axis[18] and, like anencephaly, is a lethal condition.

Closed NTDs

Closed NTDs include a range of conditions (e.g. occult spinal dysraphism, meningocele, lipomeningocele, encephalocele, iniencephaly, sacral agenesis)[19] that are generally less severe than the open NTDs (Table 1). However, iniencephaly, a rare closed NTD that is characterized by severe spinal defects and retroflexion (backward bending) of the head, is a lethal condition,[17, 20] and encephaloceles, which are characterized by herniation of the brain and/or meninges through a defect in the skull, are frequently associated with neurological impairments.[17]

Due to their prevalence and severity, epidemiological investigations have overwhelmingly focused on the common open NTDs, spina bifida (i.e. myelomeningocele) and anencephaly.[21] Hence, the remainder of this chapter focuses on these two conditions and, hereafter, the acronym, NTD(s), refers specifically to these two malformations.

Etiologic Heterogeneity

NTDs are known to be etiologically heterogeneous, and are often sub-grouped based on knowledge regarding known or suspected causes. As spina bifida and/or anencephaly can occur as part of over 50 identifiable syndromes or sequences of chromosomal (e.g. trisomy 13, trisomy 18, and triploidy), genetic (e.g. Meckel and Waardenburg syndromes), teratogenic, or unknown origin, common subgroups include the syndromic and nonsyndromic NTDs. Within the subgroup of syndromic NTDs, cases are often further differentiated based on the underlying cause of the syndrome.

Syndromic NTDs

Chromosomal: Chromosome abnormalities, including several aneuplodies, cytogenetic duplications/deletions, ring chromosomes, and microdeletions[22-24] are reported to occur in 2-10% of infants with NTDs, and appear to be more common among spontaneous abortions and fetal losses with NTDs.[25-29] Chromosome abnormalities also appear to be more common among infants with spina bifida than in those with anencephaly.[30]

Genetic: A small proportion of NTDs occur in association with Mendelian (i.e. single-gene) syndromes. Although these conditions are extremely rare, the recurrence risk (for the syndrome with or without an NTD) for siblings of an affected individual can be as high as 50%. Rare families, in which apparently, nonsyndromic forms of spina bifida and/or anencephaly segregate in an X-linked or autosomal recessive fashion, have also been identified.[1, 31-33]

Teratogenic: Teratogenic exposures that give rise to malformation syndromes that include NTDs are discussed in subsequent sections of this chapter.

Non-Syndromic NTDs

In the majority of individuals with an NTD (approximately 70-94%), no underlying syndrome or sequence can be identified. Such cases are referred to as non-syndromic NTDs. Within the subgroup of non-syndromic NTDs, cases are often further differentiated based on the presence or absence of non-secondary (i.e. independent) malformations.

Associated: NTDs that occur in association with other malformations that, collectively, do not form a recognizable syndrome and are not secondary to the NTD are often referred to as "associated" or "multiple" NTDs. Birth defects that are commonly observed with non-syndromic NTDs include facial clefting, cardiac defects, limb reduction defects, abdominal wall defects, renal anomalies, anophthalmia/microphthalmia, and anotia/microtia.[34]

Isolated: The majority of nonsyndromic NTDs occur as isolated malformations. Although individuals with isolated NTDs may have other conditions, such as hydrocephalus or club foot, these conditions are thought to be secondary to the NTD.

The extent to which the etiologies of isolated and associated NTDs overlap is not clear.[35] However, there is evidence that at least some of the epidemiological characteristics of these two subgroups of NTDs differ, suggesting that there may well be some etiologic differences.[35]

Familial Aggregation

Non-syndromic NTDs demonstrate familial aggregation with co-segregation of spina bifida and anencephaly within the same family. Such co-segregation provides strong evidence of a shared genetic contribution to the risk of spina bifida and anencephaly. However, the observed familial aggregation patterns, which include a sibling recurrence risk of 3-8%, and increased risks to monozygotic as compared to dizygotic co-twins,[36, 37] are not consistent with simple Mendelian inheritance,[38, 39] and strongly suggest that NTDs are complex conditions determined by the effects of multiple genetic and environmental factors. As nonsyndromic NTDs are more prevalent among consanguineous as compared to non-consanguineous matings,[40-42] it is likely that at least some of these genes act in an autosomal recessive manner.

Methodologic Issues in Epidemiologic Studies of NTDs

Ascertainment

A fundamental challenge in birth defect epidemiology is the assessment of occurrence. Early pregnancy loss directly affects the ability to study many birth defects, such that complete ascertainment of cases as well as delineation of the "at-risk" population is not possible. Incomplete ascertainment may occur as a result of unrecognized and unreported pregnancy loss as well as medical terminations of pregnancy that may not be captured by vital record or other surveillance systems.[29, 43, 44] For example, in California (1989-1991), the birth prevalence of anencephaly among live births and stillbirths was almost 52% lower than the total prevalence, which included live births, stillbirths, and elective terminations.[45] Hence, the number of cases lost to elective terminations may be quite substantial.

Because neither the numerator (i.e. cases) nor the denominator (i.e. at risk pregnancies) can be accurately estimated, birth defect epidemiologists prefer to express the frequency of occurrence of NTDs as a birth prevalence, usually as the total number of ascertained cases divided by the number of live births, rather than an incidence.[46] Variations in inclusion/exclusion of early fetal deaths and/or medical terminations, mechanisms of disease surveillance (e.g. passive vs. active) and clinical criteria for defining cases all impact the extent to which prevalence estimates approximate the true disease incidence.

Incomplete ascertainment of potential cases will bias estimates of prevalence and may also lead to selection bias in studies of potential disease risk factors. Such bias can arise because the cases that are ascertained (e.g. those that survive to birth) may be different than those that are not ascertained.[45, 47] For example, if access or beliefs regarding elective termination and prenatal diagnosis differ across maternal sociodemographic groups and the cases include only live births affected by an NTD, the observed associations between maternal sociodemographics and risk of having an NTD-affected pregnancy may be biased.

Case Definition

As discussed above, defects of the neural tube are a heterogeneous group of malformations that can be classified in multiple ways (e.g. open/closed; syndromic/nonsyndromic). Most epidemiological investigations of NTDs are restricted to include open, nonsyndromic NTDs. However, there are studies that include encephaloceles or other closed NTDs with the common open NTDs, anencephaly and spina bifida. In addition, there is considerable variability across studies with regard to the inclusion/exclusion of associated NTDs. Such differences in case definitions across studies reflect the current uncertainties regarding the relationship between the various subcategories of NTDs. As understanding of the etiology of these various malformations improves, more refined strategies for sub-grouping cases are likely to emerge.

Within studies that are restricted to nonsyndromic anencephaly and spina bifida, it is unclear whether these two conditions should be "lumped" or "split" for analysis. Use of composite end points (lumping) has the advantage of increasing statistical power, relative to analyses based on the individual components (splitting), when the exposure of interest has a similar effect on each of the component outcomes. However, if the exposure effects are variable across end points, power can be reduced and differences between the component end points, which might help to clarify disease mechanisms, can be obscured. The use of polytomous logistic regression, which can be used to formally assess heterogeneity of the exposure effect across the different components of a composite end point,[48] may help to resolve the lumping versus splitting issues in studies of anencephaly and spina bifida. Given the wealth of epidemiological data available for these conditions, such analyses are feasible, but have yet to be applied.

Maternal Effects

In general, etiological studies consider the genotype, characteristics, and exposure histories of case individuals. However, for birth defects, the exposure history of interest is that of the mother of the case and the effect of such exposures may well be modulated by the maternal genotype and other maternal characteristics. The need to account for maternal characteristics and exposures is well recognized in the field of birth defect epidemiology. Less recognized is the need to account for the maternal genotype, which, in addition to contributing to the offspring genome, governs the *in utero* environment of the developing offspring. Given the strong correlation between the maternal and embryonic (i.e. case) genotypes, it is important to account for both genotypes when modeling the effect of genetic variants on disease risk.[49]

Despite the many challenges, there are several features of NTDs (and birth defects in general) that simplify epidemiological studies relative to other conditions. Since the neural tube closes around week four of gestation, there is a narrow window in which exposures could result in an NTD (i.e. there is a short induction period). In addition, given that the time of ascertainment for cases is relatively close to the time of birth, parents, and possibly grandparents of the case may be recruited for participation in a study. This is particularly useful for studies that have a genetic focus. Furthermore, NTDs have a remarkably obvious, consistent phenotype making the diagnostics very straightforward and, finally, existing birth defects registries provide a convenient resource for case ascertainment.

Study Design

Although NTDs are considered a common birth defect, they are relatively rare. This is an important factor when selecting a design for studies of NTDs. Several traditional, observational, population-based epidemiologic study designs, as well as clinical/community trials, have been used in the study of NTDs (Table 2). In addition, family-based approaches have been used for studies that focus on genetic risk factors related to NTDs.

Table 2. Strengths and weaknesses of designs commonly used in epidemiological studies of neural tube defects.

Study Design	Strengths	Weaknesses
Population-based		
Cross-sectional	Relatively quick and inexpensive Hypothesis generating	Temporal sequence hard to establish Summary measures of previous exposure may not be accurate
Case-control	Permits study of a wide range of exposures (genetic and/or environmental) and outcomes Appropriate for studying rare outcomes	Not appropriate for studying rare exposures Difficult to identify valid control group Inability to assess maternal genetic effects
Clinical and community trials	Considered the "gold-standard" when assessing causation Robust against potential confounding factors Allows for the "control" of exposure levels	Ethical considerations Relatively expensive Difficult for rare outcomes
Family-based		
Case-parent triad	Appropriate for studying maternal and embryonic genetic effects Robust to population stratification bias when assessing embryonic genetic effects	Cannot study main effect of environmental exposures Increased cost of genotyping relative to case-control studies

Population-Based Studies

Cross-sectional: In a cross-sectional study (or prevalence study), a sample of a reference population is assessed at a given point in time, proving a "snapshot" of the population. For example, maternal characteristics, geographic patterns, and temporal trends can be determined with cross-sectional studies. These studies are often quicker, easier, and more economical than other epidemiologic study designs. However, this design is limited by its inability to clearly establish the temporal sequence between exposure and outcome.

Cross-sectional studies have been used to characterize the occurrence of NTDs. For example, cross-sectional studies have been used to assess the impact of folic acid fortification, as well as prenatal diagnosis and elective pregnancy termination on the birth prevalence of NTDs.[50-52] Issues regarding temporal sequence are generally less of a concern for cross-sectional studies of birth defects than for conditions with later onset, given the relatively narrow window during which an exposure might influence NTD occurrence. Moreover, temporal sequence was not an issue in the studies that assessed the impact of folic acid fortification or prenatal diagnosis on NTD prevalence, as this sequence was easily established (e.g. folic acid fortification preceded a decline in the birth prevalence of NTDs).

Case-control: Case-control studies are the most common epidemiologic study design used to evaluate potential risk factors (both environmental and genetic) associated with NTDs. Many such studies rely on birth defects surveillance data and/or birth certificates to identify both case and control groups. In the case-control design, the odds of exposure to a suspected risk factor are compared between cases (i.e. those with the outcome of interest) and controls (i.e. those without the outcome of interest). This study design is particularly useful when studying rare outcomes, such as NTDs, and is often used in studies of genetic risk factors. Case-control studies of genetic risk factors are, however, vulnerable to a type of confounding referred to as "population stratification bias", in which a false association between a genotype and disease, or the masking of a genotypic effect, is induced by the existence of subgroups within a population (e.g. different racial or ethnic groups) that have different genetic profiles (i.e. genotypes) and frequencies of disease.[53] In addition, the retrospective nature of this approach often limits the ability to adequately reconstruct exposure history, although this is not an issue for studies of potential genetic risk factors.

The National Birth Defects Prevention Study (NBDPS) is a large, ongoing case-control study of birth defects that has provided a tremendous amount of information about NTDs and other structural malformations.[54, 55] Although the traditional case-control design does not allow for the assessment of maternal genetic effects, the NBDPS has overcome this limitation by collecting biological samples from cases/controls as well as their parents.[56]

Variations of the case-control design, such as case-only,[57, 58] case-crossover,[59] and case-time-control[59] studies may also prove useful in the study of NTDs and other structural malformations, but have not been widely applied in this field.

Clinical/Community Trials: Randomized clinical trials, in which individuals are randomly assigned to a treatment group, are often considered to be the gold-standard of epidemiologic study designs. Clinical trials may also be non-randomized (i.e. subjects self-select into treatment groups) or may involve the randomization of entire communities to treatment groups. Although the use of clinical trials is rare in the field of birth defect epidemiology, randomized, non-randomized and community trials all contributed to delineation of the NTD protective effect of maternal, periconceptional use of folic acid[60-62], as discussed later in this chapter.

Family Studies

While a relatively recent addition to the field of epidemiology, family-based studies have been central to genetic epidemiology for many years. Such studies can be used to estimate familial recurrence risks and assess inheritance patterns, as previously described for NTDs. Family-based studies can also be used to identify genes that are linked to or associated with a disease. Linkage-based approaches have not, however, been extensively applied to NTDs due to the rarity of families with multiple, available affected relatives.[63] Indeed only one small linkage analysis has been conducted for NTDs.[63] In contrast, family-based genetic association studies, which do not require the presence of multiple affected family members, are well suited to the study of NTDs.

The basic family-based study design used in genetic association studies is referred to as the case-parent triad design. The triad for which this design is named is composed of the affected (i.e. case) individual and his or her biological parents. This design is particular useful for studies of birth defects and conditions with early disease onset, since parents are generally available. Several methods for analyzing the data generated in a case-parent triad study have been developed, including the transmission disequilbrium test[64, 65] and approaches using log-linear models.[66] The case-parent triad design has the advantage (as compared to case-control studies) of being immune to population stratification bias when assessing the effects of the case genotype. In addition, this design can be used to assess maternal genetic effects without incurring additional genotyping expenses (i.e. in the case-control design, evaluation of the maternal and case genotype would require genotyping cases and controls as well as the mothers of these individuals). Variations on the triad design include the pent-design, which incorporates genotype data from maternal grandparents, and hybrid-designs, which incorporate aspects of both case-control and family based designs.[67, 68]

Epidemiology

NTDs are among the most common, serious malformations, occurring in about 2-5 in 10,000 births in the U.S.[69, 70] However, there are many factors that are known to be associated with variations in the prevalence of these conditions. In addition, many potential NTD risk factors have been identified (Table 3). Suspected etiologic factors include maternal nutritional status, maternal diseases and characteristics, maternal use of certain drugs and medications, parental exposure to occupational and environmental toxicants, and genetic factors that may act through the embryonic or the maternal genotype.

Table 3. Known and strongly suspected neural tube defect risk factors.

Risk Factor	Relative Risk
Demographics	
Female infant sex	1.4-1.7
Hispanic ethnicity	1.2-1.5
Nutrition	
Folate deficiency	2-8
Family history	
Sibling of affected individual	10-30
Maternal illnesses and conditions	
Pre-gestational diabetes	2-10
Maternal obesity	2-4
Hyperthermia	2
Gestational diabetes	2-3
Medications	
Antiepileptic drugs	3-20

Descriptive Epidemiology

Location: Geographical differences in the prevalence of NTDs have been clearly demonstrated. Among Caucasian populations, the highest prevalence is seen in Ireland, where the prevalence is 5-10 per 10,000 births.[71, 72] Worldwide, the highest prevalence is seen in some areas of Northern China, were the prevalence is as high as 140/10,000 and the distribution of defects is shifted to more severe phenotypes.[73, 74] High prevalences have also been observed in Guatemala, India and some eastern Mediterranean populations.[75]

Race/Ethnicity: The prevalence of NTDs also differs by race and ethnicity. In the U.S. the prevalence of NTDs in offspring is higher in Hispanic and lower in black women, as compared to Caucasian women.[52, 76-79] Compared to offspring of non-Hispanic Caucasian mothers, the prevalence ratios for anencephaly and spina bifida among offspring of Hispanic mothers in the U.S. were reported to be 1.5 (95% confidence interval: 1.3-1.8) and 1.2 (95% confidence interval: 1.1-1.4), respectively.[78] It is not clear to what extent differences in the prevalence of NTDs across race and ethnicity are driven by genetic, nutritional, social, or other factors. However, some (although not all) studies have found that the risk of NTDs is higher for Mexican-born Hispanics in the U.S. compared to those born in the U.S.,[80-82] suggesting that environmental factors are likely to play a role.

Sex: The prevalence of NTDs is higher among females than males,[81, 83-86] and this effect is slightly more pronounced among infants with anencephaly than spina bifida (i.e. sex ratios of 0.6 and 0.7, respectively).[87]

Other: The prevalence of NTDs has also been suggested to vary with a number of additional factors, including altitude and season of conception.[81, 82, 84, 85, 88-91] However, the relationships between these factors and NTD prevalence have not been consistently corroborated.

Nutritional Risk Factors

Maternal Folate Status: Maternal folate status appears to be the most common modifier of NTD risk in the human population.[92, 93] Decades of research, including several community/clinical trials, have convincingly demonstrated the NTD-protective role of maternal folic acid supplementation.[61, 94] (Note: Folic acid is the oxidized and synthetic form of the B vitamin folate. It is more bio-available than natural dietary folates and is used in nutritional supplements and food fortification programs.) This body of work indicates that maternal periconceptional folic acid supplementation can reduce the prevalence of NTDs by 30 to 70%, and provides the basis for the U.S. Public Health Service recommendations that women capable of becoming pregnant should consume 400 µg of folic acid a day and women who have previously had a child with an NTD should consume 4000 µg of folic acid a day when planning a new pregnancy.[95] In addition, this work has lead to the implementation of mandatory folic acid fortification of the food supply in several countries. Emerging data from these programs indicate that mandatory food fortification (~200 µg/day) is associated with a subsequent 30-50% reduction in the prevalence of NTDs.[96, 97]

Although the exact mechanism by which folate decreases NTD risk is not understood, many consider the detection of this association and subsequent fortification of the U.S. food supply with folic acid one of the greatest modern triumphs of epidemiology. However, as it is has been estimated that the current food fortification programs are only able to prevent 6.8% of folate-sensitive NTDs worldwide,[98] the full public health impact of this work has yet to be realized.

Folate Related Genes: Based on the evidence that maternal folate status influences the risk of NTDs, much of the research on the genetics of NTDs has focused on candidate genes that are involved in folate-related pathways. Although many such candidate genes (e.g. *CBS*, *MTR*, *MTHFD1*, *MTRR*, *RFC-1*, *SHMT*, *FR-α* and *FR-β*) (reviewed in[99]) have been proposed, no single gene has been consistently identified as a risk factor for NTDs.

The most widely studied variant in a folate related gene is the C677T, single nucleotide polymorphism (SNP) in the *MTHFR* gene. This variant has been found to be associated with NTD risk in several studies. However, there are studies that have failed to confirm this association. Moreover, the majority of the published studies on this association have failed to adequately account for the potential effects of both the maternal and the case genotype, and only a small proportion of these studies have considered the impact of potential effect modifiers, such as maternal folate status.[100-106] As both maternal genetic effects[106] and gene-nutrition interactions,[101, 102] have been reported to affect the relationship between folate-related genes and NTD risk, future studies of this and other variants should include a more thorough interrogation of the disease-gene relationships.

Folate Receptor Autoantibodies: Maternal autoantibodies to the folate receptor have recently been associated with the occurrence of NTD-affected pregnancies.[107, 108] Though the evidence for such an association remains preliminary, the potential involvement of maternal immune responses in the development of NTDs provides a novel direction for future research.

Other Nutritional Factors: A variety of nutritional factors other than folic acid have been evaluated as risk factors for NTDs, however none have as a compelling effect as folic acid.

Several epidemiologic studies have examined the association between maternal zinc levels, but the results of such studies have been inconsistent.[109-111] In addition, there is at least some evidence that vitamins such as B12, choline and methionine, which provide methyl groups for a range of important physiological reactions (e.g. DNA synthesis, cell membrane integrity, and methyl metabolism) and have the ability to affect genomic stability and regulation of gene function through methylation of DNA, may be related to NTD risk.[112] For example, based on a review of 17 epidemiologic studies, it was concluded that there is a moderate association between maternal B12 levels and risk of NTDs.[113] Moreover, both periconceptional intake of dietary choline and maternal dietary methionine intake have been found to be associated with the risk of NTDs, independent of the effects of maternal folate status.[114, 115]

Associations between NTD risk and maternal inositol levels or intake of the dietary form of this vitamin (i.e. myo-inositol) have also been studied. These studies suggest that women carrying NTD-affected pregnancies may have lower blood inositol concentrations than women with unaffected pregnancies, and that the outcome of pregnancies subsequent to an NTD affected pregnancy may be better in women who take both folic acid and inositol as compared to those who do not.[109, 116-118] However, an association between inositol and NTD risk has not been firmly established, and there are currently no recommendations regarding maternal use of inositol comparable to those that have been made regarding folic acid.

Maternal Illnesses and Characteristics

The composition and state of the maternal habitus have been associated with the risk of having an NTD-affected pregnancy (e.g. obesity, low prepregnancy weight, and inadequate weight gain or famine exposure during pregnancy) (reviewed in [119]). In addition, maternal illnesses such as diabetes and those with constitutional symptoms resulting from exogenous exposures (e.g. hyperthermia/febrile illnesses, diarrhea) have also been associated with increased risk of NTDs (reviewed in [120]). There are, however, only three firmly established maternal illnesses/characteristics that are associated with the risk of NTDs: diabetes, obesity and hyperthermia.

Maternal diabetes: Women with pre-gestational diabetes (type 1 and type 2) are at increased risk of having offspring with NTDs and other types of structural birth defects. Studies have suggested that, among these women, there is a two-fold to ten-fold higher risk of having a child with a central nervous system malformation.[121, 122] Using data from the National Birth Defects Prevention Study, maternal pre-gestational diabetes was found to be associated with isolated anencephaly (odds ratio = 3.4, 95% confidence interval: 1.1-10.3) and spina bifida with multiple defects (odds ratio = 8.0, 95% confidence interval: 1.6-39.7).[55] Although associations were not found with isolated spina bifida or anencephaly with multiple defects, this may be attributable to the small numbers of exposed cases in these categories (i.e. 2 and 0, respectively). The risk of NTDs in the offspring of women with gestational diabetes is not as great as those with pre-gestational diabetes; however, it does appear to be greater than the general population (reviewed in [122]).

Although pre-gestational diabetes is an established risk factor for congenital malformations, the mechanism underlying its effect has not been clearly determined. Data from murine models suggest the teratogenic effect of diabetes is likely to be the result of elevated glucose concentrations. These studies suggest that excess glucose induces oxidative stress and inositol depletion and may alter the expression of genes involved in embryonic development.[123-126] The risk of NTDs might also be determined by genetic variation in metabolic pathways related to the development of diabetes,[122] although no such genes have been convincingly shown to be associated with the risk of NTDs.

Maternal obesity: Maternal obesity has emerged as a consistent risk for NTDs and other structural malformations. Women in the highest body mass index (BMI) categories (i.e. obese or BMI > 29 kg/m^2) have a 1.5- to 3.5-fold higher risk of having an NTD affected pregnancy than do women in lower categories.[127-129] A recent analysis of prepregnancy obesity in the National Birth Defects Prevention Study confirmed the association between maternal obesity and spina bifida; however the association was not present among those with anencephaly.[130] Although the mechanism is not entirely understood, obesity is associated with metabolic abnormalities, including impaired insulin metabolism. Data from one study suggest hyperinsulinemia may be the driving force for the observed risk of NTDs in obese women.[127] Since hyperinsulinemia might precede or coexist with obesity and diabetes, this metabolic state may provide a link between these two risk factors.[122]

Interestingly, the risk of having a child with an NTD seems to be increased in women who have undergone gastric bypass surgery for the treatment of morbid obesity. However, as similar risks have not been observed following intestinal bypass surgery,[131-133] this association may be attributable to reduced absorption of nutrients, which is less of an issue after intestinal bypass than it is after gastric bypass, rather than the underlying obesity.[134]

Hyperthermia: There is substantial evidence that hyperthermia as a result of maternal fever increases the risk of having a child with an NTD.[135-137] In one population-based case-control study, maternal fever (odds ratio = 1.9; 95% confidence interval: 1.4-2.7) and febrile illness (odds ratio = 2.0; 95% confidence interval: 1.2-3.4) were both associated with having a NTD-affected pregnancy.[138] Although it is difficult to determine whether this association is attributable to raised body temperature or the underlying disorder, studies in animals demonstrate that maternal hyperthermia is teratogenic (reviewed in [122]).

Other: A range of additional maternal characteristics have been implicated as potential risk factors for NTDs, including: age, stress, socioeconomic status,[139] social networks,[140] diarrhea,[141] and dieting behavior.[142] These exposures require further investigation to establish their relationships with NTDs.

Maternal use of Drugs and Medications

Anticonvulsants: Many anticonvulsant drugs are known teratogens. In a study assessing these drugs as a group (including carbamazepine, phenobarbital, phenytoin, primidone, sulfasalazine, triamterene, and trimethoprim), the adjusted odd ratio of NTDs related to exposure was 2.8 (95% confidence interval: 1.7-4.6).[143] Similar associations have also been reported for individual drugs in this class. For example, in a Dutch study, the risk for NTDs among carbamazepine exposed infants was 4.9 (95% confidence interval: 1.6-15.0)[144] and a study in France revealed the odds ratio between maternal valproic acid use and spina bifida was 20.6 (95% confidence interval: 8.2-47.9).[145] It is of note that women who use these drugs for indications other than epilepsy (e.g. bipolar disease, migrane) are also at increase of having a child with an NTD.[122]

The mechanism by which anticonvulsants cause birth defects has not been established. Potential mechanisms include folic acid antagonism[143] and the formation of free radicals as byproducts of drug metabolism.[122] In either case, such potential mechanisms support the importance of studying genetic variants related to folate and drug metabolism in order to better characterize the effects of these exposures.

Other drugs and medications: In a population-based study assessing 121 drugs, other than common anticonvulsants, the only drug associated with NTDs among offspring was oxytetracycline, an antimicrobial medication.[146] An association between NTDs and maternal use of drugs that are folic acid antagonists (e.g. aminopterin, phenobarbital, and methotrexate) (odds ratio = 2.8; 95% confidence interval: 1.7-4.6) has also been reported [143].

In addition to medicinal drug use, illegal drug use is a suspected risk factor for NTDs. However, a study conducted among Mexican American woman found no association between maternal use of street drugs and NTDs after adjustment was made for cigarette smoking.[147] While maternal smoking has itself been suggested as a risk factor for NTDs, the evidence for such an association remains equivocal.[148]

Parental Occupational and Environmental Exposures

Organic solvents: Occupational exposure to organic solvents is relatively common.[149] Studies of the association between both maternal and paternal exposure to organic solvents and congenital malformations have provided conflicting results. Two studies have reported no association between maternal occupational solvent exposures and NTDs.[148, 150] However, a recent study assessing maternal exposure to benzene reported an odds ratio of 5.3 (95% confidence interval: 1.4-21.1) for neural crest malformations (including NTDs).[151] In addition, among Mexican Americans, mothers exposed to solvents were 2.5 times more likely (95% confidence interval: 1.3-4.7) to have NTD-affected pregnancies than control mothers.[152] In a meta-analysis, mothers of infants with "major malformations" (including NTDs) had 1.6 greater odds of exposure (95% confidence interval: 1.2-2.3) to organic solvents than control mothers.[153]

Paternal occupational exposures have also been hypothesized to increase NTD risk via genetic damage to germ cells or indirect exposure to the mother from "carry-home" exposures.[119] Although studies of the association between paternal exposure to organic solvents and NTD risk have also provided conflicting results,[154-157] a meta-analysis of such studies, reported odds ratios of 1.9 (95% confidence interval: 1.4-2.5) for all NTDs and 2.2 (95% confidence interval: 1.5-3.1) for anencephaly.[149]

Hazardous waste sites: It is assumed that people living near hazardous waste sites are exposed to chemicals released from the site into the air, water, or soil.[158] The pollutants found most frequently in the air at hazardous waste sites, in decreasing order, are: benzene, toluene, perchloroethylene, and trichloroethylene.[159] Several studies have reported an increased risk of NTDs among the offspring of women living near hazardous waste sites.[160, 161] In a study conducted in five European countries (Belgium, Denmark, France, Italy, and the UK) and including 21 landfills, living within 3 km of a landfill with airborne toxic chemical waste was reported to be a significant risk factor for NTDs after adjustment for socioeconomic status (odds ratio = 3.8, 95% confidence interval: 1.0-14.4).[162] However, other studies have failed to identify similar associations.[163, 164]

For both occupational studies assessing organic solvent exposure, and studies assessing exposure to hazardous waste sites, equivocal findings regarding an association with NTD risk may be due to several variables: differences in exposure assessment, inadequate adjustment for potential confounders, and small sample sizes. Nonetheless, there is evidence that chemicals found in the work place and at hazardous waste sites are associated with NTDs.

Other: Other environmental factors and pollutants are suspected of being associated with NTDs (see Table 3). For example, by-products of water disinfection (e.g. trihalomethane), fumonisins (a mycotoxin produced by the fungus *Fusarium verticillioides* found in corn), as well as arsenic and other heavy metals have been associated with NTDs in some studies but not others (reviewed in [15]).[165] Other exposures (e.g. polycyclic aromatic hydrocarbons and ambient air pollution), which are suspected to be NTD risk factors based on studies in animals or other types of birth defects, have yet to be adequately studied as NTD risk factors in humans.[166-170]

There is a need for well-designed studies to determine if these factors are associated with NTDs. In such studies, it may be important to account for genetic variation that influences individual susceptibility to these exposures. For instance, genes responsible for phase-I or phase-II metabolism (e.g. cytochrome P450 and glutathione conjugation, respectively) are important in the biotransformation of these environmental toxicants. Furthermore, if genotoxicity after exposure to environment pollution is a potential mechanism of teratogenesis, variation in DNA repair mechanism genes may be important to assess in conjunction with such exposures.

Genetic Risk Factors (Other than Folate-Related Genes)

Though more than 190 mouse models and strains with NTDs exist,[171] few human homologues of these genes have been assessed as NTD risk factors,[15] and none have been identified to be major NTD genes.[172] Three non-folate genes that are of some interest as NTD risk factors are *T(brachyury)*, *PAX3*, and *VANGL1*.

T(brachyury): The *T* gene encodes a transcription factor required for mesodermal differentiation and normal axial development, and has been implicated as an NTD risk factor in mouse studies.[173] The human *T* gene contains an intronic variant (i.e. *TIVS7* T/C) that has been associated with NTDs in several studies. However, this association remains to be convincingly established.[63, 174-176]

PAX3: Mutations of *PAX3* have been identified in humans with Waardenburg syndrome type I. Individuals with this genetic disorder often have congenital sensorineural deafness and partial albinism, and occasionally have spina bifida. In mice, mutations in *Pax3* have also been shown to lead to a phenotype which includes NTDs. In the human studies conducted to date, *PAX3* does not seem to be strongly associated with spina bifida.[176-179] However, these studies have been conducted using relatively small sample sizes, and have not provided a thorough interrogation of the variation with *PAX3*. Hence, definitive conclusions regarding an association between this gene and NTD risk in humans are precluded at this time.

VANGL1: Genes involved in the planar cell polarity pathway, including *VANGL1*, have been implicated as NTD risk factors by studies in animals, and may be good candidates for further studies in humans.[180] Signals from this pathway direct cell polarity during convergent extension, which is a cellular rearrangement process important to normal neural tube closure. However, associations with genes in this pathway have not yet been well studied within human populations.

As for other complex human disease, identifying genetic risk factors for NTDs has proven difficult and no major causative gene has been identified. Many of the genetic association studies in humans have had relatively small sample sizes and might not have had adequate power to detect modest associations (particularly in subgroup analyses). It is suspected that given the complex nature of NTDs, many modest associations are likely to exist rather than few strong associations. This effect may consist of both independent effects of specific genes, as well as interaction between genes. Furthermore, both embryonic (i.e. inherited) genetic effects and maternal genetic effects may exist. Thus, future studies should be based on large sample sizes and be designed to account for both independent maternal and embryonic genetic effects, and interactions.

Future Directions

In the future, new technologies and methodologies will likely provide improved tools for identifying NTD risk factors (both environmental and genetic). There are currently a myriad of available biomarkers for environmental exposures, none of which have proven to be the most reliable for epidemiologic studies.[181] As investigators agree upon the most reliable biomarkers of exposure, concerns over exposure misclassification will be reduced and estimates of effect for various risk factors will become more valid. Likewise, genomewide association studies have already proven helpful in identifying genes associated with human disease and likely will be utilized in human NTD studies in the future. Also on the horizon are studies assessing copy number variants and epigenetic gene expression modification as potentially important sources of genetic variation.[182, 183] Further in the future, genomewide sequencing and epigenomic studies may also become feasible.[184] As research in this field advances, well-designed studies, appropriate analysis techniques, and replication of results will continue to be critical.

References

[1]   Christianson A, Howson CP, Modell B. March of Dimes Global Report on Birth Defects. White Plains, New York: *March of Dimes Research Foundation;* 2006.

[2]   Yoon PW, Olney RS, Khoury MJ, Sappenfield WM, Chavez GF, Taylor D. Contribution of birth defects and genetic diseases to pediatric hospitalizations. A population-based study. *Arch Pediatr Adolesc Med* 1997;151:1096-103.

[3]   Martin JA, Kochanek KD, Strobino DM, Guyer B, MacDorman MF. Annual summary of vital statistics--2003. *Pediatrics* 2005;115:619-34.

[4]   California Birth Defects Monitoring Program. *The National Cost of Birth Defects;* 1995.

[5]   De Marco P, Merello E, Mascelli S, Capra V. Current perspectives on the genetic causes of neural tube defects. *Neurogenetics* 2006;7:201-21.

[6]   Nievelstein RA, Hartwig NG, Vermeij-Keers C, Valk J. Embryonic development of the mammalian caudal neural tube. *Teratology* 1993;48:21-31.

[7]   O'Rahilly R, Muller F. Minireview: summary of the initial development of the human nervous system. *Teratology* 1999;60:39-41.

[8]   Lowery LA, Sive H. Strategies of vertebrate neurulation and a re-evaluation of teleost neural tube formation. *Mech Dev* 2004;121:1189-97.

[9]   Mersereau P, Kilker, K., Carter, H., Fassett, E., Williams, J., Flores, A., Prue, C., Williams, L., Mai, C., Mulinare, J.,. Spina bifida and anencephaly before and after folic acid mandate--United States, 1995-1996 and 1999-2000. *MMWR Morb Mortal Wkly Rep* 2004;53:362-5.

[10]   Moore CA. Classification of Neural Tube Defects. *In: Wyszynski DF, ed. Neural Tube Defects: From Origin to Treatment.* New York City: Oxford University Press; 2006:66-75.

[11]   Bol KA, Collins JS, Kirby RS. Survival of infants with neural tube defects in the presence of folic acid fortification. *Pediatrics* 2006;117:803-13.

[12]   Bowman RM, McLone DG, Grant JA, Tomita T, Ito JA. Spina bifida outcome: a 25-year prospective. *Pediatr Neurosurg* 2001;34:114-20.

[13]   Singhal B, Mathew KM. Factors affecting mortality and morbidity in adult spina bifida. *Eur J Pediatr Surg* 1999;9 Suppl 1:31-2.

[14]   McDonnell GV, McCann JP. Why do adults with spina bifida and hydrocephalus die? A clinic-based study. *Eur J Pediatr Surg* 2000;10 Suppl 1:31-2.

[15]   Mitchell LE, Adzick NS, Melchionne J, Pasquariello PS, Sutton LN, Whitehead AS. Spina bifida. *Lancet* 2004;364:1885-95.

[16]   Ouyang L, Grosse SD, Armour BS, Waitzman NJ. Health care expenditures of children and adults with spina bifida in a privately insured U.S. population. *Birth Defects Res A Clin Mol Teratol* 2007;79:552-8.

[17]   Sanders RC, ed. Structural Fetal Abnormalities: *The Total Picture.* St. Louis: Mosby-Year Book, Inc.; 1996.

[18]   Greene NDE, Copp AJ. The Embryonic Basis of Neural Tube Defects. *In: Wyszynski DF, ed. Neural Tube Defects: From Origin to Treatment.* New York City: Oxford University Press; 2006:15-28.

[19] Lemire RJ. Neural tube defects. *JAMA* 1988;259:558-62.

[20] Jeanne-Pasquier C, Carles D, Alberti EM, Jacob B. [Iniencephaly: four cases and a review of the literature]. *J Gynecol Obstet Biol Reprod* (Paris) 2002;31:276-82.

[21] Mitchell LE. Epidemiology of neural tube defects. *Am J Med Genet C Semin Med Genet* 2005;135C:88-94.

[22] Lynch SA. Non-multifactorial neural tube defects. *Am J Med Genet C Semin Med Genet* 2005;135C:69-76.

[23] Ballarati L, Rossi E, Bonati MT, et al. 13q Deletion and central nervous system anomalies: further insights from karyotype-phenotype analyses of 14 patients. *J Med Genet* 2007;44:e60.

[24] Chen CP. Chromosomal abnormalities associated with neural tube defects (II): partial aneuploidy. *Taiwan J Obstet Gynecol* 2007;46:336-51.

[25] Creasy MR, Alberman ED. Congenital malformations of the central nervous system in spontaneous abortions. *J Med Genet* 1976;13:9-16.

[26] Byrne J, Warburton D. Neural tube defects in spontaneous abortions. *Am J Med Genet* 1986;25:327-33.

[27] McFadden DE, Kalousek DK. Survey of neural tube defects in spontaneously aborted embryos. *Am J Med Genet* 1989;32:356-8.

[28] Coerdt W, Miller K, Holzgreve W, Rauskolb R, Schwinger E, Rehder H. Neural tube defects in chromosomally normal and abnormal human embryos. *Ultrasound Obstet Gynecol* 1997;10:410-5.

[29] Philipp T, Kalousek DK. Neural tube defects in missed abortions: embryoscopic and cytogenetic findings. *Am J Med Genet* 2002;107:52-7.

[30] Chen CP. Chromosomal abnormalities associated with neural tube defects (I): full aneuploidy. *Taiwan J Obstet Gynecol* 2007;46:325-35.

[31] Baraitser M, Burn J. Brief clinical report: neural tube defects as an X-linked condition. *Am J Med Genet* 1984;17:383-5.

[32] Toriello HV, Bauserman SC, Higgins JV. Sibs with the fetal akinesia sequence, fetal edema, and malformations: a new syndrome? *Am J Med Genet* 1985;21:271-7.

[33] Farag TI, Teebi AS, Al-Awadi SA. Nonsyndromal anencephaly: possible autosomal recessive variant. *Am J Med Genet* 1986;24:461-4.

[34] Seaver LH, Stevenson RE. Syndromes with Neural Tube Defects. *In: Wyszynski DF, ed. Neural Tube Defects: From Origin to Treatment.* New York City: Oxford University Press; 2006:76-83.

[35] Rasmussen SA, Frías JL. Genetics of Syndromic Neural Tube Defects. *In: Wyszynski DF, ed. Neural Tube Defects: From Origin to Treatment.* New York City: Oxford University Press; 2006:185-97.

[36] Windham GC, Sever LE. Neural tube defects among twin births. *Am J Hum Genet* 1982;34:988-98.

[37] Jorde LB, Fineman RM, Martin RA. Epidemiology and genetics of neural tube defects: an application of the Utah Genealogical Data Base. *Am J Phys Anthropol* 1983;62:23-31.

[38] Drainer E, May HM, Tolmie JL. Do familial neural tube defects breed true? *J Med Genet* 1991;28:605-8.

[39] Garabedian BH, Fraser FC. Upper and lower neural tube defects: an alternate hypothesis. *J Med Genet* 1993;30:849-51.

[40] Zlotogora J. Genetic disorders among Palestinian Arabs: 1. Effects of consanguinity. *Am J Med Genet* 1997;68:472-5.

[41] Zlotogora J. Genetic disorders among Palestinian Arabs. 2. Hydrocephalus and neural tube defects. *Am J Med Genet* 1997;71:33-5.

[42] Mahadevan B, Bhat BV. Neural tube defects in Pondicherry. *Indian J Pediatr* 2005;72:557-9.

[43] Ethen MK, Canfield MA. Impact of including elective pregnancy terminations before 20 weeks gestation on birth defect rates. *Teratology* 2002;66 Suppl 1:S32-5.

[44] Correa-Villasenor A, Satten GA, Rolka H, Langlois P, Devine O. Random error and undercounting in birth defects surveillance data: implications for inference. *Birth Defects Res A Clin Mol Teratol* 2003;67:610-6.

[45] Velie EM, Shaw GM. Impact of prenatal diagnosis and elective termination on prevalence and risk estimates of neural tube defects in California, 1989-1991. *Am J Epidemiol* 1996;144:473-9.

[46] Mason CA, Kirby RS, Sever LE, Langlois PH. Prevalence is the preferred measure of frequency of birth defects. *Birth Defects Res A Clin Mol Teratol* 2005;73:690-2.

[47] Borman B, Cryer C. Fallacies of international and national comparisons of disease occurrence in the epidemiology of neural tube defects. *Teratology* 1990;42:405-12.

[48] Glynn RJ, Rosner B. Methods to evaluate risks for composite end points and their individual components. *J Clin Epidemiol* 2004;57:113-22.

[49] Mitchell LE, Weinberg CR. Evaluation of offspring and maternal genetic effects on disease risk using a family-based approach: the "pent" design. *Am J Epidemiol* 2005;162:676-85.

[50] Williams LJ, Mai CT, Edmonds LD, et al. Prevalence of spina bifida and anencephaly during the transition to mandatory folic acid fortification in the United States. *Teratology* 2002;66:33-9.

[51] Honein MA, Paulozzi LJ, Mathews TJ, Erickson JD, Wong LY. Impact of folic acid fortification of the US food supply on the occurrence of neural tube defects. *JAMA* 2001;285:2981-6.

[52] Cragan JD, Roberts HE, Edmonds LD, et al. Surveillance for anencephaly and spina bifida and the impact of prenatal diagnosis--United States, 1985-1994. *MMWR CDC Surveill Summ* 1995;44:1-13.

[53] Campbell CD, Ogburn EL, Lunetta KL, et al. Demonstrating stratification in a European American population. *Nat Genet* 2005;37:868-72.

[54] Reefhuis J, Honein MA, Schieve LA, Correa A, Hobbs CA, Rasmussen SA. Assisted reproductive technology and major structural birth defects in the United States. *Hum Reprod* 2008.

[55] Correa A, Gilboa SM, Besser LM, et al. Diabetes mellitus and birth defects. *Am J Obstet Gynecol* 2008;199:237 e1-9.

[56] Shi M, Umbach DM, Vermeulen SH, Weinberg CR. Making the most of case-mother/control-mother studies. *Am J Epidemiol* 2008;168:541-7.

[57] Khoury MJ, Flanders WD. Nontraditional epidemiologic approaches in the analysis of gene-environment interaction: case-control studies with no controls! *Am J Epidemiol* 1996;144:207-13.

[58] Albert PS, Ratnasinghe D, Tangrea J, Wacholder S. Limitations of the case-only design for identifying gene-environment interactions. *Am J Epidemiol* 2001;154:687-93.

[59] Hernandez-Diaz S, Hernan MA, Meyer K, Werler MM, Mitchell AA. Case-crossover and case-time-control designs in birth defects epidemiology. *Am J Epidemiol* 2003;158:385-91.

[60] Smithells RW, Nevin NC, Seller MJ, et al. Further experience of vitamin supplementation for prevention of neural tube defect recurrences. *Lancet* 1983;1:1027-31.

[61] MRC. Prevention of neural tube defects: results of the Medical Research Council Vitamin Study. MRC Vitamin Study Research Group. *Lancet* 1991;338:131-7.

[62] Berry RJ, Li Z, Erickson JD, et al. Prevention of neural-tube defects with folic acid in China. China-U.S. Collaborative Project for Neural Tube Defect Prevention. *N Engl J Med* 1999;341:1485-90.

[63] Speer MC, Melvin EC, Viles KD, et al. T locus shows no evidence for linkage disequilibrium or mutation in American Caucasian neural tube defect families. *Am J Med Genet* 2002;110:215-8.

[64] Schaid DJ, Sommer SS. Genotype relative risks: methods for design and analysis of candidate-gene association studies. *Am J Hum Genet* 1993;53:1114-26.

[65] Spielman RS, McGinnis RE, Ewens WJ. Transmission test for linkage disequilibrium: the insulin gene region and insulin-dependent diabetes mellitus (IDDM). *Am J Hum Genet* 1993;52:506-16.

[66] Weinberg CR, Wilcox AJ, Lie RT. A log-linear approach to case-parent-triad data: assessing effects of disease genes that act either directly or through maternal effects and that may be subject to parental imprinting. *Am J Hum Genet* 1998;62:969-78.

[67] Vermeulen SH, Shi M, Weinberg CR, Umbach DM. A hybrid design: case-parent triads supplemented by control-mother dyads. *Genet Epidemiol* 2008.

[68] Weinberg CR, Umbach DM. A hybrid design for studying genetic influences on risk of diseases with onset early in life. *Am J Hum Genet* 2005;77:627-36.

[69] Lary JM, Edmonds LD. Prevalence of spina bifida at birth--United States, 1983-1990: a comparison of two surveillance systems. *MMWR CDC Surveill Summ* 1996;45:15-26.

[70] Mathews TJ, Honein MA, Erickson JD. Spina bifida and anencephaly prevalence--United States, 1991-2001. *MMWR Recomm Rep* 2002;51:9-11.

[71] International Clearinghouse for Birth Defects Monitoring S. Annual report 2007 with data for 2005. Rome, Italy; *International Centre for Birth Defects*; 2007

[72] Botto LD, Lisi A, Bower C, et al. Trends of selected malformations in relation to folic acid recommendations and fortification: an international assessment. *Birth Defects Res A Clin Mol Teratol* 2006;76:693-705.

[73] Li Z, Ren A, Zhang L, et al. Extremely high prevalence of neural tube defects in a 4-county area in Shanxi Province, China. *Birth Defects Res A Clin Mol Teratol* 2006;76:237-40.

[74] Moore CA, Li S, Li Z, et al. Elevated rates of severe neural tube defects in a high-prevalence area in northern China. *Am J Med Genet* 1997;73:113-8.

[75] Rampersaud E, Melvin EC, Speer MC. Nonsyndromic Neural Tube Defects: Genetic Basis and Genetic Investigations. *In: Wyszynski DF, ed. Neural Tube Defects: From Origin to Treatment.* New York City: Oxford University Press; 2006:165-75.

[76] Boulet SL, Yang Q, Mai C, et al. Trends in the postfortification prevalence of spina bifida and anencephaly in the United States. *Birth Defects Res A Clin Mol Teratol* 2008;82:527-32.

[77] Harris JA, Shaw GM. Neural tube defects--why are rates high among populations of Mexican descent? *Environ Health Perspect* 1995;103 Suppl 6:163-4.

[78] Canfield MA, Honein MA, Yuskiv N, et al. National estimates and race/ethnic-specific variation of selected birth defects in the United States, 1999-2001. *Birth Defects Res A Clin Mol Teratol* 2006;76:747-56.

[79] Feuchtbaum LB, Currier RJ, Riggle S, Roberson M, Lorey FW, Cunningham GC. Neural tube defect prevalence in California (1990-1994): eliciting patterns by type of defect and maternal race/ethnicity. *Genet Test* 1999;3:265-72.

[80] Shaw GM, Velie EM, Wasserman CR. Risk for neural tube defect-affected pregnancies among women of Mexican descent and white women in California. *Am J Public Health* 1997;87:1467-71.

[81] Hendricks KA, Simpson JS, Larsen RD. Neural tube defects along the Texas-Mexico border, 1993-1995. *Am J Epidemiol* 1999;149:1119-27.

[82] Canfield MA, Annegers JF, Brender JD, Cooper SP, Greenberg F. Hispanic origin and neural tube defects in Houston/Harris County, Texas. II. Risk factors. *Am J Epidemiol* 1996;143:12-24.

[83] Canfield MA, Annegers JF, Brender JD, Cooper SP, Greenberg F. Hispanic origin and neural tube defects in Houston/Harris County, Texas. I. Descriptive epidemiology. *Am J Epidemiol* 1996;143:1-11.

[84] McDonnell RJ, Johnson Z, Delaney V, Dack P. East Ireland 1980-1994: epidemiology of neural tube defects. *J Epidemiol Community Health* 1999;53:782-8.

[85] Whiteman D, Murphy M, Hey K, O'Donnell M, Goldacre M. Reproductive factors, subfertility, and risk of neural tube defects: a case-control study based on the Oxford Record Linkage Study Register. *Am J Epidemiol* 2000;152:823-8.

[86] Lary JM, Paulozzi LJ. Sex differences in the prevalence of human birth defects: a population-based study. *Teratology* 2001;64:237-51.

[87] Shaw GM, Carmichael SL, Kaidarova Z, Harris JA. Differential risks to males and females for congenital malformations among 2.5 million California births, 1989-1997. *Birth Defects Res A Clin Mol Teratol* 2003;67:953-8.

[88] Owen TJ, Halliday JL, Stone CA. Neural tube defects in Victoria, Australia: potential contributing factors and public health implications. *Aust N Z J Public Health* 2000;24:584-9.

[89] Castilla EE, Lopez-Camelo JS, Campana H. Altitude as a risk factor for congenital anomalies. *Am J Med Genet* 1999;86:9-14.

[90] Castilla EE, Orioli IM, Lugarinho R, et al. Monthly and seasonal variations in the frequency of congenital anomalies. *Int J Epidemiol* 1990;19:399-404.

[91] Khoury MJ, Erickson JD, Cordero JF, McCarthy BJ. Congenital malformations and intrauterine growth retardation: a population study. *Pediatrics* 1988;82:83-90.

[92] Shaw GM, Schaffer D, Velie EM, Morland K, Harris JA. Periconceptional vitamin use, dietary folate, and the occurrence of neural tube defects. *Epidemiology* 1995;6:219-26.

[93] Finnell RH, Greer KA, Barber RC, Piedrahita JA. Neural tube and craniofacial defects with special emphasis on folate pathway genes. *Crit Rev Oral Biol Med* 1998;9:38-53.

[94] Czeizel AE, Dudas I. Prevention of the first occurrence of neural-tube defects by periconceptional vitamin supplementation. *N Engl J Med* 1992;327:1832-5.

[95] Centers for Disease Control. Recommendations for the use of folic acid to reduce the number of cases of spina bifida and other neural tube defects. *MMWR* 1992;41:RR-14.

[96] De Wals P, Tairou F, Van Allen MI, et al. Reduction in neural-tube defects after folic acid fortification in Canada. *N Engl J Med* 2007;357:135-42.

[97] Mills JL, Signore C. Neural tube defect rates before and after food fortification with folic acid. *Birth Defects Res A Clin Mol Teratol* 2004;70:844-5.

[98] Bell KN, Oakley GP, Jr. Tracking the prevention of folic acid-preventable spina bifida and anencephaly. *Birth Defects Res A Clin Mol Teratol* 2006;76:654-7.

[99] Boyles AL, Hammock P, Speer MC. Candidate gene analysis in human neural tube defects. *Am J Med Genet C Semin Med Genet* 2005;135:9-23.

[100] Wilson A, Platt R, Wu Q, et al. A common variant in methionine synthase reductase combined with low cobalamin (vitamin B12) increases risk for spina bifida. *Mol Genet Metab* 1999;67:317-23.

[101] Shaw GM, Lammer EJ, Zhu H, Baker MW, Neri E, Finnell RH. Maternal periconceptional vitamin use, genetic variation of infant reduced folate carrier (A80G), and risk of spina bifida. *Am J Med Genet* 2002;108:1-6.

[102] Volcik KA, Shaw GM, Lammer EJ, Zhu H, Finnell RH. Evaluation of infant methylenetetrahydrofolate reductase genotype, maternal vitamin use, and risk of high versus low level spina bifida defects. *Birth Defects Res Part A Clin Mol Teratol* 2003;67:154-7.

[103] Gueant-Rodriguez RM, Rendeli C, Namour B, et al. Transcobalamin and methionine synthase reductase mutated polymorphisms aggravate the risk of neural tube defects in humans. *Neurosci Lett* 2003;344:189-92.

[104] De Marco P, Calevo MG, Moroni A, et al. Reduced folate carrier polymorphism (80A-->G) and neural tube defects. *Eur J Hum Genet* 2003;11:245-52.

[105] Shields DC, Kirke PN, Mills JL, et al. The "thermolabile" variant of methylenetetrahydrofolate reductase and neural tube defects: An evaluation of genetic risk and the relative importance of the genotypes of the embryo and the mother. *Am J Hum Genet* 1999;64:1045-55.

[106] Doolin MT, Barbaux S, McDonnell M, Hoess K, Whitehead AS, Mitchell LE. Maternal genetic effects, exerted by genes involved in homocysteine remethylation, influence the risk of spina bifida. *Am J Hum Genet* 2002;71:1222-6.

[107] Cabrera RM, Shaw GM, Ballard JL, et al. Autoantibodies to folate receptor during pregnancy and neural tube defect risk. *J Reprod Immunol* 2008;79:85-92.

[108] Rothenberg SP, da Costa MP, Sequeira JM, et al. Autoantibodies against folate receptors in women with a pregnancy complicated by a neural-tube defect. *N Engl J Med* 2004;350:134-42.

[109] Groenen PM, Peer PG, Wevers RA, et al. Maternal myo-inositol, glucose, and zinc status is associated with the risk of offspring with spina bifida. *Am J Obstet Gynecol* 2003;189:1713-9.

[110] Velie EM, Block G, Shaw GM, Samuels SJ, Schaffer DM, Kulldorff M. Maternal supplemental and dietary zinc intake and the occurrence of neural tube defects in California. *Am J Epidemiol* 1999;150:605-16.

[111] Milunsky A, Morris JS, Jick H, et al. Maternal zinc and fetal neural tube defects. *Teratology* 1992;46:341-8.

[112] Van den Veyver IB. Genetic effects of methylation diets. *Annu Rev Nutr* 2002;22:255-82.

[113] Ray JG, Blom HJ. Vitamin B12 insufficiency and the risk of fetal neural tube defects. *Qjm* 2003;96:289-95.

[114] Shaw GM, Velie EM, Schaffer DM. Is dietary intake of methionine associated with a reduction in risk for neural tube defect-affected pregnancies? *Teratology* 1997;56:295-9.

[115] Shoob HD, Sargent RG, Thompson SJ, Best RG, Drane JW, Tocharoen A. Dietary methionine is involved in the etiology of neural tube defect-affected pregnancies in humans. *J Nutr* 2001;131:2653-8.

[116] Cavalli P, Copp AJ. Inositol and folate resistant neural tube defects. *J Med Genet* 2002;39:E5.

[117] Cavalli P, Tedoldi S, Riboli B. Inositol supplementation in pregnancies at risk of apparently folate-resistant NTDs. *Birth Defects Res A Clin Mol Teratol* 2008;82:540-2.

[118] Shaw GM, Carmichael SL, Yang W, Schaffer DM. Periconceptional dietary intake of myo-inositol and neural tube defects in offspring. *Birth Defects Res A Clin Mol Teratol* 2005;73:184-7.

[119] Wyszynski DF. Maternal exposure to selected environmental factors and risk for neural tube defects in the offspring. *In: Wyszynski DF, ed. Neural tube defects: from origin to treatment.* New York City: Oxford University Press; 2006.

[120] Cabrera RM, Hill DS, Etheredge AJ, Finnell RH. Investigations into the etiology of neural tube defects. *Birth Defects Res C Embryo Today* 2004;72:330-44.

[121] McLeod L, Ray JG. Prevention and detection of diabetic embryopathy. *Community Genet* 2002;5:33-9.

[122] Mitchell LE. Epidemiology of Neural Tube Defects. *Am J Med Genet C Semin Med Genet* 2005;135C(1):88-94.

[123] Fine EL, Horal M, Chang TI, Fortin G, Loeken MR. Evidence that elevated glucose causes altered gene expression, apoptosis, and neural tube defects in a mouse model of diabetic pregnancy. *Diabetes* 1999;48:2454-62.

[124] Hiramatsu Y, Sekiguchi N, Hayashi M, et al. Diacylglycerol production and protein kinase C activity are increased in a mouse model of diabetic embryopathy. *Diabetes* 2002;51:2804-10.

[125] Wentzel P, Wentzel CR, Gareskog MB, Eriksson UJ. Induction of embryonic dysmorphogenesis by high glucose concentration, disturbed inositol metabolism, and inhibited protein kinase C activity. *Teratology* 2001;63:193-201.

[126] Weigensberg MJ, Garcia-Palmer FJ, Freinkel N. Uptake of myo-inositol by early-somite rat conceptus. Transport kinetics and effects of hyperglycemia. *Diabetes* 1990;39:575-82.

[127] Hendricks KA, Nuno OM, Suarez L, Larsen R. Effects of hyperinsulinemia and obesity on risk of neural tube defects among Mexican Americans. *Epidemiology* 2001;12:630-5.

[128] Werler MM, Louik C, Shapiro S, Mitchell AA. Prepregnant weight in relation to risk of neural tube defects. *JAMA* 1996;275:1089-92.

[129] Waller DK, Mills JL, Simpson JL, et al. Are obese women at higher risk for producing malformed offspring? *Am J Obstet Gynecol* 1994;170:541-8.

[130] Waller DK, Shaw GM, Rasmussen SA, et al. Prepregnancy obesity as a risk factor for structural birth defects. *Arch Pediatr Adolesc Med* 2007;161:745-50.

[131] Haddow JE, Hill LE, Kloza EM, Thanhauser D. Neural tube defects after gastric bypass. *Lancet* 1986;1:1330.

[132] Knudsen LB, Kallen B. Gastric bypass, pregnancy, and neural tube defects. *Lancet* 1986;2:227.

[133] Martin L, Chavez GF, Adams MJ, Jr., et al. Gastric bypass surgery as maternal risk factor for neural tube defects. *Lancet* 1988;1:640-1.

[134] Moliterno JA, DiLuna ML, Sood S, Roberts KE, Duncan CC. Gastric bypass: a risk factor for neural tube defects? Case report. *J Neurosurg Pediatrics* 2008;1:406-9.

[135] Milunsky A, Ulcickas M, Rothman KJ, Willett W, Jick SS, Jick H. Maternal heat exposure and neural tube defects. *JAMA* 1992;268:882-5.

[136] Lynberg MC, Khoury MJ, Lu X, Cocian T. Maternal flu, fever, and the risk of neural tube defects: a population-based case-control study. *Am J Epidemiol* 1994;140:244-55.

[137] Chambers CD, Johnson KA, Dick LM, Felix RJ, Jones KL. Maternal fever and birth outcome: a prospective study. *Teratology* 1998;58:251-7.

[138] Shaw GM, Todoroff K, Velie EM, Lammer EJ. Maternal illness, including fever and medication use as risk factors for neural tube defects. *Teratology* 1998;57:1-7.

[139] Rouhani P, Fleming LE, Frias J, Martinez-Frias ML, Bermejo E, Mendioroz J. Pilot study of socioeconomic class, nutrition and birth defects in Spain. *Matern Child Health J* 2007;11:403-5.

[140] Carmichael SL, Shaw GM, Neri E, Schaffer DM, Selvin S. Social networks and risk of neural tube defects. *Eur J Epidemiol* 2003;18:129-33.

[141] Felkner M, Hendricks K, Suarez L, Waller DK. Diarrhea: a new risk factor for neural tube defects? *Birth Defects Res Part A Clin Mol Teratol* 2003;67:504-8.

[142] Carmichael SL, Shaw GM, Schaffer DM, Laurent C, Selvin S. Dieting behaviors and risk of neural tube defects. *Am J Epidemiol* 2003;158:1127-31.

[143] Hernandez-Diaz S, Werler MM, Walker AM, Mitchell AA. Neural tube defects in relation to use of folic acid antagonists during pregnancy. *Am J Epidemiol* 2001;153:961-8.

[144] Samren EB, van Duijn CM, Koch S, et al. Maternal use of antiepileptic drugs and the risk of major congenital malformations: a joint European prospective study of human teratogenesis associated with maternal epilepsy. *Epilepsia* 1997;38:981-90.

[145] Valproic acid and spina bifida: a preliminary report--France. *MMWR Morb Mortal Wkly Rep* 1982;31:565-6.

[146] Medveczky E, Puho E, Czeizel EA. The use of drugs in mothers of offspring with neural-tube defects. *Pharmacoepidemiol Drug Saf* 2004;13:443-55.

[147] Suarez L, Felkner M, Brender JD, Canfield M, Hendricks K. Maternal exposures to cigarette smoke, alcohol, and street drugs and neural tube defect occurrence in offspring. *Matern Child Health J* 2008;12:394-401.

[148] Grewal J, Carmichael SL, Ma C, Lammer EJ, Shaw GM. Maternal periconceptional smoking and alcohol consumption and risk for select congenital anomalies. *Birth Defects Res A Clin Mol Teratol* 2008;82:519-26.

[149] Logman JF, de Vries LE, Hemels ME, Khattak S, Einarson TR. Paternal organic solvent exposure and adverse pregnancy outcomes: a meta-analysis. *Am J Ind Med* 2005;47:37-44.

[150] Blatter BM, Roeleveld N, Zielhuis GA, Mullaart RA, Gabreels FJ. Spina bifida and parental occupation. *Epidemiology* 1996;7:188-93.

[151] Wennborg H, Magnusson LL, Bonde JP, Olsen J. Congenital malformations related to maternal exposure to specific agents in biomedical research laboratories. *J Occup Environ Med* 2005;47:11-9.

[152] Brender J, Suarez L, Hendricks K, Baetz RA, Larsen R. Parental occupation and neural tube defect-affected pregnancies among Mexican Americans. *J Occup Environ Med* 2002;44:650-6.

[153] McMartin KI, Chu M, Kopecky E, Einarson TR, Koren G. Pregnancy outcome following maternal organic solvent exposure: a meta-analysis of epidemiologic studies. *Am J Ind Med* 1998;34:288-92.

[154] Fear NT, Hey K, Vincent T, Murphy M. Paternal occupation and neural tube defects: a case-control study based on the Oxford Record Linkage Study register. *Paediatr Perinat Epidemiol* 2007;21:163-8.

[155] Shaw GM, Nelson V, Olshan AF. Paternal occupational group and risk of offspring with neural tube defects. *Paediatr Perinat Epidemiol* 2002;16:328-33.

[156] Brender JD, Suarez L. Paternal occupation and anencephaly. *Am J Epidemiol* 1990;131:517-21.

[157] Magnusson LL, Bonde JP, Olsen J, Moller L, Bingefors K, Wennborg H. Paternal laboratory work and congenital malformations. *J Occup Environ Med* 2004;46:761-7.

[158] Upton AC, Kneip T, Toniolo P. Public health aspects of toxic chemical disposal sites. *Annu Rev Public Health* 1989;10:1-25.

[159] Fay RM, Mumtaz MM. Development of a priority list of chemical mixtures occurring at 1188 hazardous waste sites, using the HazDat database. *Food Chem Toxicol* 1996;34:1163-5.

[160] Evans DM, Gillespie NA, Martin NG. Biometrical genetics. *Biol Psychol* 2002;61:33-51.

[161] Suarez L, Brender JD, Langlois PH, Zhan FB, Moody K. Maternal exposures to hazardous waste sites and industrial facilities and risk of neural tube defects in offspring. *Ann Epidemiol* 2007;17:772-7.

[162] Vrijheid M, Dolk H, Armstrong B, et al. Hazard potential ranking of hazardous waste landfill sites and risk of congenital anomalies. *Occup Environ Med* 2002;59:768-76.

[163] Croen LA, Shaw GM, Wasserman CR, Tolarova MM. Racial and ethnic variations in the prevalence of orofacial clefts in California, 1983-1992. *Am J Med Genet* 1998;79:42-7.

[164] Dummer TJ, Dickinson HO, Parker L. Adverse pregnancy outcomes around incinerators and crematoriums in Cumbria, north west England, 1956-93. *J Epidemiol Community Health* 2003;57:456-61.

[165] Brender JD, Suarez L, Felkner M, et al. Maternal exposure to arsenic, cadmium, lead, and mercury and neural tube defects in offspring. *Environ Res* 2006;101:132-9.

[166] Dodds L, Seviour R. Congenital anomalies and other birth outcomes among infants born to women living near a hazardous waste site in Sydney, Nova Scotia. *Can J Public Health* 2001;92:331-4.

[167] Devesa V, Adair BM, Liu J, et al. Arsenicals in maternal and fetal mouse tissues after gestational exposure to arsenite. *Toxicology* 2006;224:147-55.

[168] Kwok RK, Kaufmann RB, Jakariya M. Arsenic in drinking-water and reproductive health outcomes: a study of participants in the Bangladesh Integrated Nutrition Programme. *J Health Popul Nutr* 2006;24:190-205.

[169] Gilboa SM, Mendola P, Olshan AF, et al. Relation between ambient air quality and selected birth defects, seven county study, Texas, 1997-2000. *Am J Epidemiol* 2005;162:238-52.

[170] Ritz B, Yu F, Fruin S, Chapa G, Shaw GM, Harris JA. Ambient air pollution and risk of birth defects in Southern California. *Am J Epidemiol* 2002;155:17-25.

[171] Harris MJ, Juriloff DM. Mouse mutants with neural tube closure defects and their role in understanding human neural tube defects. *Birth Defects Res A Clin Mol Teratol* 2007;79:187-210.

[172] Detrait ER, George TM, Etchevers HC, Gilbert JR, Vekemans M, Speer MC. Human neural tube defects: developmental biology, epidemiology, and genetics. *Neurotoxicol Teratol* 2005;27:515-24.

[173] Wilson V, Rashbass P, Beddington RS. Chimeric analysis of T (Brachyury) gene function. *Development* 1993;117:1321-31.

[174] Morrison K, Papapetrou C, Attwood J, et al. Genetic mapping of the human homologue (T) of mouse T(Brachyury) and a search for allele association between human T and spina bifida. *Hum Mol Genet* 1996;5:669-74.

[175] Morrison K, Papapetrou C, Hol FA, et al. Susceptibility to spina bifida; an association study of five candidate genes. *Ann Hum Genet* 1998;62:379-96.

[176] Trembath D, Sherbondy AL, Vandyke DC, et al. Analysis of select folate pathway genes, PAX3, and human T in a Midwestern neural tube defect population. *Teratology* 1999;59:331-41.

[177] Chatkupt S, Hol FA, Shugart YY, et al. Absence of linkage between familial neural tube defects and PAX3 gene. *J Med Genet* 1995;32:200-4.

[178] Hol FA, Geurds MP, Chatkupt S, et al. PAX genes and human neural tube defects: an amino acid substitution in PAX1 in a patient with spina bifida. *J Med Gene*t 1996;33:655-60.

[179] Volcik KA, Blanton SH, Kruzel MC, et al. Testing for genetic associations with the PAX gene family in a spina bifida population. *Am J Med Genet* 2002;110:195-202.

[180] Kibar Z, Capra V, Gros P. Toward understanding the genetic basis of neural tube defects. *Clin Genet* 2007;71:295-310.

[181] Wu T, Willett WC, Rifai N, Rimm EB. Plasma fluorescent oxidation products as potential markers of oxidative stress for epidemiologic studies. *Am J Epidemiol* 2007;166:552-60.

[182] Freeman JL, Perry GH, Feuk L, et al. Copy number variation: new insights in genome diversity. *Genome Res* 2006;16:949-61.

[183] Jablonka E. Epigenetic epidemiology. *Int J Epidemiol* 2004;33:929-35.

[184] Mardis ER. Next-generation DNA sequencing methods. *Annu Rev Genomics Hum Genet* 2008;9:387-402.

In: Textbook of Perinatal Epidemiology
Editor: Eyal Sheiner, pp. 439-452

ISBN: 978-1-60741-648-7
© 2010 Nova Science Publishers, Inc.

Chapter XXII

Epidemiology of Intrauterine Growth Restriction

Vered Kleitman, Reli Hershkovitz and Eyal Sheiner[*]

Department of Obstetrics and Gynecology, Soroka University Medical Center, Faculty of
Health Sciences, Ben-Gurion University of the Negev, Be'er-Sheva, Israel

Definitions

- Intrauterine fetal growth restriction (IUGR): a condition in which the fetus is smaller than expected for the number of weeks of pregnancy (less than the 10th and 5th percentiles or less than 2 standard deviations from the mean).
- Small for gestational age (SGA): newborns whose *actual* weight fell below the 10th percentile.
- Low birth weight: birth weight below 2500 g.
- Very low birth weight: birth weight below 1500 g.
- Extremely low birth weight: birth weight below 1000 g.

Introduction

The definition of intrauterine fetal growth restriction (IUGR) and the patterns of growth restriction have evolved significantly over the last century. The incidence of morbidity and mortality among IUGR fetuses is high and second only to the incidence of complications among premature neonates [1].

---

[*] For Correspondence: Eyal Sheiner, MD, PhD, Department of Obstetrics and Gynecology, Soroka University Medical Center, P.O. Box 151, Be'er-Sheva 84105, Israel. Tel: +972-8-640-0774; Fax: +972-8-627-5338; E-mail: sheiner@bgu.ac.il

The etiology of IUGR is diverse and important to identify in each case. The decision-making analysis for treatment is based on each patient's specific pathophysiology. Therefore, patient-tailored management is performed. The complications among IUGR fetuses are not only short-term but also long-term complications. The adult sequelae of IUGR are known as the Barker hypothesis and are associated with an increased risk of death from cardiovascular disease and stroke. This theory was published on a cohort of men and women born in Hertfordshire, England, between 1911 and 1930, suggesting the idea of fetal programming as an explanation for adult origin of disease [2].

Approaches in the Diagnosis of IUGR

Growth is classified as low birth weight, which is birth weight below 2500 g; very low birth weight (i.e., weight < 1500 g), extremely low birth weight (i.e., weight < 1000 g); or, on the other side, macrosomia (defined as weight above the 97th percentile or above 4000 g).

The classification and understanding of abnormal fetal growth has evolved dramatically over the last century. Before the early 1960s, it was assumed that a newborn with a birth weight less than 2500 g was "premature". Lubchenco et al. [3] in 1963 published their classic paper showing an increased risk for neonatal mortality when birth weight fell below the 10th percentile. These findings were the first to emphasize the importance of this subject. Overall, term IUGR infants have an increased incidence of perinatal morbidity and mortality 5–30 times greater in comparison to adequate for gestational age neonates [4].

A new approach demonstrated that only comparison of the actual birth weight to the expected weight in the population identifies neonates at risk for adverse outcome. The diagnosis of IUGR is more accurate when using specific population representative curves. These population-based growth curves took gestational age and sex into consideration and set the normal range for fetal weight in the United States to be between 2 standard deviations (SD) from the mean or between the 10th and 90th centiles at any given gestational age. The term small for gestational age (SGA) is frequently used to describe newborns whose *actual* (and not estimated) weights fell below the 10th centile and is often used interchangeably with IUGR. However, there are many newborns whose weights are around or below the 10th percentile who are constitutionally small but normal and have none of the complications associated with suboptimal fetal growth [5]. When their growth and function are evaluated by ultrasound across gestation, they exhibit normal growth curves and amniotic fluid volume, and have normal umbilical artery flow as measured by Doppler. Conversely, some newborns have birth weights well within the normal range and would not be classified as SGA but have many of the metabolic, hematologic, and neurologic alterations seen in growth-restricted infants whose weight is less than the 10th centile [6]. These observations formed the basis for the development of customized rather than population-based fetal growth standards [7]. In contrast to population-based growth standards, customized fetal growth standards utilize optimal birth weight as the endpoint of a growth curve and are based on the ability of any individual fetus to achieve its growth potential determined prospectively, independent of maternal pathology, and with consideration of variables such as maternal ethnicity, parity, height, and weight in early pregnancy as well as fetal sex [8]. In summary, diagnosis of

IUGR was initially based on absolute weight, thereafter percentiles were used; the latest concept is individual growth.

Diagnostic Tools in Fetal Growth Restriction

Ideally, the diagnosis of IUGR is a three-step procedure:

1) Recognition of the growth restriction by ultrasonography.
2) Identification of a specific cause (etiologies of IUGR).
3) Management of IUGR (or specifically deciding when to deliver).

Recognition of the Growth Restriction

Fundal height was used for estimation of fetal weight in the past. Fetal sonographic biometry has emerged as the standard for diagnosis of IUGR. Measurements of fetal bony and soft structures are related to reference ranges for gestational age and are used for calculating the sonographic estimated fetal weight. Fetal weight is estimated in the second and third trimesters using measurements of the biparietal diameter, head circumference, abdominal circumference, and femur length. Estimated fetal weight may obviously not be accurate. Estimates are usually most accurate using multiple parameters. Nomograms are also available for other fetal structures and may help in identifying specific organ system abnormalities or syndromes. These findings underline the importance of focusing on early growth, potentially to prevent irreparable damage later in pregnancy [9,10].

Etiologies of Intrauterine Growth Restriction

With approximately 4 million births per year in the United States, 400,000 neonates will have a birth weight below the 10th percentile, but not all are at risk for an adverse outcome; some are constitutionally small but otherwise normal infants [11]. Understanding that a considerable number of those diagnosed as IUGR are actually normal and healthy infants, we can start working on the diagnosis of those with the true pathology.

The first step would be proper *dating* of the pregnancy. After excluding the most common cause for IUGR, which is a mistake in calculating the gestational age and unknown last menstrual period, differential diagnosis of IUGR can be performed. The differential diagnosis, like anything else in obstetrics, is divided into maternal, fetal, and placental causes. However, it is important to remember that in clinical practice there is considerable overlap between the conditions.

Maternal Causes

Maternal causes of fetal growth restriction include any chronic uncontrolled disease [12-17]. Important examples are vascular diseases such as hypertensive disorders of pregnancy, diabetic vasculopathy [12], chronic renal disease, collagen vascular disease, and thrombophilia [13]. The associated decrease in uteroplacental blood flow is responsible for the majority of clinically recognized cases of IUGR. Poor maternal volume expansion has also been reported to compromise placental blood flow by reducing the circulating blood volume. In addition, reduction of maternal oxygenation found in women living at high altitude, or with cyanotic heart disease, parenchymal lung disease, or reduced oxygen carrying capacity, as observed with certain hemoglobinopathies and anemias, may be responsible for the cases of IUGR described in these conditions [14]. Indeed, our group found maternal anemia [15], specifically thalassemia [16], as well as asthma [17] to be independent risk factors for IUGR. Using a multiple logistic regression model, the association between IUGR and thalassemia minor remained significant with an odds ratio (OR) of 2.4, 95% CI 1.4%, 4.2% [16]; the OR for asthma was 1.5, 95% CI 1.1–1.9 [17]. Because higher rates of IUGR were found, we recommended ultrasound surveillance of fetal weight for early detection of IUGR in such cases.

It is conceivable that malnutrition due to gastrointestinal syndromes such as Crohn's disease, ulcerative colitis, or bypass surgery [18] can result in lower birth weight. However, an association with IUGR is infrequent in these conditions [14]. Higher rates of IUGR (6.3 versus 2.1%; $p = 0.042$) were found among patients with celiac disease, compared to patients without known celiac disease [19]. Accordingly, careful observation is necessary for early detection of IUGR in patients with celiac disease, and further, prospective studies should focus on screening for celiac disease among patients presenting with IUGR of unknown etiology [20].

Maternal drug ingestion may result in IUGR by a direct effect on fetal growth as well as through inadequate dietary intake. Smoking produces a symmetrically smaller fetus through reduced uterine blood flow and impaired fetal oxygenation, and is a major cause of growth restriction in developed countries. The consumption of alcohol and the use of coumadin or hydantoin derivatives are now well known to produce particular dysmorphic features in association with impaired fetal growth. Alcohol was also associated with IUGR without the dysmorphic features [21]. Maternal use of cocaine has been associated with IUGR in general and with reduced head circumference in particular [22]. Multiple risk factors can act synergistically on fetal growth. For example, the adverse impact of smoking is doubled in thin white women and further potentiated by poor maternal weight gain [23].

Preeclampsia and IUGR are two obstetric syndromes that are generally associated with increased perinatal and maternal morbidities [24]. Preeclampsia is defined as the onset of hypertension and proteinuria after 20 weeks' gestation, and it complicates 3% to 5% of all pregnancies (chapter 19). Preeclampsia and IUGR share similar pathophysiologic abnormalities, such as reduced uteroplacental blood flow, exaggerated inflammatory response, endothelial cell dysfunction, and a state of imbalance between proangiogenic and antiangiogenic factors [25]. These pathophysiologic abnormalities are presumed to be the result of a cascade of events secondary to shallow trophoblast invasion and defective remodeling of the uterine spiral arteries. However, the etiologies of preeclampsia and IUGR are multifactorial, and only IUGR and preeclampsia related to placental insufficiency probably share abnormal placentation as a common pathway. Women with a history of preeclampsia in a previous pregnancy are at increased risk for preeclampsia and/or IUGR in subsequent pregnancies [26]. The magnitude of the above risks depends on gestational age at onset of preeclampsia in the index pregnancy (the earlier in gestation the onset of preeclampsia, the higher the rates of IUGR and recurrent preeclampsia) [26,27]. In addition, women who are born growth restricted are at increased risk of severe preeclampsia and IUGR when they get pregnant [28], and they are at increased risk for cardiovascular disease later in life (fetal origin of adult disease) [24,29].

Fetal Causes

Chromosomal abnormalities, congenital malformations, and genetic syndromes have been associated with less than 10% of cases of IUGR [30]. Similarly, intrauterine infection, although long recognized as a cause of growth restriction, also accounts for less than 10% of all cases. However, genetic and infectious etiologies are of special importance because perinatal and long-term outcome are ultimately determined by the underlying condition, with little potential impact through perinatal interventions [14].

Growth restriction has been observed in 53% of cases of trisomy 13, and 64% of cases of trisomy 18 [31]; this may be visible from the first trimester. Other conditions that may present with fetal growth restriction include skeletal dysplasia and Cornelia de Lange syndrome. The online database of inheritance in humans lists more than 100 genetic syndromes that may be associated with fetal growth restriction. Of the infectious agents, Syphilis, Toxoplasma gondii, Rubella, Cytomegalovirus, and Herpes virus (STORCH) are all documented causes of IUGR [14].

Twin gestation is also associated with IUGR. It was observed that the growth curve of twins deviated from that of singletons, with a progressive fall in growth after 32 weeks [32]. This finding implies relative placental insufficiency as opposed to intrinsic fetal compromise, and suggests that the longer the twin pregnancy continues, the greater the delay in intrauterine growth, with "catch-up" growth observed after birth. Thus, twins and higher order multiples represent a group of fetuses at high risk for IUGR. The appropriate growth standard to apply to twin fetuses would appear to be the same as that for singletons [33].

Placental Causes

Abnormal placental development with subsequent placental insufficiency is a relatively common problem affecting about one-third of patients with IUGR, or about 3% of all pregnancies. Placental insufficiency accounts for the vast majority of IUGR in singleton pregnancies [34]. An absolute or relative decrease in placental mass affects the quantity of substrate the fetus receives and antedates the development of IUGR. Thus, abnormal placental vascular development, circumvallate placenta, partial placental abruption, placenta accreta, placental infarction, or hemangioma may result in growth restriction [35]. Intrinsic placental pathology, such as a single umbilical artery and placental mosaicism, has been identified in some cases of growth restriction. Placental implantation in the lower uterine segment in placenta previa is considered suboptimal for nutrient exchange and, therefore, may result in IUGR even in the absence of chronic hemorrhage [36].

Management of IUGR

From all surveillance tools such as cardiotocography, biophysical profile (BPP), umbilical artery Doppler (UA Doppler), and estimation of amniotic fluid volume, the uterine artery Doppler has a value in predicting poor perinatal outcome, particularly in high-risk cases [36].

Doppler ultrasonography of the umbilical and middle cerebral artery (MCA), in combination with biometry, provides the best tool to identify small fetuses at risk for adverse outcome [37]. Moreover, Doppler studies of the fetal cardiovascular system allow assessment of the blood flow redistribution observed in IUGR. This process is mainly characterized by an increased umbilical artery, and a decreased MCA pulsatility index (PI) [38], which suggests increased vascular resistance of the umbilical artery and cerebral vasodilatation [11]. Meta-analysis of randomized controlled trials [39] has shown that the use of umbilical artery Doppler velocimetry can improve perinatal outcome in high risk pregnancies. Thus, many clinicians consider reversed umbilical-end diastolic flow velocities after 32 weeks of gestation and absent end-diastolic flow velocities at 34 weeks or more as an indication for prompt delivery if it occurs in a tertiary center with a neonatal intensive care unit. However, in cases of reversed diastolic flow in the umbilical artery before 32 weeks, management is less straightforward [11].

Nevertheless, if a woman is screened and uterine artery Doppler is positive (presence of bilateral notches, increased resistance index), this is expected to increase the frequency of antenatal visits. For the constitutionally small fetus, the BPP and the UA Doppler are usually normal, while in a fetus with structural abnormality, abnormal karyotype, or fetal infection the BPP may be variable with a normal UA Doppler. The cardiotocography has not been shown to improve the perinatal morbidity and mortality.

How to deliver is another question being debated. There are insufficient data to justify an elective Cesarean section for all SGA fetuses [40]. A trial of labor may be considered if the UA Doppler is normal [41]. Especially in pregnancies with a constitutionally small fetus a term delivery may be anticipated. On the contrary, in a fetus with abnormality or infection, the surveillance and the time of delivery are dependent on the etiology or the fetal well-being. In cases with known poor prognosis such as trisomy 18, when the parent did not opt for pregnancy termination, there is no need for intervention due to fetal indication during labor. However, if the pregnancy progresses with ambiguous diagnosis, the intrapartum cardiotocography can reduce perinatal death rates. Delivery should take place in a unit with relevant facilities and neonatal expertise [42].

Growth Curves

Growth curves are basically population-based. While the debate of where to cross the cutoff line for IUGR (10th, 5th or 3rd percentile) was discussed previously in this chapter, here we can become familiar with another debate of what curve should be used.

Whereas perinatologists base their management on sonographic reference charts derived from normal fetuses proceeding to term delivery, neonatologists tend to rely on growth charts derived from the birth weights of preterm infants. These different approaches result in considerable discrepancies. Sonographic reference charts were once discouraged for use in newborns because they were based on estimates rather than on direct measurement. However, technical progress has since made sonographic estimates highly precise and accurate, especially in preterm fetuses [43]. At the same time, the use of growth charts derived from preterm birth weights appears problematic in that the growth of a fetus delivered preterm cannot generally be considered normal, and IUGR per se may contribute to preterm delivery [44]. As a consequence, abnormal fetal growth may be missed by the neonatologist at the cost of increased morbidity and mortality. Differentiation between IUGR and genetic small size often remains difficult. To narrow the diagnosis, perinatologists use discriminators such as Doppler ultrasound, amniotic fluid index, and biophysical profiles, whereas neonatologists, in addition to newborn weight, can use the ponderal index (PI) that combines body weight with length [45].

Numerous standard curves for fetal growth have been published. An example of one of the standard growth curves is presented in figure 1. Nevertheless, it is well recognized that growth may be influenced by factors such as race, sex, socioeconomic environment, and altitude. For example, the Denver Intrauterine Growth Curves published by Lubchenco et al. [3], widely used in the 1960s and 1970s, were obtained from a relatively small sample size (n=5635) of predominately white and Hispanic neonates born at altitude. In contrast, growth curves derived from California birth data [4], or US national data using more than 4 million births [7], demonstrated disparate weight cutoffs at the 10th percentile. Currently, there is no consensus as to how a standard population should be selected to construct a growth curve.

It would thus seem prudent to use a single standard for all racial groups within a specific geographic area. An example of the different curve weights of the 50th percentile comparing the Jewish and the Bedouin populations is given in figure 2. Data represent the whole population of births at the Soroka University Medical Center, (more than 200,000 deliveries) between 1990 and 2008. We can see that the main difference can be found at term (weeks 38 and further) as the Bedouin curve slopes, but there is no fundamental difference in the pre-term weeks (for example week 30), as shown in figures 3 and 4.

Finally, it is helpful for the clinician to be familiar with the normal variation in rates of growth across gestation. Fetal growth accelerates from about 5 g per day at 14–15 weeks' gestation to 10 g per day at 20 weeks, peaking at 30–35 g per day at 32–34 weeks, after which growth rates decrease [8,46].

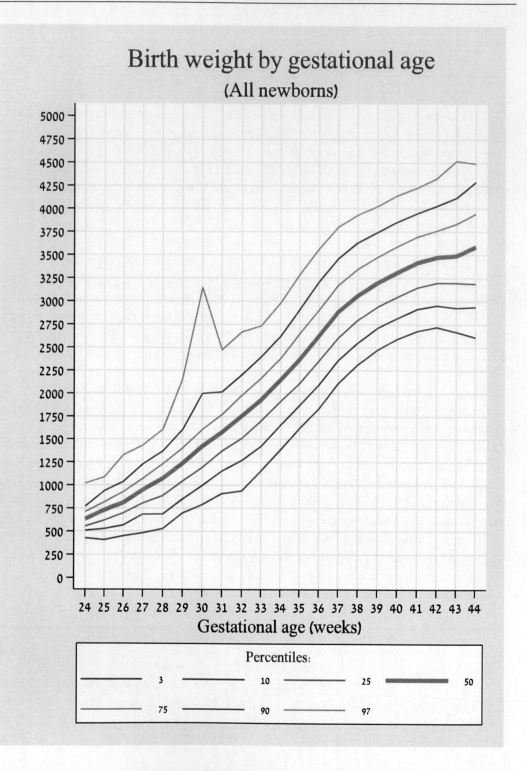

Figure 1. Growth chart representing birth weight per gestational week. Data represent the whole population of births at the Soroka University Medical Center (more than 200,000 deliveries) between 1990 and 2008.

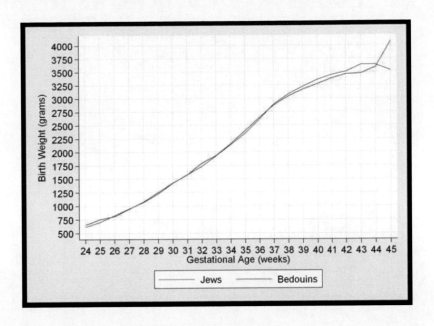

Figure 2. Growth chart of the 50th percentile of Jewish and Bedouin newborns (1990–2008).

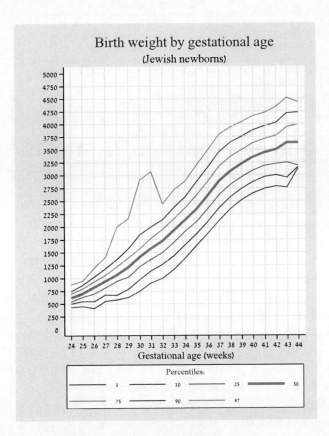

Figure 3. Growth chart of Jewish newborns divided by percentiles.

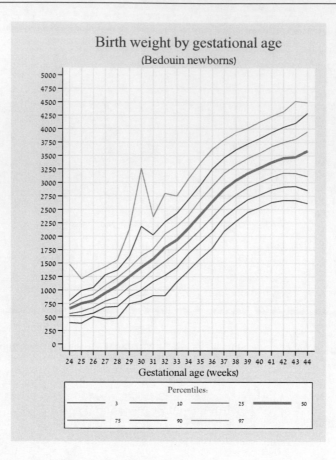

Figure 4. Growth chart of Bedouin newborns divided by percentiles.

Outcome and Future Studies

Given the multiple causes of IUGR, it is not surprising that the outcomes will be variable and related to the specific etiology of growth failure. Excluding those with aneuploidy, congenital malformations, and fetal infection, the remainder of fetuses may exist in a state of mild-to-moderate chronic oxygen and substrate deprivation, which may result in antepartum or intrapartum/neonatal hypoxia and neonatal ischemic encephalopathy, meconium aspiration, polycythemia, hypoglycemia, and other metabolic abnormalities. Consequently, it is imperative to optimize the timing of delivery, avoid progressive hypoxia during labor, and provide immediate skilled neonatal care. As noted earlier, IUGR infants have a higher risk of neonatal morbidity and mortality, particularly among those born preterm [47]. With respect to long-term outcome, the ultimate growth potential of these infants appears to be good. Several studies suggest that these infants are expected to have normal growth curves.

The issue of long-term neurological sequelae is still questionable; studies have shown a broad range of outcomes ranging from normal to small decreases in IQ (which are statistically but not clinically significant) [48] to a sharply increased risk of cerebral palsy. As might be anticipated, the worst outcomes have been observed in the more severely growth-restricted infants who are preterm, and those who exhibit the most overt evidence of impaired umbilical flow [49]. Other factors found to have an obvious impact on neurological sequelae are small head circumference, the gestational age of the infant at birth, and the post-natal environment. The prognosis for intact neurological function is quite favorable in the IUGR fetus when the cause is related to substrate deprivation, the timing of delivery is carefully selected, the fetus remains well oxygenated intrapartum, and receives skilled neonatal care [46].

Recent studies focus on placental causes for IUGR and adverse perinatal outcome [50,51]. During the past decade, several epidemiologic and case control studies evaluated the association between preeclampsia and the development of cardiovascular disease in later life. These studies were the subject of a recent systemic review and meta-analysis that revealed a relative risk for chronic hypertension of 3.7 after 14.1 years average follow-up, a relative risk of 2.2 for ischemic heart disease after 11.7 years of follow-up, and a relative risk of 1.8 for ischemic stroke after 10.4 years of follow-up [2,52].

Conclusions

Intrauterine growth today is one of the most important challenges for identification and treatment in the common obstetrical practice. It is important not only to truly diagnose the difference from expected growth, through good sonographic surveillance and use of the right growth chart for the population, but it is also important to know the exact cause of IUGR in each case in order to make a true diagnosis. Placental causes are the main goal in diagnosis for the right timing in intervention and prevention of intrauterine death. There is no doubt about the short-term consequences of growth restriction, but the long-term impact is still a matter of hypothesis and subject for further study. Growth as a model type for fetal origin of adult diseases opened a new road for further studies including intrauterine and placental investigations, as well as population studies and genetics.

References

[1]   Wolfe HM, Gross TL, Sokol RJ. Recurrent small for gestational age birth: perinatal risks and outcomes. *Am J Obstet Gynecol* 1987;157(2):288-93.

[2]   Barker DJ, Osmond C, Golding J, Kuh D, Wadsworth ME. Growth in utero, blood pressure in childhood and adult life, and mortality from cardiovascular disease. *BMJ* 1989;298(6673):564-7.

[3]   Lubchenco LO, Hansman C, Dressler M, Boyd E. Intrauterine growth as estimated from liveborn birth- weight data at 24 to 42 weeks gestation. *Pediatrics* 1963;32:793-800.

[4]   Williams RL, Creasy RK, Cunningham GC, Hawes WE, Norris FD, Tashiro M. Fetal growth and perinatal viability in California. *Obstet Gynecol* 1982;59(5):624-32.

[5]   Groom KM, Poppe KK, North RA, McCowan LME. Small-for-gestational-age infants classified by customized or population birthweight centiles: impact of gestational age at delivery. *Am J Obstet Gynecol* 2007;197(3):239.e1-e5.

[6]   Ego A, Subtil D, Grange G, Thiebaugeorges O, Senat MV, Vayssiere C, Zeitlin J. Customized versus population-based birth weight standards for identifying growth restricted infants: A French multicenter study. *Am J Obstet Gynecol* 2006;194(4):1042-9.

[7]   Zhang X, Platt RW, Cnattingius S, Joseph KS, Kramer MS. The use of customised versus population-based birthweight standards in predicting perinatal mortality. *BJOG* 2007;114(4):474-7.

[8]   Resnik R. One size does not fit all. Am J Obstet Gynecol 2007;197(3):221-2.

[9]   Källén K. Increased risk of perinatal/neonatal death in infants who were smaller than expected at ultrasound fetometry in early pregnancy. *Ultrasound Obstet Gynecol* 2004;24(1):30-4.

[10] Pedersen NG, Wøjdemann KR, Scheike T, Tabor A. Fetal growth between the first and second trimesters and the risk of adverse pregnancy outcome. *Ultrasound Obstet Gynecol* 2008;32(2):147-54.

[11] Mari G, Hanif F. Intrauterine Growth Restriction: How to Manage and When to Deliver. *Clin Obstet Gynecol* 2007;50(2):497-509.

[12] Haeri S, Khoury J, Kovilam O, Miodovnik M. The association of intrauterine growth abnormalities in women with type 1 diabetes mellitus complicated by vasculopathy. *Am J Obstet Gynecol* 2008;199(3):278.e1-e5.

[13] Weintraub AY, Sheiner E, Levy A, Yerushalmi R, Mazor M. Pregnancy complications in women with inherited thrombophilia. *Arch Gynecol Obstet* 2006;274(3):125-9.

[14] Baschat AA, Galan HL, Ross MG, Gabbe SG. Intrauterine Growth Restriction. In: Gabbe SG, Simpson JL, Niebyl JR, Galan H, Goetzl L, Jauniaux ERM, Landon M. *Obstetrics: Normal and Problem Pregnancies*. 5th ed. Oxford, UK: Churchill Livingstone; 2007:771-814.

[15] Levy A, Fraser D, Katz M, Mazor M, Sheiner E. Maternal anemia during pregnancy is an independent risk factor for low birthweight and preterm delivery. *Eur J Obstet Gynecol Reprod Biol* 2005;122(2):182-6.

[16] Sheiner E, Levy A, Yerushalmi R, Katz M. Beta-Thalassemia Minor During Pregnancy. *Obstet Gynecol* 2004;103(6):1273-7.

[17] Sheiner E, Mazor M, Levy A, Wiznitzer A, Bashiri A. Pregnancy outcome of asthmatic patients: A population-based study. *J Matern Fetal Neonatal Med* 2005;18(4):237-40.

[18] Sheiner E, Levy A, Silverberg D, Menes TS, Levy I, Katz M, Mazor M. Pregnancy after bariatric surgery is not associated with adverse perinatal outcome. *Am J Obstet Gynecol* 2004;190(5):1335-40.

[19] Sheiner E, Peleg R, Levy A. Pregnancy outcome of patients with known celiac disease. *Eur J Obstet Gynecol Reprod Biol* 2006;129(1):41-5. Epub 2005 Nov 28.

[20] Pope R, Sheiner E. Celiac disease during pregnancy: to screen or not to screen? *Arch Gynecol Obstet* 2009;279(1):1-3. Epub 2008 Sep 26.

[21] Mills JL, Graubard BI, Harley EE, Rhoads GG, Berendes HW. Maternal alcohol consumption and birth weight. How much drinking during pregnancy is safe? *JAMA* 1984;252(14):1875-9.

[22] Little BB, Snell LM, Klein VR, Gilstrap LC 3rd. Cocaine abuse during pregnancy: maternal and fetal implications. *Obstet Gynecol* 1989;73(2):157-60.

[23] Cliver S, Goldenberg R, Cutter G, Hoffman H, Davis R, Nelson K. The effect of cigarette smoking on neonatal anthropometric measurements. *Obstet.Gynecol* 1995;85(4):625-30.

[24] Sibai BM. Intergenerational Factors: A Missing Link for Preeclampsia, Fetal Growth Restriction, and Cardiovascular Disease? *Hypertension* 2008;51(4):993-4. Epub 2008 Feb 7.

[25] Gotsch F, Romero R, Friel L, Kusanovic JP, Espinoza J, Erez O, Than NG, Mittal P, Edwin S, Yoon BH, Kim CJ, Mazaki-Tovi S, Chaiworaponqsa T, Hassan SS. CXCL10/IP-10: A missing link between inflammation and anti-angiogenesis in preeclampsia? *J Matern Fetal Neonatal Med* 2007;20(11):777-92.

[26] Hnat MD, Sibai BM, Caritis S, Hauth J, Lindheimer MD, MacPherson C, VanDorsten JP, Landon M, Miodovnik M, Paul R, Meis P, Thurnau G, Dombrowski M; National Institute of Child Health and Human Development Network of Maternal-Fetal Medicine-Units. Perinatal outcome in women with recurrent preeclampsia compared with women who develop preeclampsia as nulliparas. *Am J Obstet Gynecol* 2002;186(3):422-6.

[27] Surkan PJ, Stephansson O, Dickman PW, Cnattingius S. Previous Preterm and Small-for-Gestational-Age Births and the Subsequent Risk of Stillbirth. *N Engl J Med* 2004;350(8):777-85.

[28] Zetterström K, Lindeberg S, Haglund B, Magnuson A, Hanson U. Being born small for gestational age increases the risk of severe pre-eclampsia. *BJOG* 2007;114(3):319-24.

[29] Smith GC, Pell JP, Walsh D. Pregnancy complications and maternal risk of ischaemic heart disease: a retrospective cohort study of 129, 290 births. *The Lancet* 2001;357(9273):2002-6.

[30] Khoury MJ, Erickson JD, Cordero JF, McCarthy BJ. Congenital malformations and intrauterine growth retardation: a population study. *Pediatrics* 1988;82(1):83-90.

[31] Eydoux P, Choiset A, Le Porrier N, Thépot F, Szpiro-Tapia S, Alliet J, Ramond S, Viel JF, Gautier E, Morichon N, et al. Chromosomal prenatal diagnosis: study of 936 cases of intrauterine abnormalities after ultrasound assessment. *Prenat Diagn* 1989;9(4):255-69.

[32] Gruenwald P. Growth of the human fetus. II. Abnormal growth in twins and infants of mothers with diabetes, hypertension, or isoimmunization. *Am J Obstet Gynecol* 1966;15;94(8):1120-32.

[33] Dollberg S, Haklai Z, Mimouni FB, Gorfein I, Gordon ES. Birth weight standards in the live-born population in Israel. *Isr Med Assoc J* 2005;7(5):311-4.

[34] Odegård RA, Vatten LJ, Nilsen ST, Salvesen KA, Austgulen R. Preeclampsia and Fetal Growth. *Obstet Gynecol* 2000;96(6):950-5.

[35] Abramowicz JS, Sheiner E. In Utero Imaging of the Placenta: Importance for Diseases of Pregnancy. *Placenta* 2007;28(Supplement 1):S14-S22.

[36] Abramowicz JS, Sheiner E. Ultrasound of the Placenta: A Systematic Approach. Part I: Imaging. *Placenta* 2008;29(3):225-40.

[37] Baschat AA, Galan HL, Bhide A, Berg C, Kush ML, Oepkes D, Thilaganathan B, Gembruch U, Harman CR. Doppler and biophysical assessment in growth restricted fetuses: distribution of test results. *Ultrasound Obstet Gynecol* 2006;27(1):41-7.

[38] Mari G, Deter RL. Middle cerebral artery flow velocity waveforms in normal and small-for-gestational-age fetuses. *Am J Obstet Gynecol* 1992;166(4):1262-70.

[39] Alfirevic Z, Neilson JP. The current status of Doppler sonography in obstetrics. *Curr Opin Obstet Gynecol* 1996;8(2):114-8.

[40] Grant A, Glazener CM. Elective caesarean section versus expectant management for delivery of the small baby. *Cochrane Database Syst Rev* 2001(2):CD000078.

[41] Williams KP, Farquharson DF, Bebbington M, Dansereau J, Galerneau F, Wilson RD, Shaw D, Kent N. Screening for fetal well-being in a high-risk pregnant population comparing the nonstress test with umbilical artery doppler velocimetry: A randomized controlled clinical trial. *Am J Obstet Gynecol* 2003;188(5):1366-71.

[42] Vrachnis N, Botsis D, Iliodromiti Z. The Fetus That Is Small for Gestational Age. *Ann N Y Acad Sci* 2006;1092:304-9.

[43] Kurmanavicius J, Burkhardt T, Wisser J, Huch R. Ultrasonographic fetal weight estimation: accuracy of formulas and accuracy of examiners by birth weight from 500 to 5000 g. *J Perinat Med* 2004;32(2):155-61.

[44] Gardosi JO. Prematurity and fetal growth restriction. *Early Hum Dev* 2005;81(1):43-9.

[45] Burkhardt T, Schäffer L, Zimmermann R, Kurmanavicius J. Newborn weight charts underestimate the incidence of low birthweight in preterm infants. *Am J Obstet Gynecol* 2008;199(2):139.e1-e6.

[46] Resnik R. Intrauterine Growth Restriction. *Obstet Gynecol* 2002;99(3):490-6.

[47] Simchen MJ, Beiner ME, Strauss-Liviathan N, Dulitzky M, Kuint J, Mashiach S, Schiff E. Neonatal outcome in growth-restricted versus appropriately grown preterm infants. *Am J Perinatol* 2000;17(4):187-92.

[48] Paz I, Laor A, Gale R, Harlap S, Stevenson DK, Seidman DS. Term infants with fetal growth restriction are not at increased risk for low intelligence scores at age 17 years. *J Pediatr* 2001;138(1):87-91.

[49] Wienerroither H, Steiner H, Tomaselli J, Lobendanz M, Thun-Hohenstein L. Intrauterine Blood Flow and Long-Term Intellectual, Neurologic, and Social Development. *Obstet Gynecol* 2001;97(3):449-53.

[50] Apel-Sarid L, Levy A, Holcberg G, Sheiner E. Placental pathologies associated with intrauterine growth restriction with and without oligohydramnios. *Arch Gynecol Obstet* 2009; 280(4):549-52.

[51] Apel-Sarid L, Levy A, Holcberg G, Sheiner E. Term and preterm (<34 and <37 weeks gestation) placental pathologies associated with fetal growth restriction. *Arch Gynecol Obstet* 2010 (in press).

[52] Bellamy L, Casas JP, Hingorani AD, Williams DJ. Pre-eclampsia and risk of cardiovascular disease and cancer in later life: systematic review and meta-analysis. *BMJ* 2007;335(7627):974.

In: Textbook of Perinatal Epidemiology
Editor: Eyal Sheiner, pp. 453-498

ISBN: 978-1-60741-648-7
© 2010 Nova Science Publishers, Inc.

Chapter XXIII

The Epidemiology of Shoulder Dystocia and Associated Neonatal Brachial Plexus Injury

Edith D. Gurewitsch and *Robert H. Allen*

Departments of Gynecology/Obstetrics and Biomedical Engineering
Johns Hopkins University School of Maryland, Baltimore, USA

Keywords: biomechanics research, birth complications, brachial plexus injury, education, fetal manipulation, injury prevention, maneuvers, McRoberts, Rubin, nerve injury, neurapraxia, obstetric palsy, patient safety, risk management, simulation, shoulder dystocia

Introduction

Shoulder dystocia, first described in 1730, is an infrequent complication of cephalic vaginal delivery wherein final expulsion of the fetal trunk following delivery of the head through the vaginal introitus is obstructed by a bony impaction of either the anterior fetal shoulder against the pubic symphysis or of both shoulders, with the posterior one also impacted against the sacral promontory [1]. One difficulty with the description, however, is that the degree of impaction varies, and shoulder dystocia ultimately is a clinical diagnosis made by applying traction to the head and discovering that "customary" traction fails to deliver the shoulders. This makes diagnosis subjective, especially for milder forms of shoulder dystocia [2]. Alternative diagnoses of the condition have been proposed, including deliveries in which specialized maneuvers are required, or where the head-to-body delivery interval is longer than 60 seconds [1,3-5]. A recent assertion remains apropos: "Shoulder dystocia has no generally accepted definition" [6].

---

*For Correspondence: Edith D. Gurewitsch, MD, Associate Professor of Gynecology/Obstetrics, Division of Maternal Fetal Medicine, The Johns Hopkins Hospital – Phipps 217, 600 North Wolfe Street, Baltimore, Maryland 21287, U.S.A. Telephone: 410-955-8297; Fax: 410-614-8305; Email: egurewi@jhmi.edu

Aside from the lack of consistent clinical definitions, comprehensive or definitive review of the epidemiology of shoulder dystocia or, separately, of its associated neonatal complications, is also confounded by such issues as non-universal classifications of the severity of either shoulder dystocia or of neonatal injury and variable use of differing denominators of "at-risk" patients for incidence calculation. Furthermore, shoulder dystocia is widely considered to be unpredictable and unpreventable [7], and an encounter with shoulder dystocia, although rightly considered an obstetrical emergency, is not a maloccurrence in and of itself since the majority are resolved uneventfully. Fortunately, when they do occur, most of the neonatal complications linked to shoulder dystocia, such as neonatal depression, brachial plexus injuries and skeletal fractures, are temporary. Although undesirable and preferably avoided, such impairments lack long-term or permanent sequelae and do not justify the obstetric intervention of elective cesarean delivery without trial of labor, the only alternative guaranteed to prevent a shoulder impaction against the bony pelvis but not necessarily guaranteed to prevent some of the complications seen more commonly with shoulder dystocia. Such seemingly facile intervention is unjustified because the surgery itself is fraught with substituted risks to the mother that are usually of greater significance than the potential risks to the neonate [8].

The science of epidemiology is the identification of patterns of disease or injury and determination of potential interventions on a public health scale for their prevention or mitigation. However, the aforementioned difficulties in identifying consistent etiological risk factors or in developing reasonable and effective interventions for the majority of incidences of either shoulder dystocia or of its associated complications beg the question: why study them from an epidemiological perspective? It is the premise of this chapter that, by limiting the scope of review specifically to *causally linked* shoulder dystocia-associated neonatal brachial plexus injury, an epidemiological approach proves especially useful. The reason for this is the specific entity of shoulder dystocia-related neonatal brachial plexus injury has the potential for permanent disability, an elucidated pathophysiology and mechanism of injury, several consistent population-based risk factors, and focal areas for specific interventions of tested efficacy.

Injury prevention researchers commonly employ a tool known as the Haddon Matrix to systematically review pre-event, event and post-event phases of injury and their intersection with the "hosts" (e.g., the persons injured), "vectors" (e.g., the equipment or "vehicle") and physical and social "environmental factors" involved [9]. Each cell of the resultant table identifies potential prevention or amelioration opportunities. Table 1 is our modified Haddon Matrix generated for shoulder dystocia-related neonatal birth injuries, which forms the organizational basis of this chapter.

Thus, the present chapter reviews the epidemiology of those neonatal complications that arise following shoulder dystocia—differentiating them from similar but *causally distinct* complications *not* associated with obstructed delivery of the shoulders. With an eye toward their interrelationship, we begin with a brief exploration of shoulder dystocia pathophysiology and review the types of mechanical birth injuries associated with it, focusing on the physical forces involved in deliveries complicated by shoulder dystocia and are most likely causative of mechanical injury based on biological and physical plausibility. Next, we address those risk factors that are consistently associated with shoulder dystocia deliveries in which mechanical birth injuries occur, concentrating on those that are potentially amenable to modification and for which policy and protocol development would likely have far-reaching public health benefits, even beyond prevention of shoulder dystocia-associated mechanical birth injuries. Finally, we consider the management of shoulder dystocia itself and its relationship to untoward outcomes, aiming to highlight those areas that demand standardization and quality assurance on a public health scale.

Table 1. Haddon Matrix for Shoulder Dystocia-Related Neonatal Complications.

	Mother	Fetus	Clinician
Antepartum	Prior shoulder dystocia Obesity/Weight Gain Diabetes	Macrosomia Postdatism	Training/Experience Prenatal Care/Assessment of Fetal Growth Delivery Planning/Informed Consent
Intrapartum	Abnormal Second Stage Expulsive Forces	Fetal Position/Asynclitism Fetal Oxygenation	Operative Vaginal Delivery Shoulder Dystocia Recognition/Management
Postpartum	Subsequent Pregnancy Planning	Natural History of Recovery	Counseling/Debriefing Coordinated Pediatric Management

Part I: Epidemiology of Shoulder Dystocia

Shoulder Dystocia Incidence

The incidence of shoulder dystocia varies in the literature by a factor of 100, reported as occurring from 1 in 7 deliveries [5] to 1 in 750 [10]. Most ranges vary between 1% and 2% of vaginal deliveries [11-16]. Although few in number, prospective studies of shoulder dystocia incidence generally report higher values, from 3.3% to 7% [5,17-20]. Reasons for the wide spread in incidence include:

- Type of study—population-based, prospective or retrospective
- Patient population
- Lack of consistent definition
- Source of records—delivery logs, discharge summaries, ICD-9 codes
- Varying denominators—all deliveries, vaginal deliveries only, cephalic deliveries only or deliveries of only the "at risk" population (>34 weeks gestation, or birth weights exceeding 2000 grams)

As a result, the actual incidence is unknown, although the higher values of the few prospective studies are probably the most accurate. This strongly suggests that the incidence among the at-risk population often goes undocumented or unrecognized. Milder forms a more difficult to diagnose.[2] In addition, since most shoulder dystocia deliveries are uneventful, they have a tendency not to be documented [10].

Before a systematic epidemiological approach to shoulder dystocia prevention or management can be undertaken, we first present the precise mechanisms and pathological antecedents that underlie the occurrence of shoulder dystocia and its potential consequences to the neonate. By reviewing the pathophysiology of shoulder dystocia, we elucidate the association *and* the potential causal link between certain risk factors that predispose to shoulder dystocia occurrence and its relationship to associated neonatal injury.

Pathogenesis of Shoulder Dystocia and Associated Mechanical Injury to the Newborn

The cardinal movements, which describe the traversal of the fetal head and body through the birth canal, can be divided into phases corresponding to before and after the head emerges through the vaginal introitus. The latter gyrations—extension, external rotation, and finally expulsion—are mechanistically associated with the aftercoming shoulders' negotiation of the maternal bony pelvis, subsequent to which expulsion of the remainder of the trunk is usually unimpeded. As the head crowns at the introitus during extension, the fetal neck becomes deflexed as it is forced through the J-shaped curvature of the maternal pelvis by uterine contractions and maternal expulsive effort. It is just as the head delivers that the fetal shoulders first come in to contact with the pelvic inlet, and in *normal* delivery, the posterior shoulder naturally will become laterally deviated from the head, sufficient to produce measurable stretch of the posterior brachial plexus [21]. Since the oblique diameter of the pelvic inlet is greater than the anteroposterior, subsequent external rotation occurs, corresponding in time sequence to restitution of the fetal head outside the mother's body. In this way, the fetal trunk is usually rotated in a screw-like forward-progressing motion to accommodate the wider (relative to the head) fetal shoulder-width dimension.

In an unobstructed delivery, the posterior shoulder usually descends first, entering the hollow of the sacrum, and the relative lateral deviation of the head and posterior shoulder is corrected toward neutral. The head and neck laterally flex slightly toward the anterior shoulder, which simultaneously rotates approximately 30° to the left or right of the pubic symphysis. Nevertheless, although the previous description is the usual case, researchers have established that passage of the shoulders is highly variable [22-24]. With continued maternal effort and often guided by down-and-outward-directed application of traction to the fetal head by the birth attendant, axial orientation of the head and shoulders is restored and the anterior shoulder delivers through the pelvic inlet. At this juncture, the posterior shoulder is propelled upward as it negotiates the J-shaped curvature of the pelvic outlet (equivalent to extension of the head prior to its emergence), which is often assisted by the upward tilting of the head and support of the trunk by the delivering clinician as the remainder of the body is expelled.

Impedance of normal traversal of birth canal by the fetal shoulders resulting from their impaction behind either or both the pubic symphysis anteriorly or the sacral promontory posteriorly after the head has emerged defines the entity of shoulder dystocia from a biomechanical perspective. Since the degree of impedance to shoulder delivery varies, some shoulder dystocia deliveries will escape clinical detection—especially by inexperienced providers [2]. Similarly, if less-than-optimal rotation of the fetal shoulders to the oblique dimension occurs during restitution and the shoulders still manage to deliver in relative anteroposterior alignment, compressive stress on the fetal clavicles *within* the pelvic inlet collapses the shoulder width before clinically-detectable impedance to shoulder delivery occurs [25]. Mechanical injury, such as neurapraxia resulting from brachial plexus stretch [26] and clavicle fracture [27] resulting from compression-induced bending are possible in these difficult to diagnose shoulder dystocia deliveries. Fortunately, these almost never have permanent sequelae.

However, as the degree of impedance to shoulder delivery increases, the chin often—though not uniformly—will retract backward and tightly against the introitus (the "turtle sign"). Subsequent restitution either is incomplete or fails to occur at all. The mechanical obstruction will become evident clinically as the birth attendant notes that usual traction fails to deliver the shoulders.

With increasing severity of shoulder dystocia, ancillary maneuvers in addition to or substituted for traction on the fetal head are needed to complete delivery of the fetal shoulders and trunk; in the most severe of cases, greater numbers of so-called shoulder dystocia maneuvers of varying types are required as time between delivery of the head and body increases. Although permanent peripheral nerve injury can occur in mild shoulder dystocia, the risk of such injury and its relative severity increases with the severity of shoulder impaction [16]. A review of the varying types of neonatal brachial plexus injury and their biomechanical mechanisms is provided later in this chapter.

How, then, does shoulder dystocia—a pathological persistence of relative anteroposterior positioning of the fetus' shoulder width relative to the mother's pelvic inlet—arise in a given parturient? Differentiating a *pre-existing* fetopelvic size discrepancy from a more dynamic and *de novo*-arising relative fetopelvic position discrepancy, though not necessarily mutually exclusive in a given instance of shoulder dystocia, is helpful to understand the problem mechanistically. With pre-existing size discrepancy, a fetus has relative head and body proportions that allow the head to fit through the pelvis but its truncal dimensions are too large to allow unimpeded delivery. Another less common pre-existing size discrepancy occurs when maternal pelvic architecture that is either measurably contracted or—despite being adequate based upon clinical pelvimetry—structurally predisposes to incomplete rotation of the shoulders and concomitant restitution of the head once it exits the introitus. By their nature, these conditions are relatively uncommon by population-based standards, yet have epidemiological risk factors potentially identifiable, and in some instances modifiable [28].

In instances of shoulder dystocia where the relative fetopelvic dimensions are more than likely to have been compatible (as may occur in a mother who previously delivered a larger fetus uneventfully), the impedance to shoulder delivery arises *de novo* intrapartum, owing to suboptimal fetopelvic positioning. One example is a compound presentation of the arm with the body, causing the trunk to be elevated within the pelvis, and the "high-riding" anterior shoulder becomes impeded by contact with the symphysis pubis [29]. Another intrapartum risk factor is asynclitic positioning of the head. This often impedes normal descent and internal rotation, which in turn may prevent optimal alignment of the shoulders as they approach the pelvic inlet. In the latter instance, lateral deviation of the head from the posterior shoulder will elongate the posterior brachial plexus prior to its incurring its normal stretch during extension, thereby predisposing to injury—even without shoulder dystocia or clinician-applied traction [26].

The aforementioned examples of position-related causes of shoulder dystocia are unpredictable prior to already-advanced active labor. However, they potentially are anatomically recognizable, thereby allowing an astute and skillful birth attendant to anticipate difficulties in delivery and/or attempt corrective maneuvers by correcting asynclitism manually or operatively, or by first delivering the posterior arm in a recognized compound presentation. However, fetopelvic positional discrepancy will arise more often—and paradoxically—*without* true anatomical position deviations. Rather, insufficient time has elapsed to accommodate and complete normal physiologic rotation of the shoulders into an oblique position at the pelvic inlet as or immediately after the head delivers. This is especially common in, though not unique to, operative vaginal deliveries [17,30] and those with a precipitous second stage [31,32].

It should also be noted that optimal fetal positioning for delivery is never solely an intrapartum occurrence. Pre-labor contractions and overall increased uterine tone in the last month of pregnancy are responsible for producing and maintaining proper alignment of the fetal axis in true longitudinal lie and cephalic presentation, even prior to the cervical ripening and thinning of the lower uterine segment that allow proper descent and engagement in the pelvis. Epidemiologically, this explains the higher—though inconsistent—association of shoulder dystocia with induction of labor [33-38] and those conditions associated with significant uterine laxity, such as grandmultiparity [39]. It also may be an alternative explanation to the paradoxical inability of early induction of labor for so-called "impending macrosomia" to reduce the incidence of severe shoulder dystocia [33]. This is counterintuitive to the notion that earlier delivery might be preventive, where smaller yet still large-for-gestational-age infant is expected to fit into a pelvis [33,35-38,40]. This clinical paradox also highlights the significance of relative *asymmetry* of accelerated fetal growth among large-for-gestational-age fetuses in predisposing them to shoulder dystocia, since induction of labor specifically for infants of diabetic mothers seems to be protective against shoulder dystocia [36].

Pathophysiology of Central Nervous System Injury from Shoulder Dystocia

The mechanism for the competing risk of central nervous system injury involves the interruption of cord blood flow during the head-to-body interval of the shoulder dystocia episode and thus depends on the variable and inconsistent vulnerability of the cord to compression within the birth canal. Mechanical obstruction to blood flow can occur in two ways: external compression resulting from the entrapment of a segment of cord between the fetal upper torso (above the umbilicus) or neck and the bony pelvis; and elongation of the cord through which the elastic intima of the blood vessels constrict. It is rare that either of these mechanisms will produce complete obstruction to blood flow; rather, as in all intrapartum occurrences of cord compression, the severity and duration of fetal circulatory effect will have a variable relationship to the presence, frequency and intensity of uterine contractions. Such erratic or incomplete circulatory effects underlie the complexity of the relationship between head-to-body interval and hypoxic ischemic encephalopathy or fatality resulting from shoulder dystocia [41].

In a medical hypothesis recently touted by Mercer et al., it appears as though an unequal compression of the umbilical vein greater than that of the artery owing to compression within the birth canal during shoulder dystocia leads to preferential transfusion of blood from the fetus to the placenta with resultant fetal hypovolemia [42]. A natural "compression trousers-like effect" from vaginal wall pressure on the fetus during the shoulder dystocia episode is protective; however, upon resolution of the shoulder dystocia and delivery of the infant, the release of this pressure and return of peripheral circulation in the face of profound hypovolemia results in cardiac asystole even moments after a normal fetal heart rate had been detected [42].

Managing shoulder dystocia with the commonly used "four-minute" head-to-body interval is likely conservative, as it is based only upon extrapolated data concerning the decline in cord pH during head-to-body interval in non-shoulder dystocia deliveries [43]. Four studies have specifically examined the effect of the head-to-body interval during shoulder dystocia on neonatal acidosis or depression, and found no clinically significant decrease in cord pH, or increase in five-minute Apgar scores below seven for up to six minutes' duration of head-to-body interval [5,13,44,45]. In fact, the two cases described by Mercer et al. each involved head to body intervals of six minutes or more [42]. Indeed, among shoulder dystocia deliveries, little change is noted in cord pH from an average of 7.24 until approximately 8 minutes into the head-to-body interval [13], only after which did any cases of permanent central nervous system sequelae occur [44,45]. Thus, although time for resolving shoulder dystocia is limited, hasty, frenetic or panicked response immediately upon its diagnosis is unwarranted and increases the risk of iatrogenic injury [46]. Similarly, nuchal cord management in *any* delivery—and especially in those already recognized as being complicated by shoulder dystocia—demands assurance of freedom of motion of the anterior shoulder prior to severing the fetus' essential lifeline [47,48]. Mercer et al. even advise a delay in clamping the cord after a long shoulder dystocia episode to allow reperfusion from the placenta once the pressure on the umbilical veins has been released [42].

Having reviewed the pathophysiology of shoulder dystocia and the mechanisms for its potential associated neonatal injury, we now address in greater depth the antepartum and intrapartum risk factors—and potential interventions—that form the backbone of an epidemiological approach to shoulder dystocia and its associated neonatal injuries.

Antepartum Risk Factors for Shoulder Dystocia

Although myriad antepartum risk factors of varying consistency and increased odds ratios for the occurrence of shoulder dystocia can be found throughout extensive and multidisciplinary literature on the subject (Table 2), the most consistent and significant antepartum risk factors for shoulder dystocia *and* its related neonatal complications are fetal macrosomia and a history of shoulder dystocia in a prior pregnancy—especially a history of shoulder dystocia in which a mechanical birth injury resulted. Pathophysiologically plausible, these two entities are consistent with mechanistically probable etiologies of shoulder dystocia related to a fetopelvic size discrepancy [49]. The other relatively consistent antepartum risk factors for shoulder dystocia—diabetes, maternal obesity and/or excessive weight gain during pregnancy, and postdatism—relate directly to their association with high birth weight and macrosomia. An awareness of prior shoulder dystocia-complicated deliveries and/or recognition and management of accelerated fetal growth regardless of other risk factors should prepare the obstetric provider for the possibility of shoulder dystocia based on fetopelvic size discrepancy.

Table 2. Risk Ratios for Shoulder Dystocia of Specific Antepartum Risk Factors*.

	Prior Shoulder Dystocia	Macrosomia (>4,000gm)	Diabetes	Obesity (>180 lbs)	Exc Wt Gain	Postdatism	Misc
Acker 1985[11]		5-10	5.20			2.12	
Benedetti 1978[30]		17	12%	54%**			
Baskett 1995[150]	2.5	2-10				3	Multiparity: NS
Bofill 1997[17]		6.5%-33%	P=0.08	P=NS		P=0.026	Multiparity: NS
Nesbitt 1998[35]		5.2%-21.1%	1.7			NS	
Sheiner 2004[61]		24.3	1.7				No prenatal care: 1.5
Sandmire 1988		4-10	6.5	2.3	NS		Multiparity: P<0.05
Gross 1987[185]		Mean 4kg	1%	10%	NS	12%	
Geary 1995[197]					yes		Prior macrosomia
Bahar 1996[62]	P<0.01		P<0.001				
Yeo 1995[198]		yes	yes	yes			Low SEC, multiparity
Smith 1994[52]	yes						
Lewis 1995[50]	7.0						

*Where risk ratios are not explicitly given or able to be calculated from available data, either percentage of shoulder dystocia cases exhibiting the specific risk factor is provided, or where percentage not available, p-value of statistical association between risk factor (vs. lack of risk factor) and shoulder dystocia is given., **Data concerning the risk factor not available for all subjects in the study; NS: non-significant, SEC: socioeconomic class

Prior Shoulder Dystocia

The risk of recurrence of shoulder dystocia in a subsequent pregnancy approaches 20% in most studies that included prior shoulder dystocia [28,50-55]. The actual recurrence rate is likely higher in that prior shoulder dystocia often is not noted in the subsequent pregnancy, an omission often attributable to the patient's not having been aware of its occurrence because there were no associated complications. Among those women with a known prior history of shoulder dystocia who undergo a trial of labor that results in a vaginal delivery, the recurrence of shoulder dystocia is approximately 10 times the incidence of shoulder dystocia in the general population [55]. This finding suggests that some women may indeed have pelvic architecture that is predisposed to shoulder dystocia, and pelvimetry obtained after the first occurrence may uncover previously unappreciated deformities or suboptimal dimensions [28].

Birth weight at the first delivery complicated by shoulder dystocia is also predictive of recurrence [55], which emphasizes the tendency among women predisposed to shoulder dystocia to reproduce larger-than-average infants. In addition, Moore et al. noted that the severity of shoulder dystocia in the original pregnancy—defined as being complicated by injury—doubles the recurrence risk [56]. These findings underscore the importance of counseling patients about the occurrence of a shoulder dystocia, even if resolved uneventfully, since the greatest predictor of injury at any shoulder dystocia, including in recurrent shoulder dystocia, is the birth weight of the infant [57-59] and the severity of the shoulder dystocia [45,51,59,60]. Each of these factors can guide delivery planning in subsequent pregnancies.

Macrosomia

Although 50% of all shoulder dystocia deliveries occurs with normal weight or even small-for-gestational-age fetuses, there is no doubt that the occurrence of shoulder dystocia is more common among higher birth weight infants [11,12,31]. Acker et al. noted that for each 500-gm increment in birth weight, the incidence of shoulder dystocia rises steadily, with a ten-fold increase from 2.3% in the median birth weight group (3,500 to 3,999 gm) to 23.9% in the highest birth weight group (≥ 4,500 gm); and a statistically significant and marked jump in incidence by nearly five-fold beyond 4,000 gm [11]. Other risk factors for shoulder dystocia, such as postdatism and excessive weight gain in pregnancy, are often surrogates or indirect markers for high birth weight. Indeed, increasing gestational age or other risk factors for shoulder dystocia will drop out of logistic regression analyses when birth weight is specifically controlled for [61].

Nevertheless, some antepartum risk factors remain significant beyond birth weight alone: By matching for exact birth weight, Bahar demonstrated in a case-control study that while macrosomia is a principal risk factor for shoulder dystocia, prior history of shoulder dystocia and diabetes were significant antepartum risk factors for shoulder dystocia that were independent of birth weight [62]. It is notable, however, that the risk for neonatal injury resulting from shoulder dystocia is directly correlated to birth weight, regardless of the presence or absence of other risk factors [46,63]. This association is addressed further in the specific review of risk factors for brachial plexus injury provided later in this chapter.

From the perspective of shoulder dystocia-related neonatal injury *prevention*, since nearly half of shoulder dystocia incidents will involve term infants of normal or even low birth weight [15,31] and since large-for-gestational-age infants occur in only 10% of term deliveries (and fetuses weighing more than 4,500 g or 5,000 g comprising even fewer deliveries), strategies for prevention of shoulder dystocia that focus solely on pre-identifying the high-birth weight infant *at term* with the aim simply to avoid vaginal birth in the latter group [4] will have no impact on the shoulder dystocia incidence [64]. Even if it did, substituting surgical risk of cesarean delivery for risk of shoulder dystocia would not be justified—particularly for patients who are diabetics or obese—because their surgical risk is above that of other normal weight and non-diabetic parturients, and such a policy will have limited effect on overall obstetric morbidity (fetal and maternal combined) in this relatively small group of at risk mother-infant dyads [64].

Furthermore, the accuracy of sonographic estimation of fetal weight—particularly at the extreme (beyond the 97th percentile)—is suboptimal to begin with, with margins of error approaching ± 500 g [65,66]. Even attempts at more sophisticated scoring schema to pre-identify the specifically macrosomic fetus (large trunk:head ratio) based upon bisacromial width and other estimation of ponderal index have been wanting in terms of their reliability in predicting subsequent shoulder dystocia at delivery [54,67,68]. These limitations of pre-delivery ultrasound diagnosis of the destined-to-be-injured high birth weight infant curtail the armamentarium, as well as the reasonable options, by which the obstetric provider might impact shoulder dystocia-related complications by the time labor ensues.

Thus, from an epidemiological perspective, the prevention of macrosomia in the first place is likely to have more significant impact not only on shoulder dystocia and its associated injury incidence, but on other obstetric morbidities [69] and even future pediatric and adult disease incidences [70,71]. Among preventive health initiatives, there has been significant attention to low birth weight and its impact on long-term neonatal survival and morbidity [72]. There is even appreciation of low birth weight's impact on adult conditions, such as high blood pressure, diabetes and cardiovascular disease [73]. A comparative focus on the implications and prevention of overnutrition and accelerated fetal growth is lacking. Yet, there is a growing body of evidence to suggest that high birth weight has significant impact on obesity in adulthood, as well as other determinants of cardiovascular and metabolic disease [70,71]. Therefore, the next sections focus on those determinants of fetal macrosomia most amenable to intervention: maternal diabetes, obesity and excess maternal weight gain.

Diabetes, Metabolic Syndrome and the Spectrum of Impaired Glucose Tolerance

Women with either pregestational or gestational diabetes are at increased risk for shoulder dystocia when carrying a fetus exhibiting accelerated growth [35]. Furthermore, per incremental increase in birth weight, delivery complications are two to three times greater among diabetic mothers than among non-diabetic mothers [74]. The macrosomic infant of a diabetic mother is at specifically increased risk for shoulder dystocia among large-for-gestational-age infants because of characteristic of asymmetry in accelerated somatic growth compared to overall growth in utero in these fetuses [49]. The particular predisposition to asymmetric growth of the trunk among fetuses of diabetic women relates more closely to fetal hyperinsulinemia than to fetal hyperglycemia (though these are usually interrelated). According to the Pedersen Hypothesis, the availability of excess fuel to the fetus caused by the insulin resistance of Type II pregestational diabetes and/or gestational diabetes revs up insulin production in the fetal pancreas. A somatic growth factor, insulin itself rather than the potential increased calories of too readily available excess fuel, contributes to rapid fetal growth and increased ponderal index in infants of diabetic mothers. It is well established that meticulous control of maternal glucose levels in diabetic pregnancy improves multiple obstetric outcomes, including a reduction in shoulder dystocia incidence among these women and their fetuses [75]. However, there are still instances of demonstrable accelerated fetal growth in spite of apparently well-maintained blood sugar levels at optimum levels. While the precise mechanism is poorly understood, there likely are other food energy sources whose proper metabolism is impaired by heightened insulin resistance in pregnancy. Indeed, empiric supplementation with exogenous insulin or oral hypoglycemic agents in diabetic gravidas with apparent optimal glycemic control on diet alone who nonetheless exhibit sonographic evidence of asymmetric accelerated fetal growth (i.e., abdominal circumference ≥ 35 cm or $\geq$ 75% for gestational age) has had a positive effect in curtailing the rate of fetal growth in randomized controlled trials [76-78].

The management of identified diabetes in pregnancy is best accomplished with close prenatal observation, counseling and motivated cooperation of the patient [75]. Indeed, when this is accomplished, adverse outcome is reduced to that of the general population [79]. However, there is another group with *subclinical* diabetes (i.e., below levels of detection by current screening cut-offs) but likely impaired glucose tolerance that consistently demonstrates an increase in untoward delivery outcome, including a higher incidence of shoulder dystocia. These are patients with a false positive glucose challenge test (where one-hour glucose screen is elevated but subsequent three-hour test is normal); they have an odds ratio for shoulder dystocia of 2.85 compared to normal (negative GCT) controls [80,81]. It is likely that such women eventually deliver higher birth weight infants than even some women with overt gestational diabetes, owing to comparatively less attention paid to diet, weight gain and overall fetal growth patterns in the former group.

Another group of women potentially underappreciated as being at risk for accelerated fetal growth and its associated impact on delivery outcome are those with other forms of glucose metabolism impairment, such as the polycystic-ovary–hirsutism-and-insulin resistance spectrum or those with the metabolic syndrome. Such women may comprise some of the aforementioned false-positive GCT group or may even have normal test results and yet may benefit from close monitoring of fetal growth during the third trimester [82].

Obesity and Excessive Weight Gain During Pregnancy

The association between obesity in pregnancy and high birth weight is a complex one, owing to the interaction of several factors. These include:

1) genetics (the fetus' own predisposition to high ponderal index derived from its parent(s)' predisposition to the same);
2) increased insulin resistance in the mother (not necessarily to diabetic range) derived from elevated adipose to lean body mass ratio; and
3) general overnutrition from both stored energy and excess calorie intake in this population.

The correlation noted in the literature between obesity and the occurrence of shoulder dystocia varies from lack of association in some studies to marked association in others (see Table 2). When studied from the perspective of outcomes in cohorts of overweight and obese parturients compared to normal weight controls, shoulder dystocia is at least twice as likely among obese mothers, yet most such women will experience uncomplicated vaginal deliveries [83-85]. However, among women who experience a shoulder dystocia, obesity appears to be a risk factor for increased severity of shoulder dystocia and greater likelihood of neonatal injury [63,86]. The interaction between obesity and high birth weight among shoulder dystocia deliveries is also varied, with some studies finding obesity to be an independent risk factor and others not (Table 2). A recorded "difficulty with delivery of the shoulders" (at times distinct from "true" shoulder dystocia) may be explained by an overall increase in impedance to normal progress of labor among obese women [29,87]. This is likely attributable to excess soft tissue rather than true bony obstruction, adding to the severity of a possible shoulder dystocia.

Aside from beginning a pregnancy with a high body mass index, even women of normal pre-pregnant weight who gain in excess of 35 lbs during the pregnancy are at increased risk of shoulder dystocia [88]. Yet, even less than this amount may be unwise: Recommended weight gain during pregnancy has increased from 8 kg (17.5 lbs) above ideal body weight for the average-sized woman in 1945 [89] to the current Institute of Medicine guidelines of between 25 and 35 lbs over non-pregnant ideal body weight in 1990. In a pointed brief communication, Spellacy proposes that the collective liberalizing of pregnancy weight gain recommendations by United States obstetric providers over the last half-century has resulted in larger infant birth weights, greater numbers of obstetric complications (especially at delivery) and obesity in children [90]. Paradoxically, this has not impacted the morbidity and mortality rates associated with poor fetal growth, which the liberalized weight gain recommendations were intended to curtail.

Perhaps an even more significant, and often ignored, consequence of this overnutrition during pregnancy is the anthropometric changes that occur in the pregnant women herself, changes that tend to be retained postpartum. Obese women in particular demonstrate a tendency toward the development of central obesity – a known risk factor for cardiovascular disease—as they gain weight during pregnancy and retain this by the postpartum period [91]. Newer research has debunked earlier fears of detrimental effects of caloric and nutrient restriction on fetal growth. In a randomized control trial of gravid primates, pregnant baboons were fed either ad libitum or they were allotted only 70% of such food consumed. While maternal weight and weight gain were reduced compared to controls, fetal weight and length were unaffected [92].

Thus, from an epidemiologic and public health perspective, preconceptional counseling and attainment of ideal body weight, as well as greater attention to weight gain during pregnancy, will have far-reaching impact not only in preventing fetal macrosomia and its attendant risks for labor and delivery complications and their potential injuries, but also preventing other scourges of overnutrition for both mother and newborn.

Intrapartum Risk Factors for Shoulder Dystocia and Related Neonatal Mechanical Injury

Aside from antepartum risk factors for shoulder dystocia, there are additional risk factors that may accrue once a trial of labor is undertaken, which will independently increase the odds of shoulder dystocia (Table 3). Those intrapartum events most strongly associated with shoulder dystocia—as well as with ensuing neonatal injury—are operative vaginal delivery and precipitous second stage of labor [11,30,57].

Table 3. Risk Ratios for Shoulder Dystocia of Specific Intrapartum Risk Factors*.

	Operative vaginal delivery	Precipitous 2nd Stage (<20 min)	Prolonged 2nd Stage	Induction of Labor	Epidural Analgesia	Misc
Acker 1985[11]	18-20%	NS	3.18			Prolonged latent phase: NS Protraction disorders: NS
Acker 1986[31]**	NS	8.5%	2.2			
Benedetti 1978[30]	28		4.6%			
Baskett 1995[150]	10		3.0			
Nesbitt 1998[35]	8.6%-29%					
Sheiner 2004[61]	5.7					
Sandmire 1988	P<0.05	NS	NS	P<0.05		
Gross 1987[185]	35%		15.4%			
Geary 1995[197]	yes					
Bahar 1996[62]	P<0.01					

*Where risk ratios are not explicitly given or able to be calculated from available data, either percentage of shoulder dystocia cases exhibiting the specific risk factor is provided, or where percentage not available, p-value of statistical association between risk factor (vs. lack of risk factor) and shoulder dystocia is given.
**Data confined to average-weight infants only; NS: non-significant

Whereas most of the antepartum risk factors reviewed contribute to fetopelvic size discrepancy as an etiology for shoulder dystocia, it is specifically these two intrapartum risk factors—unlike prolonged second stage or need for augmentation—that are time-dependent (rather than size-dependent) precursors of relative positional discrepancies between fetal shoulder and maternal pelvic dimensions. Simply stated, with either a precipitous second stage or an operative vaginal delivery, the interval between emergence of the head and subsequent restitution and simultaneous shoulder rotation is shortened. Hurried completion of fetal expulsion, usually by the birth attendant but even spontaneously, may not allow sufficient time for the shoulders to rotate and occupy the oblique dimensions of the pelvis before descent, culminating in impaction behind the bony prominences of the anteroposterior pelvic dimensions. Often, patience and/or a non-interventionist approach can avert or mitigate the likelihood of fetal injury simply by reducing the occurrence or severity of shoulder dystocia in these settings [93]. Several authors have espoused the importance of awaiting the next contraction after the head delivers, which allows time for proper suctioning of the oro- and nasopharynx, assessment of cord position and assessment (and even adjustment) of the oblique positioning of the shoulders, and produces a documented reduction in the incidence of shoulder dystocia [29,94, 95,96].

As previously discussed, there may be fetopelvic positional discrepancies predisposing to shoulder dystocia that may be exacerbated by induction of labor or use of epidural analgesia, perhaps related to these interventions' potential impact on uterine and/or abdominal tone and their effect on fetal descent during labor. However, since these effects are relative, which may explain their weaker association specifically with shoulder dystocia [97], and since induction of labor and use of epidural analgesia are multi-purposeful, exceedingly common, and frequently indicated, curtailment of their use solely for avoidance shoulder dystocia is perhaps only justified for the intentional induction of labor solely for "impending" or suspected macrosomia, which is ineffective in reducing shoulder dystocia incidence [33,38,59,98]. Other somewhat weaker associations of shoulder dystocia with such risk factors as abnormalities of the first stage or prolonged second stage are more likely related to these being markers of a larger-than-average fetus causing protraction disorders in general (several of which will end up with absolute cephalopelvic disproportion and subsequent cesarean deliveries) and *all* types of high birth weight-related dystocias rather than causing shoulder dystocia in particular.

Two intrapartum risk factors for shoulder dystocia in particular—operative vaginal delivery and precipitous second stage—have a coincident greater association with subsequent injury. The reasons for this are addressed next.

Operative Vaginal Delivery

In the United States, the incidence of operative vaginal delivery in general is about 15% [99]. In most studies of shoulder dystocia births, the incidence of an antecedent operative delivery reach double that rate, ranging from 8.2%–35% [1,11,16,30,32,100,101]. In the original paper to demonstrate the link between shoulder dystocia and operative delivery, mid-pelvic procedures conferred 28 times the risk, especially when performed following a prolonged stage [30]. In a prospective sense, the decision to use an instrument in a particular delivery should be made with the knowledge that doing so at least doubles the risk of shoulder dystocia. For a patient who already has antenatal risk factors for shoulder dystocia (e.g., diabetes, obesity, prior shoulder dystocia), the attempt at operative delivery should always be made with anticipation of the possibility of having to manage an iatrogenically generated encounter with shoulder dystocia.

Nowhere is this more prudent advice than in the face of a suspected large-for-gestational-age infant: A California-based population study of all newborns weighing 3,500 gm or more also emphasizes the importance of the cumulative effect of operative vaginal delivery with other antepartum risk factors and rising incidence of shoulder dystocia [35]. For every 250-gm increment in birth weight above 4,000 gm, the percentage of infants delivered using either forceps or vacuum who subsequently experienced shoulder dystocia rises steadily from 8.6% to 29% (compared to unassisted deliveries in similar birth weight categories of between 5.2% to 21.1%; however, the percentage of shoulder dystocia deliveries occurring following a combination of diabetes and operative vaginal delivery among the same birth weight categories were 12.2% to 34.8% [35].

Contrary to the belief that the traction forces of the operative delivery itself are causative in neonatal brachial plexus injury [99,102], forceps and vacuum traction far beyond the range needed to produce fetal brachial plexus injury are well tolerated during operative delivery without incident [103,104]. This force magnitude is tolerated because of the anatomical relationship of the brachial plexus to the cervicothoracic spine and the typically axially-directed nature of the traction forces applied during instrumented deliveries. Furthermore, although shoulder dystocia is more likely to occur with operative vaginal deliveries, those shoulder dystocia deliveries in which an injury occurs are no more likely to have been operative deliveries than non-operative. In studies of obstetric antecedents of brachial plexus injuries, incidences of operative delivery are also double the national average; however these deliveries also resulted in shoulder dystocia. If the instrument were etiologic for injury, we would expect a higher incidence of injuries in operative deliveries independent of shoulder dystocia.

However, the severity of injury that occurs following shoulder dystocia in these settings appears to be impacted by the use *and type* of instrumented delivery. In the only randomized controlled trial of the type of instrumented delivery to analyze a potential difference in the risk of subsequent shoulder dystocia, Bofill et al. demonstrated a higher rate of shoulder dystocia among vacuum deliveries compared to forceps (4.7% vs.1.9%, respectively) [17]. More importantly, they found a direct relationship between the length of time needed to complete an operative vaginal delivery and the subsequent occurrence of shoulder dystocia, with only one instance of shoulder dystocia occurring in 195 operative deliveries completed in under two minutes compared to nearly 4% among those taking between two and six minutes to complete (12/304), and nearly twice that (7.9%) among 76 operative deliveries lasting longer than six minutes. This rise in incidence of shoulder dystocia among operative deliveries was also evident with increasing birth weight above 3,500 gm, though a much more marked increase in occurrence (from 6.5% to 33%) was demonstrated among macrosomic infants (>4,000 gm) [17]. These findings emphasize the relationship between the difficulty of operative delivery and relative fetopelvic size discrepancy, and the potential cumulative effect of operative delivery and macrosomia in the pathophysiology of shoulder dystocia. As a result, it may be prudent to avoid operative delivery in a patient that exhibits shoulder dystocia risk factors.

Abnormalities of the Second Stage of Labor

Since Benedetti and Gabbe first implicated prolonged second stage as a risk factor for shoulder dystocia, the focus on slowly progressing labors has pervaded the shoulder dystocia literature landscape [1,4,30,37,105-109]. The focus on prolonged second stage as a significant risk factor for shoulder dystocia is likely the result of the ability to manipulate it— by augmenting labor, using an instrument, or delivering by cesarean section. As noted above, the first two of these possible interventions increases the risk of shoulder dystocia, especially when used with the larger than average fetus. It should be remembered that prolonged second stage is likely a marker for the large-for-gestational-age infant; in fact, in some series, if birth weight is controlled for, the association of shoulder dystocia with prolonged second stage is eliminated. In the final analysis, the incidence of prolonged second stage among shoulder dystocia deliveries is only about 10% (Table 3). A more significant second stage abnormality associated with both shoulder dystocia and injury is the opposite problem: precipitous second stage, usually defined as less than 20 minutes' duration, regardless of parity.

Acker et al. first identified precipitous second stage as a risk factor for shoulder dystocia with temporary injury [11]. They attributed this to two causes: insufficient time for the shoulders to rotate into the oblique pelvic dimension and insufficient time for the providers to prepare. In the only case-controlled study on intrapartum risk factors for permanent injury among shoulder dystocia deliveries, Poggi et al., after controlling for birth weight, diabetes and parity, found that (1) operative delivery or abnormal second stage (either prolonged or precipitous) incidences were similar in the uninjured group and the injured group, and (2) precipitous second stage is the most prevalent intrapartum risk factor for shoulder dystocia, complicating 30% of shoulder dystocia deliveries in that series [32]. From the perspective of injury prevention, since precipitous delivery is often unexpected and certainly outside the control of the birth attendant, little can be done to modify it as a risk factor for shoulder dystocia; however, as a risk factor for injury, there is potential for mitigation, since the awareness of a potential for shoulder dystocia should alert personnel who might otherwise be expecting rapid expulsion of the fetal trunk following a precipitous descent of the fetal head to anticipate the opposite.

Having completed a review of antepartum and intrapartum risk factors for shoulder dystocia, it is appropriate and noteworthy to remind the reader that about half of shoulder dystocia incidents occur without any identifiable risk factors. Additionally, even those shoulder dystocia deliveries noted retrospectively to have had risk factors either failed to be appreciated antepartum (owing to limitations of estimation of fetal weight or lack of knowledge of prior shoulder dystocia) or were recognized but did not reach thresholds for which avoidance of vaginal delivery would be justified. Thus, all obstetric providers must be prepared for encounters with the complication, as they are inevitable in any practice setting. Furthermore, although some risk factors for shoulder dystocia will confer greater risk of an injurious result, by far the greatest determinant of neonatal injury is the actual management of shoulder dystocia, once it occurs. Thus, any epidemiologic review of shoulder dystocia and its relationship to fetal injury must necessarily devote attention to review and critical evaluation of existing treatments. However, before these are addressed, a general review of neonatal brachial plexus injury epidemiology is needed.

Part II: Epidemiology of Neonatal Brachial Plexus Injury

Brachial plexus injuries diagnosed at birth often have different modifiers: obstetric, birth, congenital, perinatal, neonatal and pediatric. The reason for the multiple descriptors is partly a function of the medical specialties interested in the problem (obstetrics, neonatology, neurology, neurosurgery, orthopedics, physical rehabilitation and medicine). Because medicine is generally not interdisciplinary, research from different fields use different terms, have different perspectives, and at times have markedly different interpretations. Another reason for the varied terminology is the current legal climate in obstetrics in countries where lawsuits are not uncommon [110]. Since obstetricians can be blamed for causing these injuries, describing the injuries as birth, congenital, perinatal or neonatal either neutralizes the issue of causation or suggests an alternative etiology thereby exonerating the accocheur [111-115].

There are, in fact, many etiologies to neonatal brachial plexus impairment*—most unrelated to shoulder dystocia—and the purpose of this section is to identify the different ones, their incidences, specific causes and, most importantly, to identify those injuries which are amenable to prevention and explain how to prevent them.

We begin by exploring the anatomy of the newborn brachial plexus and the types and mechanisms of injury it may sustain. We then discuss injury classification, incidence, obstetric risk factors, and etiology. Although necessary to appreciate preventing injuries, we state at the outset that this is only a cursory review by non-treating injury researchers and the interested reader wanting to delve further can do so with a number of specialized texts and articles by treating clinicians [116-119].

Brachial Plexus Anatomy

To understand the clinical presentation and provide anticipatory guidance for families affected by neonatal brachial plexus injury, the treating clinician must have a grasp of, and be able to articulate neonatal peripheral nerve anatomy. As seen in Figure 1, the brachial plexus consists of a network of five nerve tracts (the ventral rami) that emanate from the fifth cervical vertebrae or C5, through the first thoracic vertebrae or T1. Although this is the

---

* Neonatal is the modifier used in this chapter, as this term accurately describes the patient at birth and not the cause.

typical anatomy, clinicians should also be aware that there is considerable variation in newborn brachial plexus anatomy [120].

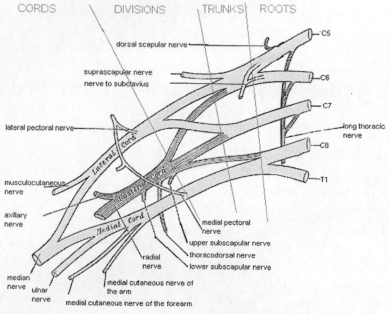

Figure 1. Brachial plexus anatomy. Erb's point is the anatomical location of the union of nerves emanating from C5 and C6, which is located about 1 centimeter from the spinal column in the newborn. The region proximal to the spine from a line emanating from Erb's point is known as the root. The nerve emanating from the seventh vertical vertebrae, or C7 becomes the middle trunk, and the nerves emanating from C8 and T1 come together and form the lower trunk. Each trunk divides into anterior and posterior divisions to create the cords, which then subdivide further into branches that supply the muscles of the arm.

Lesions and Impairments of the Brachial Plexus

Injuries and impairments of the brachial plexus may be mild, with only temporary sequelae, or be devastating, resulting in lifelong paralysis of the affected arm that remains flaccid, withered and lacks sensory perception [118]. The number of nerves involved and the degree to which each level is disrupted determines the severity of the effect [117,119,121-123]. The basic types of brachial plexus palsies include the following:

- Erb-Duchenne palsy or upper trunk injury is defined by its affecting only the nerves emanating from C5 and C6.
- Upper-middle trunk brachial plexus palsy involves nerve fibers emanating from C5, C6, and C7 levels.
- Klumpke palsy results in deficits at levels C8 and T1; however isolated C8-T1 injuries almost never occur in newborns delivered vaginally in cephalic presentation. If otherwise identified at birth, they are concomitant with spinal cord injury or some other neurological anomaly.
- Complete and/or panplexus neonatal brachial plexus injury affects nerves of at least four vertebral levels, either C5-C8 or C5-T1.

As primary peripheral nerve impairments, almost all brachial plexus lesions evident at birth are ipsilateral, or one sided, unless their etiology is secondary to a central lesion affecting the brain or spinal cord. Bilateral neonatal brachial plexus injury does occur rarely, primarily in breech deliveries, but the severity of impairment in each injured plexus is always different. Those who treat neonatal brachial plexus palsy have discovered a host of non-traumatic etiologies for neonatal brachial plexus impairment. These include aplasia of brachial plexus roots, humerus head osteomylitis, idiopathic atrophy, overfolding of the scapha helix, premature telarche, neoplasms, congenital cervical rib, varicella infection, and vascular insult causing neonatal gangrene [124-130]. Rarely, prolonged severe fetal intrauterine maladaptation caused by distorted uterine anatomy (e.g., maternal uterine malformation, uterine fibroids) or anhydramnios may be causative; classically, a neglected persistent transverse lie, shoulder presentation or asynclitism in labor, with otherwise catastrophic consequences for both mother and fetus have also been reported [131]. Notably, these impairments are *all* case reports indicating that these conditions are too rare to be able to perform a study on their incidence, and that nothing prenatally can be done to prevent most of them. However, if incidentally detected prenatally via ultrasound, the treating obstetrician should counsel the patient appropriately and obtain a pediatric neurological or orthopedic consultation.

By far, the overwhelming majority of neonatal brachial plexus impairments evident at birth result from a mechanical stretch sustained at some time during the final stages of delivery. As such they are termed as injuries. From an epidemiological perspective, this terminology is not intended to imply negligence or malfeasance, but simply etiology. It is this form of neonatal brachial plexus impairment that we consider in detail.

Stretch Injury Classification

Seddon defines three grades of nerve injury (neurapraxia, axonotmesis, and neurotmesis) based on the extent of damage to the structural components of the peripheral nerve tracts [132]. Although not technically damage to the structural component of the nerve itself, avulsion of the nerve root from the spinal cord is a fourth type of injury that can occur in a newborn [119].

Neurapraxia is the mildest grade of nerve injury, and is characterized by a reduction of conduction across a segment of nerve. Axonal continuity is maintained and nerve conduction is preserved both proximal and distal to the lesion, but not across it. Neonatal neurapraxia occurs when the nerve is stretched enough to disrupt axonal flow but not sufficient to induce non-recoverable mechanical damage. Conduction is restored when remyelination occurs. Neurapraxic injuries are always reversible and a full recovery can occur in hours, days, weeks or months.

Axonotmesis represents the least severe grade of persistent nerve injury and is characterized by interruption of the axons with preservation of the surrounding connective tissue, which can support axonal regeneration. Distal Wallerian degeneration (axon and myelin degeneration distal to site of injury) of the axons occurs over a few days' interval (much shorter than adults), after which direct electrical stimulation of the disconnected distal nerve stump will not give rise to a nerve conduction or muscle response [133]. Some recovery usually can occur through axonal regeneration owing to the preservation of the connective tissue, which includes Schwann cells that can form longitudinal conduits through which axons regenerate. However, in the newborn, axonotmetic injuries usually recover to an extent, but incompletely. The scar tissue or neuroma that develops during healing will limit conduction through the nerve, thereby inducing clinical limitations in the shoulder, arm or both.   This is the most common permanent injury in the newborn.

Neurotmesis is the severest grade of injury to the nerve itself. Neurotmetic injuries are characterized by disruption of the axon, myelin, and connective tissue components of the nerve. Because of the damage to structurally supportive connective tissue, recovery through regeneration cannot occur. This grade of injury may encompass nerve lesions where external continuity of the nerve can be preserved but fibrosis occurs and blocks axonal regeneration. Neurotmetic injuries also include nerves whose continuity has been completely interrupted. Since the there is no tissue for axonal regeneration, surgery is needed to remove intervening scar tissue and to re-establish continuity of the nerve usually via autologous nerve graft. This type of injury is commonly referred to as a rupture.

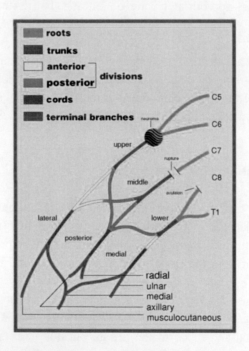

Figure 2. Pattern of traction-induced brachial plexus injury with increasing lateral deviation of the head from the contralateral shoulder. Described in the late nineteenth century, forcible lateral deviation of the head produces a consistent pattern of injury to the brachial plexus: nerve roots C5 and C6 are injured before damage to C7 occurs. Lower root injuries (often avulsions) occur as total plexopathies, after C5-C7 are injured.

Avulsion injury is the most severe because it involves dislocation of the nerve roots from the spinal cord, thereby permanently and irreversibly eliminating conduction through the affected nerve completely. Surgery for this type injury will only attempt to reinnervate the muscles affected by the loss of conduction through rerouting of those brachial plexus nerve roots that have retained continuity with the spinal cord. This is accomplished either via grafts between healthy nerves on the ipsilateral side to the distal portion of the affected nerve or, if too distant, the grafting procedure may involve transfer of fibers from the healthy nerve fibers from the contralateral side [134]. Figure 2 depicts a brachial plexus schematic with an upper neuroma, a middle rupture and a lower root avulsion. In pan plexus injuries, this is a typical injury pattern.

Although the severity and permanence of injury the nerve is not diagnosable at birth, it is important to evaluate which nerves are affected by clinical exam, even in the newborn. Although muscles in the shoulder and arm are innervated by more than one nerve of the brachial plexus, individual nerves primarily innervate individual muscles. Specifically, C5 innervates the bicep, C6 the deltoid, C7 the tricep, C8 the hand, and T1 the fourth and fifth digit. Rarely, injury to the phrenic nerve (which arises from C4) can lead to hemidiaphragm paralysis on the affected side. The lower roots, if avulsed, may also affect the sympathetic system at that level and induce ophthalmologic abnormities, such as ptosis and Horner's syndrome. However, clinicians should be aware that these neonatal eye disorders are more often *not* associated with concomitant brachial plexus injury [135].

The clinician treating newborns must also recognize the uniqueness of neonatal brachial plexus injuries as distinct from traumatic brachial plexus injuries sustained by children and adults. The damage in neonates usually results from slow traction injuries, unlike the high-energy, shearing type of trauma seen in older individuals [117]. Not only are the latter injuries often more severe, but, even with injuries of similar extent, infants show a better functional outcome [136]. This clinical observation was observed in 14 infants and 19 adults with surgical evidence of complete avulsion of the upper trunk roots (C5-C6). Electromyelogram (EMG) results showed normal recruitment of biceps and deltoid in the infants and complete denervation in the older individuals. However, when C7 was also torn, the infants demonstrated complete denervation. Vredeveld et al. attribute this observation to neonatal C7 innervation of the biceps and deltoid that is absent if C5-C6 roots are functional [136].

Incidence of Neonatal Brachial Plexus Injury

The incidence of neonatal brachial plexus injury is difficult to assess because it varies with population, place, time, data source and the medical specialty examining the issue. In addition, because the impairment is an infrequent event, millions of births are needed to generate a sizeable population of injuries. Even with these limitations, four population-based studies, shown in Table 4, have reported injury incidence in a general population: neonatal brachial plexus injury occurs between one in 2000 deliveries and one in 500. When distinguished from temporary neurapraxias, permanent neonatal brachial plexus injury has a reported incidence of less than 1 in over 50000 deliveries to one in 786 cephalic deliveries [137,138]. In the largest study to date, Foad et al. examined over 11,000,000 deliveries and 17,000 neonatal brachial plexus injuries in the United States over a six-year period and discovered rates decreasing from 0.17% in 1997 to 0.16% in 2000 to 0.13% in 2003 (p<0.01) [114]. On the other hand, Bager et al. discovered increasing incidence over time in a Swedish study [139]. Why the variation in incidence? One reason is the lack of a consistent denominator representing the "at-risk" population. Specifically, the population studies often do not provide data on the various types of deliveries: cephalic, breech, spontaneous, operative, cesarean, term-only, singleton-only or all deliveries. Another reason is variation in the source of data, with some studies assessing incidence in specific networks of hospitals, others using state or national birth records, others reviewing the incidence in pediatric centers and specialized brachial plexus clinics.

Table 4. Incidence of Neonatal Brachial Plexus Injury Derived from Population-Based Studies.

Study, Year	Years, Location	Data Source	Total Deliveries	NBPI	NBPI Incidence*
Bager, 1997[139]	15, Sweden	Med. Birth Registry	1,564,307	2694	0.17% (0.13%-0.22%)**
Cristoffersson, 2002[10]	9, Sweden	Med. Birth Registry	1,076,545	2132	0.20%
Foad, 2008[114]	3, United States	Pediatric database	11,540,000	17334	0.15%
Gilbert, 1999[199]	2, California	Birth certificates	1,094,298	1611	0.15%
McFarland, 1986[59]	3, Washington St	Birth certificates	210, 947	106	0.05%

NBPI: neonatal brachial plexus injury;

*The incidence of NBPI during cesarean section is usually not reported. However, the number for section-associated NBPI is as follows: 643 in the Foad report, 60 in the Gilbert report, 46 in the Christoffersson report, and 4 in the McFarland report.

**Bager evaluated the incidence of NBPI annually and reported a generally increasing trend. Values presented are for 1980 and1994.

However, even when we explore incidence within individual hospitals, the incidence of neonatal brachial plexus injury also varies by at risk population defined and/or time period reviewed: with incidence reports of between one in 1500 deliveries to one in 188 deliveries [10,14,16,57,137,139-143]. A sampling of the dozens of such papers is listed in Table 5. Unique among these is a 1967 study by Adler and Patterson, two New York City-based pediatric neurologists who treated children with neonatal brachial plexus injuries at New York Hospital for Special Surgery for close to 40 years. They observed from 1922 though 1938, the incidence of neonatal brachial plexus injury was 1.6 per 1000 births; and from 1939 though 1962, the incidence dropped 400% to 0.38 neonatal brachial plexus injury per 1000 deliveries. Of note, this was during an era when cesarean section incidence was 2%, and birth weights were increasing. This was the first report to attribute a reduction in neonatal brachial plexus injury incidence to improved obstetrical technique [144]. Indeed, historically corresponding to the time period and locale under study, two shoulder dystocia management techniques that had been reintroduced during the 1940s in New York were Woods maneuver [145] and delivery of the posterior arm [146].

Thus, careful examination of Table 5 reveals that (1) neonatal brachial plexus injury occurs in infants delivered by cesarean section; (2) neonatal brachial plexus injury likely occurs during routine deliveries without shoulder dystocia; and, most importantly, (3) that neonatal brachial plexus injury incidence variation can be significant and is attributable not only to obstetrical population but to obstetrical technique, which varies over time and from place to place. This last factor is especially true concerning persistent injuries, and provides clinical evidence to support the epidemiological assertion made here that many injuries are likely amenable to prevention. Most notable, therefore, is the link between permanent neonatal brachial plexus injury and antecedent shoulder dystocia, which we address next.

Table 5. Sampling of Incidences of Neonatal Brachial Plexus Injury Derived at Individual Institutions.

Study, Year	Years, Location	Data Source	Total Deliveries (TD) Vaginal Deliveries (VD)	NBPI	NBPI Incidence/ VD NBPI incidence*
Acker, 1988[57]	2, Harvard	Maternal Records	32,468	22	0.07%
Bager, 1997[139]	10, Skarabough County, Sweden	Pediatric Records	33,160	52	0.16%
Chauhan 2005[142]	23, Spartanburg Reg. Med. Center, Mississippi	ICD codes	89,978	85	0.09%
Gherman, 1998**[12]	2, USC Medical Center, California	Neonatal records	9,071 VD	40	0.44%
Graham, 1997[141]	4.5, University of Pennsylvania Hosp	Maternal & Neonatal Records	14,358 TD 11,484 VD	15	0.10% 0.13%
Jennett, 1992[137]	4, St. Joseph's Hospital, Arizona	Neonatal records	57,597	39	0.07%
Nocon, 1993[14]	4.5, Wishard Memorial Hospital, Indiana	Maternal & neonatal records	14,297 TD 12,532 VD	33	0.23% 0.26%
Wolf, 2000[143]	9, Amsterdam Medical Center, Netherlands	Amsterdam	13,366 9,912 (vaginal, cephalic, singleton)	62 61	0.46% 0.56%

NBPI: neonatal brachial plexus injury;

*Persistent BPI incidences, if reported, are as follows: Bager reports 18, Chauhan 11, Gherman 9, Jennett none, Nocon 2 and Wolf 16.

**Gherman et al. report incidence for an additional seven NBPI incidence studies not listed here with incidences varying from 0.07% up to 0.44%.[200-205]

Risk Factors for Neonatal Brachial Plexus Injury

The most consistent risk factor for either transient or permanent neonatal brachial plexus injury is antecedent shoulder dystocia [19,113,147,148]. It is no surprise, then, that both antenatal and intrapartum risk factors for neonatal brachial plexus injury are identical to those of shoulder dystocia discussed earlier. These are: prior shoulder dystocia, diabetes, macrosomia, obesity, weight gain, post-dates, induction for macrosomia, prolonged second stage, operative delivery, and precipitous second stage [30,57]. Studies aimed at determining whether any of these risk factors for transient or permanent neonatal brachial plexus injury are independent of shoulder dystocia have been negative [32,149]. Even more significant is that the single biggest risk factor for neonatal brachial plexus injury is clinician-applied traction at deliveries complicated by shoulder dystocia [3,19,150-154], *the* factor most mechanistically plausible, as we now demonstrate.

Mechanism of Neonatal Brachial Plexus Injury

Traumatic neonatal brachial plexus stretch injuries can *only* result when a mechanical hyperextension of one side of the neck is forcibly induced; nothing else can cause the nerves of the right or left brachial plexus to stretch beyond the limit at which injury occurs. The mechanism is a mechanical event, not a biological one. The magnitude and duration of applied forces to (1) the head when the shoulders are fixed, or (2) to the trunk when the head is fixed usually determines the severity or grade of a neonatal brachial plexus injury [123,154]. The most common circumstance in which such mechanical stress is induced in newborns occurs when the head deviates laterally away from one shoulder, or is rotated beyond 90 degrees, or both, during shoulder dystocia. This fact has been established over a century ago [155], and has since been confirmed by many [23,123,131,156,157], with three being especially noteworthy:

In his classic paper on shoulder dystocia, Morris dissected the necks of a series of stillborns and made the following observations about the brachial plexus when he manipulated the head relative to the trunk:

1) Brachial plexus stretch is greatest when the head is deviated laterally to the side (i.e., ear to shoulder).
2) Brachial plexus is least affected when the head is extended directly from the trunk.
3) Head rotation produces an intermediate amount of brachial plexus stretch.
4) Brachial plexus injury is more easily produced when head motion is induced rapidly rather than slowly [23].

Only one quantitative study specifically simulated shoulder dystocia to explore the effect of lateral head deviation via the external application of known force loads to the head. Resultant injury thresholds were observed in the exposed but *in-situ* brachial plexi of newborn cadavers [123]. Increasing lateral load placed on the head while keeping the shoulders fixed produced the following results:

1) The upper plexus (C5-C6) was always the first to be damaged, followed sequentially by injury to C7, C8 and then T1, as loads increased.

2) Injury patterns typically involved ruptures of the upper roots and avulsions of the lower roots; this is a consequence of greater mechanical strength of the corresponding ligaments that maintain and protect the nerve roots' connection to the spinal cord at individual intraforamenal levels.

3) The threshold for visible mechanical injuries varied from 44 lbs (upper roots only) to 88 lbs (pan plexus injuries with lower root avulsions) of laterally-applied external traction [123].

The only study to explore the mechanical limits specifically of fetal nerve was performed by Kalmin, who divided 51 fetal and newborn cadavers into three gestational age groups: 28–32 weeks, 33–36 weeks and 37–40 weeks [158]. Vagal and phrenic nerves were tested mechanically in all three groups. The results demonstrated that despite differences in geometric and strength properties among the groups, the ultimate strain beyond which rupture of the nerve tract occurs was about the same for each group: 47%–52% beyond original length. This result confirms those of others who find that pediatric nerve tissue is generally far more elastic than that of adults, which will rupture at only 15%–20% strain [159].

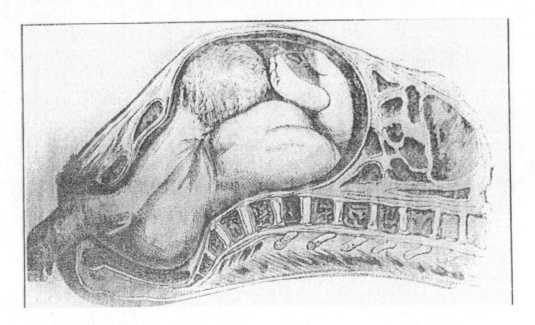

Figure 3. Example of mechanisms of traumatic neonatal brachial plexus injury. A neglected shoulder presentation, which was ultimately fatal, resulted in hyperextension of the left brachial plexus.

How does hyperextension of the neck sufficient to cause injury occur clinically in a newborn? Figure 3 shows how this may occur either *in utero* or during delivery in much the way described in these experiments. Brachial plexus injuries also occur in breech deliveries, though by different mechanisms. One way is when the trunk is deviated from the undelivered aftercoming head, which stretches one side of the neck and can injure the brachial plexus.

However, the typical injury pattern in this circumstance is different from cephalic deliveries in that most often it is the upper roots that are avulsed rather than the lower ones [160]. Another antecedent for injury during breech delivery occurs with nuchal arm(s), when the fetal arm(s) is(are) outstretched *in utero*, and can be hyperextended, which can lead to lower brachial plexus injury during descent. When this occurs, it is not possible to prevent injury.

Brachial plexus evident after delivery in cephalic presentation may also occur in the absence of recorded or probable shoulder dystocia or in the absence of traction altogether [14,26,31,137,141]. However, these newborns often exhibit evidence of a tendency to maladaptation, such as asynclitism, acidosis or other abnormalities [16,26,161]. While injuries such as these are not amenable to prevention, they constitute only a small percentage of all neonatal brachial plexus injuries and are almost always temporary in an otherwise healthy newborn [14,26,31,137].

Controversies Concerning the Obstetric Etiology of Neonatal Brachial Plexus Injury

Within the obstetric literature of the last 18 years, whether hyperextension of the fetal neck sufficient to cause injury occurs in utero, during labor or with "normal" application of delivery traction has been a major issue of contention. Understandably, great interest has been generated in alternative causes besides clinician-applied traction, because of the implication that if actions undertaken by birth attendants are contributory, they potentially can be held liable. Curiously, litigation only started to seriously affect providers since the early 1990s, when this controversy began [162]. Since Jennett and Tarby's retrospective study in 1992 first suggested that since neonatal brachial plexus "impairment" occurs without shoulder dystocia (N.B. such cases were only among the *temporary* injuries observed in that series), the injury itself should not be taken as "prima fascia evidence of birth process injury" [137], dozens of obstetric authors have published retrospective reports asserting that neonatal brachial plexus injuries occur independently of obstetrical technique, including neonatal brachial plexus injury occurring without shoulder dystocia during routine vaginal delivery, permanent brachial plexus injury occurring during cesarean section [161], severe permanent neonatal brachial plexus injury in the posterior shoulder [163,164], complete neonatal brachial plexus injuries having a different mechanism than Erb-Duchenne palsy [165] and shoulder dystocia itself being responsible for injury [166,167]. However, most of these reports fail to distinguish permanent from temporary injury.

As previously stated, despite the aforementioned delivery circumstances culminating in neonatal brachial plexus injury where shoulder dystocia was not a factor, most injuries in fact occur during a shoulder dystocia. This is especially true for the most clinically relevant injury, the permanent neonatal brachial plexus injury, which is almost universally associated with shoulder dystocia delivery and, more specifically, with clinician-applied traction to the head during such delivery [15,16,19,147,154,168]. To understand this association, we next focus on the role of clinician-applied traction during delivery.

Clinician Forces of Delivery

Although qualitative attempts have been made to estimate traction during delivery, this concept has not gained wide acceptance in practice yet [150,154,169]. Nonetheless, more than 10 quantitative research studies have reported on clinician-applied forces in over 500 clinical and simulated deliveries during the last twenty years [25,152,170-172]. These included routine, difficult and shoulder dystocia deliveries in the simulated and clinical environments. The principal findings from these studies are listed below:

1) The typical traction used for a routine delivery varies from 0 to 10 pounds; this can be increased to 20 pounds or more during shoulder dystocia delivery [19;170].
2) Clinicians can generally distinguish between three types of delivery (routine, difficult and shoulder dystocia) [173].
3) More difficult delivery often results in additional traction being applied in subsequent delivery attempts [173].
4) Training with simulated shoulder dystocia deliveries reduces clinician traction in subsequent simulated deliveries by the same provider [174].

One clinical study quantified traction applied during a shoulder dystocia delivery that resulted in a clavicle fracture and temporary brachial plexus injury [19]. This is the only clinical data to quantify a possible injury limit of 22 lbs applied laterally and quickly to the head.

In a recent study, Mollberg et al. developed a visual analog scale for quantifying traction in a prospective study that included 16 permanent brachial plexopathies. In *all* of them, they found forceful downward traction to have been used with delivery. This led to their conclusion: "Forceful downward traction applied to the head after the fetal third rotation represents an important risk factor of obstetric brachial plexus palsy in vaginal deliveries in cephalic presentation" [154].

With this background on the etiology of neonatal brachial plexus injury, we are now able to explore shoulder dystocia management with an eye toward minimizing traction to prevent neonatal brachial plexus injury in a way that still accomplishes delivery without asphyxia. We next focus on maneuvers and their efficacy in minimizing the risk of injury where possible.

Part III: Management of Shoulder Dystocia to Prevent Neonatal Brachial Plexus Injury

To avoid injury, traction applied to the head during difficult or shoulder dystocia deliveries should not be greater than normal, or even not used at all [19,95,96,152,175-177]. However, as presented earlier, this is not readily done in practice: traction during shoulder dystocia is on average increased, sometime to amounts that cause with permanent injury [123,154,173]. Beyond the increased magnitude, clinician-applied traction during shoulder dystocia is often off-axis of the fetal spine; to the extent possible, it should be directed axially more than laterally to reduce the risk of injury [23,152].

Awaiting the Next Contraction

Also not commonly practiced, simply awaiting the next contraction during a shoulder dystocia has been shown to be beneficial. This is especially true during a precipitous second stage, in which the only cause of shoulder dystocia may be insufficient time for normal-sized shoulders to assume their physiologic oblique orientation [29,93,95]. Studies have shown that awaiting the next contraction actually lowers the incidence of shoulder dystocia [29,93].

However, if these principles are meticulously observed, the obstruction to delivery resulting from true shoulder dystocia often will not be overcome either by patience or by gentle traction alone; specialized maneuvers will have to be employed to successfully deliver the infant without injury or asphyxia.

A Review of Maneuvers

The objective of any shoulder dystocia maneuver is to compensate for the incompatible fetal shoulder and maternal pelvic dimensions. This is done by changing the relative positions of the maternal pelvis and the fetal shoulders, shrinking the shoulder width, and/or manually performing a rotational movement of the shoulders within the birth canal. Some maneuvers simultaneously involve more than one of these manipulations. The most familiar and commonly practiced maneuvers for shoulder dystocia can be divided into two broad categories: those that involve external manipulation of the mother and those that involve manipulation of the fetus within the birth canal. Five principal maneuvers are reviewed in detail here: McRoberts' positioning and suprapubic pressure (maternal maneuvers), and Rubin's maneuver, posterior arm delivery and Woods maneuver (fetal maneuvers). Although other maneuvers exist, such as the all fours maneuver, Zavanelli maneuver and symphysiotomy, we focus on the aforementioned five because of their efficacy, as well as their avoidance of difficult repositioning of the patient and/or surgery. Although maneuver descriptions and procedures are presented briefly here, a more comprehensive review can be found elsewhere [45].

McRoberts' Positioning

Sharp flexion of the maternal thighs against the abdomen, was first proposed in 1899 in France and was adopted in the United States as early as 1914, although the technique seemed to have been lost for several generations thereafter [178]. The maneuver is usually accomplished with the aid of one or two assistants who remove the mother's legs from the footrests and, by flexing the hips, manually tilt the pelvis cephalad by about 15 degrees [179]. Although McRoberts' positioning does not actually widen the pelvic bones, it does raise the pubic symphysis anteriorly about 9 mm and cephalad 28 mm, as shown in Figure 4. The effect of McRoberts' maneuver is to flatten the sacrum by flexing the spine and compressing the vertebral joints just above the sacral promontory, allowing the posterior shoulder to descend further into the pelvis. Traction is then usually applied to the fetal head by the birth attendant to complete the delivery [19,152].

In a laboratory study, for some mild shoulder dystocia deliveries, McRoberts' positioning resulted in fewer clavicle fractures, less traction and less brachial plexus stretch than the same size fetal model delivered through lithotomy positioning, as shown in Table 6 [152]. However, as shoulder dystocia became more severe (bisacromial diameter > 12.5 cm), the effect of McRoberts' position was negated: more traction was necessary and fracture incidence increased and more brachial plexus stretch occurred. This is why McRoberts' positioning only resolves shoulder dystocia atraumatically about 40% of the time [60,180]. In addition, in a randomized control trial, prophylactic use of McRoberts' maneuver in anticipation of possible shoulder dystocia did not result in less traction being applied to the head to accomplish delivery [20].

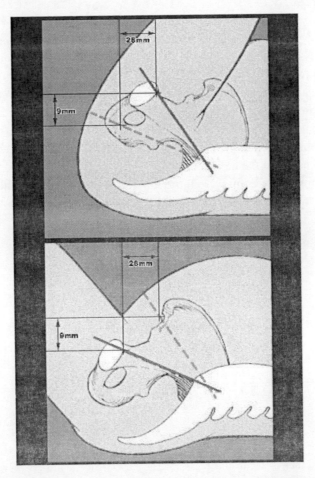

Figure 4. Mechanical effect of McRoberts' positioning. Pelvic rotation of approximately 15° lifts the pubic symphysis about 9 mm in a gynecoid pelvis. In about ½ of shoulder dystocia deliveries, this is sufficient to clear the obstructed anterior shoulder.[180] Reprinted with permission.[206]

Table 6. Peak Force and Clavicle Fracture Incidences for Lithotomy and McRoberts Positioning for Four Classes of Shoulder Dystocia Severity.

Bisacromial Diameter (cm)	Number of Deliveries *	Peak Force, McRoberts **	Peak Force, Lithotomy **	P	Fracture incidence (%), McRoberts	Fracture incidence (%), Lithotomy
11.5	5	63.8 + 3.2	73.0 + 2.4	<.01	0	0
12.0	7	80.2 + 2.4	91.6 + 4.7	<.05	0	63[□]
12.5	6	102.0 + 5.4	106.2 + 7.1	NS	83	100
13.0	1	98.4	104.8		100	100

* For lithotomy positioning, N was 8 and 4 for 12.0 cm and 12.5 cm, respectively.
** Units measured in Newtons. A Newton is equivalent to 0.1 kg or 0.225 lbs.
[□] P < .025. All other P values for fracture incidence are not significant.

Suprapubic Pressure

First published in 1959, and depicted in Figure 5, suprapubic pressure involves an assistant applying fisted pressure near the anatomical location of the symphyisis pubis [181]. Its purposes are three-fold: (1) By applying significant pressure *laterally* from behind the *posterior* aspect of the anterior shoulder (at a 45-degree downward direction) the shoulders can potentially rotate into the oblique; (2) the shoulders can potentially adduct, reducing the bisacromial diameter; and (3) soft tissue should compress thereby increasing the clearance for the shoulders. The birth attendant confirms the orientation of the shoulder by direct palpation of the fetal shoulder behind the delivered head [182]. He or she then instructs the assistant as to which side to apply the pressure: from the mother's right side when the fetus is in ROA or ROT presentation, or from the left side in an LOA or LOT position. After the pressure is applied, the attendant attempts traction.

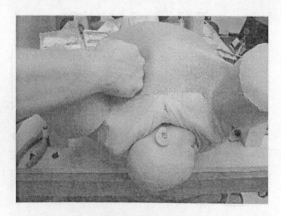

Figure 5. Correct application of suprapubic pressure. The closed-fisted, obliquely oriented downward pressure is applied just above the pubic symphysis. In an attempt to rotate (adduct) or facilitate rotation of the fetal shoulders, firm pressure is applied behind the posterior aspect of the anterior shoulder. The firm application also has the effect of compressing soft tissue, which is likely to decrease the level of impaction.

Suprapubic pressure and McRoberts' maneuver are often performed concommitantly, followed by traction to the head by the attendant. The prudent birth attendant must be mindful of the tendency to apply more traction than is customary. It is during this time that stretching and possible injury to brachial plexus can take place. As a result, if McRoberts' maneuver and suprapubic pressure with traction do not completely succeed within one traction attempt that lasts for *less* than 10 seconds, traction should be abandoned and fetal maneuvers should be attempted.

The Advantage of Fetal Maneuvers

Unfortunately, epidemiological evaluation of shoulder dystocia management has led to a misguided notion that manipulation of the fetus within the birth canal during shoulder dystocia increases the risk of injury. Three retrospective studies relating shoulder dystocia maneuvers and outcome concluded that either no maneuver was superior to another or that fetal maneuvers were the damaging ones [14,60,183]. The authors reached these conclusions because they assumed the injury occurred during the final maneuver in shoulder dystocia deliveries where multiple maneuvers were needed. However, in all of the deliveries involving fetal maneuvers, McRoberts' and suprapubic were always tried first, unsuccessfully. As described above, these maneuvers most often involved traction to the head, usually greater traction than normal.

Table 7. Correlation between Number and Type of Maneuvers and Neonatal Injury Rate.

Study	# Maneuvers Used	BPP Rate
McFarland, 1996[60]	1-2	7.7%
	≥3	25%
Gherman, 1998[12]	1-2	11-22%
	3 + proctoepisiotomy	31%
Study	Maneuvers Used	BPP Incidence
Gross, 1987[185]	SPP, DPA, Woods	1/1
	Woods only	0/5
	DPA only	0/4
Baskett, 1995[150]	Traction Only	12/48
	McRoberts, Woods, DPA	3/15
	Woods Only	2/32
	DPA Only	0/9

SPP: Suprapubic Pressure; DPA: Delivery of the Posterior Arm

However, the effective difference between maternal and fetal maneuvers is that in the former, traction is applied *during* the impaction in an attempt to relieve it, whereas in the latter, traction to the head (if necessary) is applied only *after* the impaction is resolved. This is true for Rubin's maneuver, Wood's maneuver and delivery of the posterior arm. Indeed, in reports where a fetal maneuver was performed first in shoulder dystocia management, fewer or no injuries were reported than when other management maneuvers were employed [150,184,185]. Table 7 presents the results of these studies.

Finally, in one of the two quantitative studies that exist, Poggi et al. published the force needed to deliver the posterior arm in a shoulder dystocia delivery was about 6 lbs compared to an 11 lb attempt during an unsuccessful McRobert's maneuver [20]. Gurewitsch et al. compared Rubin's maneuver with McRoberts' maneuver in a laboratory study of 30 simulated shoulder dystocia deliveries. In general, deliveries using Rubin's maneuver followed by traction resulted in ½ as much traction being required as in those deliveries in which McRoberts positioning was employed; more importantly, brachial plexus stretch was 1/3 as much [172].

We recommend fetal maneuvers for reducing the risk of injury when managing a shoulder dystocia in progress, in part because of the studies cited above and in part because of the biomechanical advantages they afford.

Rubin's Maneuver

In Rubin's maneuver, an attempt is made to re-establish the proper oblique orientation of the bisacromial diameter within the pelvis. The clinician performs a ~30° rotation of the fetal trunk by placing a hand within the vagina and applying pressure to the posterior aspect of the anterior shoulder, much the same was suprapubic pressure tries to do, as shown in Figure 6 [186]. If successful, the rotation from the anterior-posterior dimension (typically, 10.5 cm) into the oblique diameter of the pelvis (typically 12.5 cm) increases the space between the shoulders and the pelvis by 20 mm, more than twice that of the McRoberts' maneuver. This is the mechanical reason that Rubin's maneuver performed better then McRoberts maneuver when objectively compared in the laboratory [172]. Rotation of the fetal shoulders should *never* be attempted by rotating the fetal head itself, as this will likely be insufficient to move the shoulders and will only twist the neck, increasing the risk for injury. If possible, the hand including the thumb, rather than just fingers should be applied to the posterior aspect of the shoulder in an effort to adduct the shoulders while rotating the trunk [174].

Most importantly, Rubin's maneuver can be used *prior* to application of traction on the fetal head as an initial maneuver for shoulder dystocia [182]. Once the anterior shoulder is disimpacted, routine traction can be applied to the head in an attempt to deliver the anterior shoulder first, or upward traction may be used to deliver the posterior shoulder first. If neither shoulder delivers at this point, or if rotation is not possible to perform, this indicates a severe dystocia. Maternal maneuvers should be *abandoned* and either a complete Woods' corkscrew maneuver or delivery of the posterior arm should be attempted.

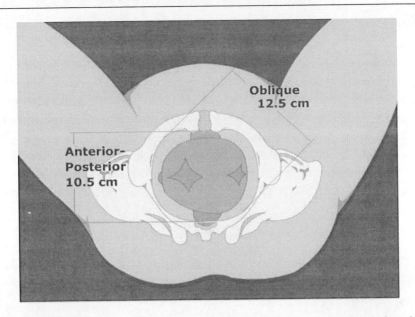

Figure 6. Mechanical effect of Rubin's maneuver. A 30° rotation of the shoulders from their pathological anteroposterior orientation to the more physiologic oblique orientation within the pelvis affords approximately 20 mm more room for passage of the shoulders. Reprinted with permission.[45]

Delivery of the Posterior Arm (Barnum)

A rather inventive method for shrinking the fetal shoulder width during shoulder dystocia was described long ago by Jacquemier and later in the United States by Barnum [146,187]. By delivering the posterior arm before the shoulders, the bisacromial diameter is reduced to the axilloacromial diameter, and the delivered arm may be used to help rotate the trunk. The technique begins similarly to Rubin's maneuver by reaching behind the head to locate and manipulate the posterior shoulder and arm. Sliding the hand along the dorsal aspect of the humerus, the clinician palpates the elbow. If the elbow is already flexed, the operator's hand is guided around the elbow to grasp the fetus' forearm and wrist. If the elbow is extended, the operator grasps the elbow and tries to flex it using his/her fingers along the dorsal aspect of the forearm. Once the elbow is flexed, the operator continues to guide the hand around the elbow to grasp the forearm and wrist as described above. After grasping the forearm and wrist, the operator pulls the forearm over the chest and across the infant's face, extending the arm at the elbow and shoulder to deliver through the introitus. All motions should be directed medially toward and across the fetal chest, supporting and pressing the humerus against the chest to avoid fracture.

Although humerus fracture is almost exclusively associated with delivery of the posterior arm, it is not common and only occurs when forcing the arm sufficiently hard to induce fracture. Even if fracture occurs, the relative morbidity must be considered. Skeletal fractures will always heal; whereas, at least 10% of brachial plexus nerve injuries result in lifelong dysfunction. After other maneuvers are attempted, delivery of the posterior arm almost always works.

Modified Woods' Corkscrew Maneuver

Woods first described using fundal pressure and rotating the shoulders in a way to abduct them [145]. In current obstetric practice, this has been changed to avoid the increased risk of injury associated with fundal pressure [185]. The modified Wood's screw maneuver does not employ fundal pressure and the trunk is rotated such that the shoulders are adducted. It is an extension of the Rubin's maneuver in that the rotation goes past 30 degrees. A forward-progressing winding motion is made, bringing the posterior shoulder nearly 180° to an anterior position, but forward of the pubic symphysis. Spontaneous delivery of the trunk usually follows [188]. If delivery does not follow spontaneously, the rotation can be repeated bringing the trunk further forward in the pelvis. As with Rubin's maneuver, the modified Woods screw maneuver should never be attempted by rotating the fetal head.

Simulation-Based Instruction and Rehearsal of Shoulder Dystocia Maneuvers

One difficulty with developing competency in fetal manipulation techniques for atraumatic resolution of shoulder dystocia is that clinical experience with them is limited because shoulder dystocia is infrequent, and most are resolved with McRoberts' maneuver, with or without suprapubic pressure, and moderate traction. Most clinicians are unwilling to practice fetal maneuvers for routine deliveries.

For injury prevention, resolving severe shoulder dystocia in a simulated clinical environment has the benefit of managing shoulder dystocia without injury risks to the patient. Medical simulation in general is a rapidly growing training and retraining tool [189]. Some success has already been reported in shoulder dystocia management using birth simulators that attempt to mimic the clinical condition [174,189-193].

Despite this, simulation reviews often focus on teamwork, communication and documentation [192,194,195]. While this is important, injury is best prevented when simulation focuses on the clinician's delivery technique. Only a few papers have addressed that issue and those are limited in that no correlation to injury has been made [171,177]. One birthing simulator captures the shoulder dystocia phenomenon and measures clinician-applied forces *and* their resultant effects on the fetus [196]. With it, we have begun to answer heretofore unanswered questions regarding manipulation of forces at delivery related to particular maneuvers [21,172]. It is our hope that simulation will advance to the point where it can be used for standardized training, certification and for recertification.

Summary

In presenting the epidemiology of shoulder dystocia and its associated neonatal brachial plexus injuries, we conveyed what we believe are the essential points. These are:

- In prospective studies, shoulder dystocia incidence among vaginal deliveries is between 3% and 7%. This most likely represents the true incidence in contrast to the lower incidences reported in retrospective studies.
- The major antepartum risk factors for shoulder dystocia are fetal macrosomia and a history of shoulder dystocia in a prior pregnancy; other antepartum risk factors (e.g., obesity, diabetes, postdatism) relate to the tendency to produce larger than average infants.
- The major intrapartum risk factors for shoulder dystocia are operative vaginal delivery and precipitous second stage; other intrapartum risk factors (e.g., prolonged second stage, induction for impending macrosomia, epidural analgesia) relate to pre-existing fetopelvic size and/or positional discrepancy.
- Although risk factors for shoulder dystocia exist, nearly half of shoulder dystocia deliveries occur in the absence of risk factors; as such, shoulder dystocia can rightly be considered unpredictable and unpreventable.
- Pre-identification of the at-risk mother-infant dyad at term prior to the onset of labor will have limited impact on shoulder dystocia incidence; preventive measures need to focus on reducing the incidence of fetal macrosomia throughout the prenatal period by monitoring maternal weight gain, carbohydrate metabolism and fetal growth.
- Instrumented delivery increases the risk of shoulder dystocia by at least a factor of 2. It is the most significant modifiable intrapartum risk factor for subsequent shoulder dystocia, as well as injury, especially among large-for-gestational-age infants.
- Neonatal brachial plexus injury denotes damage to the structural components of the peripheral nerve tracts conferred by forcible hyperextension of one side of the fetal neck; although several etiologies exist, the single greatest risk factor for neonatal brachial plexus injury is clinician-applied traction during antecedent shoulder dystocia.
- Qualitative and quantitative studies in laboratory and actual shoulder dystocia deliveries have established consistent correlations between magnitude, direction and rate of clinician-applied traction and degree and extent of resultant neonatal brachial plexus injury.
- Shoulder dystocia maneuvers that minimize or eliminate direct application of traction to the fetal head have greater mechanical advantage in reducing the risk of neonatal brachial plexus injury compared to those maneuvers that still employ such traction. These should be prioritized in shoulder dystocia management algorithms.
- Training in and rehearsal of fetal maneuvers for management of shoulder dystocia is best accomplished in the safe environment of medical simulation; objective metrics correlating clinician-applied force with resultant fetal mechanical response holds promise for standardization of universal competency assessment among obstetric providers.
- Contrary to the popular notion that nothing can be done to prevent neonatal brachial plexus injuries, an epidemiological approach, such as one outlined through generation of a Haddon matrix, highlights those areas amenable to prevention and mitigation.

References

[1] Dildy GA, Clark SL. Shoulder dystocia: risk identification. *Clin Obstet Gynecol* 2000;43:265-82.

[2] Cohen AW, Otto SR. Obstetric clavicular fractures: A three-year analysis. *J Reprod Med* 1980;25:119-22.

[3] American College of Obstetricians and Gynecologists. Shoulder dystocia. *ACOG Practice Patterns* No. 7. 1997. Washington (DC), ACOG.

[4] American College of Obstetricians and Gynecologists. Shoulder dystocia. *Practice Bulletin* No.40 100(5), 1045-50. 2002. Washington (DC), ACOG.

[5] Spong CY, Beall M, Rodrigues D, Ross MG. An objective definition of shoulder dystocia: prolonged head to body delivery intervals and/ or the use of ancillary obstetric maneuvers. *Obstet Gynecol* 1995;86:433-6.

[6] Ramieri J, Iffy L. Shoulder dystocia. In: Apuzzio JJ, Vintzileos AM, Iffy L, editors. *Operative Obstetrics*. London: Taylor & Francis; 2006: 253-64.

[7] Gherman RB, Chauhan S, Ouzounian JG, Lerner H, Gonik B, Goodwin TM. Shoulder dystocia: The unpreventable obstetric emergency with empiric management guidelines. *Am J Obstet Gynecol* 2006;195:-657.

[8] Hankins GD, Clark SM, Munn MB. Cesarean section on request at 39 weeks: impact on shoulder dystocia, fetal trauma, neonatal encephalopathy and intrauterine demise. *Semin Perinatol* 2006;30:276-87.

[9] Barnett DJ, Balicer RD, Blodgett D, Fews AL, Parker CL, Links JM. The application of the Haddon matrix to public health readiness and response planning. *Environ Health Perspect* 2005;113:561-66.

[10] Christoffersson M, Rydhstroem H. Shoulder dystocia and brachial plexus injury: a population-based study. *Gynecol Obstet Invest* 2002;53:42-7.

[11] Acker DB, Sachs BP, Friedman EA. Risk factors for shoulder dystocia. Obstet Gynecol 1985;66:762-8.

[12] Gherman RB, Goodwin TM. Shoulder dystocia. *Curr Opin Obstet Gynecol* 1998;10:459-63.

[13] Stallings SP, Edwards RK, Johnson JWC. Correlation of head-to-body delivery intervals in shoulder dystocia and umbilical artery acidosis. *Am J Obstet Gynecol* 2001;185:268-74.

[14] Nocon JJ, McKenzie DK, Thomas LJ, Hansell RS. Shoulder dystocia: An analysis of risks and obstetric maneuvers. *Am J Obstet Gynecol* 1993;168:1732-9.

[15] Morrison JC, Sanders JR, Magann EF, Wiser WL. The diagnosis and management of dystocia of the shoulder. *Surg Gynecol Obstet* 1992;175:515-22.

[16] Gurewitsch ED, Johnson E, Hamzehzadeh S, Allen RH. Risk factors for brachial plexus injury with and without shoulder dystocia. *Am J Obstet Gynec* 2006;194:486-92.

[17] Bofill JA, Rust OA, Devidas M, Roberts WE, Morrison JC, Martin JN. Shoulder dystocia and operative vaginal delivery. *J Matern Fetal Med* 1997;6:220-4.

[18] Beall MH, Spong C, McKay J, Ross M. Objective definition of shoulder dystocia: a prospective evaluation. *Am J Obstet Gynecol* 1998;179:934-7.

[19] Allen R, Sorab J, Gonik B. Risk factors for shoulder dystocia: An engineering study of clinician-applied forces. *Obstet Gynecol* 1991;77:352-5.

[20] Poggi S, Spong C, Patel C, Ghidini A, Pezzullo J, Allen RH. Randomized trial of prophylactic McRobers versus lithotomy ro decrease force applied to fetus during delivery. *Am J Obstet Gynecol* 2004;191:874-8.

[21] Allen RH, Cha SL, Kranker LM, Johnson TL, Gurewitsch ED. Comparing mechanical fetal response during descent, crowning, and restitution among deliveries with and without shoulder dystocia. *Am J Obstet Gynecol* 2007;196:539.e1-5.

[22] Rydberg E. *The Mechanism of Labour*. Springfield, Illinois, USA: Charles C Thomas, 1954.

[23] Morris WIC. Shoulder dystocia. *J Obstet Gynecol Br Empire* 1955;62:302-6.

[24] Borell U, Fernström I. The movements at the sacro-iliac joints and their imporance to changes in the pelvic dimensions during parturition. *Acta Obstet Gynecol Scand* 1957;35:42-57.

[25] Bankoski BR, Allen RH, Nagey DA, Miller F. Measuring clavicle strength and modeling birth: towards understanding birth injury. In: *Vossoughi J*, editor. Proc 13th Southern Biomed Engng Conf, Washington, DC. 1994; 586-9.

[26] Allen RH, Gurewitsch ED. Temporary Erb-Duchenne palsy without shoulder dystocia or traction to the fetal head. *Obstet Gynecol* 2005;105:1210-2.

[27] Gilbert WM, Tchabo JG. Fractured clavicle in newborns. *Int Surg* 1988;73:123-5.

[28] Gurewitsch ED, Johnson TL, Allen RH. After shoulder dystocia: Managing the subsequent pregnancy and delivery. *Sem Perinatol* 2007;31:185-95.

[29] Mortimore VR, McNabb M. A six-year retrospective analysis of shoulder dystocia and delivery of the shoulders. *Midwifery* 1998;14:162-73.

[30] Benedetti TJ, Gabbe SG. Shoulder dystocia: a complication of fetal macrosomia and prolonged second stage of labor with midpelvic delivery. *Obstet Gynecol* 1978;52:526-9.

[31] Acker DB, Sachs BP, Friedman EA. Risk factors for shoulder dystocia in the average-weight infant. *Obstet Gynecol* 1986;67:614-8.

[32] Poggi SH, Stallings SP, Ghidini A, Spong CY, Deering SH, Allen RH. Intrapartum risk factors for permanent brachial plexus injury. *Am J Obstet Gynecol* 2003;189:725-9.

[33] Gonen O, Rosen DJ, Dolfinn Z, Tepper R, Markov S, Fejgin MD. Induction of labor versus expectant management in macrosomia: A randomized study. *Obstet Gynecol* 1997;89:913-7.

[34] Conway DL. Delivery of the macrosomic infant: cesarean section versus vaginal delivery. *Semin Perinatol* 2002;26:225-31.

[35] Nesbitt T, Gilbert W, Herrchen B. Shoulder dystocia and associated risk factors with macrosomic infants born in California. *Am J Obstet Gynecol* 1998;179:476-80.

[36] Lurie S, Insler V, Hagay ZJ. Induction of labor at 38-39 weeks of gestation reduces the incidence of shoulder dystocia in gestational diabetic patients class A2. *Am J Perinatol* 1996;13:293-6.

[37] McFarland M, Hod M, Piper JM, Xenakis EMJ, Langer O. Are labor abnormalities more common in shoulder dystocia? *Am J Obstet Gynecol* 1995;173:1211-4.

[38] Sanchez-Ramos L, Bernstein S, Kaunitz AM. Expectant management versus labor induction for suspected fetal macrosomia: a systematic review. *Obstet Gynecol* 2002;100:997-1002.

[39] Gurewitsch ED, Johnson E, Allen RH, Diament P, Fong J, Weinstein D et al. The descent curve of the grand multiparous woman. *Am J Obstet Gynecol* 2003;189:1036-41.

[40] Conway DL, Langer O. Elective delivery of infants with macrosomia in diabetic women: Reduced shoulder dystocia versus increased cesarean deliveries. *Am J Obstet Gynecol* 1998;178:922-5.

[41] Hope P, Breslin S, Lamont L, Lucas A, Martin D, Moore I et al. Fatal shoulder dystocia: a review of 56 cases reported to the Confidential Enquiry into Stillbirths and Deaths in Infancy. *Br J Obstet Gynaecol* 1998;105:1256-61.

[42] Mercer J, Erickson-Owens D, Skovgaard R. Cardiac asystole at birth: Is hypovolemic shock the cause? *Medical Hypotheses* 2008;72:458-63

[43] Wood C, Ng KH, Hounslow D. Time - an important variable in normal delivery. *J Obstet Gynaecol Br Commonwealth* 1973;80:295-300.

[44] Allen RH, Rosenbaum TC, Ghidini A, Poggi SH, Spong CY. Correlating head-to-body delivery intervals with neonatal depression in vaginal births that result in permanent brachial plexus injury. *Am J Obstet Gynecol* 2002;187:839-42.

[45] Gurewitsch ED, Allen RH. Fetal manipulation for management of shoulder dystocia. *Fetal Matern Med Rev* 2006;17:185-204.

[46] Iffy L, Varadi V, Jakobovits A. Common intrapartum denominators of shoulder dysocia related birth injuries. *Zentralbl Gynaekol* 1994;116:33-7.

[47] Iffy L, Gittens-Williams LN. Shoulder dystocia and nuchal cord. *Acta Obstet Gynecol Scand* 2007;86:253.

[48] Cunningham FG, MacDonald PC, Grant NF, Leveno KJ, Gilstrap LC, Hankins GDV et al. *Williams Obstetrics*, 20th Edition. Norwalk, CT: Appleton & Lange, 1997:855-9.

[49] McFarland MB, Trylovich CG, Langer O. Anthropometric differences in macrosomic infants of diabetic and nondiabetic mothers. *J Matern Fetal Med* 1998;7:292-5.

[50] Lewis D, Raymond RC, Perkins MB, Brooks GG, Heymann AR. Recurrence rate of shoulder dystocia. *Am J Obstet Gynecol* 1995;172:1369-71.

[51] Baskett TF, O'Connell CM, Allen A. Antecedents, prevalence, and recurrence of shoulder dystocia and brachial plexus injury. *Obstet Gynecol* 2006;107:63S.

[52] Smith RB, Lane C, Pearson JF. Shoulder dystocia: what happens at the next delivery? *Br J Obstet Gynecol* 1994;101:713-5.

[53] Ginsberg NA, Moisidis C. How to predict recurrent shoulder dystocia. *Am J Obstet Gynecol* 2001;184:1427-30.

[54] Johnstone FD, Myerscough PR. Shoulder dystocia. *Br J Obstet Gynecol* 1998;105:811-5.

[55] Mehta SH, Blackwell SC, Chadha R, Sokol RJ. Shoulder dystocia and the next delivery: Outcomes and management. *J Matern Fetal Neonatal Med* 2007;20:729-33.

[56] Moore HM, Reed SD, Batra M, Schiff MA. Risk factors for recurrent shoulder dystocia, Washington state, 1987-2004. *Am J Obstet Gynecol* 2008; 198:e16-24.

[57] Acker DB, Gregory KD, Sachs BP, Friedman EA. Risk factors for Erb-Duchenne palsy. *Obstet Gynecol* 1988;71:389-92.

[58] Christoffersson M, Kannisto P, Rydhstroem H, Stale H, Walles B. Shoulder dystocia and brachial plexus injury: a case-control study. *Acta Obstet Gynecol Scand* 2003;82:147-51.

[59] McFarland LV, Raskin M, Daling J, Benedetti TJ. Erb-Duchenne's palsy: A consequence of fetal macrosomia and method of delivery. *Obstet Gynecol* 1986;68:784-8.

[60] McFarland MB, Langer O, Piper JM, Berkus MD. Perinatal outcome and the type and number of maneuvers in shoulder dystocia. *Int J Gynaecol Obstet* 1996;55:219-24.

[61] Sheiner E, Levy A, Hershkovitz R, Hallak M, Hammel RD, Katz M, Mazor M. Determining factors associated with shoulder dystocia: a population-based study. *Eur J Obstet Gynecol Reprod Biol* 2006;126:11-15.

[62] Bahar AM. Risk factors and fetal outcome in cases of shoulder dystocia compared with normal deliveries of similar birthweight. *Br J Obstet Gynaecol* 1996;103:868-72.

[63] Iffy L, Brimacombe M, Apuzzio JJ, Varadi V, Portuondo N, Nagy B. The risk of shoulder dystocia related permanent fetal injury in relation to birth weight. *Eur J Obstet Gynecol Reprod Biol* 2008;136:53-60.

[64] Rouse DJ, Owen J, Goldenberg RL, Cliver SP. The effectiveness and costs of elective cesarean delivery for fetal macrosomia diagnosed by ultrasound. *J Am Med Assoc* 1996;276:1480-6.

[65] Chauhan SP, Hendrix NW, Magann EF, Morrison JC, Kenney SP, Devoe LD. Limitations of clinical sonographic estimates of birth weight: Experience with 1034 parturients. *Obstet Gynecol* 1998;91:72-7.

[66] Weiner Z, Ben-Shlomo I, Beck-Fruchter R, Goldberg Y, Shalev E. Clinical and ultrasonographic weight estimation in large for gestational age fetus. *Eur J Obstet Gynecol Reprod Biol* 2002;105:20-4.

[67] Jazayeri A, Heffron JA, Phillips R, Spellacy WN. Macrosomia prediction using ultrasound fetal abdominal circumference of 35 centimeters or more. *Obstet Gynecol* 1999;93:523-6.

[68] Cohen BF, Penning S, Ansley D, Porto M, Garite T. The incidence and severity of shoulder dystocia correlates with a sonographic measurement of asymmetry in patients with diabetes. *Am J Perinatol* 1999;16:197-201.

[69] Ray JG, Vermeulen MJ, Shapiro JL, Kenshole AB. Maternal and neonatal outcomes in pregestational and gestational diabetes mellitus, and the influence of maternal obesity and weight gain: the DEPOSIT study. Diabetes Endocrine Pregnancy Outcome Study in Toronto. *QJM* 2001;94:347-56.

[70] Barker DJP. Fetal and infant origins of adult disease. BMJ 1990;301:1111.

[71] Oken E, Gillman MW. Fetal origins of obesity. *Obesity Res* 2003;11:496-506.

[72] Spong CY. Recent developments in preventing recurrent preterm birth. *Obstet Gynecol* 2003;101:1153-4.

[73] Fernandez-Twinn DS, Ozanne SE. Mechanisms by which poor early growth programs type-2 diabetes, obesity and the metabolic syndrome. *Physiol Behav* 2006;88:234-43.

[74] Langer O, Berkus MD, Huff RW, Samueloff A. Shoulder dystocia: Should the fetus weighing ≥ 4000 grams be delivered by cesarean section? *Am J Obstet Gynecol* 1991;165:831-7.

[75] Langer O, Rodriguez DA, Xenakis MJ, McFarland MB, Berkus MD, Arredondo F. Intensified versus conventional management of gestational diabetes. *Am J Obstet Gynecol* 1994;170:1036-47.

[76] Bonomo M, Cetin I, Pisoni MP, Faden D, Mion E, Taricco E et al. Flexible treatment of gestational diabetes modulated on ultrasound evaluation of intrauterine growth: a controlled randomized clinical trial. *Diabetes Metab* 2004;30:237-44.

[77] Kjos SL, Schaefer-Graf U, Sardesi S, Peters RK, Buley A, Xiang AH et al. A randomized controlled trial using glycemic plus fetal ultrasound parameters versus glycemic parameters to determine insulin therapy in gestational diabetes with fasting hyperglycemia. *Diabetes Care* 2001;24:1904-10.

[78] Schaefer-Graf UM, Kjos SL, Fauzan OH, Buhling KJ, Siebert G, Buhrer C et al. A randomized trial evaluating a predominantly fetal growth-based strategy to guide management of gestational diabetes in Caucasian women. *Diabetes Care* 2004;27:297-302.

[79] Langer O, Yogev Y, Xenakis EM, Rosenn B. Insulin and glyburide therapy: dosage, severity level of gestational diabetes and pregnancy outcome. *Am J Obstet Gynecol* 2005;192:134-39.

[80] Stamilio DM, Olsen T, Ratcliffe S, Sehdev HM, Macones GA. False-positive 1-hour glucose challenge test and adverse perinatal outcomes. *Obstet Gynecol* 2004;103:148-56.

[81] Grotegut CA, Tatineni H, Dandolu V, Whiteman VE, Katari S, Geifman-Holtzman O. Obstetric outcomes with a false-positive one-hour glucose challenge test by the Carpenter-Coustan criteria. *J Matern Fetal Neonatal Med* 2008;21:315-20.

[82] De Reu PA, Smits LJ, Oosterbaan HP, Nijhuis JG. Value of a single early third trimester fetal biometry for the prediction of birth weight deviations in a low risk population. *J Perinat Med* 2008;36:324-29.

[83] Yogev Y, Langer O. Pregnancy outcome in obese and morbidly obese gestational diabetic women. *Eur J Obstet Gynecol Reprod Biol* 2008;137:21-26.

[84] Jensen DM, Damm P, Sorensen B, Molsted-Pedersen L, Westergaard JG, Ovesen P. et al. Pregnancy outcome and prepregnancy body mass index in 2459 glucose-tolerant Danish women. *Am J Obstet Gynecol* 2003;189:239-44.

[85] Cedergren MI. Maternal morbid obesity and the risk of adverse pregnancy outcome. *Obstet Gynecol* 2004;103:219-24.

[86] Gurewitsch E, Donithan M, Moore P, Allen L, Petersen S, Allen R. Outcomes of mild versus severe shoulder dystocia. *Am J Obstet Gynecol* 2003;189:S208.

[87] Gross TL, Sokol RJ, Williams T, Thompson K. Shoulder dystocia: A fetal-physician risk. *Am J Obstet Gynecol* 1987;156:1408-18.

[88] Geary M. Risk factors and fetal outcome in cases of shoulder dystocia compared with normal deliveries of a similar birthweight. *Br J Obstet Gynecol* 1997;104;121.

[89] Dieckmann WJ, Turner DF, Ruby BA. Diet regulation and controlled weight in pregnancy. *Am J Obstet Gynecol* 1945;50:701-12.

[90] Spellacy WN. Obstetric practice in the United States of America may contribute to the obesity epidemic. *J Reprod Med* 2008;53:955-56.

[91] Soltani H, Fraser RB. A longitudinal study of maternal anthropometric changes in normal weight, overweight and obese women during pregnancy and postpartum. *Br J Nutr* 2000;84:95-101.

[92] Schlabritz-Loutsevitch NE, Dudley CJ, Gomez JJ, Nevill CH, Smith BK, Jenkins SL et al. Metaboloic adjustments to moderate maternal nutrient restriction. *Br J Nutr* 2007;98:276-84.

[93] Iffy L, Apuzzio J, Ganesh V. A randomized controlled trial of prophylactic maneuvers to reduce head-to-body delivery time in patients at risk for shoulder dystocia. *Obstet Gynecol* 2003;102:1089-90.

[94] Iffy L. Perinatal implications of shoulder dystocia. Obstet Gynecol 1996;87:638-9.

[95] Hart G. Waiting for shoulders. *Midwifery Today* 1997;42:32-4.

[96] Bottoms SF, Sokol RJ. Mechanisms and conduct of labor. In: Iffy L, Kaminetzky HA, editors. *Principles and practice of obstetrics & perinatology.* New York: John Wiley & Sons; 1981. p. 815-37.

[97] Sandmire HF, O'Halloin TJ. Shoulder dystocia: Its incidence and associated risk factors. *Int J Gynaecol Obstet* 1988;26:65-73.

[98] Combs CA, Singh NB, Khoury JC. Elective induction versus spontaneous labor after sonographic diagnosis of fetal macrosomia. *Obstet Gynecol* 1993;81:492-6.

[99] Towner D, Castro MA, Eby-Wilkens E, Gilbert WM. Effect of mode of delivery in nulliparous women on neonatal intracranial injury. *N Eng J Med* 1999;341:1709-14.

[100] Mollberg M, Hagberg H, Bager B, Hakan L, Lilja H, Ladfors L. Risk factors for obstetric brachial plexus palsy among neonates delivered by vacuum extraction. *Obstet Gynecol* 2005;106:913-8.

[101] Gurewitsch ED, Johnson E, Hamzehzadeh S, Allen RH. Risk factors for brachial plexus injury with and without shoulder dystocia. *Am J Obstet Gynecol* 2006;194:486-92.

[102] Towner DR, Ciotti MC. Operative vaginal delivery: a cause of birth injury or is it? *Clin Obstet Gynecol* 2007;50:563-81.

[103] Pearse WH. Electronic recording of forceps delivery. *Am J Obstet Gynecol* 1963;86:43-51.

[104] Allen RH. On the mechanical aspects of shoulder dystocia and birth injury. *Clinical Obstetrics and Gynecology* 2007;50:607-23.

[105] Collins D. Prolonged second stage results in shoulder dystocia (Legally Speaking). *Contemp OB/GYN* 2006;51:41.

[106] Myles TD, Santolaya J. Maternal and neonatal outcomes in patients with a prolonged second stage of labor. *Obstet Gynecol* 2003;102:52-8.

[107] Gemer O, Bergman M, Segal S. Labor abnormalities as a risk factor for shoulder dystocia. *Acta Obstet Gynecol Scand* 1999;78:735-6.

[108] Mehta SH, Hamilton E, Bujold E, Berman S, Sockol ER, Blackwell SC. Shoulder dystocia is associated with protracted active labor in nulliparous women. *Am J Obstet Gynecol* 2003;189:5211.

[109] Bowes WA, Thorp JM. Clinical aspects of normal and abnormal labor. In: Creasy RK, Resnik R, editors. *Maternal-Fetal Medicine: Principles and Practice*. Philadelphia, Pa.: Saunders; 2004. p. 671.

[110] Gurewitsch ED, Allen RH. Shoulder Dystocia. *Clin Perinatol* 2007;34:365-85.

[111] Piatt JH. Birth injuries of the brachial plexus. *Pediatr Clin N Am* 2004;51:421-40.

[112] Evans-Jones G, Kay SPJ, Weindling AM, Cranny G, Ward A, Bradshaw A et al. Congenital brachial plasy: incidence, causes, and outcome in the United Kingdom and Republic of Ireland. *Arch Dis Child Fetal Neonatal Ed* 2003;88:F185-F189.

[113] Anderson J, Watt J, Olson J, Van Erde J. Perinatal brachial plexus injury. *Paediat Child Health* 2006;11:93-100.

[114] Foad SC, Mehlman CT, Ying J. The epidemiology of neonatal brachial plexus injury. *J Bone Joint Surg Am* 2008;90:1258-64.

[115] Donnelly V, Foran A, Murphy J, McParland P, Keane D, O'Herlihy C. Neonatal brachial plexus palsy: An unpredictable injury. *Am J Obstet Gynecol* 2002;187:1209-12.

[116] Alfonso I, Alfonso DT, Papazian O. Focal upper extremity neuropathy in neonates. *Sem Ped Neuro* 2000;7:4-14.

[117] Leffert RD. Congenital brachial palsy. In: Leffert RD, editor. *Brachial Plexus Injuries*. New York: Churchill Livingstone; 1985. p. 91-120.

[118] Volpe JJ. Injuries of extracranial, cranial, intracranial, spinal cord, peripheral nervous system structures. In: Volpe JJ, editor. *Neurology of the newborn*. St. Louis: W.B. Saunders Company; 1995.

[119] Nath RK. Obstetric Brachial Plexus Injuries. Houston: Texas Nerve & Paralysis, 2006.

[120] Uysal II, Seker M, Karabulut AK, Buyukmumcu M, Zlylan T. Brachial plexus variations in human fetuses. *Neurosurgery* 2003;53:676-84.

[121] Sunderland S. The anatomy and physiology of nerve injury. *Muscle Nerve* 1990;13:771-84.

[122] Shenaq SM, Berzin E, Lee R, Laurent JP, Nath R, Nelson MR. Brachial plexus birth injuries and current management. *Clin Plast Surg* 1998;25:527-36.

[123] Metaizeau JP, Gayet C, Plenat F. [Brachial plexus injuries: An experimental study]. *Chirug Ped* 1979;20:159-63.

[124] Alfonso I, Diaz-Arca G, Alfonso DT, Shuhaiber H, Papazian O, Price AE et al. Fetal deformations: A risk factor for obstetrical brachial plexus palsy? *Pediatr Neurol* 2006;35:246-9.

[125] Alfonso I, Papazian O, Prieto G, Alfonso DT, Melnick SJ. Neoplasm as a cause of brachial plexus palsy in neonates. *Pediatr Neurosurg* 2000;22:309-11.

[126] Al-Qattan MM, Thompson HG. Congenital varicella of the upper limb: A preventable disaster. *J Hand Surg (Br)* 1995;20:115-7.

[127] Lucas JW, Holden KR, Purohit DM, Cure JK. Neonatal hemangiomatosis associated with brachial plexus palsy. *J Child Neuro* 1995;10:411-3.

[128] Sinclair S, Murray PM, Terkonda SP. Combined intrauterine vascular insufficiency and brachial plexus palsy: A case report. *Hand* 2008;3:135-8.

[129] Paradiso G, Granana N, Maza E. Prenatal brachial plexus paralysis. *Neurology* 1997;49:261-2.

[130] Dunn DW, Engle WA. Brachial plexus palsy: Intrauterine onset. *Pediatr Neurol* 1985;1:367-9.

[131] Sever JW. Obstetric paralysis: Its etiology, pathology, clinical aspects and treatment, with a report of four hundred and seventy cases. *Am J Dis Child* 1916;12:541-78.

[132] Seddon HJ. Classification of nerve injuries. *BMJ* 1942;2:237.

[133] Gonik B, McCormick EM, Verweij BH, Rossman KM, Nigro MA. The timing of congenital brachial plexus injury: A study of electromyography findings in the newborn piglet. *Am J Obstet Gynecol* 1998;178:688-95.

[134] Belzberg AJ, Dorsi MJ, Storm PB, Moriarity JL. Surgical repair of brachial plexus injury: a multinational survey of experienced peripheral nerve surgeons. J *Neurosurg focus* 2004;161:365-76-11.

[135] Jeffrey AR, Ellis FJ, Repka MX, Buncic JR. Pediatric Horner syndrome. *J AAPOS* 1998;2:159-67.

[136] Vredeveld JW, Blaauw G, Slooff BACJ, Richards R, Rozeman SCAM. The findings in paediatric obstetric brachial palsy differ from those in oler patients: a suggested explanation. *Dev Med Child Neurol* 2000;42:158-61.

[137] Jennett RJ, Tarby T, Kreinick CJ. Brachial plexus palsy: An old problem revisited. *Am J Obstet Gynecol* 1992;166:1673-7.

[138] Hoeskma AF, Wolf H, Qei SL. Obstetric brachial plexus injuries: incidence, natural course and shoulder contracture. *Clin Rehab* 2000;14:523-6.

[139] Bager B. Perinatally acquired brachial plexus palsy: a persisting challenge. *Acta Paediatr* 1997;86:1214-9.

[140] Gherman RB, Ouzounian JG, Goodwin TM. Brachial plexus palsy: An in utero injury? *Am J Obstet Gynecol* 1999;180:1303-7.

[141] Graham EM, Forouzan I, Morgan MA. A retrospective analysis of Erb's palsy cases and their relation to birth weight and trauma at delivery. *J Matern Fetal Med* 1997;6:1-5.

[142] Chauhan SP, Rose CH, Gherman R, Magann EF, Holland MW, Morrison JC. Brachial plexus injury: A 23-year experience from a tertiary center. *Am J Obstet Gynecol* 2005;192:1795-802.

[143] Wolf H, Hoeksma AF, Oei SL, Bleker OP. Obstetric brachial plexus injury: risk factors related to recovery. *Eur J Obstet Gynecol Reprod Biol* 2000;88:133-8.

[144] Adler J, Patterson RL. Erb's palsy: long term results of treatment in eighty-eight cases. *J Bone Jt Surg* 1967;49-A:1052-64.

[145] Woods CE. A principle of physics as applicable to shoulder dystocia. *Am J Obstet Gynecol* 1943;45:796-804.

[146] Barnum CG. Dystocia due to the shoulders. *Am J Obstet Gynecol* 1945;50:439-42.

[147] Mollberg M, Hagberg H, Bager B, Lilja H, Ladfors L. High birthweight and shoulder dystocia: the strongest risk factors for obstetrical brachial plexus palsy in a Swedish population-based study. *Acta Obstet Gynecol Scand* 2005;84:654-9.

[148] Allen RH, Edelberg SC. Brachial plexus palsy causation. *Birth* 2003;30:141-6.

[149] Gherman RB, Ouzounian JG, Satin AJ, Goodwin TM, Phelan JP. A comparison of shoulder dystocia-associated transient and permanent brachial plexus palsies. *Obstet Gynecol* 2003;102:544-8.

[150] Baskett TF, Allen AC. Perinatal implications of shoulder dystocia. *Obstet Gynecol* 1995;86:14-7.

[151] Gonik B, Hollyer VL, Allen RH. Shoulder dystocia recognition: Differences in neonatal risks for injury. O'Sullivan MJ. Abstract No. 164. 1988. Las Vegas, NV. Eighth Annual Clinical, Scientific and Business Meeting for the Society of Perinatal Obstetricians. 1930.

[152] Gonik B, Allen R, Sorab J. Objective evaluation of the shoulder dystocia phenomenon: Effect of maternal pelvic orientation on force reduction. *Obstet Gynecol* 1989;74:44-8.

[153] American College of Obstetricians and Gynecologists. P*recis—An update in obstetrics and gynecology*. Washington, DC: American College of Obstetricians and Gynecologists, 1998:95-7.

[154] Mollberg M, Wennergren M, Bager B, Ladfors L, Hagberg H. Obstetric brachial plexus palsy: a prospective study on risk factors related to manual assistance during the second stage of labor. *Acta Obstet Gynecol Scand* 2007;86:198-204.

[155] Fieux G. Pathogenesis of brachial paralyses in the neonate. Obstetrical paralyses. *Ann Gynecol Obstet* 1897;47:52-64.

[156] Thorburn W. Obstetrical paralysis. *J Obstet Gynecol Br Empire* 1903;3:454-8.

[157] Clark LP, Taylor AS, Prout TP. A study on brachial birth palsy. *Am J Med Sci* 1905;130:670-707.

[158] Kalmin OV. Structural based for tensile strength properties of nerves. *Morfologiia* 1997;111:39-43.

[159] Sunderland S, Bradley KC. Stress-strain phenomena in human peripheral nerve trunks. *Brain* 1961;84:102-19.

[160] Geutjens G, Gilbert A, Helsen K. Obstetric brachial plexus palsy associated with breech delivery - A different pattern of injury. *J Bone Jt Surg Br* 1996;78-B:303-6.

[161] Gherman RB, Goodwin TM, Ouzounian JG, Miller DA, Paul RH. Brachial plexus palsy associated with cesarean section-An in utero injury? *Am J Obstet Gynecol* 1997;177:1162-4.

[162] Leigh TH, James CE. Medicolegal commentary: Shoulder dystocia. *Br J Obstet Gynecol* 1998;105:815-7.

[163] Hankins GDV, Clark SL. Brachial plexus palsy involving the posterior shoulder at spontaneous vaginal delivery. *Am J Perinatol* 1995;12:44-5.

[164] Ouzounian JG, Korst LM, Phelan JP. Permanent Erb palsy- A traction-related injury? *Obstet Gynecol* 1997;89:139-41.

[165] Jennett RJ, Tarby TJ, Krauss RL. Erb's palsy contrasted with Klumpke's and total palsy: Different mechanisms are involved. *Am J Obstet Gynecol* 2002;186:1216-20.

[166] Gonik B, Walker A, Grimm M. Mathematical modeling of forces associated with shoulder dystocia: A comparison of endogenous and exogenous sources. *Am J Obstet Gynecol* 2000;182:689-91.

[167] Gonik B, Zhang N, Grimm MJ. Defining forces that are associated with shoulder dystocia: The use of a mathematic dynamic computer model. *Am J Obstet Gynecol* 2003;188:1068-72.

[168] Ubachs JMH, Slooff ACJ, Peeters LLH. Obstetric antecedents of surgically treated obstetric brachial-plexus injuries. *Br J Obstet Gynecol* 1995;102:813-7.

[169] Acker DB. A shoulder dystocia intervention form. *Obstet Gynecol* 1991;78:150-1.

[170] Sorab J, Allen RH, Gonik B. Tactile sensory monitoring of clinician-applied forces during delivery of newborns. *IEEE Trans Biomed Eng* 1988;35:1090-3.

[171] Crofts JF, Ellis D, James M, Hunt LP, Fox R, Draycott TJ. Pattern and degree of forces applied during simulation of shoulder dystocia. *Am J Obstet Gynecol* 2007;197.

[172] Gurewitsch ED, Kim EJ, Yang JH, Outland KE, McDonald MK, Allen RH. Comparing McRoberts' and Rubin's maneuvers for initial management of shoulder dystocia: An objective evaluation. *Am J Obstet Gynecol* 2005;192:153-60.

[173] Allen RH, Bankoski BR, Butzin CA, Nagey DA. Comparing clinician-applied loads for routine, difficult, and shoulder dystocia deliveries. *Am J Obstet Gynecol* 1994;171:1621-7.

[174] Crofts JF, Bartlett C, Ellis D, Hunt LP, Fox R, Draycott TJ. Management of shoulder dystocia - Skill retention 6 and 12 months after training. *Obstet Gynecol* 2007;110:1069-74.

[175] Allen RH, Bankoski BR, Nagey DA. Simulating birth to investigate clinician-applied loads on newborns. *Med Eng Phys* 1995;17:380-4.

[176] Tam W, Hoe YSG, Huang S, Gurewitsch ED, Fox HE, Allen RH. Measuring hand-applied forces during vaginal delivery without instrumenting the fetus or interfering with grasping function. *J Soc Gynecal Investig* 2004;11:S205A.

[177] Crofts JF, Bartlett C, Ellis D, Hunt LP, Fox R, Draycott TJ. Training for shoulder dystocia - A trial of simulation using low-fidelity and high-fidelity mannequins. *Obstet Gynecol* 2006;108:1477-85.

[178] Bonnaire C, Bue E. Influence of the position on the shape and dimensions of the pelvis. *Annales de Gynecologie et d'Obstetrique* 1899;Tome L11:296-310.

[179] Gonik B, Stringer C, Held B. An alternate maneuver for management of shoulder dystocia. *Am J Obstet Gynecol* 1983;145:882-4.

[180] Gherman RB, Goodwin M, Souter I, Neumann K, Ouzounian JG, Paul RH. The McRoberts' maneuver for the alleviation of shoulder dystocia: how successful is it? *Am J Obstet Gynecol* 1997;176:656-61.

[181] Mazzanti GA. Delivery of the anterior shoulder- A neglected art. *Obstet Gynecol* 1959;13:603-7.

[182] Reid DE. Conduct of normal labor and the puerperium. In: Reid DE, editor. *Textbook of Obstetrics*. Philadelphia: W.B. Saunders Company; 1962. p. 448-89.

[183] Gherman RB, Ouzounian JG, Goodwin TM. Obstetric maneuvers for shoulder dystocia and associated fetal morbidity. *Am J Obstet Gynecol* 1998;178:1126-30.

[184] Schwartz BC, Dixon DM. Shoulder dystocia. *Obstet Gynecol* 1958;11:468-71.

[185] Gross SJ, Shime J, Farine D. Shoulder dystocia: Predictors and outcome. *Am J Obstet Gynecol* 1987;156:334-6.

[186] Rubin A. Management of shoulder dystocia. J Am Med Assoc 1964;189:835-7.

[187] Beer E. Shoulder dystocia and posture for birth: a history lesson. *Obstet Gynecol Survey* 2003;58:697-9.

[188] Woods CE. A principle of physics as applicable to shoulder delivery. *Am J Obstet Gynecol* 1943;45:796-804.

[189] Gardner R, Walzer TB. Obstetric simulation: State of the art in 2005. *Cont Obstet Gynecol* 2005;24-32.

[190] Crofts JF, Attilakos G, Read M, Sibanda T. Shoulder dystocia training using a new birth training mannequin. *BJOG* 2005;112:997-9.

[191] Macedonia CR, Gherman RB, Satin AJ. Simulation laboratories for training in obstetrics and gynecology. *Obstet Gynecol* 2003;102:388-92.

[192] Deering S, Poggi S, Macedonia C, Gherman R, Satin AJ. Improving resident competency in the management of shoulder dystocia with simulation training. *Obstet Gynecol* 2004;103:1224-8.

[193] Goffman D, Heo H, Pardanani S, Merkatz IR, Bernstein PS. Improving shoulder dystocia management among resident and attending physicians using simulations. *Am J Obstet Gynecol* 2007;197:S185.

[194] Deering S, Poggi S, Hodor J, Macedonia C, Satin AJ. Evaluation of residents' delivery notes after a simulated shoulder dystocia. *Obstet Gynecol* 2004;104:667-70.

[195] Goffman D, Heo H, Chazotte C, Merkatz I, Bernstein P. Using simulation training to improve shoulder dystocia documentation. *Obstet Gynecol* 2008;111:3S.

[196] Allen RH, Gurewitsch ED, Gilka P, Kim E, Theprungsirikul P. Birthing Simulator.. United States Patent 7,465,168; 16 December 2008.

[197] Geary M, McParland P, Johnson H, Stronge J. Shoulder dystocia- Is it predictable? *Eur J Obstet Gynecol* 1995;62:15-8.

[198] Yeo GSH, Lim YW, Yeong CT, Tan TC. An analysis of risk factors for the prediction of shoulder dystocia in 16471 consecutive births. *Ann Acad Med Singapore* 1995;24:836-40.

[199] Gilbert WM, Nesbitt TS, Danielsen B. Associated factors in 1611 cases of brachial plexus injury. *Obstet Gynecol* 1999;93:536-40.

[200] Lipscomb KR, Gregory K, Shaw K. The outcome of macrosomic infants weighing at least 4500 grams: Los Angeles county + University of Southern California experience. *Obstet Gynecol* 1995;85:558-64.

[201] Perlow JH, Wigton T, Hart J, Strassner HT, Nageotte MP, Wolk BM. Birth trauma- A five year review of incidence and associated perinatal factors. *J Reprod Med* 1996;41:754-60.

[202] Gonik B, Hollyer VL, Allen R. Shoulder dystocia recognition: Differences in neonatal risks for injury. *Am J Perinatol* 1991;8:31-4.

[203] Levine MG, Holroyde J, Woods JR, Siddiqi TA, Scott M, Miodovnik M. Birth trauma: Incidence and predisposing factors. *Obstet Gynecol* 1984;63:792-5.

[204] Sandmire HF, DeMott RK. The Green Bay cesarean section study. *Am J Obstet Gynecol* 1996;174:1557-64.

[205] Peleg D, Hasnin J, Shalav E. Fractured clavicle and Erb's palsy unrelated to birth trauma. *Am J Obstet Gynecol* 1997;177:1038-40.

[206] Poggi SH, Spong CY, Allen RH. Prioritizing posterior arm delivery during severe shoulder dystocia. *Obstet Gynecol* 2003;101:1068-72.

In: Textbook of Perinatal Epidemiology
Editor: Eyal Sheiner, pp. 499-521

ISBN: 978-1-60741-648-7
© 2010 Nova Science Publishers, Inc.

Chapter XXIV

Epidemiology of Cerebral Palsy

Steven J. Korzeniewski[1] and Nigel Paneth[2]*
Departments of Epidemiology and Pediatrics & Human Development,
Michigan State University USA[2]

Introduction

Cerebral palsy (CP), first described in the latter half of the 19th century as a clinical syndrome by the orthopedic practitioner William John Little,[1] and first classified into subgroups by the then-neurologist Sigmund Freud,[2] is defined as "a group of developmental disorders of movement and posture causing activity limitation or disability that are attributed to disturbances occurring in the fetal or infant brain and that may be accompanied by a seizure disorder or by disturbance of sensation, cognition, communications and/or behavior".[3]

The reason for including a chapter on CP in a textbook of perinatal epidemiology is that no other neurodevelopmental disorder bears as close a causal relationship to the hazards of intrauterine and perinatal life as does CP. Yet, in spite of significant improvements in perinatal care in recent decades – including both more intensive labor surveillance and improved neonatal care, especially for premature infants - the prevalence of CP has remained for the most part quite stable at about two per thousand school-age children. While recent epidemiologic research has elucidated a range of risk factors for cerebral palsy, particularly among low birthweight infants, the major causes of CP still remain largely obscure.

CP is a very important health outcome. Compared to most severe threats to childhood health – for example, the muscular dystrophies and cystic fibrosis – CP is relatively common. At the same time, it places substantial burdens on affected children, their families and

---
* For Correspondence: Steven J. Korzeniewski Ph.D Candidate MA MSc, MPRO- Michigan's Peer Review Organization, 22670 Haggerty Rd Ste. 100, Farmington Hills, MI 48335, Telephone: (248) 465-7365, Email: skorzeniewski@mpro.org

societies. About 30% of children with CP cannot walk, and nearly 20% walk only with an assistive device.[4] CP is often accompanied by other neurodevelopmental disabilities, most commonly a seizure disorder, impairment of cognitive capacity, or difficulties with hearing or vision.[5] The CDC has estimated that each of the estimated 12,000 new cases of CP each year in the US will incur lifetime direct and indirect costs of nearly $1 million. Each annual US birth cohort thus incurs about $11.5 billion in lifetime health care, education and social service expenditures and lost economic opportunity costs because of CP.[6]

Definition of Cerebral Palsy

CP is clinically defined, its central construct being impairment of motor function that clearly interferes with ordinary tasks such as walking, running, jumping and/or climbing stairs. No laboratory test, tissue histology, or neuroimaging pattern defines the presence or absence of CP. An international committee has provided, in two recent publications, a careful definition of CP, a detailed explanation of the definition, and a discussion of the several ways in which CP may be classified.[3, 7]

The age at which a child is diagnosed with CP is an important aspect of its definition.[8] The diagnosis should not be assigned until the child is old enough for motor-related developmental milestones – especially walking – to be observed. Clinicians and family members alike can be surprised by how some severe motor neurological signs can resolve in infancy. For this reason, the diagnosis of CP before 24 months of age (corrected for degree of prematurity) should be viewed with suspicion.

CP is generally described as a non-progressive disorder, to differentiate it from a variety of clearly progressive, degenerative diseases affecting motor ability that are generally of genetic origin. However, as noted in the recent definitional documents cited above, the motor dysfunction of CP may worsen over time. This worsening, though still incompletely understood, seems to reflect the interaction of the aberrant motor mechanisms in CP with aging and its accompanying stresses on bones, joints and muscles. Such "progression" is very different from the progression in the degenerative disorders, because the pathophysiologic process underlying the damage, which in CP results from an injury that occurred, by definition, at a fixed time in the prenatal or perinatal period, is no longer an active process as it is in neurodegenerative disorders.

Typology of Cerebral Palsy

The simplest way to classify CP is by number of affected limbs. Thus the commonest classification terminology is to distinguish monoplegia, diplegia, and quadriplegia. It should be noted that some authorities doubt that true monoplegias exist; rather, subtle hemiplegias masquerade as monoplegias. The type of motor abnormality- spasticity, dystonia, dyskinesia, hypotonia, ataxia- is also used commonly in classification.

To an epidemiologist, the principal reason to classify CP into sub-groups is in case these sub-groups have different etiologies. In fact, it is likely that they do. Perinatal ischemic stroke, to be discussed later, is a much more prominent antecedent of hemiplegic CP than of other forms. Diplegia is particularly associated with premature birth. Dyskinetic CP can be characteristic of infants who have suffered bilirubin encephalopathy in the newborn period. These observations, however, are not sufficient to conclude that there are not common etiologies to CP as well, with severity of insult, or individual host response variation accounting for some of the differences in the CP pattern seen.

The degree of interference of the motor disability with normal activities is also useful for classification purposes, especially for rehabilitative efforts. A major advance in this effort has been the development of the Gross Motor Function Classification System (GMFCS).[9] The GMFCS categorizes severity of motor impairment by self-initiated functional abilities in sitting and walking and the need for assistive devices and has been rigorously assessed across multiple settings around the world. Similar efforts are underway to classify manual ability (Manual Ability Classification System- MACS) [10] and communication impairment (Communication Function Classification System- CFCS), [11] though these have yet to be studied in as much detail as the GMFCS.

Recent advances in neuroimaging have led some researchers to propose categorization of CP by image patterns, although no accepted system has been proposed as yet. The most common abnormality found by neuroimaging of CP cases is white matter damage, particularly among children born prematurely and children with spastic, athetoid or ataxic CP, while the least common finding is isolated grey matter damage.[12] As many as 10-15% of children with CP are found to have an underlying malformation of the brain, and a similar proportion have no detectable anatomic lesion on MRI or CT.

Prevalence

The frequency of a disease at a given time in a population, or its prevalence, is among the first things assessed during epidemiologic investigation. Knowledge of disease prevalence facilitates resource allocation by providing a context for competing public health priorities. Counting cases of disease in a population requires having a good operational case definition, sound sources of information about cases and at risk populations, and a system for collection and systematizing that information. Such systems are not universal and are particularly lacking in the Western Hemisphere, which does not have any ongoing CP registry. In marked contrast, Europe has many registries, and these registries now pool much of their data for analysis. We have recently reviewed the work of CP registries internationally and the prevalence data they have produced.[13]

The 'at risk population' is an important epidemiologic concept, as it is the appropriate denominator for prevalence calculations. Naturally, those not at risk for a disease should not populate the denominator of a prevalence estimate. Accordingly, because newborns and infants are the only population at risk of CP (children acquiring brain damage later in life are excluded from the CP rubric by definition), it makes sense to use the birth cohort from whence the cases arose as the denominator. While birth cohorts are the commonly used denominator among many CP registries, this practice is not universal, and children of school age have sometimes served as denominator populations.

Because the risk of CP occurs only once in a lifetime, the important epidemiologic dimension of "time at risk" has no application. It follows then, that like birth defects, CP frequency can only be described as a prevalence and not as an incidence. This is true whether the denominator is live births, children or adults.

Questions about the appropriate denominator for CP prevalence have also included whether to use live births or neonatal survivors. It can be argued that infants who die during the neonatal period are not at risk of the disease. In countries where the infant mortality rate is relatively low (~8/1,000) the difference between the two denominators is trivial. However, among very low birth weight infants (VLBW) the difference can be substantial. We think that public health is better served by examining CP rates per live births in VLBW small infants, because this rate takes account of the contribution of improving survival to the prevalence of CP in the population when survival rates are rapidly improving, as they have been in the US and developed countries for the past thirty years. During the last quarter of the 20th century, there was evidence that the improvement in survival in premature infants was in fact contributing to a modest risk in the overall prevalence of CP.[14] This may now be leveling off.[13, 15, 16]

The prevalence of CP is remarkably similar in developed countries varying between 1.5 and 2.5 per thousand live births or child survivors. A recent tristate US study, however, found considerably higher prevalences – from 3.3 to 3.8 per thousand.[17] This latter study denominatored CP to eight-year-old children, but whether this factor explains the unusually high prevalence found is not clear.

Risk Factors

While approximately half of all CP cases occur among infants born after 37 weeks of gestation, the other half occur in the 10% or so of babies born preterm. The risk of CP increases steadily with decreasing gestational age at birth. In fact, the risk of CP at the lowest gestational ages at which survival now occurs – 23 to 26 weeks of gestation - is around 10%, or about fifty times the risk of infants born at term. In children who are born very preterm, the frequency of both cognitive and neuromotor impairments, assessed at age five years, increase with decreasing gestational age.[18] There is also evidence that the more premature the infant, the more severe the degree of motor and cognitive disability.[19] Due to the distinctive difference in risk, risk factors for CP are often considered separately in term-born and preterm-born children.

Term Infants

Birth Asphyxia

While the idea that reduced oxygen and blood flow to the brain is a major cause of CP has persisted since first proposed by Little in 1862, [1] epidemiologic evidence suggests otherwise, indicating that hypoxia-ischemia or asphyxia – as assessed clinically - have only a modest role in the etiology of CP. The classic reports of the National Collaborative Perinatal Project, a study of more than 50,000 children born in the US from 1959 to 1966 and followed to age seven, showed that clinical measures reflective of birth asphyxia (fetal bradycardia, low Apgar score, delayed time to first breath, etc.) occurred in only a minority of children with CP. Among 189 cases of cerebral palsy in the study, just 17 could clearly be attributed to birth asphyxia.[20] While it might be thought that where professional facilities for the management of labor and delivery are not available the fraction of CP attributable to perinatal asphyxia would be higher, it must be remembered that survival of perinatally asphyxiated babies is compromised by the lack of clinical facilities for newborns that parallels lack of obstetrical services.

The best neonatal predictor of CP is an abnormal neurological examination, and that relationship probably holds regardless of the cause of the abnormal neurological findings. Infants with newborn encephalopathy, who exhibit a range of signs from poor feeding and lethargy all the way to coma, respiratory arrest and convulsions are at high risk of CP.[21] If these findings are preceded either by dramatic intrauterine events such as severe persistent bradycardia, or by clear evidence of severe metabolic acidosis, it might be reasonable to consider the possibility that the findings are due to a hypoxic-ischemic insult and to label the child as having hypoxic-ischemic encephalopathy. But it is also important to consider the fact that a surprising fraction of newborns with encephalopathic findings have background factors *other* than those suggesting hypoxia or ischemia.[22, 23]

Malformations

Congenital malformations of many organ systems are more common among children with CP than among controls,[20] suggesting that factors operating early in gestation may be important etiologic factors of CP. The inclusion of brain malformations under the diagnostic rubric of CP has historically been controversial: brain malformation syndromes such as neural tube defects are usually not classified as CP, even when motor findings compatible with CP are present. However, because malformations can not be excluded from CP without brain imaging, the most recent international definition of CP includes brain malformations in the CP category if they produce the clinical motor findings characteristic of the disorder.[3]

The brain malformations that lead to CP are often due to interruptions in neuronal migration, when the presumed neurologic insult interferes with the process of grouping local and distant synaptic connections into cylindrical columns and layers to form the cortex.[24] Migrational disorders can produce varying levels of abnormal gyral and sulcal development (cortical dysplasia); those commonly found in CP range from lissencephaly and heterotopias to polymicrogyria/pachygyria schizencephaly (agenetic porencephaly), and hemi-megalencephaly. [12] Malformations are more common among term than pre-term born children with CP, and in hemiplegic forms of the disease.[25, 26, 27, 28]

Infections

Although congenital rubella was historically the cause of an occasional case of CP prior to widespread rubella vaccination, the conventional view is that viral infections produce only occasional cases of CP. [29, 30] Newer molecular diagnostic tools have made it possible to identify the footprints of perinatally acquired viral infections such as cytomegalovirus (CMV) [31, 32, 33] (whose role in CP has been suggested in at least two studies [34, 35]) and Herpes viruses (HSV) via PCR-based analysis of archived newborn blood spots.[36] Gibson et al have examined viral DNA in newborn blood spots and shown that evidence of exposure to viruses of Herpes group B was associated with elevated CP risk.[37] A possible role for enteroviruses [38, 39, 40] and pestiviruses [41, 42] in causing CP has been suggested recently. The protozoan *Toxoplasma Gondi* characteristically produces an infection in the fetus that leads to hydrocephalus via aqueductal obstruction, which can lead to CP.

Meta-analyses of the relationship between chorioamnionitis and CP in term-born infants have yielded a pooled odds ratio (OR) of 4.6.[43, 44] A case-control study, published after the meta-analysis, of CP in children born after 36 weeks of gestation found a similar multivariate OR of 4.1 for the presence of chorioamnionitis.[45]

Nelson et al [46] and Grether et al [47] reported on the results of a case-control study of 31 term-born children with spastic CP and 65 matched controls. Investigating proteins assayed on frozen archived newborn blood spots from California, they found higher levels of interleukins, interferons, chemokines and colony-stimulating factors in the CP cases, as well as higher levels of certain coagulation abnormalities.

Thyroid Hormone and Iodine

While post-natal infant hypothyroidism produces mental retardation and severely retarded development of many organ systems, prenatal exposure to maternal iodine-deficiency hypothyroidism often leaves the fetus with an intact thyroid gland (and therefore euthyroid), but with major neurologic deficits (referred to as neurologic cretinism) that include a neurologic syndrome which may be considered a form of CP, with spasticity of the legs being a particularly common finding.[48] Affected children are also mentally retarded with sensorineural hearing loss, and some imaging studies suggest damage to basal ganglia.[49] Iodine supplementation in the form of iodized salt, or, where the indigenous salt market cannot be penetrated, by iodized oil injections to women of child-bearing age can prevent this form of CP.[50, 51, 52] While most cases of cretinism in the *developed* world are due to malformations affecting fetal and neonatal thyroid hormone production, *in iodine deficient regions,* cretinism, generally with neurological deficits, is produced by in-utero maternal hypothyroxinemia resulting from severe lack of dietary iodine. An unanswered question is whether milder levels of iodine deficiency in developed countries may currently contribute to neurodevelopmental disorders. The NCPP found CP more often when mothers had thyroid abnormalities during or prior to pregnancy.[20] The aforementioned study by Grether et al found lower levels of thyroid hormone at birth in spastic CP cases than in matched controls .[47]

Hyperbilirubinemia

Unconjugated bilirubin exposure in the perinatal period is known to cause brain damage, specifically kernicterus, a condition in which yellow (icteric) staining of specific brain nuclei surrounding the basal ganglia is found.[53] According to a recent evidence-based review of this topic, kernicterus is associated with at least a 10% risk of mortality and a 70% risk of long term morbidity including hearing loss, low IQ, and CP. [54]

In developed countries, the specific form of dyskinetic CP that can occur in survivors of exposure to very severe hyperbilirubinemia is now mainly of historical interest, because of the successful use of Rh immune globulin to control rhesus hemolytic disease, and careful attention to, and management of, neonatal hyperbilirubinemia via phototherapy and exchange transfusion.[55] However, the practice of very early discharge of babies from hospital, which may be unaccompanied by an appropriate plan to monitor the baby for jaundice, may have placed some US infants at risk of kernicteric brain damage and potentially dyskinetic CP.[56, 57] Evidence for this proposition has been reported in a paper documenting over-representation of mildly premature infants managed as term infants (i.e. without special attention to their increased risk of bilirubin induced encephalopathy) in a registry of children with kernicteric brain damage.[58] At the same time, a recent population-based study of near-term infants in Nova Scotia reported no association between peak total serum bilirubin levels of $\geq$325 μmol/L (19 mg/dL) and CP, although the study found suggestions of an association with developmental delay, attention-deficit disorder, and autism.[59]

Perinatal Stroke, Thrombophillias

Perinatal stroke (PS) is defined as a cerebrovascular event occurring between 28 weeks of gestation and 28 days of postnatal age, often involving the middle cerebral artery, and commonly the result of thromboembolism from an intracranial or extracranial vessel, the heart, or the placenta. [60] Acute neonatal illnesses, congenital heart disease, birth asphyxia and sickle cell anemia can each play a role in PS, and several studies suggest associations as well with inherited thrombophilias, such as Factor V Leiden heterozygosity and antithrombin-III deficiency and, for hemorrhagic strokes, protein-C and protein-S deficiencies. [61] Maternal antiphospholipid antibodies, including lupus anticoagulant and anticardiolipin, are not rare, and since they interfere with normal coagulation, they can also increase the risk for PS. While some studies have found such polymorphisms in children with CP, it is not yet firmly established that the frequency is higher than in the background population.[62, 63] Golomb et al. assessed the frequency of CP in children in an arterial PS database and reported that 68% of the 111 children had CP, most commonly hemiplegic (87%).[64] A recent commentary estimated that ischemic PS might be responsible for up to 30% of hemiplegic CP cases.[65]

Family History and Genetics

In general, genetic factors are thought to play a minor role in CP etiology, with occasional case reports of familial clustering or evidence of a mutation.[66, 67] However, a relative risk of 4.8 for CP recurrence in siblings was found in a recent large Swedish study. [68] A CP case-control study in Western Australia between 1980 and 1986, on the other hand, failed to find recurrence of cerebral palsy, congenital malformations or reproductive loss in cerebral palsy families. [69] Two case-control studies have found a higher prevalence of certain less common apolipoprotein E alleles in CP than controls. [70, 71] This genetic polymorphism, which is shared with Alzheimer's disease, may reflect general brain repair and injury-response mechanisms. [72]

Multiple Births and Vanishing Twins

Multiple birth infants are at increased risk of CP. Yokoyama et al. found a steadily increasing prevalence of CP from 0.9% among twins, to 3.1% among triplets, to 11.1% among quadruplets. [73] Similarly Pharoah reported a gradient in prevalence from 0.23% in singletons to 1.3% in twins to 4.5% in triplets. [74]

While it appears that the relationship between multiparous birth and CP is mediated by the lower gestational age and birthweight seen in multiple births, two circumstances unique to twins – a common circulation (twin-twin transfusion syndrome) and death of a co-twin in utero (the vanishing twin syndrome) – may elevate risk of CP. [75] The risk of CP has been estimated to be 14 times higher when a co-twin is known to have died in utero, [76] likely as a result of toxic products of decomposition. [77] Pharoah has hypothesized that in some cases of CP in apparent singletons, a co-twin died in utero early in pregnancy before twinning could be diagnosed. Support for this concept comes from a careful study of early pregnancy that found that a twin died in utero in 71% of twin pregnancies diagnosed before the 10th week of pregnancy. [78] This figure, if generalizable, would imply that for every set of twins diagnosed at birth, 2.45 singletons are born who were former twins (71%/29%). With a singleton birth/twin births ratio of 88:1, as many as 2.8% of singletons might be former twins, and at elevated risk of CP. However, the relative risk of CP in infants whose co-twin died very early in utero remains unknown. Newton et al. conducted a small case-control study of vanishing twin as a risk factor for CP in women who had an obstetric ultrasound during pregnancy and reported one of 86 mothers of cases had evidence of vanishing twin compared to two of 381 controls (OR 2.2, CI 0.2-24.8). Clearly, there was insufficient statistical power to draw firm conclusions. [79]

Methylmercury (Mehg)

Consumption of foods contaminated by MeHg by pregnant mothers has produced spastic quadriplegia with mental retardation in Japan (where the food source was fish contaminated with industrial effluent containing MeHg) and Iraq (where grain was accidentally contaminated). [80, 81] There is as yet no evidence of an association of CP with the lesser levels of MeHg exposure occurring in the US (principally via fish consumption), although this topic has not been thoroughly studied.

Fetal Growth Pattern

Fetal growth restriction (FGR) has been shown to be a risk factor for cerebral palsy both in singletons, [82, 83] and twins. [84] A variety of mechanisms can be implicated in this relationship because several maternal conditions and behaviors (e.g. pre-eclampsia, smoking, cocaine use) are associated with FGR. FGR may also be a marker for pre-existing brain damage, since microcephaly, itself a risk factor for CP, [85] occurs significantly more commonly in SGA infants. Uvebrant and Hagberg [86] found that CP risk in small-for-gestational age (SGA) infants was increased more than six-fold at term, and nearly four-fold in preterm infants. Blair et al reported, from a population-based registry in Western Australia, that FGR interacted strongly with gestational age in its association with CP; the largest OR's were seen in term or mildly premature infants. [87]

The Surveillance of Cerebral Palsy in Europe (SCPE) group pooled data from several European CP registries to conduct the largest study of CP cases (N = 4,503). [83] The study reported an excess of CP in children below the 10th percentile in fetal growth for all gestational ages above 32 weeks. The finding that some term-born infants with CP have periventricular white matter loss similar to that of premature infants [88] suggests the hypothesis that injury to developing oligodendrocytes in the late second/early third trimester may not always lead to preterm delivery, but may be marked by poor fetal growth subsequent to the injury. A surprising result of the SCPE study was that an increased risk of CP was also seen in children above the 97th percentile of birthweight for gestational age.

CP Risk Factors in Preterm Infants

Fetal Growth

The relationship of fetal growth to CP in preterm infants is less clear and more complex than in term-born infants. Two of the better-controlled studies failed to find an excess risk of CP in growth retarded preterm-infants, [89, 90] while the above-cited SCPE study also did not find an excess of CP in growth retarded babies under 32 weeks unless fetal (rather than neonatal) growth standards were used to define IUGR. [83] The relationship between fetal growth and CP in preterm infants is particularly complex because some risk factors for preterm birth associated with impaired fetal growth, such as pre-eclampsia, might actually convey diminished risk for CP. [91]

Infection and Inflammation

Premature infants have both a high risk of CP and a high prevalence of bacterial invasion of the placenta, and associated chorioamnionitis. CP was found to be 3.4 times more common among low birthweight National Collaborative Perinatal Project (NCPP) survivors who had experienced chorionitis. [92] However, in Wu et al's meta-analysis of 21 studies, the pooled OR for clinical chorioamnionitis and CP in preterm infants, while statistically significant, was only 1.9. [44] A review of this topic by Willoughby and Nelson was more skeptical of the chorioamnionitis-CP relationship in preterm infants, seeing it as "equivocal". [93] Papers published since Wu's meta-analysis reinforce the weak association of chorioamnionitis and CP in preterm infants. [94, 95, 96]

Chorioamnionitis is defined as an inflammatory response of the fetal membranes. It is possible that more intense levels of inflammation of the placenta may be more closely related to perinatal brain damage. In infants <1,500 g at birth, Leviton et al found that late parenchymal echolucent lesions on cranial ultrasound (strong predictors of CP) were not associated with membrane inflammation, but were strongly linked to placental fetal vasculitis (OR = 10.8) when membranes were not ruptured for ≥ I hour prior to birth. [97] This finding implies that brain damage only occurs when the fetus mounts an inflammatory response, a theme pursued by Dammann, Leviton and colleagues in a series of papers, [98, 99, 100, 101, 102] that argue that products of the fetal inflammatory response, such as chemokines and cytokines, are critical brain damage promoters. The mechanism by which these inflammatory products contribute to CP may be through damage to immature or pre-myelinating oligodendrocytes, which then fail to participate in the myelination required for normal white matter development. [103, 104]

Pro-inflammatory cytokines in newborn blood, cord blood and amniotic fluid have indeed been linked to CP, and a pathophysiologic sequence from infection product (lipopolysaccharide) to fetal brain inflammation to white matter injury has been shown in experimental animals. [105, 106] Minagawa et al found, in infants < 35 weeks, that cord blood IL-18 was strongly linked to CP, [107] a finding partially replicated in a Finnish cord blood study. [108] Yoon, Romero and colleagues have linked elevation of several cytokines in amniotic fluid to CP (significant OR's ranging from 5.9 - 6.4) in preterm infants.[109, 110, 111] Grether and Nelson, however, were unable to replicate, in preterm infants, the association they found of CP in term infants with inflammatory markers retrieved from newborn blood spots. [112]

Mycoplasmas (*M.hominis, U urealyticum*), vaginal microbes implicated in chorioamnionitis, may be important fetal inflammatory stimuli. Studies linking such organisms to brain damage or CP have found mixed results. [113, 114, 115]

Transient Hypothyroxinemia of the Premature

Premature infants frequently experience very low thyroid hormone (TH) levels in the first post-natal weeks, termed Transient Hypothyroxinemia of Prematurity (THOP). A comprehensive overview of this clinical problem is provided in a recent special issue of

Seminars in Perinatology.[116] Although once viewed as a *"benign relative delay in the maturation of the HPA axis"*, [117] Reuss et al have shown that infants of < 33 weeks gestation with T_4 levels more than 2.6 SD's below the mean of term infants had a relative odds of CP of 4.4 in a multivariate model which adjusted for 22 potential confounding variables. [118] Cerebral palsy has not been much studied in relation to THOP in other settings, but two large European cohort studies have found impaired neurodevelopment in relation to low thyroid hormone levels in prematures. [119, 120]

Corticosteroids

Premature infants exposed to corticosteroids in labor appear to have lower risks of forms of brain damage, such as PVL, that often represent cerebral palsy, [121, 122] One possible mechanism for this effect is suggested by the observation that a full course of steroids in the 48 hours before birth in infants < 28 weeks gestation raises thyroxine levels in the infants. [123]

The EPIPAGE study is an observational population-based cohort study that included all births at gestational age between 22 and 32 weeks in 1997 in nine regions of France and assessed survivors at age 5 years. The study found that antenatal steroids, while contributing to improved survival, had no effects on the risk of CP. [124] However, several smaller studies, summarized in a Cochrane review, suggest that the risk of CP may increase if prematures are exposed to corticosteroids post-natally. [125] This observation is reinforced by a recently published randomized trial discussed below. [126]

Hypocapnia/ Hyperoxia

Several studies have suggested that hypocapnia (low levels of PCO_2) may be associated with periventricular leukomalacia in premature infants [127, 128] and with CP. [129] There is increasing evidence that it is prudent to aim to maintain PCO_2 levels above 35 mm Hg by judicious mechanical ventilation practices. Hyperoxia was also found to increase risk of CP in one study, and maintaining PaO_2 levels between 60-70 mm Hg may likewise be prudent. [129]

Magnesium (Mg)

Magnesium is usually provided as $MgSO_4$ to mothers in labor for tocolysis or preeclampsia management. Since Mg is a blocker of the NMDA receptor in the brain, and since the NMDA receptor is implicated in the excitotoxic amino acid cascade that contributes to asphyxial brain damage, two case-control studies that linked CP to magnesium exposure in labor were received with considerable interest. The protective odds ratios for magnesium were very large in each study – 0.14 (95% confidence interval 0.05 - 0.51) [130] and 0.11 (95% confidence interval 0.02 - 0.81). [131] A subsequent cohort study found a much more modest protective association that was not statistically significant (adjusted OR, 0.63; 95% confidence interval, 0.32 to 1.24). [132]

Recent Contributions to CP Epidemiology from Randomized Clinical Trials

The rarity of CP as an outcome would seem to make it an unlikely candidate for a disorder whose etiology might be studied through randomized controlled trials (RCTs). However, in the last few years, a number of prevention trials that have used CP as an end-point have found significant or nearly significant effects. Not surprisingly, all of these trials have been in neonates at very high risk of CP.

A promising line of research suggests that cooling a baby to below 36 degrees C (either by whole body cooling or by head cooling) may reduce the risk of brain damage that follows hypoxic-ischemic encephalopathy (HIE). Unfortunately, all studies have chosen to study composite outcomes in which death and disability are combined. This has made it difficult to determine whether this intervention can prevent CP. Schulzke et al conducted a systematic review of neuroprotection cooling trials in neonates with HIE, and found, among five trials including 552 neonates, a significant effect on the composite outcome of death or disability (RR: 0.78, 95% CI: 0.66, 0.92) as well as on the single outcomes of mortality (RR: 0.75, 95% CI: 0.59, 0.96) and neurodevelopmental disability at 18 to 22 months (RR: 0.72, 95% CI: 0.53, 0.98). [133] However, methodological differences among the trials, wide confidence intervals, and failure to distinguish CP clearly from other forms of disability prevent us from firmly concluding that this treatment modality can prevent CP.

In premature infants, three different interventions have recently been found to result in significantly fewer cases of CP in randomized trials. These are high-frequency ventilation (HIFI); [134] $MgSO_4$; [135, 136, 137] and caffeine. [138] At the same time, one intervention, postnatal dexamethasone, has been found in an RCT to increase the risk of CP. [136]

Truffert et al's study of HIFI found the largest effect on CP; nearly four times as many children conventionally ventilated had CP than did children in the intervention arm (16/95 in the conventional arm vs. 4/97 in the HIFI arm). Remarkably, the initial report of this trial showed a considerably higher frequency of severe intraventricular hemorrhage in the HIFI arm. [139]

The findings for $MgSO_4$ given to the mother in preterm labor are bolstered by the replication of a trend towards reduced risk of CP in three separate trials. Crowther et al found a modest and non-significant reduction in CP (RR = 0.83; 95% CI, 0.54-1.27) that was accompanied, however, by a significant halving of the risk of "substantial neurologic dysfunction" at age two. [135] A more recent trial by Rouse et al found a more robust reduction in CP (RR = 0.55; 95% CI, 0.32 to 0.95). [136] Yet the Rouse et al trial found four more deaths in the $MgSO_4$ arm, and, since the trial end-point was the combination of death and CP, and because in this trial deaths outnumbered CP by more than four to one, the overall result of the trial was null (RR = 0.97; 95% confidence interval, 0.77 to 1.23). The third trial, conducted in France by Marret et al found a non-significant RR for CP of 0.63 (CI 0.35 – 1.15) [137] and, unlike the Rouse et al trial, was accompanied by a non-significant reduction in mortality in the Mg arm and a significant reduction in the combined outcome of death and disability.

The mean RR for CP in the Mg arms of the three trials is 0.67 ([0.83 + 0.55 + 0.63]/3), surprisingly close to the OR of 0.63 found in the single cohort study. Taken together with the observational data, the possibility that $MgSO_4$ provided in labor can prevent some cases of CP cannot be dismissed.

Caffeine and other methylxanthines (aminophylline, theophylline) have been administered to premature infants as respiratory stimulants for over 30 years as a therapy for apnea of prematurity. [140] Until recently, this practice had not been evaluated beyond short-term outcomes. Schmidt et al. conducted a large, international, randomized, placebo-controlled trial to study both short and long-term efficacy of caffeine therapy in infants with very low birthweight and reported a significant protective effect on CP. [138] CP was found in 4.4% of the intervention group and in 7.3% of the placebo group; the adjusted odds ratio of CP was 0.58 (95% CI, 0.39 to 0.87; P=0.009).

Conclusions

The persistence of CP as a health problem of considerable frequency and severity indicates a pressing need for research into causation. The prevalence of CP does not appear to vary significantly among Western nations, though data from the Americas are sparse. Over the past forty years the overall CP prevalence has remained stable; however, a modest increase in prevalence, likely attributable to increased survival of VLBW infants, probably occurred in the last decades of the 20th century.

New paradigms of CP etiology are emerging that move away from seeing birth asphyxia as the central cause to a more complex approach that examines the roles of hormonal, thrombotic and inflammatory pathways and genetic polymorphisms. In term-born infants, a modest fraction of CP is contributed by congenital malformations of the brain. Fetal growth retardation, neonatal encephalopathy (sometimes, but not always, caused by birth asphyxia), prenatal infection and perinatal stroke may be contributors to CP in term infants. In preterm infants, ventilator management, post-natal corticosteroid use, perinatal infection/inflammation, and transient thyroid hormone deficiency may be important risk factors.

Recent randomized trials provide optimism that some post-natal interventions might help reduce the CP burden. In term infants with HIE, head and/or body cooling has now been shown to prevent some cases of CP. In preterm infants, MgSO4 treatment in labor, caffeine administration and HIFI ventilation have each been shown in at least one randomized trial to reduce the frequency of CP.

Establishing the role of risk factors in the pathogenesis and etiology of CP is a necessary first step before prevention efforts. With excess lifetime costs of more than $1 million per individual, and an annual excess cost to the US economy of nearly $12 billion, if a risk factor can be identified that can be translated into an intervention that reduces CP prevalence by even as little as 5%, the societal benefit would be very substantial.

References

[1] Little WJ. On the influence of abnormal parturition, difficult labors, premature birth, and asphyxia neonatorum, on the mental and physical condition of the child, especially in relation to deformities. *Transactions of the Obstetrical Society of London*. 1861: III: 293-344.

[2] Freud S. *Die Infantile Cerebrallähmung*. Vienna: Alfred Holder, 1897

[3] Rosenbaum P, Paneth N, Leviton A, Goldstein M, Bax M, Damiano D, Dan B, Jacobsson B. A report: the definition and classification of cerebral palsy April 2006. *Dev Med Child Neurol Suppl*. 2007;109:8-14.

[4] Beckung E, Hagberg g, Uldall P, Cans C; Surveillance of cerebral palsy in Europe. Probability of walking in children with cerebral palsy in Europe. *Pediatrics*. 2008;121:e187-92.

[5] Beckung E, Hagberg G. Neuroimpairments, activity limitations, and participation restrictions in children with cerebral palsy. *Dev Med Child Neurol*. 2002;44:309-16.

[6] Centers for Disease Control and Prevention (CDC). Economic costs associated with mental retardation, cerebral palsy, hearing loss, and vision impairment--United States, 2003. *MMWR Morb Mortal Wkly Rep*. 2004;53(3):57-9

[7] Bax M, Goldstein M, Rosenbaum P, Leviton A, Paneth N, Dan B, Jacobsson B, Damiano D. Executive Committee for the Definition of Cerebral Palsy. Proposed definition and classification of cerebral palsy, April 2005. *Dev Med Child Neurol*. 2005;47(8):571-6.

[8] Voss W, Neubauer A-P, Wachtendorf M, Verhey JF, Kattner E. Neurodevelopmental outcome in extremely low birth weight infants: what is the minimum age for reliable developmental prognosis? *Acta Paediatr* 2007;96:342-347

[9] Palisano R, Rosenbaum P, Walter S, Russell D, Wood E, Galuppi B. Development and reliability of a system to classify gross motor function in children with cerebral palsy. *Dev Med Child Neurol* 1997;39:214–223.

[10] Eliasson AC, Krumlinde-Sundholm L, Rösblad B, Beckung E, Arner M, Ohrvall AM, Rosenbaum P. The Manual Ability Classification System (MACS) for children with cerebral palsy: scale development and evidence of validity and reliability. *Dev Med Child Neurol* 2006;48:549–554.

[11] Hidecker MJC, Paneth N, Rosenbaum P, Kent RD, Lillie J, Johnson B, Chester K. Developing a classification tool of functional communication in children with cerebral palsy. *Dev Med Child Neurol* 2008;50(Suppl.4), 43.

[12] Korzeniewski S, Birbeck G, DeLano MC, Potchen MJ, Paneth N. A Systematic Review of Neuroimaging for Cerebral Palsy. *J Child Neurol* 2008;23:216-227.

[13] Paneth N, Hong T, Korzeniewski S. The Descriptive Epidemiology of Cerebral Palsy. *Clinics in Perinatology*, 2006; 33 (2):251-265.

[14] Bhushan V, Paneth N, Kiely JL. Recent secular trends in the prevalence of cerebra palsy. *Pediatrics* 1993;91:1094-1100.

[15] Platt MJ, Cans C, Johnson A, Surman G, Topp M, Torrioli MG, Krageloh-Mann I. Trends in cerebral palsy among infants of very low birthweight (<1500 g) or born

prematurely (<32 weeks) in 16 European centres: a database study. *Lancet* 2007;6;369:43-50.

[16] Wilson-Costello D, Friedman H, Minich N, Siner B, Taylor G, Schluchter M, Hack M. Improved neurodevelopmental outcomes for extremely low birth weight infants in 2000-2002. *Pediatrics.* 2007;119:37-45.

[17] Yeargin-Allsopp M, Van Naarden Braun K, Doernberg NS, Benedict RE, Kirby RS, Durkin MS. Prevalence of cerebral palsy in 8-year-old children in three areas of the United States in 2002: a multisite collaboration. *Pediatrics.* 2008;121(3):547-54.

[18] Larroque, B, Ancel, PY, Marret, S, Marchand L, Andre M, Arnaud C, Pierrat V, Roze JC, Messer J, Thiriez G, Burguet A, Picaud JC, Breart G, Kaminski M; the EPIPAGE Study group. Neurodevelopmental disabilities and special care of 5-year-old children born before 33 weeks of gestation (the EPIPAGE study): a longitudinal cohort study. *Lancet* 2008;371(9615):813-820.

[19] Hemming K, Colver A, Hutton JL. The Influence of Gestational Age on Severity of Impairment in Spastic Cerebral Palsy. *J Pediatr* 2008;153:203-208.e4.

[20] Nelson KB, Ellenberg JH. Antecedents of cerebral palsy. Multivariate analysis of risk. *N Engl J Med* 1986;10;315:81-6.

[21] Collins M, Paneth N. The Relationship of Birth Asphyxia to Later Motor Disability. *In Donn SM, Sinha SK, Chiswick ML, eds. Birth Asphyxia and the Brain: Basic Science and Clinical Implications,* Armonk, NY: Futura Publishing, 2002.

[22] Adamson SJ, Alessandri LM, Badawi N, Burton PR, Pemberton PJ, Stanley F. Predictors of neonatal encephalopathy in full-term infants BMJ. 1995;311(7005):598-602.

[23] Badawi N, Kurinczuk JJ, Keogh JM, Alessandri LM, O'Sullivan F, Burton PR, Pemberton PJ, Stanley FJ. Antepartum risk factors for newborn encephalopathy: the Western Australian case-control study. *BMJ.* 1998;5;317(7172):1549-53.

[24] Grant PE, Barkovich AJ. Neuroimaging in CP: Issues in pathogenesis and diagnosis. *Mental Retardation and Developmental Disabilities Research Reviews* 1997;3(2):118-128.

[25] Hyakawa K, Kanda T, Hashimoto K, Okuno Y, Yamori Y. MR of Spastic Tetraplegia. *AJNR* 1997;18:247-253.

[26] Candy EJ, Hoon AH, Capute AJ, Bryan RN. MRI in Motor Delay - Important Adjunct to Classification of Cerebral-Palsy. *Pediatric Neurology* 1993;9(6):421-429.

[27] Jaw T, Jong Y, Sheu R, Liu G, Chou M, Yang R. Etiology, Timing of Insult, and Neuropathology of Cerebral Palsy Evaluated with Magnetic Resonance Imaging. *Journal of the Formos Medical Association* 1998;97(4):239-246.

[28] Kragelohmann I, Petersen D, Hagberg G, Vollmer B, Hagberg B, Michaelis R. Bilateral Spastic Cerebral-Palsy - MRI Pathology and Origin - Analysis from a Representative Series of 56 Cases. *Developmental Medicine and Child Neurology* 1995;37(5):379-397.

[29] Stanley F, Blair E, Alberman E. Cerebral Palsies: *Epidemiology and Causal Pathways*. London: MacKeith Press, 2000, p.55.

[30] Paneth N. The causes of cerebral palsy. Recent evidence. *Clin Invest Med.*1993;16:95-102.

[31] Binda S, Caroppo S, Dido P, Primache V, Veronesi L, Calvario A, Piana A, Barbi M. Modification of CMV DNA detection from dried blood spots for diagnosing congenital CMV infection. *J Clin Virol*. 2004;30(3):276-9.

[32] Haginoya K, Ohura T, Kon K, Yagi T, Sawaishi Y, Ishii KK, Funato T, Higano S, Takahashi S, Iinuma K. Abnormal white matter lesions with sensorineural hearing loss caused by congenital cytomegalovirus infection: retrospective diagnosis by PCR using Guthrie cards. *Brain Dev*. 2002;24(7):710-4.

[33] van der Knaap MS, Vermeulen G, Barkhof F, Hart AA, Loeber JG, Weel JF. Pattern of white matter abnormalities at MR imaging: use of polymerase chain reaction testing of Guthrie cards to link pattern with congenital cytomegalovirus infection. *Radiology*. 2004;230(2):529-36.

[34] Madden C, Wiley S, Schleiss M, Benton C, Meinzen-Derr J, Greinwald J, Choo D. Audiometric, clinical and educational outcomes in a pediatric symptomatic congenital cytomegalovirus (CMV) population with sensorineural hearing loss. *Int J Pediatr Otorhinolaryngol*. 2005;69(9):1191-8.

[35] Pass RF, Fowler KB, Boppana SB, Britt WJ, Stagno S. Congenital cytomegalovirus infection following first trimester maternal infection: symptoms at birth and outcome. *J Clin Virol*. 2006;35(2):216-20.

[36] Lewensohn-Fuchs I, Osterwall P, Forsgren M, Malm G. Detection of herpes simplex virus DNA in dried blood spots making a retrospective diagnosis possible. *J Clin Virol*. 2003;26(1):39-48.

[37] Gibson CS, MacLennan AH, Goldwater PN, Haan EA, Dekker GA. Neurotropic viruses and cerebral palsy: population based case-control study. *BMJ* 2006;332:76-80.

[38] Verboon-Maciolek MA, Groenendaal F, Cowan F: White matter damage in neonatal enterovirus meningoencephalitis. *Neurology* 2006;66:1267-9.

[39] Jaidane H, Chouchane C, Gharbi J, Chouchane S, Merchaoui Z, Ben Meriem C, Aouni M, Guediche MN. Neuromeningeal enterovirus infections in Tunisia: epidemiology, clinical presentation, and outcome of 26 pediatric cases] *Med Mal Infect*. 2005;35(1):33-8.

[40] Yang TT, Huang LM, Lu CY. Clinical features and factors of unfavorable outcomes for non-polio enterovirus infection of the central nervous system in northern Taiwan, 1994-2003. *J Microbiol Immunol Infect*. 2005;38(6):417-24.

[41] Dammann O, Hori A, Szentiks C, Hewicker-Trautwein M. Absence of pestivirus antigen in brains with white matter damage. *Dev Med Child Neurol* 2006;48: 290-3.

[42] Rennie J, Peebles D. Pestivirus as a cause of white matter damage - down but not out. *Dev Med Child Neurol* 2006;48: 243.

[43] Wu YW, Colford JM. Chorioamnionitis as a risk factor for cerebral palsy: A meta-analysis. *JAMA* 2000;284:1417-24.

[44] Wu YW. Systematic review of chorioamnionitis and cerebral palsy. *Mental Retardation and Developmental Disabilities Research Reviews* 2002;8:25-9.

[45] Wu YW, Escobar GJ, Grether JK, Croen LA, Greene JD, Newman TB. Chorioamnionitis and cerebral palsy in term and near-term infants. *JAMA* 2003;290:2677-2684.

[46] Nelson KB, Dambrosia JM, Grether JK, Phillips TM. Neonatal cytokines and coagulation factors in children with cerebral palsy. *Ann Neurol.* 1998;44:665-75.

[47] Grether JK, Nelson KB, Dambrosia JM, Phillips TM. Interferons and cerebral palsy. *J Pediatr* 1999;134:324-32.

[48] Hong T, Paneth N. Maternal and infant thyroid disorders and cerebal palsy. *Seminars in Perinatology* 2008;32:438-445.

[49] Halpern JP, Boyages SC, Maberly GF, Collins JK, Eastman CJ, Morris JG. The neurology of endemic cretinism. A study of two endemias. *Brain* 1991;114 (Pt 2):825-41.

[50] Delange F. Iodine deficiency as a cause of brain damage. *Postgraduate Medical Journal* 2001;77:217-220.

[51] Hetzel BS. Iodine and neuropsychological development. *Journal of Nutrition* 2000 130:493S-495S.

[52] Pharoah POD, Connolly KJ. Iodine and Brain-Development. *Developmental Medicine and Child Neurology* 1995;37:744-748.

[53] Blackmon LR, Fanaroff AA, Raju TN. Research on prevention of bilirubin-induced brain injury and kernicterus. National institute of Child Health and Human Development conference executive summary. *Pediatrics* 2003 114:229-33.

[54] Ip S, Chung M, Kulig J, O'Brien R, Sege R, Glicken S, Maisels J, Lau J; Subcommitte on Hyperbilirubinemia. An evidence-based review of important issues concerning neonatal hyperbilirubinemia. *Pediatrics* 2004;114(1):E130-E153.

[55] Maisels MJ, Baltz RD, Bhutani VK, Subcommittee on Hyperbilirubinemia. Management of hyperbilirubinemia in the newborn infant 35 or more weeks of gestation. *Pediatrics* 2004;114:297-316.

[56] Watchko JF, Maisels MJ. Jaundice in low birthweight infants: pathobiology and outcome. *Archives of Disease in Childhood* 2003;88:F455-F458.

[57] Maisels MJ, Watchko JF. Treatment of jaundice in low birthweight infants. *Archives of Disease in Childhood* 2003;88:F459-F463.

[58] Bhutani VK, Johnson L: Kernicterus in late preterm infants cared for as term healthy infants. *Semin Perinatol* 2006;30:89-97.

[59] Jangaard KA, Fell DB, Dodds L, Allen AC. Outcomes in a population of healthy term and near-term infants with serum bilirubin levels of >or=325 micromol/L (>or=19 mg/dL) who were born in Nova Scotia, Canada, between 1994 and 2000. *Pediatrics* 2008;122(1):119-24.

[60] Raju TN, Nelson KB, Ferriero D, Lynch JK. NICHD-NINDS Perinatal Stroke Workshop Participants. Ischemic perinatal stroke: summary of a workshop sponsored by the National Institute of Child Health and Human Development and the National Institute of Neurological Disorders and Stroke. *Pediatrics.* 2007;120:609-16.

[61] Debus O, Koch H, Kurlemann G, Strater R, Vielhaber H, Weber P, Nowak-Gottl U. Factor V Leiden and genetic defects of thrombophilia in childhood porencephaly. *Archive of Disease in Childhood.* 1998;78:121-24.

[62] Lynch JK, Nelson KB, Curry CJ, Grether JK. Cerebrovascular disorders in children with the factor V Leiden mutation. Journal of Child *Neurology* 2001;16:735-744.

[63] Lynch JK, Nelson KB. Epidemiology of perinatal stroke. *Current Opinion in Pediatrics* 2001;13:499-505.

[64] Golomb MR, Garg BP, Saha C, Azzouz F, Williams LS. Cerebral palsy after perinatal arterial ischemic stroke. *J Child Neurol.* 2008;23(3):279-86.

[65] Raju TN. Ischemic perinatal stroke: challenge and opportunities. *Int J Stroke.* 2008;3(3):169-72.

[66] Amor DJ, Craig JE, Delatycki MB, Reddihough D. Genetic factors in athetoid cerebral palsy. *Journal of Child Neurology* 2001;16:793-797.

[67] Fryer A, Appleton R, Sweeney MG, Rosenbloom L, Harding AE. Mitochondrial-DNA-8993 (Narp) Mutation Presenting with a Heterogeneous Phenotype Including Cerebral-Palsy. *Archives of Disease in Childhood* 1994;71:419-422.

[68] Hemminki, K., Li, X., Sundquist, K., Sundquist, J. High familial risks for cerebral palsy implicate partial heritable aetiology. Paediatric and Perinatal *Epidemiology.* 2007;21(3):235-41.

[69] Palmer L, Petterson B, Blair E, Burton P. Family Patterns of Gestational-Age at Delivery and Growth in-Utero in Moderate and Severe Cerebral-Palsy. *Developmental Medicine and Child Neurology* 1994;36:1108-1119.

[70] Pessoa de Barr MK, Rodrigues CJ, de Barros TE, Bevilacqua RG. Presence of apolipoprotein E epsilon4 allele in cerebral palsy. *Pediatr Orthop.* 2000;20:786-9.

[71] Kuroda MM, Weck ME, Sarwark JF, Hamidullah A, Wainwright MS. Association of apolipoprotein E genotype and cerebral palsy in children. *Pediatrics* 2007;119:306-13.

[72] Laskowitz DT, Vitek MP. Apolipoprotein E and neurological disease: therapeutic potential and pharmacogenomic interactions. *Pharmacogenomics.* 2007;8(8):959-69.

[73] Yokoyama Y, Shimizu T, Hayakawa K. Prevalence of cerebral palsy in twins, triplets and quadruplets. *Int J Epidemiol* 1995;24:943-8.

[74] Pharoah PO, Cooke T. Cerebral palsy and multiple births. *Arch Dis Child Fetal Neonatal Ed* 1996;75:F174-7.

[75] Pharoah POD, Adi Y. Consequences of in-utero death in a twin pregnancy. *Lancet* 2000;355:1597-1602.

[76] Aslan H, Gul A, Cebeci A, Polat I, Ceylan Y. The outcome of twin pregnancies Complicated by single fetal death after 20 weeks of gestation. *Twin Research* 2004;7:1-4.

[77] Benirschke K. Intrauterine death of a twin: Mechanisms, implications for surviving twin, and placental pathology. *Semin Diagn Pathol* 1993;10:222.

[78] Levi S. *Ultrasonic assessment of the high rate of human multiple pregnancy in the first trimester.* 1976;4.

[79] Newton R, Casabonne D, Johnson A, Pharoah P. A case-control study of vanishing twin as a risk factor for cerebral palsy. *Twin Res.* 2003;6(2):83-4.

[80] Kondo K. Congenital Minamata disease: Warnings from Japan's experience. *Journal of Child Neurology* 2000;15:458-464.

[81] Amin-Zaki L, Majeed MA, Elhassani SB, Clarkson TW, Greenwood MR, Doherty RA. Prenatal methylmercury poisoning. Clinical observations over five years. *Am J Dis Child* 1979;133:172-7.

[82] Kyllerman M. Dyskinetic cerebral palsy. II. Pathogenetic risk factors and intra-uterine growth. *Acta Paediatr Scand*. 1982;71:551-8.

[83] Jarvis S, Glinianaia SV, Torrioli MG, Platt MJ, Miceli M, Jouk PS, Johnson A, Hutton J, Hemming K, Hagberg G, Dolk H, Chalmers J. Surveillance of Cerebral Palsy in Europe (SCPE) collaboration of European Cerebral Palsy Registers: Cerebral palsy and intrauterine growth in single births: European collaborative study. *Lancet*. 2003;362:1106-11

[84] Glinianaia SV, Jarvis S, Topp M, Guillem P, Platt MJ, Pearce MS, Parker L; SCPE Collaboration of European Cerebral Palsy Registers. Intrauterine growth and cerebral palsy in twins: a European multicenter study. *Twin Res Hum Genet* 2006;9:460-6

[85] Watemberg N, Silver S, Harel S. Significance of microcephaly among children with developmental disabilities. *J Child Neurol*. 2002;17:117-22.

[86] Uvebrant P, Hagberg G. Intrauterine growth in children with cerebral palsy. *Acta Paediatrica* 1992;81:407-12.

[87] Blair E, Stanley F. Intrauterine growth and spastic cerebral palsy. I. Association with birth weight for gestational age.*Am J Obstet Gynecol*. 1990;162:229-37.

[88] Truwit C, Barkovich A, Koch T, Ferriero D. Cerebral palsy: MR findings in 40 patients. *AJNR Am J Neuroradiol* 1992;13:67-78.

[89] Dammann O, Dammann CE, Alfred EN, Veelken N. Fetal growth restriction is not associated witih a reduced risk for bilateral spastic cerebral palsy in very-low-birthweight infants. *Early Hum Dev* 2001;64:79-89.

[90] Topp M, Langhoff-Roos J, Uldall P, Kristensen J. Intrauterine growth and gestational age in preterm infants with cerebral palsy. *Early Hum Dev* 1996;44:27-36.

[91] Collins M, Paneth N. Preeclampsia and cerebral palsy: are they related? *Developmental Medicine and Child Neurology* 1998;40:207-211.

[92] Nelson KB, Ellenberg JH. Predictors of low and very low birth weight and the relation of these to cerebral palsy. *JAMA* 1985;254:1473-9.

[93] Willoughby RE, Nelson KB. Chorioamnionitis and brain injury. *Clin Perinatol*. 2002;29:603-21.

[94] Gray PH, Jones P, O'Callaghan MJ. Maternal antecedents for cerebral palsy in extremely preterm babies: a case-control study. *Dev Med Child Neurol*. 2001;43:580-5.

[95] Fung G, Bawden K, Chow P, Yu V. Chorioamnionitis and outcome in extremely preterm infants. *Ann Acad Med Singapore*. 2003;32:305-10.

[96] Constantine MM, How HY, Coppage K, Maxwell RA, Sibai BM. Does peripartum infection increase the incidence of cerebral palsy in extremely low birthweight infants? *AJOG* 2007; e6-e8.

[97] Leviton A, Paneth N, Reuss ML, Susser M, Allred EN, Dammann O, Kuban K,Van Marter LJ, Pagano M, Hegyi T, Hiatt M, Sanocka U, Shahrivar F, Abiri M, Disalvo D, Doubilet P, Kairam R, Kazam E, Kirpekar M, Rosenfeld D, Schonfeld S, Share J, Collins M, Genest D, Shen-Schwarz, S. Maternal infection, fetal inflammatory response and brain damage in very low birthweight infants. *Pediatr Res* 1999;46:566-575.

[98] Dammann O, Leviton A. Maternal intrauterine infection, cytokines, and brain damage in the preterm newborn. *Pediatr Res*. 1997;42(1):1-8.

[99] Dammann O, Leviton A. Role of the fetus in perinatal infection and neonatal brain damage. *Curr Opin Pediatr*. 2000;12:99-104.

[100] Dammann O, Leviton A. Possible strategies to protect the preterm brain against the fetal inflammatory response. *Dev Med Child Neurol Suppl*. 2001; 86:18-20.

[101] Dammann O, Kuban KC, Leviton A. Perinatal infection, fetal inflammatory response, white matter damage, and cognitive limitations in children born preterm. *Ment Retard Dev Disabil Res Rev*. 2002;8:46-50

[102] Dammann O, Leviton A. Inflammatory brain damage in preterm newborns--dry numbers, wet lab, and causal inferences. *Early Hum Dev*. 2004 ;79:1-15.

[103] Folkerth RD. Periventricular leukomalacia: overview and recent findings. *Pediatr Dev Pathol* 2006; 9:3-13.

[104] Back SA. Perinatal white matter injury: the changing spectrum of pathology and emerging insights into pathogenetic mechanisms. *Ment Retard Dev Disabil Res Rev*. 2006;12: 129-40.

[105] Rousset CI, Chalon S, Cantagrel S, Bodard S, Andre C, Gressens P, Saliba E. Maternal exposure to LPS induces hypomyelination in the internal capsule and programmed cell death in the deep gray matter in newborn rats. *Ped Research* 2006; 59:428-33.

[106] Wang X, Rousset CI, Hagberg H, Mallard C. Lipopolysaccharide-induced inflammation and perinatal brain injury. *Semin Fetal Neonatal Med*. 2006 19 [epub]

[107] Minagawa K, Tsuji Y, Ueda H, Koyama K, Tanizawa K, Okamura H, Hashimoto-Tamaoki T. Possible correlation between high levels of IL-18 in the cord blood of preterm infants and neonatal development of periventricular leukomalacia and cerebral palsy. *Cytokine*. 2002;17:164-70.

[108] Kaukola T, Satyaraj E, Patel DD, Tchernev VT, Grimwade BG, Kingsmore SF, Koskela P, Tammela O, Vainionpaa L, Pihko H, Aarimaa T, Hallman M. Cerebral palsy is characterized by protein mediators in cord serum. *Ann Neurol*. 2004; 55:186-94.

[109] Yoon BH, Jun JK, Romero R, Park KH, Gomez R, Choi JH, Kim IO: Amniotic fluid inflammatory cytokines (interleukin-6, interleukin-1beta, and tumor necrosis factor-alpha), neonatal brain white matter lesions, and cerebral palsy. *Am J Obstet Gynecol*. 1997;177:19-26.

[110] Yoon BH, Romero R, Park JS, Kim CJ, KimSH, Choi JH, Han TR. Fetal exposure to an intra-amniotic inflammation and the development of cerebral palsy at the age of three years. *Am J Obstet Gynecol*. 2000;182:675-81.

[111] Moon JB, Kim JC, Yoon BH, Romero R, Kim G, Oh SY, Kim M, Shim SS. Amniotic fluid matrix metalloproteinase-8 and the development of cerebral palsy. *J Perinat Med*. 2002;30(4):301-6.

[112] Grether JK, Nelson KB, Walsh E, Willoughby RE, Redline RW: Intrauterine exposure to infection and risk of cerebral palsy in very preterm infants. *Arch Pediatr Adolesc Med* 2003;157:26-32.

[113] Dammann O, Allred EN, Genest DR, Kundsin RB, Leviton A. Antenatal mycoplasma infection, the fetal inflammatory response and cerebral white matter damage in very-low-birthweight infants. *Paediatr Perinat Epidemiol*. 2003;17(1):49-57.

[114] Ollikainen J, Hiekkaniemi H, Korppi M, Katila ML, Heinonen K. Ureaplasma urealyticum cultured from brain tissue of preterm twins who died of intraventricular hemorrhage. *Scand J Infect Dis.* 1993;25:529-31.

[115] Berger A, Witt A, Haiden N, Kaider A, Klebermasz K, Fuiko R, Langgartner M, Pollak A. Intrauterine infection with Ureaplasma species is associated with adverse neuromotor outcome at 1 and 2 years adjusted age in preterm infants. *J Perinatal Medicine* 2009;37:72–78.

[116] LaGamma EF, ed. Transient Hypothyroxinemia of Prematurity. *Seminars in Neonatology* 2008;32:377-446.

[117] Hadeed AJ, Asay LD, Klein AH, Fisher DA. Significance of transient postnatal hypothyroxinemia in premature infants with and without respiratory distress syndrome. *Pediatrics* 1981;68:494-8.

[118] Reuss L, Paneth N, Pinto-Martin JA, Lorenz JM, Susser M. Transient hypothyroxinemia in preterm infants and neurodevelopment at age two. *N Eng J Med* 1996;334:821-827.

[119] Den Ouden AL, Kok JH, Verkerk PH, Brand R, Verloove-Vanhorick SP. The relation between neonatal thyroxine levels and neurodevelopmental outcome at age 5 and 9 years in a national cohort of very preterm and/or very low birth weight infants. *Pediatr Res.* 1996;39:142-5.

[120] Lucas A, Morley R, Fewtrell MS. Low triiodothyronine concentration in preterm infants and subsequent intelligence quotient (IQ) at 8 year follow up. *BMJ.* 1996;312:1132-3.

[121] Agarwal R, Chiswick ML, Rimmer S, Taylor GM, McNally RJ, Alston RD, D'Souza SW. Antenatal steroids are associated with a reduction in the incidence of cerebral white matter lesions in very low birthweight infants. *Arch Dis Child Fetal Neonatal Ed.* 2002;86:F96-F101.

[122] Kent A, Lomas F, Hurrion E, Dahlstrom JE. Antenatal steroids may reduce adverse neurological outcome following chorioamnionitis: neurodevelopmental outcome and chorioamnionitis in premature infants. *J Paediatr Child Health.* 2005;41:186-90.

[123] Martin CR, Van Marter LJ, Allred L, Leviton A; Developmental Epidemiology Network. Antenatal glucocorticoids increase early total thyroxine levels in premature infants. *Biol Neonate* 2005;87(4):273-80

[124] Foix-L'Hélias L, Marret S, Ancel PY, Marchand L, Arnaud C, Fresson J, Picaud JC, Rozé JC, Theret B, Burguet A, Larroque B, Kaminski M. EPIPAGE Study Group. Impact of the use of antenatal corticosteroids on mortality, cerebral lesions and 5-year neurodevelopmental outcomes of very preterm infants: the EPIPAGE cohort study. *BJOG.* 2008;115(2):275-82.

[125] Halliday HL, Ehrenkranz RA, Doyle LW. Early postnatal (<96 hours) corticosteroids for preventing chronic lung disease in preterm infants. *Cochrane Database Syst Rev* 2003;(1):CD001146..

[126] O'Shea TM, Washburn LK, Nixon PA, Goldstein DJ. Follow-up of a randomized, placebo-controlled trial of dexamethasone to decrease the duration of ventilator dependency in very low birth weight infants: neurodevelopmental outcomes at 4 to 11 years of age. *Pediatrics* 2007;120:594-602.

[127] Salokorpi T, Rajantie I, Vititala J, Rita H, Von Wendt L. Does perinatal hypocarbia play a role in the pathogenesis of cerebral palsy? *Acta Paediatr* 1999;88:571-5.

[128] Griesen G, Munck H, Lou H. Severe hypocarbia in preterm infants and neurodevelopmental deficits. *Acta Paediatr Scand* 1987;76.

[129] Collins MP, Lorenz JM, Jetton JR, Paneth N. Hypocapnia and other ventilation-related risk factors for cerebral palsy in low birth weight infants. *Pediatric Research* 2001;50:712-719.

[130] Nelson KB, Grether JK. Can magnesium sulfate reduce the risk of cerebral palsy in very low birthweight infants? *Pediatrics*. 1996 May;97(5):780-2

[131] Schendel DE, Berg CJ, Yeargin-Allsopp M, Boyle CA, Decoufle P. Prenatal magnesium sulfate exposure and the risk for cerebral palsy or mental retardation among very low-birth-weight children aged 3 to 5 years. *JAMA.* 1996;276(22):1805-10.

[132] Paneth N, Jetton J, Pinto-Martin J, Susser M and the NBH Study Team. Magnesium sulfate in labor and risk of neonatal brain lesions and cerebral palsy in low birthweight infants. *Pediatrics* 1997; 97:723.

[133] Schulzke, S.M., Rao, S., Patole, S.K. A systematic review of cooling for neuroprotection in neonates with hypoxic ischemic encephalopathy- are we there yet? *BMC Pediatr.* 2007(7):30.

[134] Truffert P, Paris-Llado J, Escande B, Magny JF, Cambonie G, Saliba E, Thiriez G, Zupan-Simunek V, Blanc T, Rozé JC, Bréart G, Moriette G. Neuromotor outcome at 2 years of very preterm infants who were treated with high-frequency oscillatory ventilation or conventional ventilation for neonatal respiratory distress syndrome. *Pediatrics.* 2007;119(4):e860-5

[135] Crowther CA, Hiller JE, Doyle LW, Haslam RR. Effect of magnesium sulfate given for neuroprotection before preterm birth: a randomized controlled trial. *JAMA* 2003;290:2669-76.

[136] Rouse DJ, Hirtz DG, Thom E, Varner MW, Spong CY, Mercer BM, Iams JD, Wapner RJ, Sorokin Y, Alexander JM, Harper M, Thorp JM Jr, Ramin SM, Malone FD, Carpenter M, Miodovnik M, Moawad A, O'Sullivan MJ, Peaceman AM, Hankins GD, Langer O, Caritis SN, Roberts JM, Eunice Kennedy Shriver NICHD Maternal-Fetal Medicine Units Network. A randomized, controlled trial of magnesium sulfate for the prevention of cerebral palsy. *N Engl J Med*. 2008;359(9):895-905.

[137] Marret S, Marpeau L, Follet-Bouhamed C, Cambonie G, Astruc D, Delaporte B, Bruel H, Guillois B, Pinquier D, Zupan-Simunek V, Bénichou J; le groupe PREMAG. [Effect of magnesium sulphate on mortality and neurologic morbidity of the very-preterm newborn (of less than 33 weeks) with two-year neurological outcome: results of the prospective PREMAG trial. *Gynecol Obstet Fertil*. 2008;36(3):278-88.

[138] Schmidt B, Roberts RS, Davis P, Doyle LW, Barrington KJ, Ohlsson A, Solimano A, Tin W. Caffeine for Apnea of Prematurity Trial Group. Long-term effects of caffeine therapy for apnea of prematurity. *New Engl J Med*. 2007;357(19):1893-902.

[139] Moriette G, Paris-Llado J, Walti H, Escande B, Magny JF, Cambonie G, Thiriez G, Cantagrel S, Lacaze-Masmonteil T, Storme L, Blanc T, Liet JM, André C, Salanave B, Bréart G. Prospective randomized multicenter comparison of high-frequency oscillatory

ventilation and conventional ventilation in preterm infants of less than 30 weeks with respiratory distress syndrome. *Pediatrics* 2001 Feb;107(2):363-72.

[140] Martin RJ, Abu-Shaweesh JM, Baird TM: Apnoea of prematurity. *Paediatr Respir Rev* 2004;5:Suppl A: s377-S382.

In: Textbook of Perinatal Epidemiology
Editor: Eyal Sheiner, pp. 523-539

ISBN: 978-1-60741-648-7
© 2010 Nova Science Publishers, Inc.

Chapter XXV

The Relationship between Fetal Gender and Pregnancy Outcomes

Gali Pariente and Eyal Sheiner[*]

Department of Obstetrics and Gynecology, Soroka University Medical Center, Faculty of
Health Sciences, Ben-Gurion University of the Negev, Be'er-Sheva, Israel

Introduction

Genesis 3:16 is the passage usually quoted by those who believe women were cursed to give birth in pain. God punished Eve with pain during labor after she was beguiled by the serpent and ate of the forbidden fruit from the tree of knowledge. God said, "I will greatly multiply your pain in childbearing; in pain you shall bring forth children".

Nevertheless, the word translated as "children" is the Hebrew word *banim*, which means "boys". Indeed, most interpreters have translated the word "boys" as "children". Yet, there is increasing scientific evidence that gender does matter [1].

Gender differences in perinatal medicine have raised the concern of many clinicians because of the simple observation and the general belief that male pregnancies are more likely to be prone to adverse pregnancy outcomes. Indeed, while reviewing the literature, there is a growing body of evidence (although not always reasonably explained) regarding differences in pregnancy aspects, outcomes and labor complications between pregnancies of male and female fetuses.

[*] For Correspondence: Eyal Sheiner, MD, PhD, Department of Obstetrics and Gynecology, Soroka University Medical Center, P.O. Box 151, Be'er-Sheva 84105, Israel. Tel: +972-8-640-0774; Fax: +972-8-627-5338; E-mail: sheiner@bgu.ac.il

Male-to-Female Ratio among Fetuses and Newborns

In a review article from 2007, Di Ranzo et al. found fetal sex-dependent differences in many aspects of pregnancy from conception through birth [2]. It is well documented that at conception the number of male embryos exceeds the number of female embryos [3]. The sex ratio of males to females at birth is, on average, 103:100, ranging from the highest male-to-female ratio in Asia (106:100) to the lowest male-to-female ratio in American Indian newborns (102:100) [4-6].

In fetuses born after very short-duration pregnancies (16–19 weeks), an extremely high male-to-female ratio of 248:100 has been found. This ratio declines to 130:100 around the 20th week, remaining almost at this level among premature births up to the 36th week, and stabilizing at term at 100:100 [7].

In the absence of manipulation, both the sex ratio at birth and the population sex ratio have been found to remain constant in human populations. Small alterations are known to occur naturally, such as an excess of male births during and after wartime [8]. This phenomenon may be attributed to a combination of threshold of intensity combined with duration that is present during wartime, which together may influence the sex ratio.

Certain biological and environmental factors may have an impact on fetal sex, but findings of seasonal, parental education, birth order and maternal age effects on the sex ratio at birth are not always in agreement, and a number of studies report minimal variation [9].

Chacon Puignau and Jaffe [10] studied the Venezuelan population, which endures extreme conditions of poverty. They observed that sex ratio at birth may be related to socioeconomic status (also known as the Trivers-Willard [T-W] effect). Sex ratio deviations varied according to socioeconomic status: higher educational level was associated with higher sex ratio at birth; extreme poverty was associated with lower sex ratio at birth and had a stronger impact on sex ratio at birth than did high socioeconomic status. The T-W effect appeared to be stronger before conception and to vary by maternal marital status. Female fetuses had a greater advantage if mothers were unmarried. The sex ratios for mortality did not differ for any of the socioeconomic status indicators, but differences were noted for type of birth and gestational age at delivery, with single births and early gestational delivery having higher male mortality [10].

Differences in Chromosomal Aberrations between the Two Sexes

Kovalena [11] reviewed of the literature on sex-specific chromosome instability and found a female prevalence in cases of mosaicism associated with uniparental disomy (UPD). This predominance was highest <16 weeks' gestation with a sex ratio of 0.36, which was significantly different from the expected ratio of 1.28. Potential correction of trisomies predominantly in females may be the reason for the decrease in this ratio at later stages of fetal development. A threefold prevalence of *46,XX/45,X* mosaicism over *46,XY/45,X* mosaicism in prenatally diagnosed cases also suggested a sex-specific post zygotic chromosome loss. Male prevalence in Prader-Willi syndrome with maternal UPD of chromosome 15, explains the sex-specific trisomy correction where loss of a maternal chromosome causes biparental inheritance and complete correction of trisomy in females (without UPD). In both prenatal and postnatal ill-defined cases a female predominance was also noted in carriers of chromosome rearrangement with pericentromere breaks. It is possible that gonadal mosaicism for aneuploidies and structural rearrangements occur more frequently in females than in males, suggesting a maternal origin bias in offspring with trisomies or structural rearrangements [11].

Gender Variations in the Different Aspects of Pregnancy

Gender Impact on Biochemical and Sonographic Markers for Down Syndrome

First-trimester free beta-human chorionic gonadotropin (hCG) is known to be significantly higher in pregnancies with a female fetus than with a male fetus. The pronounced gender impact found for free beta-hCG, is 16% higher for female fetuses than for males [12]. It appears that the sex of the fetus does not affect the regulation of cytotrophoblast cell proliferation; that is, the difference in maternal serum and cord blood hCG levels in correlation with fetal sex is not associated with cytotrophoblast cell activity in the human placenta [13].

Bazzett and co-authors [14] described the fetal gender impact on biochemical screening for prenatal diagnosis. They showed that maternal serum alfa-fetoprotein (AFP) levels in women carrying female fetuses were consistently lower than in those carrying males contrary to the previously mentioned higher hCG levels in pregnancies with female fetuses as compared with males. It is noteworthy that no gender- related difference was documented for unconjugated estriol [14]. Contradicting results were found in another study, using an amniotic fluid AFP cut-off level of >1.9 MoM, in which the screen-positive result risk of AFP-associated malformations was significantly higher for female fetuses than for males (29% versus 15%) [14]. In pregnant women aged <35 years, increase in nuchal translucency a sonographic marker for Down syndrome was observed more commonly in gestations with a male fetus [15]. Looking for differences in other 'soft markers' for Down syndrome (i.e., sonographic markers without any clinical significance other than being a marker for Down syndrome), differences between the two sexes can also be found. Wax et al. [16] checked differences in frequency of soft sonographic aneuploidy markers between fetal sexes. All singleton fetuses with known sex undergoing genetic sonography at 17 weeks' to 21 weeks 6 days' gestation in a single perinatal center were identified. Markers studied were biparietal diameter/femur length, transcerebellar diameter, ear length, echogenic bowel, femur length, humerus length, absent middle fifth phalanx, nuchal fold, renal pelvis dilatation, echogenic cardiac focus, and choroid plexus cysts. Additional information extracted from the prospectively ascertained database included maternal age, referral indications, and chromosomal analyses. In total, 4057 eligible fetuses, 2103 male and 1954 female, were examined at 18.9 ± 0.9 weeks (mean $\pm$ SD). Overall, male fetuses exhibited echogenic fetal bowel (odds ratio, 1.76; 95% confidence interval [CI], 1.14–2.72; $P = .009$) and renal pelvis dilatation (odds ratio, 2.00; 95% CI, 1.30–3.09; $P = .001$) more frequently than female fetuses. However, when fetuses were evaluated for single isolated markers, only male predominance of renal pelvis dilatation persisted (odds ratio, 2.32; 95% CI, 1.32–4.09; $P = .003$). No markers increased frequency in females. It is speculated that in the majority of male fetuses the presence of pyelectasis represents either a normal physiologic variant or occurs secondary to anatomic abnormalities such as a posterior urethral valve. Consequently, some investigators have hypothesized that the presence of pyelectasis in a female fetus is indicative of a greater risk of aneuploidy [17, 18]. On the other hand, in a retrospective analysis of about 750,000 amniocentesis results, fetal pyelectasis was reported in 671 cases. Male predominance, with a male-to-female ratio of 2.14:1 (457 versus 214), was statistically significant ($P < 0.001$); a major trisomy was detected in 26 (5.7%) male fetuses. It suggests that the prevalence of major trisomies among fetuses with pyelectasis is unlikely to be dependent on fetal sex, and that sex-specific adjustment of sonographically-derived aneuploidy risk is not yet indicated [19].

Pregnancy Complications and Morbidity

A number of diagnoses during pregnancy have been noted to occur more frequently with a particular fetal sex. Pregnant women with a diagnosis of hyperemesis gravidarum in the first trimester give birth to a higher proportion of females than do all mothers [20]. This finding is consistent with the increase in serum hCG mentioned earlier in pregnancies with a female fetus [12].

With regard to differences in the development or the effect of infectious disease organisms in fetuses, the high prevalence of *Toxoplasma gondii* in the human population may considerably affect the sex ratio. Sex ratio for boys and girls born to women with the highest concentration of anti-Toxoplasma antibodies is 260:100 respectively. The survival of male embryos may be enhanced by the immunosuppression or immunomodulation associated with toxoplasmosis [21]. Amniotic fluid cytomegalovirus DNA load, on the other hand, has not been found to be significantly higher in males than in females, and was also similar in severely and non severely infected fetuses [22]. Female infants may be more susceptible to HIV infection both before and after birth even when controlling for viral load as a measure of infectiousness and for birth weight which was significantly lower among female infants. Two explanations are possible: (1) HIV infection may preferentially target female offspring in utero (from conception to birth). The factors involved may be genetic, immunologic, hormonal, or environmental. (2) In utero mortality rates of HIV-infected males may be disproportionately higher than the infected females, therefore more HIV-infected females may be born [23].

Significant differences in male-to-female ratio at birth in pregnant women with placenta previa were also observed.In a meta-analysis of seven articles the preponderance of male sex at birth in pregnancies with and without placenta previa was evaluated [24]. This meta-analysis found that the male-to-female ratio at birth was significantly higher in women with placenta previa (1.19) than in those without placenta previa (1.05) (p<0.001). The association of placenta previa with male gender persisted when the analysis was either stratified or adjusted for the effects of maternal age, maternal parity, maternal smoking during the index pregnancy, race/ethnicity, the infant's gestational age, and the infant's birth weight. The meta-analytic results from the fixed-effect and random-effects models showed a 14% excess of placenta previa when women were carrying a viable male fetus as compared with a viable female fetus during pregnancy [24].

On the contrary, in a large population-based retrospective study performed by our group, no significant differences were documented in the gender distribution of placenta previa. Nevertheless, there was a non-significant tendency towards male distribution, with 55% of placenta previa cases noted among males and only 45% among females (P=0.214) [25].

Pre-eclamptic women were reported to have lower third trimester hemoglobin values and less frequent proteinuria in those carrying male fetuses versus females. Excessive syncytial knots, hypothetically caused by the greater maternal blood plasma volume expansion associated with male than with female fetuses in pre-eclamptic pregnancies, were also observed less frequently with males than with females [26]. A sex disadvantage has been noted in infants of diabetic mothers, with male fetuses having higher morbidity rates compared with females, owing to a higher incidence of hypoglycemia and the need for neonatal intensive care for more than two days [27].

Pre-Term Births and Premature Rupture of Membranes

A higher incidence of pre-term births and premature pre-term rupture of membranes (PROM) has been observed in different populations among mothers of male newborns compared with mothers of females [28]. This observation, however, is not consistent for PROM since contradictory results have recently been documented [29]. National figures from Sweden show that boys are more likely to be delivered prematurely, accounting for 55% to 60% of all newborns between 23 and 32 gestational weeks [30]. It has been speculated that this higher incidence may be linked to the relatively greater proportion of lower gestational age in male newborns versus females. Others have suggested that the greater incidence of preterm births and premature PROM is caused by an increased vulnerability to infection in women carrying male fetuses [28]. Cooperstock et al. [31] examined the interactions of race, gestational age, and births of multiples. They observed a highly significant racial difference: a 7.2% excess of males was found among white singleton pre-term births but only a 2.8% excess among comparable blacks (P < 0.001) an approximately constant effect for 20 to 37 weeks gestation. Being married increased this effect for white, but not black women, and a similar effect was found in white fetal deaths.

Male excess in pre-term births for white twins occurred only at 20 to 33 weeks gestation. A mechanism of pre-term birth influenced by fetal sex may possibly create an excess of males in selected groups. Pre-term births in blacks and in twins >33 weeks may be more often caused by alternative mechanisms independent of fetal sex [31]. Male fetuses appear to be more susceptible to pre-term labor, and pregnancies carrying female infants appear to have a greater predisposition to the indicated very-preterm births associated with hypertension [32]. The study evaluated fetal sex, onset of labor (spontaneous vs. induced), and causes of preterm birth and showed that male infants had a greater incidence of spontaneous preterm birth (relative risk [RR] = 1.42; 95% CI, 1.21–1.66), but less risk of the indicated pre-term births associated with hypertensive disorders, with and without growth restriction (RR = 0.73; 95% CI, 0.55–0.97 and RR = 0.77; 95% CI, 0.60–0.97, respectively). Nevertheless, while analyzing data acquired from the Soroka University Medical Center, a higher number of male as compared to female fetuses were born in all gestational ages (figure 1).

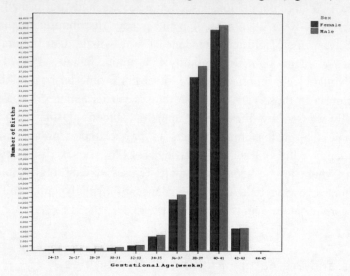

Figure 1. Number of births according to gestational age in male vs. female neonates.

No association was noted between fetal sex and lesions of acute inflammation, intra-placental vascular pathology, or utero-placental vascular pathology in premature deliveries at <32 weeks. However, lesions of chronic inflammation were significantly more evident in male fetuses than in females (P = 0.001). In severe prematurity, male fetal sex was associated with chronic inflammatory placental lesions that may develop from a maternal immune response against the invading interstitial trophoblast [33]. Another study checked risk factors for pulmonary hypoplasia after second-trimester PROM at <28 weeks gestation. In this study, two thirds of the infants who developed pulmonary hypoplasia were males [34].

Gender and Multiple Pregnancies

Association between fetal sex and discordant growth in pregnancy with twins has not been documented [35]. Nevertheless, females appear predominant in pregnancies complicated by severe twin-to-twin transfusion syndrome. The reasons for this are unclear, but may be related to placental or fetal sex-specific differences for a subset of monochorionic twin pregnancies [36, 37].

Gender mix, in particular, whether a hormone transfer occurs in utero between the male fetus and his female co-twin, although has been shown in animals, has not been incontrovertibly proven in humans. The Belgian East Flanders Prospective Twin Survey

(EFPTS) [38] started in 1964, is a population based survey. The twins (and higher order births) are ascertained at birth, basic perinatal data are collected, chorion type is established and, when appropriate, genetic markers including DNA finger prints, are determined. It was observed in this survey that the female's birth weight is not affected by her male co-twin, but the female twin slightly enhances the birth weight of the male by prolonging gestation. However, the cognitive development of the female twin rises, compared with controls, if her birth weight surpasses that of her male co-twin.

Post-Term Pregnancies

Divon et al. [39] checked gender differences in post date pregnancies. Male sex was shown to predispose the prolongation of pregnancy. By 43 weeks' gestation, the sex ratio at birth is 3 males to 2 females. The mean (SD) gestational age at birth was significantly higher for males (280.6 [8.9] days versus 279.8 [8.6] days for females; $P < 0.01$). Moreover, the percentage of pregnancies that surpassed term was significantly higher for male fetuses than for females (26.5% versus 22.5% at >41 weeks gestation and 7.6% versus 5.5% at >42 weeks gestation, respectively) [39].

The mechanisms involved in the initiation of labor are complexed and not fully understood. One explanation for the male-to-female excess in post term pregnancies can be provided by the X-linked recessive deficiency of the placental steroid sulfatase. This enzymatic deficiency leads to abnormally low estrogen production in the affected male fetus, with a subsequent prolongation of pregnancy. An X-linked disease results in a higher proportion of male fetuses delivered after term [40]. Sonographic overestimation of gestational age among males can provide an alternative explanation for the male-to-female excess observed in post-term pregnancies. Davis et al. [41] studied the impact of fetal sex on the accuracy of sonographic estimates of gestational age and found that sonographic dates tended to be higher than last menstrual period dates in male fetuses, while, sonographic dates underestimated gestational age in the female fetuses. It is unlikely,however, that sonographic overestimation of gestational age in male fetuses is the sole explanation for these results. The fact that the likelihood of delivering a male infant increases in a linear fashion at each successive week beyond 40 weeks' gestation is evidence against the possibility of a male-related fixed error in gestational dating. Thus, gender-specific mechanisms may be involved in the initiation of labor and delivery in humans [39]. Kitlinski et al. [42] found an uncorrected OR for having a male infant at >42 weeks of 1.41 (95% CI, 1.33–1.49). After adjusting gestational age by +0.75 days (i.e., adding 0.75 days to menstrual age at ultrasound fetometry in male fetus pregnancies and subtracting 0.75 days from the female- fetus pregnancies), the OR decreased to 0.90 (95% CI, 0.84–0.95). When gestational age was corrected for fetal sex, the risk for labor induction was significantly above unity in male fetus pregnancies delivered after 41 weeks. In the same series male fetus pregnancies were more likely to be induced post date when recognized as post term, thereby making a calculation of the true gender distribution in prolonged pregnancy uncertain [42].

Stillbirths and Perinatal Mortality

Jakobovits et al. in their article showed that during pregnancy male gender is significantly associated with either spontaneous abortions or stillbirths [43].

Others have estimated a 30% increased risk for male fetuses in chromosomally normal spontaneous abortions [44].

The rate of stillbirth taken from the Sweden National Birth Registry [30] shows that the stillbirth rate was similar among male fetuses (3.8 per 1000) as compared with females (3.9 per 1000). Likewise, in a population-based study comparing all singleton pregnancies of patients carrying male and female fetuses performed by our group, the rate of perinatal mortality did not differ between males (1.3%) and females (1.4%; P=0.160). In our study, deliveries occurred between the years 1988 and 1999 in the Soroka University Medical Center, which is the sole hospital in the Negev (the southern part of Israel) and thus receives the entire Negev obstetrical population. Hence, the study was based on non-selective data [45]. However, in the Sweden National Birth Registry [30] there was a >50% increase in the number of post-partum death of males infants. In 1993, the overall 1-year mortality rate (including all gestational weeks) in Sweden was 5.4% for boys and 4.1% for girls. Neonatal deaths between 23 and 32 gestational weeks were more common among boys. The difference in infant mortality within 1 year was most pronounced at extremely early births (23-24 gestational weeks): 60% for boys versus 38% for girls [30]. In total, the rate of mortality up to 1 year was 3.44 per 1000 for males as versus 2.18 per 1000 for females (based on 175,382 newborns) [46].

Sami and Baloch [47], in a small cross-sectional hospital-based study during the year 2002, found fetal sex to be a statistically significant risk factor for perinatal mortality. Out of 16 early neonatal deaths, 11 were of male infants. Obviously, this study had several limitations based on the small sample size and short duration. Nevertheless, the authors concluded that it should pave the way for future community-based studies to confirm such an association, after adjusting for confounders. Interestingly, in another small study of 70 cases of placental abruption, stillbirth was more frequent in male fetuses than in females [48].

Differences in Labor and Delivery

Sheiner et al. [45], in a large population-based retrospective study, compared labor characteristics and perinatal outcomes of 55,891 pregnancies of male fetuses versus 53,104 pregnancies of female fetuses. Higher rates of labor complications and adverse pregnancy outcomes appeared in male pregnancies. While there were no significant differences between the groups regarding maternal age, birth order, gestational age and the rate of hypertensive disorders, male pregnancies had higher rates of failure to progress during the 1st stage of labor (870 of male fetuses vs. 683 of female fetuses, p<0.001) and 2nd stages of labor (1057 of male fetuses vs. 733 of female fetuses, p<0.001), cord prolapse, nuchal cord and true umbilical cord knots, and non-reassuring FHR patterns (4.0% of male fetuses vs. 2.9% of female fetuses OR of 1.4 with 95% CI 1.3–1.7) (Table 1). In addition, the males were more likely to weigh >4 kg than the females. Males were more likely to grade lower 1- and 5-min Apgar scores than the females [45,49].

Table 1. Clinical and labor characteristics and outcomes of pregnancies of male vs. female fetuses.

Characteristics	Males (n=55,891)	Females (n= 53,104)
Gestational diabetes mellitus*	3,433 (6.1%)	3,070 (5.8%)
Cord prolapse*	229 (0.4%)	170 (0.3%)
Non reassuring FHR*	2,208(4.0%)	1,535 (2.9%)
Shoulder dystocia*	147 (0.3%)	87 (0.2%)
Birth weight >4 kg*	3,270 (5.9%)	1,629(3.1%)
Apgar <7 ,1 min*	2,512 (4.6%)	1,797 (3.5%)
Apgar <7 ,5 min*	335 (0.6%)	241 (0.5%)

* p<0.05 Adopted from Sheiner et al. [45]

Differences in Modes of Delivery

Sheiner and coauthors have also shown that male fetus pregnancies had higher rates of cesarean, vacuum and forceps deliveries [45]. Even after controlling for confounding factors, such as birth weight and gestational age, male gender was still found as an independent risk factor for CS.

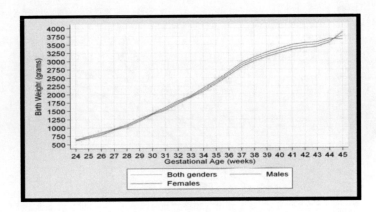

Figure 2. Birth weight according to gestational age in males vs. females; the figure represents the 50th percentile.

Comparing modes of delivery, Lieberman et al. found a 17%–40% increase in cesarean sections for low-risk, term, and nulliparous women carrying male fetuses compared with similar women with female fetuses [50]. The rate of cesarean section for both failure to progress and fetal distress was higher among women carrying male fetuses. The increase in cesarean sections for failure to progress can be explained on the basis of the larger size of male fetuses.

Male infants have a significantly larger head size than female infants, and this may account for to the longer duration of labor and the higher incidence of operative deliveries

[51]. Males are also heavier than females, i.e., higher birth weight, higher percentage of fetal macrosomia (birth weight > 4 kg) and large-for-gestational-age newborns [45,52]. Fetal macrosomia is an important risk factor for prolonged and operative deliveries [53,54]. Moreover, fetal macrosomia contributes greatly to the occurrence of shoulder dystocia [55-58] which is also more frequent among males. Gestational diabetes accounts for excessive fetal weight, which leads to an increased risk for difficult deliveries and shoulder dystocia [55-57]. Gestational diabetes is also more common among patients carrying male fetuses [45]. Looking at birth weights collected from a data base from Soroke hospital, a tertiary medical center, higher birth weights were seen in male fetuses compared to female fetuses in all gestational ages (figure 2).

Figures 3 and 4 show the median percentile of average birth weight for every gestational age. This data can be used as a reference in similar populations for growth evaluation, which might differ between genders. While analyzing growth restriction the curves might even change management.

Intrauterine Growth Restriction

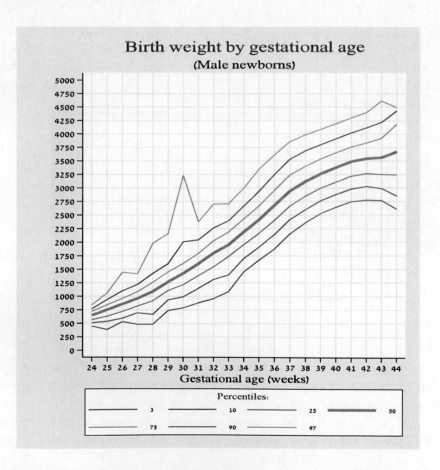

Figure 3. Birth weight by gestational age in male newborns.

Looking at the other side of the birth weight spectrum, i.e, the intrauterine growth-restricted fetuses (i.e., estimated fetal weight of <5 percentile for gestational age), Spinillo et al. found that fetal gender can affect the magnitude of the classic risk factors for fetal growth restriction. Although fetal growth restriction is more frequent in female than male fetuses, a low (< 50 kg) maternal pre-pregnancy weight and a low maternal (< 18) body mass index (BMI; kg/m2) were significant risk factors for fetal growth restriction in male fetuses. Even though maternal smoking in pregnancy was a significant risk factor for growth restriction in both male and female fetuses, its effect was significantly stronger for male fetuses [59].

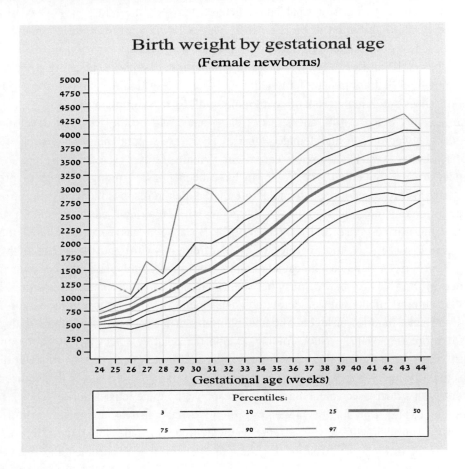

Figure 4. Birth weight by gestational age in female newborns.

Fetal Distress during Labor

As mentioned before, an increase in cesarean sections due to fetal distress is higher among women carrying male fetuses than female fetuses. Moreover, male infants delivered by cesarean section for fetal distress also have lower Apgar scores than female fetuses delivered by cesarean section for the same indication [50]. At 1 minute, 45.7% of male infants had an Apgar score of <7 compared with 15% of female infants (risk ratio 3.1, 95% CI 1.0 to 9.2). At 5 minutes, 17.1% of males compared with 5% of female infants continued to have an Apgar score of <7. The association at 5 minutes was not statistically significant (risk ratio of 3.4, 95% CI 0.4–26.5) but this could be the result of small numbers of infants with low Apgar scores at 5 minutes. Several studies have found abnormal fetal heart rate patterns to be more common among male fetuses [60-62]. In a prospective study analyzing the significance of abnormal fetal heart rate patterns during the second stage of labor, male gender was found to be an independent risk factor affecting the occurrence of abnormal second-stage fetal heart rate patterns (OR 1.5; 95% CI 1.01–2.2) [60]. Although Oguch et al. found that fetal sex does not affect fetal heart rate and heart rate variation [63], others reported that the response to normal labor differed between the sexes [61]. They observed differences in the distribution of baseline fetal heart rate, in short term variation [52] and in the occurrence of decelerations in traces during labor and delivery between male and female fetuses. These differences were not present antepartum, thereby suggesting an increased incidence of fetal distress in male fetuses during labor. These findings support the conclusion that male fetuses are at higher risk of developing fetal distress during labor.

The reason for these differences is not clear but could be the result of developmental differences between male and female fetuses. There are animal data suggesting that the sympatho-adrenal system develops earlier in female fetuses [64,65]. In humans, sex differences in catecholamine levels at birth have been noted. Among a group of pre-term fetuses, females produced more catecholamine than males in response to asphyxia [66]. It has also been demonstrated in a number of species that the fetal adrenal gland produces catecholamines in response to hypoxia [67-69]. Because it has been postulated that this catecholamine surge may improve the ability of a fetus to withstand the effects of hypoxia [70,71], such sex differences in catecholamine response could plausibly be related to a difference in the rates of fetal distress between male and female fetuses. In addition, it was found that among infants with moderate acidosis (mean pH 7.16), those infants with Apgar scores less than 7 had lower levels of catecholamines at birth than those infants with Apgar scores of more than 7 [72]. Such findings support a positive effect of catecholamines on newborn status. The finding that male infants delivered by cesarean section for fetal distress more frequently had lower Apgar scores than female infants delivered for that indication is consistent with a decreased catecholaminergic response by male fetuses during labor.

Another explanation for the higher rate of male fetal distress compared to the female fetus can be found in differences in energy metabolism in male and female fetuses [73]. Growth rate is influenced, possibly, by the presence of the Y chromosome because the growth rate of blastocysts and embryos is higher in XY than in XX chromosome bearers, which suggests a higher metabolic rate in male fetuses. At the same time, there are arguments to suggest an inverse relationship between life span and metabolic rate [74]. Therefore, an increased metabolic rate might cause increased vulnerability of the male fetus during critical stages of development.

Cord Problems and Male Gender

The association between true umbilical cord knots and male gender has been documented previously. There is a statistically significant correlation between male fetuses and true umbilical cord knot [75,76]. Hershkovitz et al. [75] found male predominance in the incidence of true knot of cord; 64% of the true knot of cord group were male fetuses compared to 38.6% female fetuses (p<0.001). The significant association that is seen between male gender and cord problems may be partially explained by longer cords in males. This could result in higher rates of prolapse, as true umbilical cord knots and nuchal cords are factors occurring more frequently in association with longer cords. Abnormal fetal heart rate patterns and specifically variable decelerations may also be more common when there are cord entanglements [60]. Unfortunately, there is little information in the literature regarding the length of the umbilical cords and differences between the two sexes. Further studies should investigate umbilical cord length differences between male and female fetuses.

Conclusion

This chapter shows that gender does matter: Male sex is an independent risk factor for adverse pregnancy outcome. This observation, however, should not lead to an alteration of the obstetric management of patients simply based on the gender of the fetus. Even though the absolute value of these studies is more academic than clinical, these findings certainly confirm higher rates of adverse pregnancy outcomes with male fetuses. It seems that there is something beyond the weight itself and the other associated risk factors that should explain the gender differences that have been described. The impact of fetal gender on birth outcome remains unclear. Further research is needed to clarify the effect of gender differences on birth outcomes. What this chapter does show is that when we say "it must be a boy" as a humorous explanation of complications of labor and delivery, we are scientifically more correct than previously supposed.

References

[1]   Sheiner E. The relationship between fetal gender and pregnancy outcome. *Arch Gynecol Obstet* 2007;275:317-9.

[2]   Di Renzo C, Rosati A, Sarti R, Cruciani L, Cutuli A: Does fetal sex affect pregnancy outcome? *Gender Medicine* 2007;4(1):19-30.

[3]   Munne S, Tang YX, Weier HUG, Stein J, Finklestein M, Grifo J. Sex distribution in arrested precompacted human embryos. *Zygote* 1993;1: 155-62.

[4]   Van der Pal-de Bruin KM, Vefloove-Vanhorick SP, Roeleveld N: Change in male: female ratio among newborn babies in Netherlands. *Lancet* 1997;349:62.

[5]   Maconochie N, Roman E: Sex ratios: Are there natural variations within the human population? *Br J Obstet Gynaecol* 1997;104: 1050-1053.

[6]   Quddus S: Fetal gender determination and the male:female population ratio in Bangladesh. *R Soc Health* 2005;125:93-94.

[7]   Jongbloet PH: Fetal sex and very preterm birth. *Am J Obstet Gynecol* 2005;193:302.

[8] Hesketh T, Xing ZW: Abnormal sex ratios in human populations: Causes and consequences. *Proc Natl Acad Sci U S A* 2006;103:13271-13275.

[9] Wallner B, Huber S, Mitterauer L, Pavlova B, Fieder M: Academic mothers have a pronounced seasonal variation in their offspring sex ratio. *Neuro Endocrinol Lett* 2005;26:759-762.

[10] Chacon-Puignau GC, Jaffe K. Sex ratio at birth deviations in modem Venezuela: The Trivers-Willard effect. *Soc Biol* 1996;43:257-270.

[11] Kovaleva NV: Sex-specific chromosome instability in early human development. *Am J Med Genet A* 2005;136:401-413.

[12] Larsen SO, Wojdemann KR, Shalmi AC, Sundberg K, Christiansen M, Tabor A: Gender impact on first trimester marker in Down syndrome screening. *Prenat Diagn* 2002;22:1207-1208.

[13] Gol M, Tuna B, Dogan E, Gulekli B, Bagci M, Altunyurt S, Saygili U: Does fetal gender affect cytotrophoblast cell activity in the human term placenta? Correlation with maternal hCG levels. *Acta Obstet Gynecol Scand* 2004;83:711-715.

[14] Bazzett LB, Yaron Y, O'Brien JE, Critchfield G, Kramer RL, Ayoub M, Johnson MP, Evans MI: Fetal gender impact on multiple-marker screening results. *Am J Med Genet* 1998;76:369-371.

[15] Drugan A, Weissman A, Avrahami R, Zamir R, Evans MI: Sonographic nuchal markers for Down syndrome are more common but less ominous in gestations with a male fetus. *Fetal Diagn Ther* 2002;17:295- 297.

[16] Wax JR, Cartin A, Pinette MG, Blackstone J: Does the frequency of soft sonographic aneuploidy markers vary by fetal sex? *J Ultrasound Med* 2005; 24:1059-1063.

[17] Chudleigh PM, Chitty LS, Pembrey M, Campbell S: The association of aneuploidy and mild fetal pyelectasis in an unselected population: the results of a multicenter study. *Ultrasound Obstet Gynecol* 2001;17:197–202.

[18] Nicolaides KH, Cheng HH, Abbas A, Snijders RJ, Gosden C: Fetal renal defects: associated malformations and chromosomal defects. *Fetal Diagn Ther* 1992;7:1–11

[19] Bornstein E, Barnhard Y, Donnenfeld A, Ferber A, Divon MY: Fetal pyelectasis: Does fetal gender modify the risk of major trisomies? *Obstet Gynecol* 2006;107: *877-879.*

[20] Del Mar Melero-Montes M, Jick H. Hyperemesis gravidarum and the sex of the offspring. *Epidemiology* 2000;12:123-124.

[21] Kankova S, Sulc J, Nouzova K, Fajfrlík K, Frynta D, Flegr J: Women infected with parasite Toxoplasma have more sons. *Naturwissenschaflen* 2007;94:122-12.

[22] Picone O, Costa JM, Dejean A, Ville Y: Is fetal gender a risk factor for severe congenital cytomegalovirus infection? *Prenat Diagn* 2005;25:34-38.

[23] Taha TE, Nour S, Kumwenda NI, Broadhead RL, Fiscus SA, Kafulafula G, Nkhoma C, Chen S, Hoover DR: Gender differences in perinatal HIV acquisition among African infants. *Pediatrics* 2005; 115:167-172.

[24] Demissie K, Breckenridge MB, Joseph L, Rhoads GG. Placenta previa: Preponderance of male sex at birth. *Am J Epidemiol* 1999;149:824-830.

[25] Sheiner E, Shoham-Vardi I, Hallak M, Hershkowitz R, Katz M, Mazor M.: Placenta previa: obstetric risk factors and pregnancy outcome. *J Matern Fetal Med* 2001;10:414-9.

[26] Naeye RL, Demers LM: Differing effects of fetal sex on pregnancy and its outcome. *Am J Med Genet Suppl* 1987; 3:67- 74.

[27] Bracero LA, Cassidy S, Byrne DW: Effect of gender on perinatal outcome in pregnancies complicated by diabetes. *Gynecol Obstet Invest* 1996;41:10- 14.

[28] McGregor JA, Leff M, Orleans M, Baron A: Fetal gender differences in preterm birth: Findings in a North American cohort. *Am J Perinatol* 1992;9: 43-48.

[29] Burstein E, Sheiner E, Mazor M, Carmel E, Levy A, Hershkovitz R: Identifying risk factors for premature rupture of membranes in small for gestational age neonates: A population-based study. *J Matern Fetal Neonatal Med* 2008; (in press).

[30] Ingemarsson I: Gender aspects of preterm birth. *BJOG* 2003;110(Suppl 20):34-38.

[31] Cooperstock M, Campbell J: Excess males in preterm birth: Interactions with gestational age, race, and multiple birth. *Obstet Gynecol* 1996;88: 189-193.

[32] Zeitlin J, Ancel PY, Larroque B, Kaminski M, for the EPIPAGE Study. Fetal sex and indicated very preterm birth: Results of the EPIPAGE study. *Am J Obstet Gynecol* 2004;190:1322-1325.

[33] Ghidini A, Salafia CM. Gender differences of placental dysfunction in severe prematurity. *BJOG* 2005; 112:140 144.

[34] Vergani P, Ghidini A, Locatelli A, Cavallone M, Ciarla I, Cappellini A, Lapinski RH: Risk factors for pulmonary hypoplasia in secondtrimester premature rupture of membranes. *Am J Obstet Gynecol* 1994;170:1359-1364.

[35] Luo YM, Fang Q, Zhuang GL, Liang RC, Chen YZ, Chen ML: Perinatal outcome of discordant twin pregnancies. *Zhonghua Fu Chart Ke Za Zhi* 2005;40:449-452.

[36] Notes J, Athanassiou A, Elkadry E, Malone FD, Craigo SD, D'Alton ME: Gender differences in twin-twin transfusion syndrome. *Obstet Gynecol* 1997;90:580-582.

[37] Hsieh YY, Chang PC, Tsai HD: Gender prevalence in twin-twin transfusion syndrome. *Chang Gung Med* J 2000;23:476-479.

[38] Derom R, Derom C, Loos RJ, Thiery E, Vlietinck R, Fryns JP: Gender mix: Does it modify birthweight-outcome association? *Paediatr Perinat Epidemiol* 2005;19(Suppl 1): 37-40.

[39] Divon MY, Ferber A, Nisell H, Westgren M: Male gender predisposes to prolongation of pregnancy. *Am J Obstet Gynecol* 2002;187:1081-1083.

[40] Rabe T, Hosch R, Runnebaum B: Sulfatase deficiency in the human placenta: Clinical findings. *Biol Res Pregnancy Perinatol* 1983;4:95-102.

[41] Davis RO, Cutter GR, Goldenberg RL, Hoffman HJ, Cliver SP, Brumfield CG: Fetal biparietal diameter, head circumference, abdominal circumference and femur length. A comparison by race and sex. *J Reprod Med* 1993;38:201- 206.

[42] Kitlinski LM, Kallen K, Marsal K, Olofsson P: Skewed fetal gender distribution inn prolonged pregnancy: A fallacy with consequences. *Ultrasound Obstet Gynecol* 2003;21:262-266.

[43] Jakobovits AA: Sex ratio of spontaneously aborted fetuses and delivered neonates in the second trimester: *Eur J Obstet Gynecol Reprod Biol* 1991;40:211-3.

[44] Hassold T, Quillen SD, Yamane JA: Sex ratio in spontaneous abortions. *Ann Hum Genet* 1983;47: 39-47.

[45] Sheiner E, Levy A, Katz M, Hershkovitz R, Leron E, Mazor M.: Gender Does Matter in Perinatal Medicine. *Fetal Diagn Ther* 2004;19 :366–369.

[46] Ingemarsson I, Amer Wahlin I, Liedman R: Cord arterial blood glucose levels. *Am J Obstet Gynecol* 1997; 176:S 164.

[47] Sami S, Baloch SN: Perinatal mortality rate in relation to gender. *J Coll Physicians Surg Pak* 2004; 14:545-548.

[48] Nwosu EC, Kumar B, El-Sayed M, Hollis S: Is fetal gender significant in the perinatal outcome of pregnancies complicated by placental abruption? *J Obstet Gynaecol* 1999;19:612-614.

[49] Bekedam DJ, Engelsbel S, Mol BW, Buitendijk SE, van der Pal-de Bruin KM.: Male predominance in fetal distress during labor. *Am J Obstet Gynecol* 2002; 187:1605 7.

[50] Lieberman E, Lang JM, Cohen AP, Frigoletto FD Jr, Acker D, Rao R: The association of fetal sex with the rate of cesarean section. *Am J Obstet Gynecol* 1997; 176: 667-71.

[51] Hindmarsh PC, Geary MP, Rodeck CH, Kingdom JC, Cole TJ: Intrauterine growth and its relationship to size and shape at birth. *Pediatr Res* 2002; 52:263-8.

[52] Maeve A Eogan, Michael P Geary, Michael P O'Connell, Declan P Keane: Effect of fetal sex on labour and delivery: retrospective review. *BMJ* 2003 volume 326.

[53] Mocanu EV, Greene RA, Byrne BM, Turner MJ: Obstetric and neonatal outcome of babies weighing more than 4.5 kg: An analysis by parity. *Eur J Obstet Gynecol Reprod Biol* 2000; 92: 229– 233.

[54] Sheiner E, Shoham-Vardi I, Silberstein T, Katz M, Mazor M: Failed vacuum extraction: Maternal risk factors and pregnancy outcome. *J Reprod Med* 2001;46: 819–824.

[55] Langer O, Berkus MD, Huff RW, Samueloff A: Shoulder dystocia: Should the fetus weighing greater than or equal to 4,000 grams be delivered by cesarean section? *Am J Obstet Gynecol* 1991;165: 831–837.

[56] Ginsberg NA, Moisidis C: How to predict shoulder dystocia. *Am J Obstet Gynecol* 2001; 184:1427– 1430.

[57] Christoffersson M, Rydhstroem H: Shoulder dystocia and brachial plexus injury: A population- based study. *Gynecol Obstet Invest* 2002; 53:42–47.

[58] McFarland M, Hod M, Piper JM, Xenakis EMJ, Langer O: Are labor abnormalities more common in shoulder dystocia? *Am J Obstet Gynecol* 1995;173: 1211–1214.

[59] Spinillo A, Capuzzo E, Nicola S, Colonna L, Iasci A, Zara C: Interaction between fetal gender and risk factors for fetal growth retardation. *Am J Obstet Gynecol* 1994;171:1273-7.

[60] Sheiner E, Hadar A, Hallak M, Katz M, Mazor M, Shoham-Vardi I: Clinical significance of fetal heart rate tracings during the second stage of labor. *Obstet Gynecol* 2001;97:747–752.

[61] Dawes NW, Dawes GS, Moulden M, Redman CWG: Fetal heart rate patterns in term labor vary with sex, gestational age, epidural analgesia, and fetal weight. *Am J Obstet Gynecol* 1999;180:181–187.

[62] Bekedam DJ, Engelsbel S, Mol BW, Buitendijk SE, van der Pal-de Bruin KM: Male predominance in fetal distress during labor. *Am J Obstet Gynecol* 2002;187:1605–1607.

[63] Oguch O, Steer P: Gender does not affect fetal heart rate variation. *Br J Obstet Gynaecol* 1998;105:1312–1314.

[64] PadburyJF, Hobel CJ, Lam RW, Fisher DA: Sex differences in lung and adrenal neurosympathetic development in rabbits. *Am J Obstet Gynecol* 1981;141:199-204.

[65] PadburyJF, Hobel CJ, Gonzalez FA, Fisher DA: Ontogenesis and sex differences in rabbit fetal adrenal phenylethanolamine N-methyltransferase. *Biol Neonate* 1983;43:205-10.

[66] Greenough A, Lagercrantz H, Pool J, Dahlin I: Plasma catecholamine levels in preterm infants. *Acta Paediatr Scand* 1987;76:54-9.

[67] Cohen WR, Piasecki GJ, Jackson BT: Plasma catecholamines during hypoxemia in fetal lamb. *Am Physiol Soc* 1982;243: 520-5.

[68] Cohen WR, Piasecki GJ, Cohn HE, Young JB, Jackson BT: Adrenal secretion of catecholamines during hypoxemia in fetal lambs. *Endocrinology* 1984;114:383-90.

[69] Comline RS, Silver M: Development of activity in the adrenal medulla of the foetus and new-born animal. *Br Med Bull* 1966;22:16-20.

[70] Lagercrantz H, Slotkin TA: The "stress" of being born. *Sci Am* 1986;254:100-7.

[71] Nylund L, Dahlin I, Lagercrantz H: Fetal catecholamines and the Apgar score. *J Perinat Med* 1987;15:340-4.

[72] Lagercrantz H: Asphyxia and the Apgar score [letter]. *Lancet* 1982;966.

[73] Clarke C, Mittwoch U.: Changes in the male to female ratio at different stages of live. *Br J Obstet Gynaecol* 1995;102:677-9

[74] Lynn CS, Wallwork C: Does food restriction retard aging by reducing metabolic rate? *J Nutr* 1992;122:1917-8.

[75] Hershkovitz R, Silberstein T, Shcincr E, Shoham- Vardi I, Holcberg G, Katz M, Mazor M: Risk factors associated with true knots of the umbilical cord. *Eur J Obstet Gynecol Reprod Biol* 2001;98:36–39.

[76] Blickstein I, Shoham-Schwartz Z, Lancet M: Predisposing factors in the formation of true knots of the umbilical cord – analysis of morphometric and perinatal data. *Int J Gynecol Obstet* 1987;25:395–398.

Peripartum Complications

In: Textbook of Perinatal Epidemiology
Editor: Eyal Sheiner, pp. 543-592

ISBN: 978-1-60741-648-7
© 2010 Nova Science Publishers, Inc.

Chapter XXVI

The Epidemiology of Preterm Birth

Offer Erez[*1], *Idit Erez-Weiss*[2], *Edi Vaisbuch*[3] *and Moshe Mazor*[1]

Department of Obstetrics and Gynecology, Soroka University Medical Center,
School of Medicine, Faculty of Health Sciences, Ben Gurion University of the Negev,
Beer Sheva, Israel[1]
Department of Family Medicine, School of Medicine, Faculty of Health Sciences,
Ben Gurion University of the Negev, Beer Sheva, Israel[2]
Department of Obstetrics and Gynecology, Kaplan Medical Center, School of Medicine,
Hebrew University, Jerusalem, Israel[3]

Introduction

Preterm delivery is the leading cause of perinatal morbidity and mortality worldwide [1]. The annual societal economic burden associated with preterm birth in the United States exceeded $26.2 billion in 2005 [1]. Preterm parturition is associated with short-and long-term maternal and fetal sequella. The mothers are at risk of recurrent preterm birth and cardiovascular disease later in life [2,3]. The premature newborn is at risk for acute (i.e., respiratory distress syndrome, necrotizing enterocolitis, and intraventricular hemorrhage) and chronic illness (i.e., retinopathy of prematurity, cerebral palsy, broncho pulmonary dysplasia), as well as social and behavioral maladjustment later in life [4].

1. Definition

Preterm birth is a delivery between fetal viability and 37 completed weeks of gestation [5]. While the upper cutoff of 37 weeks according to menstrual age is well accepted [6,7],

* For Correspondence: Offer Erez, MD. Department of Obstetrics and Gynecology, Soroka University Medical Center, School of Medicine, Faculty of Health SciencesE-mail: oerez@med.wayne.edu

there is a debate regarding the lower cutoff which is currently defined as the limit of viability, a point at which the risk for neonatal death does not exceed 50%. According to this definition the cutoff should be set at 24 weeks of gestation and/or birth weight of ≥500g, regardless of ethnicity or race.

2. Prevalence

The prevalence of preterm birth varies from 6% to 15% of all deliveries depending on the geographical and demographical characteristics of the population tested [6-8]. In Europe, the rate of preterm deliveries varies from 5% to 9% [8], while the rate of preterm birth in the United States reached 12.8% by 2006 [7], 20% higher than in 1990. While the rate of early (<34 weeks) preterm birth remained relatively constant (2.9% among singleton and 3.3% to 3.6% among multiple gestations), the rate of late preterm birth (34–37 weeks) increased among singleton births by 19.1% (from 6.1% to 8.1%) and by 24.7% among all pluralities from 1990 to 2005 (Figure 1) [9]. Moreover, the increased incidence of "indicated" preterm births of singleton and multiple gestations, as well as the rise in the rate of older parturients, were additional contributors to the increasing preterm delivery rate [10]. It is noteworthy that within the United States the proportion of preterm deliveries varies among different states, from 6.2% in Vermont up to 12.6% in Alabama [11].

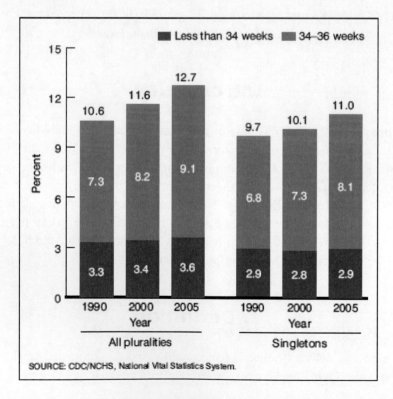

Figure 1. The rate of early (<34 weeks of gestation) and late (34–36 weeks) preterm birth in the USA between the years 1990, 2000, 2005. According to the CDC Birth: final data 2005 [9] with permission.

3.0 Subtypes of Preterm Births

Preterm delivery is classified by gestational age at delivery and the type of preterm birth:

3.0.1 Classification by Gestational Age at Delivery

The gestational age at which preterm delivery occurs has a direct effect on neonatal morbidity and mortality. Several cutoffs have been proposed to differentiate early from late preterm birth. The most commonly used cutoffs are 32 or 34 weeks of gestation. The Centers for Disease Control and Prevention (CDC) has defined 34 weeks of gestation to distinguish between early and late preterm delivery [7,9]. However, the survival rate of neonates born after 32 weeks of gestation is nearly 100%, and neonatal morbidity substantially declines at this gestational age [12]. Thus, the use of 32 weeks of gestation as the cutoff for early preterm birth has been proposed [8]. Although this cutoff may seem appealing, not all countries have well-developed neonatal intensive care units, and their survival rate at 32 weeks of gestation is lower. Hence, the CDC approach to the definition of early preterm birth as a delivery before 34 weeks may serve as a better cutoff for clinical and comparative epidemiological studies.

Alternatively, preterm delivery can be defined by the severity of prematurity: (1) extreme prematurity—a delivery before 28 weeks of gestation that accounts for 5% of preterm deliveries; (2) severe prematurity—delivery from 28 to $31^6/_7$ weeks, accounting for 15% of all preterm deliveries; (3) moderate prematurity—delivery between 32 to $33^6/_7$ weeks of gestation, occurring in about 20% of preterm births; and (4) near term—birth that occurs from 34 to $36^6/_7$ weeks of gestation, comprising the largest group at 60–70% of all preterm deliveries [1].

3.0.2 Classification by Type—Spontaneous Vs. Indicated Preterm Birth

Preterm delivery can be either spontaneous or medically induced (indicated) regardless of the gestational age at delivery. Spontaneous preterm birth accounts for 75% of all preterm deliveries [13-15] and can be the end result of three main clinical presentations: (1) preterm labor with intact membranes, (2) preterm prelabor rupture of membranes (preterm PROM), and (3) cervical insufficiency [16]. Indicated preterm birth results from medical intervention due to maternal or fetal complications that necessitate medical intervention [5,14,17-19]. Although many studies have focused on the rate of preterm birth [20-22], an important consideration is whether these deliveries are the result of spontaneous labor or "indicated" preterm deliveries. The need for this distinction is based on the premise that the risk factors for recurrent preterm PROM, preterm labor with intact membranes, preeclampsia, and/or SGA are different. However, recent observations suggest that these conditions may overlap [17,19], so that a patient with an "indicated" preterm birth may also be at risk for spontaneous preterm birth [17,19]. The converse may also be true (i.e., that a patient with a spontaneous preterm birth is at risk for an "indicated" preterm birth in a subsequent pregnancy).

3.1 Spontaneous Preterm Birth

Spontaneous Preterm Birth is defined as a labor that begins without prior medical intervention and can present either as a preterm contraction with intact, ruptur of the chorioamniotic membranes, or related diagnoses such as incompetent cervix that leads to preterm delivery. Preterm labor, preterm prelabor ruptured membranes, and cervical insufficiency are all obstetrical syndromes [23-26]. Each of these pathologies can be derived from several underlying mechanisms including infection, thrombosis, hormonal, autoimmunity, allergy and others [23-26].

The risk factors for spontaneous preterm birth change according to gestational age at delivery and parity. Previous preterm birth, vaginal bleeding during the first or second trimester, positive fetal fibronectin test, and cervical length < 25 mm are risk factors for preterm birth before 37, 35 and 32 weeks of gestation [27-29]. Bacterial vaginosis and maternal body mass index (BMI) <19.8 kg/m^2 are associated with an increased risk for preterm birth before 32 weeks of gestation, while African-American ethnicity is a risk factor for preterm delivery before 37 weeks of gestation. When the risk is stratified according to parity a low BMI (<19.8) and an increased Bishop score were significantly associated with spontaneous preterm delivery in nulliparous and multiparous women. Black race, poor social environment, and working during pregnancy were associated with increased risk for nulliparous women. However, among multiparous patients a prior preterm birth overshadows the socioeconomic risk factors and is associated with a twofold increase in the odds of spontaneous preterm delivery for each prior spontaneous preterm birth. Finally, multiple gestations are an independent risk factor for preterm birth regardless to gestational age at delivery or parity [27-29].

3.1.1 Preterm Labor with Intact Membranes

Preterm labor with intact membranes is defined as uterine contractions before 37 completed weeks of gestation that lead to cervical effacement and/or dilatation without rupture of the membranes [24]. Preterm labor with intact membranes accounts for 40–45% of all preterm deliveries [1]. Regarding singleton gestation in the US, the rate of spontaneous preterm labor declined between the years 1989 to 2000 by 6.5%, from 6.1% in 1989 to 5.7% in 2000. However, when these changes were studied according to ethnic origin, the rate of spontaneous preterm labor leading to preterm birth increased by 2% in Caucasian (from 4.9% in 1989 to 5.0% in 2000) and decreased by 24.8% in African-Americans (from 12.1% in 1989 to 9.1% in 2000) [30].

3.1.2 Preterm PROM

Preterm PROM is defined as a spontaneous rupture of the chorioamniotic membranes before 37 completed weeks of gestation without labor, and it accounts for 25% of all preterm deliveries. Among singleton gestation in the USA, the rate of preterm PROM declined between the years 1989 to 2000 by 30.8%, from 1.3% in 1989 to 0.9% in 2000. The rate of preterm PROM has declined in both Caucasians (a 27.2% decrease from 1.1% in 1989 to

0.8% in 2000) and African-Americans (a 34.8% decrease from 2.3% in 1989 to 1.5% in 2000) [30]. The three factors that were prominently associated with preterm PROM include the following: (1) a previous preterm delivery [31;32]; (2) a history of vaginal bleeding during the index pregnancy [31-33]; and (3) cigarette smoking [32,33]. Mercer et al. [34] differentiated the risk factors for preterm PROM before 35 weeks of gestation according to parity. Cervical length≤ 25 mm was an independent risk factor in nulliparous (OR 9.9, 95% CI 3.8–25.9) as well as in multiparous (OR 4.2, 95% CI 2.0–8.9) women [34]. Independent risk factors for preterm PROM among nulliparous patients included working during pregnancy and medical complications, while the independent risk factors for this syndrome among multiparous patients were previous preterm PROM, spontaneous preterm delivery with intact membranes, positive fetal fibronectin in the absence of bacterial vaginosis, and the presence of bacterial vaginosis with a negative fetal fibronectin test [34].

3.2 Indicated Preterm Deliveries

Indicated preterm birth, are preterm deliveries in which the medical team has decided to deliver the patient before term as a result of maternal or fetal indications. Indicated preterm births account for about 30–35% of all preterm births [1]. In the US, from 1989 to 2000, there was a 46% increase in the rate of indicated preterm births (from 2.6% in 1989 to 3.8% in 2000). During this period the rate of indicated preterm deliveries increased by 56.5% in Caucasians and by 36.6% in African-Americans (Figure 2) [19, 30].

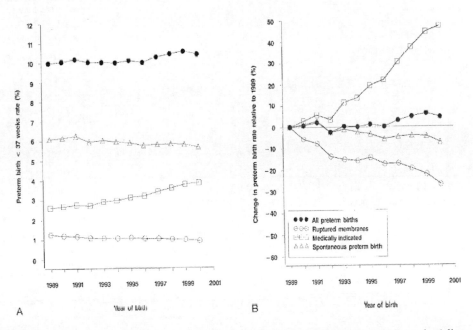

Figure 2. Rates (A) and relative temporal changes since 1989 (B) of preterm birth <37 weeks (all races), as well as those resulting from ruptured membranes, medically indicated, and spontaneous preterm birth: United States, 1989 through 2000. Adopted from Ananth et al. [30] with permission.

The most common diagnoses that precede an indicated preterm birth are pre-eclampsia (40%), fetal distress (25%) intrauterine growth restriction (10%), placental abruption (7%), and fetal demise (7%) [15]. Illicit drug use in pregnancy, especially cocaine ingestion, has been associated with indicated preterm birth (Table I) [35].

Ananth et al. [30] calculated that from 1989 to 2000, the perinatal mortality rate among preterm birth <37 weeks of gestation in Caucasians decreased by 29%. However, the authors reported that after stratification according to the type of preterm delivery, if indicated preterm births were not included, the decrease in the perinatal mortality rate was only 21%. Thus, the increase in the rate of indicated preterm deliveries was associated with a reduction in the rate of perinatal death. Of note, among African-Americans the major contributors to the reduction in perinatal mortality rate were the reduction in the rate of spontaneous preterm labor and preterm PROM and not the increase in the rate of indicated preterm deliveries [30].

Table I. Distribution of preeclampsia, SGA, fetal distress and abruption among medically indicated preterm birth at <35 weeks and among term/near-term birth*.

Maternal-fetal conditions	Rate among term/near term birth at ≥35 weeks (%)	Medically indicated preterm birth at <35 weeks	
		Rate (%)	Adjusted RR(95% CI)
Preeclampsia only	2.9	10.4	6.4 (5.9,7.0)
Preeclampsia + SGA	0.6	5.6	16.8 (15.1,18.7)
Preeclampsia + fetal distress	0.3	3.1	20.6 (17.8,23.8)
Preeclampsia + SGA+ fetal distress	0.1	2.6	44.5 (37.7,52.6)
Preeclampsia + abruption	0.02	0.8	63.1 (45.8,86.8)
Preeclampsia + SGA+ abruption	0.02	0.5	38.2 (23.2,62.9)
Preeclampsia + fetal distress+ abruption	0.01	0.3	83.9 (49.9,141.0)
Preeclampsia + SGA+ fetal distress+ abruption	0.01	0.2	58.6 (30.2,113.8)
Fetal distress only	4.6	11.4	4.2 (3.8,4.5)
Fetal distress + SGA	0.9	3.3	5.5 (4.8,6.3)
Fetal distress + abruption	0.1	1.6	32.0 (26.1,39.3)
Fetal distress + SGA + abruption	0.02	0.5	29.0 (20.1,42.0)
SGA only	7.9	5.0	0.9 (0.8,1.0)
SGA + abruption	0.1	1.4	21.5 (17.3,26.8)
Placental abruption only	0.3	6.8	37.6 (33.8,41.8)

CI, confidence interval; SGA, small for gestational age. Relative risks (RR) are adjusted for the confounding effect of period of birth, maternal age, parity, maternal race/ethnicity, marital status, maternal education, smoking and alcohol use during pregnancy, and pre-pregnancy body mass index. *The data shown in this table are reproduced (with modification) from Ananth and Vintzileos with the permission of the publisher (Reference 19).

4. Risk Factors for Preterm Birth

Identification of patients at risk for preterm delivery has a major role in the primary and secondary prevention of preterm birth. Since preterm delivery is a syndrome that results from several underlying mechanisms, there is no single diagnostic test that will enable the clinician to identify patients at risk for preterm delivery. Thus, the current risk assessment for preterm birth is based upon clinical risk factors.

4.1 Obstetric History

A previous preterm birth is an independent risk factor for a subsequent preterm delivery before 32, 35 and 37 weeks of gestation [28]. Indeed, preterm births tend to reoccur, and women with a previous preterm delivery have a higher chance to deliver preterm than women with a previous term delivery. All types of preterm births are associated with an increased risk of preterm delivery in subsequent pregnancies [5,17]. Moreover, patients with indicated preterm delivery are at increased risk for spontaneous as well as indicated preterm delivery in a subsequent pregnancy. [5,12,14,15,17,29].

4.1.1 The Effect of Previous Pregnancy Outcome on Recurrent Preterm Delivery with Intact Membranes

Medicine network (NICHD MFMU) reported that the rate of spontaneous preterm birth (<35 weeks) was 13–15% in patients with a prior history of preterm delivery or late abortion, and only 3% in patients who previously delivered at term [36]. Similarly, Mercer et al. [29] reported that the rate of spontaneous preterm birth (<37 weeks) was 21.7% in patients with a prior preterm delivery and 8.8% among those with a previous term delivery. Thus, a prior preterm delivery conferred a 2.5-fold risk for a subsequent preterm birth.

Gestational age at delivery of a previous preterm birth affects the likelihood of preterm delivery in subsequent pregnancies [28,29]. A spontaneous preterm birth between 23–27 weeks of gestation is associated with an odds ratio of 22.1 for a recurrent preterm delivery <28 weeks of gestation in comparison to women without a prior preterm birth [17] (Table II).

The highest rate of recurrent preterm birth (65%) was among patients with a prior preterm delivery who had a sonographicaly short cervix (<25 mm) and a positive fetal fibronectin test at mid trimester [29] of the index pregnancy, while the rate of recurrent preterm delivery among patients with a cervical length >35 mm and a negative fetal fibronectin test was only 7% [29].

4.1.2 The Effect of Previous Pregnancy Outcome on Recurrent Preterm Delivery in Patients with Preterm PROM

Preterm delivery after preterm PROM is a risk factor for subsequent preterm PROM and delivery. Indeed, a study conducted by the NICHD MFMU [34] reported that preterm PROM in a previous pregnancy was independently associated with a recurrent preterm delivery due to preterm PROM (<37 weeks: odds ratio [OR] 3.1, 95% CI 18–5.4; <35 weeks: OR 4.1, 95% CI 2.–8.7). In addition, patients with a previous preterm delivery after preterm labor with intact membrane were also at risk for preterm delivery due to preterm PROM in a subsequent pregnancy (<37 weeks: OR 1.8, 95% CI 1.1–3.1; <35 weeks: OR 2.6, 95% CI 1.2–5.3). Multiparous patients with a previous preterm PROM, a mid trimester ultrasonographic short cervix (<25 mm), and a positive fetal fibronectin test had a 7.8-fold increased risk for preterm PROM<37 weeks and a 31.3-fold increased risk for preterm PROM <35 weeks of gestation in comparison with those who had none of these risk factors [34].

Table II. Recurrence of preterm birth based on timing and clinical subtypes in the second pregnancy in relation to severity and clinical subtypes of previous preterm birth: Missouri, 1989–1997*

First pregnancy	Adjusted odds ratio (95% confidence interval) for preterm birth in the second pregnancy							
	<28 weeks		28-31 weeks		32-33 weeks		34-36 weeks	
	Spont.	Med.	Spont.	Med.	Spont.	Med.	Spont.	Med.
<28 weeks								
Spont.	13.2 (8.8, 19.8)	12.6 (7.0, 22.7)	6.0 (3.9, 9.2)	6.4 (3.6, 11.3)	3.2 (1.9, 5.3)	3.4 (1.6, 7.3)	3.1 (2.4, 3.9)	2.1 (1.3, 3.4)
Med.	10.4 (5.0, 21.7)	22.7 (11.3, 46.0)	3.6 (1.4, 8.8)	19.9 (11.5, 34.3)	1.6 (0.5, 5.1)	14.1 (7.5, 26.3)	1.2 (0.7, 2.1)	14.4 (10.5, 19.8)
28-31 weeks								
Spont.	4.5 (2.8, 7.2)	5.1 (3.6, 7.2)	6.1 (3.3, 11.5)	3.0 (1.6, 5.7)	3.8 (2.7, 5.4)	2.1 (1.0, 4.4)	2.9 (2.4, 3.5)	2.1 (1.4, 3.1)
Med.	1.3 (0.3, 5.1)	14.7 (7.8, 27.6)	3.4 (1.7, 6.7)	15.3 (9.8, 24.0)	1.7 (0.7, 3.8)	12.8 (7.8, 20.9)	0.9 (0.6, 1.4)	9.6 (7.4, 12.6)
32-33 weeks								
Spont.	4.8 (3.1, 7.4)	2.3 (1.0, 5.8)	5.8 (4.2, 8.0)	2.7 (1.5, 5.0)	5.9 (4.6, 7.2)	2.6 (1.4, 4.8)	3.0 (2.5, 3.5)	1.7 (1.2, 2.4)
Med.	0.7 (0.1, 5.2)	12.5 (6.3, 24.8)	1.7 (0.6, 4.5)	8.2 (4.5, 14.7)	0.9 (0.3, 2.8)	11.9 (7.3, 19.3)	1.1 (0.7, 1.7)	10.2 (7.9, 13.1)
34-36 weeks								
Spont.	2.1 (1.6, 2.8)	1.4 (0.9, 2.4)	3.0 (2.4, 3.6)	2.1 (1.6, 2.9)	3.1 (2.6, 3.6)	1.9 (1.4, 2.6)	3.0 (2.8, 3.2)	1.0 (0.8, 1.2)
Med.	1.4 (0.7, 2.7)	4.5 (2.7, 7.6)	1.9 (1.2, 2.9)	5.3 (3.8, 7.5)	0.8 (0.4, 1.4)	6.2 (4.6, 8.5)	0.8 (0.6, 1.0)	5.8 (5.0, 6.7)

Spont., spontaneous preterm birth; Med., medically-indicated preterm birth. Odd ratios were adjusted for period of birth, maternal age, parity, maternal race/ethnicity, marital status, maternal education, smoking and alcohol use during pregnancy, and pre-pregnancy body mass index. *The data shown in this Table are reproduced from Ananth et al. with the permission of the publisher (Reference 19)
The National Institute of Child Health and Human Development Maternal Fetal

4.1.3 The Effect pf Previous Indicated Preterm Birth on the Risk for Recurrent Preterm Delivery

The risk of subsequent preterm birth (induced or spontaneous) among women who were induced prematurely due to maternal or fetal indication increases according to the gestational age in which the patient was delivered.[17] The odds ratio for recurrent indicated preterm birth increases from 7.7 for women who were delivered <37 weeks to 11.3 for those who were delivered before 32 weeks of gestation (Table II) [17].

4.1.4 The Effect of Previous Pregnancy Outcome on Recurrent Preterm Delivery in Patients with Twins

There are conflicting reports regarding the risk for subsequent preterm delivery in patients who had a twin gestation and delivered preterm. Patients with a twin pregnancy have an overall increased risk for a subsequent preterm singleton delivery (RR 2.8, 95% CI 1.02–8.09) [37]. However, when the patients were further stratified according to the gestational age at delivery, only those who delivered twins before 34 weeks of gestation were at increased risk for subsequent preterm birth. Other investigators suggested that women who had a preterm singleton delivery but not during a twins gestation had an increase risk for a subsequent preterm birth in singleton and twins [38,39].

4.2 Cervical Insufficiency

The classic definition of cervical insufficiency is a painless dilatation and/or shortening of the cervix, not accompanied by uterine contraction, resulting in pregnancy loss or preterm delivery. There is not a uniform definition regarding the minimal cervical dilatation needed for diagnosis, Lee et al. [40] defined it as ≥ 1.5 cm, and McElrath et al. [16] as greater than 2 cm. The diagnosis was traditionally based of a history of recurrent late second trimester or early third trimester deliveries. The efforts thus far for the identification of patients at risk for cervical insufficiency in non-pregnant women [41-44] yielded inconclusive scientific evidence reading their value in predicting the outcome of a subsequent pregnancy. Thus, currently there are no objective diagnostic tests for the diagnosis of cervical insufficiency.

The incidence rate of cervical insufficiency in the US [45], Australia [46] and Denmark [47] is between 2 to 5/1000 birth; while McElrath et al. [16] reported that 5% of patients who delivered a live newborn before 28 weeks had cervical insufficiency. The discrepancy between these reports is derived from the differences in the definition of cervical insufficiency (some included bulging of the membranes through the cervical os while others defined only as cervical dilation).

Cervical insufficiency is syndromic in nature [48] and it is the clinical presentation of several underlying mechanisms including the following: (1) congenital disorder such as cervical hypoplasia after diethylstilbestrol exposure [49-52]; (2) loss of cervical connective tissue after cervical surgery [53-55]; (3) intrauterine infection [56,57]; (4) suspension of progesterone action—indeed, among patients with preterm labor the rate of cervical shortening was lower in those who were treated with 17-hydroxy progesterone caproate than in those allocated to placebo [58,59]; and (5) patients with intrinsic cervical disorder that present as cervical insufficiency.

4.2.1 The Effect of Previous Pregnancy Outcome on Recurrent Preterm Delivery in Patients with Cervical Insufficiency

The exact effect of cervical insufficiency and the risk for subsequent late abortion or preterm birth is not well documented. Even though the definition of cervical insufficiency includes recurrent early second trimester losses, there is a lack of information regarding the recurrence rate of this obstetric syndrome in subsequent pregnancies. Harger et al. [60] used patients with cervical insufficiency as their own control and demonstrated that infant viability was 25% in pregnancies before the placement of cerclage and 75% following pregnancies in which a cerclage was placed. The introduction of sonographic measurements of cervical length during gestation led to the proposal that cervical sufficiency/insufficiency is a continuum [61]. Indeed, Iames et al. [61] detected a strong relationship, nearly linear, between cervical length in the index pregnancy and gestational age at delivery in the first pregnancy. Patients with a typical history of a cervical insufficiency (painless dilation) do not constitute a separate group from those with a history of spontaneous preterm delivery (preterm labor or preterm PROM) [61]. Similar results have been reported by Guzman et al. [62]. Thus, patients with a history of cervical insufficiency should be consulted regarding their risk for a subsequent preterm birth.

4.3 Infection

Systemic and subclinical infections are a leading cause of preterm birth. Indeed, pyelonephritis and pneumonia are frequently associated with the onset of premature labor and delivery [63-75]. Similarly, subclinical intrauterine infection is a frequent and important mechanism of disease leading to premature contraction, preterm labor and preterm delivery [76-90]. Microbiological and histo-pathological studies suggest that infection-related inflammation may account for 25 to 40% of cases of preterm delivery [91].

4.3.1 Infection as a Risk Factor for Preterm Delivery with Intact Membranes

Goncalves et al. [76] studied the rate of positive amniotic fluid cultures for microorganisms in women with preterm labor and intact membranes. The authors reviewed the results of amniotic fluid cultures from 33 studies and the prevalence of microbial invasion of amniotic fluid among patients with preterm labor was 12.8% [76,92], the rate of polymicrobial invasion of the amniotic cavity was 50% (Table III). The most common microbial organisms isolated from the amniotic fluid of women with preterm labor and intact membranes were Ureaplasma urealyticum, Fusobacterium species and Mycoplasma hominis [93]. Other microorganisms that have been found in the amniotic fluid include Streptococcus agalactiae, Petostreptococcus spp., Fusobacterium spp., Staphylococcus aureus, Gardenerella vaginalis, Streptococcus viridans, and Bacterioides spp. Occasionally, Lactobacillus spp., Escherichia coli, Enterococcus faecalis, Neisseria gonorrhea, and Peptococcus spp. have been encountered. Haemophilus influenzae, Capnocytophaga spp., Stomato coccus spp., and Clostridium spp. were only rarely identified [94,95]. The rate of microbial invasion of the amniotic cavity in patients with preterm labor and intact membrane is gestational age dependant. It is as high as 45% at 23–26 weeks and decreases to 11.5% at 31–34 weeks of gestation [96]. Thus, the earlier the gestational age at preterm birth, the more likely that microbial invasion of the amniotic cavity is present [96].

Table III. Microbial invasion of the amniotic cavity in women with preterm labor and intact membranes as determined by amniotic fluid studies obtained by transabdominal amniocentesis.

Author	Ref. Year	No. Patients	Positive Cultures No. (%)	Mycoplasma Culture	Clinical Chorioamnionitis No. (%)	Preterm Delivery in Patients with Positive Cultures (%)	Relative Risk [95% CI]
Miller et al.	1980	23	11 (47.8)	No	8 (72. 7)	—	—
Bobbitt et al.	1981	31	8 (25.8)	No	6 (75. 0)	7 (87. 5)	—
Wallace and Herrick	1981	25	3 (12.0)	No	1 (33.3)	—	—
Hameed et al.	1984	37	4 (10.8)	No	3 (75.0)	3 (75. 0)	3.7 [0.7, 20]
Wahbeh et al.	1984	33	7 (21.2)	No	2 (28. 5)	5 (71.4)	—
Wieble and Randall	1985	35	1 (2.9)	No	1 (100)	—	—
Leight and Garite	1986	59	7 (11.9)	No	4 (57. 1)	7 (100)	—
Gravett et al.	1986	54	13 (24.1)	Yes	5 (38. 5)	5 (38. 5)	—
Iams et al.	1987	5	0 (0.0)	Yes	—	—	—
Duff and Kopelman	1987	24	1 (4.2)	No	0 (0)	0 (0)	—
Romero et al.	1988a	41	4 (9.8)	Yes	1 (14. 3)	—	—
Skoll et al.	1989	127	7 (5.5)	No	3 (12.5)	7 (100)	1.57 [1.2, 1.9]
Romero et al.	1989a	264	24 (9.1)	Yes	—	24 (100)	2.75 [2.3, 3.2]
Romero et al.	1990 b	109	15 (13.8)	Yes	—	15 (100)	—
Romero et al.	1990c	168	23 (13.7)	Yes	4 (17. 4)	—	—
Gauthier et al.	1991	113	18 (15.9)	Yes	—	—	—
Romero et al.	1991 b	195	25 (12.8)	Yes	4 (16.0)	25 (100)	1.97 [1.6, 2.3]
Coultrip et al.	1992	107	12 (11.2)	Yes	7 (63. 6)	—	—
Watts et al.	1992	105	20 (19.0)	Yes	—	17 (85. 0)	—
Romero et al.	1993a	120	11 (9.2)	Yes	2 (18.2)	11 (100)	—
Coultrip et al.	1994	89	12 (13.5)	Yes	7 (58.3)	—	—

Yoon et al.	1996	102	11 (10.8)	Yes	2 (18. 2)	—	—
Markenson	1997	54	5 (9.3)	Yes	—	5 (100)	2.64 [0.3, 20.9]
Gomez	1998	103	11 (10.7)	Yes	—	—	—
Hussey	1998	127	16 (12.6)	Yes	—	—	—
Kara	1998	74	25 (33.8)	Yes	—	—	—
Oyarzun	1998	50	6 (12)	Yes	—	4 (66.7)	1.33 [0.3, 6.6]
Rizzo	1998	144	18 (12.5)	Yes	—	—	—
Greci	1998	103	9 (8.7)	Yes	—	—	—
Yoon	1998	181	21 (11.6)	Yes	—	—	—
Elimian	1998	104	12 (11.5)	Yes	—	—	—
Gonzalez-Bosquet	1999	113	13 (11.5)	Yes	—	—	—
Locksmith	1999	44	6 (13.6)	Yes	—	—	—
Total		2963	379 (12.8)		60 (37.5)	110 (85.3)	2.00 [1.2, 1.9]

* Clinical chorioamnionitis is expressed as percentage of patients with positive amniotic fluid culture. The data shown in this Table are reproduced from Goncalves et al. with the permission of the publisher (Reference 76).

4.3.2 Infection as a Risk Factor for Preterm PROM

In preterm PROM, the prevalence of a positive amniotic fluid culture for microorganisms is approximately 32.4% [76,92]. However, when amniocenteses were performed at the time of the onset of labor, 75% of patients had microbial invasion of the amniotic cavity [97], suggesting that some patients are already infected prior to the clinical rupture of membranes, while others are infected after the membranes have ruptured. The most common microorganisms detected in the amniotic fluid of women with preterm PROM are the following: genital mycoplasmas (*Ureaplasma urealyticum* and Mycoplasma hominis) followed by Streptococcus agalactiae, Fusobacterium species, and Gardnerella Vaginalis; polymicrobial infection is found in 26.7% of cases (Table IV) [97-103].

4.3.3 Intra-Amniotic Infection in Patients with Cervical Insufficiency

The rate of microbial invasion of amniotic cavity among women presenting with a cervical insufficiency in the midtrimester is around 33% (range 13%–52%) [57,104] and 45% to 51% in the early third trimester [104]. The most common microorganisms were: Ureaplasma urealyticum, Gardnerella vaginalis, Candida albicans, and Fusobacterium species [57]. In addition, a recent study has demonstrated that while only 8% of patients with cervical insufficiency had a positive amniotic fluid culture, 80% have an intra-amniotic inflammation determined by a positive rapid MMP-8 kit [40]. Patients with intra-amniotic inflammation and negative amniotic fluid culture had a shorter amniocentesis-to-delivery interval and a lower gestational age at delivery than patients without intra-amniotic infection/inflammation. In twin gestations, microbial invasion of the amniotic cavity occurs in 11.9% of patients presenting with preterm labor and deliver preterm [105,106].

Table IV. Microbial invasion of the amniotic cavity in women with preterm PROM as determined by amniotic fluid studies obtained by trans-abdominal amniocentesis.

Author	Ref. Year	No. of Patients	Positive Culture No. (%)	Mycoplasma Culture	Success Rate (%)	Clinical Chorioamnionitis No. (%)	Neonatal Infection No. (%)
Garite et al.	1979	59	9/30 (30. 0)	No	51	6 (66.6)	2 (22.2)
Garite and Freeman	1982	207	20/86 (23. 3)	No	42	11 (55.0)	5 (25.0)
Cotton et al.	1984	61	6/41 (14. 6)	No	67	6 (100.0)	1 (16.6)
Broekhuizen et al.	1985	79	15/53 (28. 3)	No	67	3 (20.0)	8 (53.3)
Vintzileos et al.	1986	54	12/54 (22. 2)	No	—	2 (16.7)	4 (33.3)
Felnstein et al.	1986	73	12/50 (20. 0)	No	68	6 (50)	5 (41.6)
Romero et al.	1988b	230	65/221 (29. 4)	Yes	96	—	5 (12.8)
Gauthier et al.	1991	91	49/91 (53. 8)	Yes	—	—	—
Coultrip et al.	1992	29	12/29 (41. 4)	Yes	—	3 (25.0)	—
Gauthier and Meyer	1992	117	56/117 (47. 9)	Yes	—	—	—
Romero et al.	1993b	110	42/110 (38.2)	Yes	—	5 (11.9)	20 (47.6)
Font et al.	1995	74	21/37 (56.8)	Yes	—	—	—
Averbuch et al.	1995	90	32/90 (35.6)	Yes	—	—	7 (21.9)
Carroll et al.	1996	97	30/97 (30.9)	Yes	—	—	—
Gomez et al.	1998	52	30/52 (57.7)	Yes	—	—	—
Hussey et al.	1998	26	4/26 (15.4)	Yes	—	—	—
Rizzo et al.	1998	124	21/124 (16.9)	Yes	—	—	—
Yoon et al.	2000	154	37/154 (24)	Yes	—	7 (18.9)	10/32 (31.2)
Total		1727	473/1462 (32.4)			49/165 (29.7)	67/277 (24.2)

The data shown in this Table are reproduced from Goncalves et al. with the permission of the publisher (Reference 76).

4.3.4 Bacterial Vaginosis and Preterm Birth

Bacterial vaginosis is a risk factor for spontaneous preterm birth with intact or ruptures membranes. The rate of bacterial vaginosis during pregnancy is 15–20%; however, 50% of these patients are asymptomatic. A meta-analysis [107] of 18 studies (20,232 patients) concluded that bacterial vaginosis was associated with an increased risk for preterm delivery < 37 weeks of gestation (OR 2.19, 95% CI 1.54–3.12), and this effect was significant among singleton gestations, as well as among low and high risk pregnancies for preterm delivery. Detection of bacterial vaginosis <16 weeks of pregnancy was associated with an increased risk for preterm birth (OR 7.55, 95% CI 1.8–31.65) [107]. Bacterial vaginosis was also found to be associated with intra-amniotic infection, histologic chorioamnionitis, preterm PROM, first trimester losses in women who conceived after in vitro fertilization, and second trimesters abortions, as well as post cesarean section endometritis and wound infection [108-114].

Randomized clinical trials for the prevention of preterm birth by antibiotic treatment of patients with bacterial vaginosis have yielded contradictory results [115-123]. The randomized placebo control trial of the NICHD MFMU network [116] included 1953 women with bacterial vaginosis who were assigned to treatment with oral metronidazol or placebo. Treatment with metronidazol was not associated with a significant reduction in the rate of preterm birth. Moreover, a sub-analysis of high risk patients for preterm delivery demonstrated a higher rate of preterm delivery and preterm PROM in the treatment group [116]. A Cochrane review [124] concluded that, overall, antibiotic treatment of bacterial vaginosis did not reduce the risk for preterm birth; however, treatment before 20 weeks of gestation may reduce the risk for preterm delivery < 37 weeks (OR 0.72, 95% CI 0.55–0.95). Among patients with a previous preterm birth, treatment for bacterial vaginosis may reduce the risk for preterm PROM and low birthweight.

4.4 Multiple Pregnancies

Twin gestation as well as higher order gestations have a strong association with preterm birth [125-138]. The twin birth rate (number of twin deliveries per 1,000 births) had risen by 70% from 1980 to 2004 (from 18.9 per 1,000 to 32.1 per 1,000 births). The triplet/+ rate (the number of triplets, quadruplets, and quintuplets and other higher order multiples per 100,000 live births) climbed more than 400 percent during the 1980s and 1990s, but it has declined by 21% since the all-time high in 1998.

Multiple pregnancies comprise 14.1% of all preterm deliveries (<37 weeks) and 19.7% of early preterm deliveries (<28 weeks of gestation). In addition to spontaneous preterm labor, multiple gestations are more commonly complicated by medical and obstetrical disorders that lead to preterm delivery. Discordant fetal growth, fetal anomalies, hypertension, placental abruption, and fetal compromise are more common in multiple gestations, and increase with the number of fetuses [139]. As the incidence of multiple gestation has increased due to assisted reproductive technology [140], the proportion of preterm births caused by multiple gestation has also increased [141]. Of 31,582 births after assited repoductive technologies (ART) in the US in 2000, 54.4% were multiple gestations [142], while in Europe only 26.3% of ART pregnancies resulted in multiple [143]. This disparity may result from the differences in embryo transfer protocols. However, changes in the embryo transfer policy in the US is one of the leading factors for the constant decline in the proportion of higher order multiples in the recent years and the stable rate of twin deliveries between 2004–2006 [7].

4.5 Vaginal Bleeding and Vascular Pathology

Vaginal bleeding during pregnancy is a risk factor for spontaneous as well as indicated preterm birth [28;144-146]. Pregnancy complications such as placenta previa, placental abruption, and idiopathic vaginal bleeding during the first and second trimester have all been associated with an increased risk for preterm delivery [28,144-146]. Unexplained vaginal bleeding has been more strongly associated with subsequent preterm birth when it is persistent and when it occurs in Caucasians [145]. Vaginal bleeding may lead to indicated preterm delivery in cases where the magnitude of bleeding places the mother and /or the fetus at risk, especially in cases of placenta previa and/or abruption. Nevertheless, vaginal bleeding may be the presenting symptom of other underlying pathologies including uterine ischemia [147-149] and intra-amniotic infection [150].

The placenta of patients who delivered preterm after preterm labor with intact membranes as well as those of patients with preterm PROM have a higher rate of vascular lesion than those who delivered at term. Indeed, the rate of placental vascular lesion was 34.1% in patients with preterm labor, 35.1% in those with preterm PROM, and only 11.8% in women with normal pregnancies who delivered at term (p=0.065, p=0.0022, respectively). Moreover "failure of physiologic transformation of the spiral arteries," atherosis, fibrinoid necrosis of the decidual vessels, and decidual vessel thrombosis consistent with decidual vasculopathy were more prevalent among patients with preterm labor and preterm PROM than those with term delivery [149].

Patients with preterm delivery either due to preterm labor with intact membranes or preterm PROM have an increased activation of the coagulation cascade as reflected by the higher concentration of thrombin anti-thrombin (TAT) III complexes both in the maternal plasma [151-154] and in amniotic fluid [155]. This is of clinical relevance since thrombin has a uterotonic property and maternal plasma TAT III complex concentration > 8 ng/ml had a positive predictive value of 80% for delivery within a week [154].

4.6 Ethnicity

The risk for preterm birth is almost double among African Americans in comparison to other ethnic origins [156-158]. The rate of preterm birth in these patients in 2006 was 18.4%, while among Asian and Pacific Islanders it was 10.9% and in Caucasians 11.7% [159]. Even among women who live in high income neighborhoods in Chicago, African-Americans had a twofold greater rate of preterm birth (< 37 weeks) than Caucasians: (relative risk [RR] 2.2, 95% CI 1.7–2.9). Of note, Ananth et al. [156] reported an overall increase in the rate of preterm birth in the US between 1975 to 1995 of 3.6% among African Americans and 22.3% among Caucasians [156]. Nevertheless, the preterm delivery rate was still higher among African Americans (16%) than among Caucasians (8.4%) [156], suggesting that other factors aside from socioeconomic status (e.g., genetic predisposition) are associated with the ethnic disparity in the preterm delivery rate. African Americans also had a higher risk for preterm PROM between 20–28 weeks of gestation than Caucasians (Hazard Ratio: 3.81, 95% CI 1.04–13.99) [160]. Among women who delivered low-birth-weight neonates, those of African-American origin had a higher risk for PROM than Caucasians (OR 1.82, 95% CI 1.45–2.28) [161].

Among other ethnic groups, Hispanic women had a lower risk for preterm birth than Caucasians (OR 0.66, 95% CI 0.54–0.8) or African Americans (OR 0.57, 95% CI 0.48–0.67) [162]. Differences in the prevalence of preterm deliveries have been reported also among Asian-American subgroups. The lowest preterm delivery rate was in Chinese (7.74%) and the highest in Hawaiian (14.33%). After adjustment for potential confounders, Filipinos (OR 1.68, 95% CI 1.56–1.80) and Hawaiians (OR 1.61, 95% CI 1.89–1.94) had a higher odds ratio for preterm birth than Chinese [163].

Outside the US, Zeitlin and colleagues reported that the French Caribbean/Indian Ocean population had an adjusted OR of 1.6 for preterm deliveries in comparison to other multiethnic populations in France [164]. Similarly, in the UK, Afro Caribbeans were more prone to deliver preterm [165]. In New Zealand, Maori and Indian women had a higher rate of preterm deliveries from 1996 to 2001 [166]. The rate of preterm delivery of Hong Kong Chinese (7.4%) between the year 1995–1996 [167] was similar to the one reported among American Chinese [163]. In southern Israel, Bedouins have a higher risk of preterm delivery than that of Jews (OR 1.22, 95% CI 1.14–1.32) [168] and a higher rate of preterm delivery was found among Ethiopian immigrant [169].

Paternal ethnicity, especially African-American, also increases the risk for preterm birth. Indeed, in a cohort of 2,845,686 singleton birth, paternal African-American race was associated with an increased risk for preterm birth (OR 1.2, 95% CI 1.1–1.3), regardless of maternal race [170]. Similarly couples of Caucasian mother and African-American father had a higher risk for preterm delivery < 35 weeks (OR 1.28, 95% CI 1.13–1.46) [158].

The disparities of racial ethnic life events before and during pregnancy were examined among 33,542 Americans. African-American and Indian/Alaska Native-American women had a higher number of stressor life events (35% more financial stressors, 163% more partner-related stressors, and 83% more traumatic stressors) compared to non-Hispanic Caucasians. In accord with other studies [157,162], after using a regression model no significant association was found between these life events and preterm birth [171]. In contrast, Caucasians but not African Americans had a higher risk for preterm birth if they reported a higher number of negative life events, or were living without their partner [172].

4.7 Müllerian Anomalies

Maternal Müllerian anomalies are associated with an increased risk for preterm birth [173]. The general rate of preterm birth (including all Müllerian anomalies) ranged from 14.9% to 25% [173-175]; however, the incidence of preterm birth is dependant on the specific Müllerian anomaly. The highest rate of preterm delivery was reported in women with uterus didelphus, uterus bicornis, or septated uterus [174 176]. In addition, the NICHD MFMU network reported that the presence of a Müllerian anomaly was an independent risk factor for indicated preterm delivery (OR 7.02, 95% CI 1.69–29.15) [15].

4.8 Genetics

There is a genetic predisposition for preterm birth, and gene environment interaction had been proposed as a mechanism of disease of preterm birth. These topics are reviewed in the next chapter.

4.9 Socioeconomic Factors

The effect of maternal occupation and work load on the risk for preterm birth has been studied extensively. The main factor that has been associated with preterm delivery is the time period spent standing during work. Indeed, jobs that demand many hours of standing (e.g., food services, shop keeper, Janitors) have been associated with a higher incident of preterm birth [177-181]. Meyer et al. [182] studied more than 26,000 women in Connecticut, and found a higher rate of preterm delivery among women with stressful occupation (OR 1.35), while workings in shifts or long hours, as well as the income were not associated with an increased risk for preterm birth [183]. In contrast, other studies reported a lower rate of preterm birth among teachers, clerks or librarians [181,183,184].

The environmental effect on the preterm birth rate was studied by Hournani et al. who reported that exposure of the father to pesticides was independently associated with preterm delivery (OR 2.52, 95% CI 1.05–6.01) [184].

Maternal education was inversely correlated with preterm birth [185⁻188]. A recent study from Denmark which included 75,890 singleton birth (1996–2002) reported that women with less than 10 years of education had a higher risk for preterm delivery than those with >12 years of eduction [189]. Similarly, a study by Auger et al. from Montreal Canada including 98,330 live births, reported that mothers lacking a high school diploma had a higher risk for preterm delivery (OR 1.67, 95% CI 1.49–1.87) [185].

5. Perinatal Mortality and Morbidity

5.1 Perinatal Mortality

Preterm birth is the leading cause for perinatal mortality and morbidity. The definition of the perinatal mortality rate by the World Health Organization (WHO) is as follows: "the number of deaths of fetuses weighing at least 500g (or, when birth weight is unavailable, after 22 completed weeks of gestation or with a crown-heel length of 25 cm or more), plus the number of early neonatal deaths, per 1000 total births. Because of the different denominators in each component, this is not necessarily equal to the sum of the fetal death rate and the **early neonatal mortality rate**" [190]. According to the WHO data the rate of perinatal mortality is decreasing worldwide [190]. In the US the National Center for Health Statistics chose to define the perinatal mortality rate as the number of late fetal deaths (after 28 weeks) plus infant deaths within 7 days of birth per 1000 total births after 28 weeks [191]. According to that definition the overall perinatal mortality rate decreased in the US from 32.5/1000 in 1950 to 6.9/1000 in 2001. However, improvements in survival and morbidity for infants born between 23 and 25 weeks have reached a limit. Between 1996 and 2000, survival rates improved from 20 to 30% at 23 weeks, 58 to 60% at 24 weeks, and 75 to 80% at 25 weeks [192].

Perinatal mortality is dependent on the gestational age at delivery and birthweight [193,194]. Indeed, the earlier the preterm birth occurred the higher the perinatal mortality rate. In the study by Mercer et al. [12], the mortality rate declined from about 80% between 22–24 weeks to 20% for those delivered after 25 weeks of gestation (Figure 3). Similarly, studies conducted in Europe [193⁻196] and Australia [197] reported that the survival rate for neonates who were born between 22–23 weeks ranged from 0–20% and increased substantially from 24 weeks to more than 80% after 28 weeks of gestation. However, the combination of gestational age at delivery and neonatal birthweight can give a better prediction of neonatal survival. Indeed, a newborn who was delivered at 25 weeks of gestation has a survival rate of 17% for a birthweight of 250–500 grams, this rate increases up to 42% if the neonate birthweight was 1000–1250 grams [193,194].

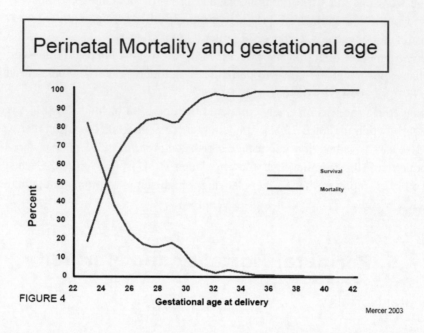

FIGURE 4

Figure 3. The rate of perinatal mortality according to gestational age. Adopted from Mercer BM [12] with permission.

Ethnic origin has its impact on perinatal survival. In the year 2000, the overall perinatal mortality rate was double among African Americans (10.8%) than among Caucasians (5.4%); this is in spit of a 27% reduction in the overall perinatal mortality among African Americans and a 30% reduction among Caucasians, from 1989 to 2000. The disparity is even greater when only preterm deliveries are taken into account. While in Caucasians the perinatal mortality rate among all preterm births declined by 28.5% during the period of 1989 to 2000, in African-Americans this rate was decreased only by 12.4% (Table V) [30].

In addition to the factors discussed above, a female neonate (OR 0.42, 95% CI 0.29–0.61), being small for gestational age (OR 0.58, 95%CI 0.38–0.88), antenatal treatment with corticosteroids (OR 0.52, 95% CI 0.36–0.76) as well as neonatal treatment with surfactant, all increase the survival of preterm neonates [198-200]. In contrast, intrauterine infection [199] and an expectation by the health care team that the infant will not survive [201,202] increase the mortality rate of preterm neonates. Of note, these rates vary among different neonatal intensive care units with similar care practices and patient demographics [203]. Therefore, local statistics are preferred when counseling patients.

Table V. Changes in rates of preterm birth clinical subtypes and perinatal mortality among singleton live birth in the U.S. between 1989 and 2000*.

Preterm birth clinical subtypes	Preterm birth rates			Perinatal mortality		
	1989	2000	RR (95% CI)	1989	2000	RR (95% CI)
White women						
All preterm births	8.3	9.4	1.14(1.13, 1.15)	50.6	36.2	0.71(0.69, 0.73)
PROM	1.1	0.8	0.77(0.76, 0.78)	60.8	42.6	0.69(0.63, 0.74)
Spontaneous preterm	4.9	5.0	1.03(1.02, 1.04)	41.6	29.3	0.70(0.67, 0.73)
Medically indicated	2.3	3.6	1.55(1.53, 1.56)	64.7	44.4	0.67(0.64, 0.70)
Black women						
All preterm births	18.5	16.2	0.85(0.84, 0.86)	54.1	47.4	0.87(0.84, 0.91)
PROM	2.3	1.5	0.63(0.62, 0.65)	74.9	70.9	0.94(0.85, 1.05)
Spontaneous preterm	12.1	9.1	0.73(0.70, 0.76)	47.2	41.1	0.87(0.82, 0.91)
Medically indicated	4.1	5.6	1.32(1.29, 1.34)	63.0	51.4	0.81(0.75, 0.87)

Relative risks (RR) denote changes in preterm birth and perinatal mortality rates between 1989 and 2000. Perinatal mortality rates are expressed per 1000 singleton birth.

*The data shown in this table are reproduced (with modification) from Ananth et al. with the permission of the publisher (Reference 30).

5.2 Perinatal Morbidity

Preterm births are associated with specific perinatal morbidities that are derived from the immaturity of the neonatal organs. This morbidity is gestational age dependent and the earlier the preterm delivery the more severe is the neonatal morbidity, especially among neonates born before 30 weeks of gestation [204]. The morbidity of preterm infants can be divided into acute and chronic. The acute neonatal morbidity of preterm infants includes the following: respiratory distress syndrome (RDS), intraventricular hemorrhage (IVH), patent ductus arteriosus (PDA), sepsis, apnea, and necrotizing enterocolitis (NEC). The rates for the most common neonatal morbidities and their change according to gestational age are shown in Figure 4. The introduction of prenatal administration of corticosteroids has lowered the rate of most acute neonatal morbidities. In addition the use of recombinant surfactant has also contributed to the substantial reduction in rate of RDS.

5.2.1 Long-Term Outcomes

The chronic morbidity of prematurity carries a lifetime burden. Evidence in support of this view include the following: (1) bronchopulmonary dysplasia (BPD) is associated with the need for oxygen supplementary during the first two years of life, and with a reversible and irreversible lung damage [194]. (2) Cerebral palsy (CP) is associated with intrauterine infection/inflammation [205-208] and intraventricular hemorrhage grades III and IV [209-212]; (3) Retinopathy of prematurity (ROP) has been associated with the administration of supplementary oxygen treatment, the length of hospitalization after delivery and neonatal birthweight. Indeed, among neonates born in New York, the incidence of ROP was higher in those who were hospitalized >28 days (14.5%) than that among all newborns (0.2%);

furthermore, even higher rates were observed in infant with birthweight <1500 gram (20.3%) and in those with birthweight <1200 gram (27.3%) [213]. (4) Growth impairment is an additional long term effect of prematurity. Indeed, almost all infants born <30 weeks will have some form of growth impairment that in very premature neonate may persist for 12 months or more [194].

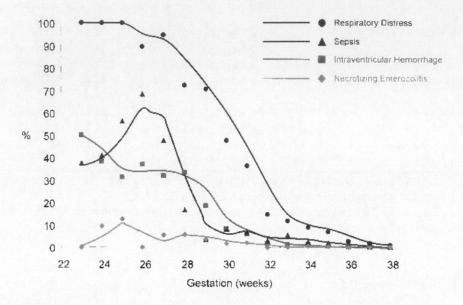

Figure 4. The rate of specific perinatal morbidity according to gestational age. Adopted from Mercer BM [12] with permission.

The neurological development of preterm infants is delayed; this observation is relatively common especially among early preterm neonates. Indeed, a study from the United Kingdom compared 78% of 308 survivors born before 25 weeks to their classmates of normal birth weight, demonstrating that almost all had some disability at age six: 22% had severe neuro-cognitive disabilities (cerebral palsy, IQ > 3 SD below mean, blindness, or deafness), 24% had moderate disabilities, 34% had mild disabilities, and 20% had no neuro-cognitive disabilities [214]. Another study compared 280 children who were born <32 weeks. A multivariate analysis detected that the IQ score at the age of 7 was associated with gestational age at delivery, the presence of persistence ductus arteriosus, and the head circumference [215]. Moreover, 176 children who were born at 33–35 weeks had a higher proportion of schooling difficulties that were associated in a multivariate analysis with a male gender, and discharge from hospital **before 36 weeks' corrected age** [216]. Similarly, self esteem among prematurely born adolescents is higher than expected. A report of self-described quality of life among 132 adolescents who weighed less than 1000 grams at birth found that although 24% had significant sensory deficits, they did not differ from controls of normal birth weight in their self-perception of global self worth, scholastic or job competence, or social acceptance [217].

The effect of prematurity on adult life was investigated in a cohort of 903,402 infants who were born alive and without congenital anomalies (1822 born at 23 to 27 weeks of gestation, 2805 at 28 to 30 weeks, 7424 at 31 to 33 weeks, 32,945 at 34 to 36 weeks, and 858,406 at 37 weeks or later). The survival rates to adult life were 17.8%, 57.3%, 85.7%, 94.6%, and 96.5%, respectively. Among the survivors, the prevalence of having a cerebral palsy was 0.1% for those born at term versus 9.1% for those born at 23 to 27 weeks of gestation (RR for birth at 23 to 27 weeks of gestation, 78.9; 95% CI 56.5–110.0); the prevalence of having mental retardation, 0.4% versus 4.4% (RR 10.3, 95% CI 6.2–17.2); and the prevalence of receiving a disability pension, 1.7% versus 10.6% (RR 7.5, 95% CI 5.5–10.0). Among those who did not have medical disabilities, the gestational age at birth was associated with the education level attained, income, receipt of Social Security benefits, and the establishment of a family, but not with rates of unemployment or criminal activity [4].

5.2.2 The Effect of Late Preterm Birth on Neonatal Mortality and Morbidity

Late preterm birth is considered by many as safe. Indeed by reviewing the data presented in Figures 3 and 4 the expected neonatal mortality and morbidity is similar to term delivery. However, recent reports suggest that this may not be the case. Neonates delivered in late preterm birth have an 8 times (95% CI 6.2–10.4) higher perinatal mortality rate and 5.5 times (95% CI 3.4–8.9) higher neonatal mortality rate than neonates delivered at term [218]. In addition, late preterm birth is associated with an increased risk for neonatal infections and respiratory morbidity in comparison to term neonates [218,219]. Thus, in spite of the low incidence of neonatal complications among those who were born from 34 to 36 weeks of gestation when compared to that of neonates who were born before 32 weeks of gestations. Late preterm delivery is still associated with a significant increase risk for neonatal morbidity and mortality in comparison to term delivery and the decision to perform an indicated preterm birth at this gestational age must be taken after careful considerations.

6. Identification of Patients at Risk for Preterm Birth

The identification of patients at risk for preterm birth has been one of the leading questions in the recent years. Since the syndrome of preterm delivery is a clinical end point of several underlying mechanisms, the identification of patients at risk can not be accomplish by a single marker. The preterm prediction study by the NICHD MFMU group investigated this question on a cohort of 2929 singleton pregnancies and 147 twin gestations from 10 medical centers. Many markers were associated with preterm birth <32 (Table VI) and <35 weeks of gestation (Table VII). The most prominent risk factors for preterm delivery in the index pregnancy were fetal fibronectin concentration, a sonographic cervical length <25 mm and a history of preterm birth [28,220]. Since a history of preterm birth is relevant only in multiparous the other two markers can be useful screening tool for the detection of patients at risk for a subsequent preterm birth also in nulliparous patients.

Table VI. Risk factors and tests for spontaneous preterm birth <32 weeks obtained or available at 24 weeks' gestational age in cases and controls.

Factor	Source of Data or Fluid	Test Cutoff	Cases % Positive n = 48	Controls % Positive n =48	OR Cases vs. Controls	Significant (P < .05)
Corticotropin releasing factor	Serum	90th %ile	10.6	4.3	2.7	No
Alpha fetoprotein	Serum	90th %ile	36.1	6.4	8.3	Yes
Alkaline phosphatase	Serum	90th %ile	22.9	4.2	6.8	Yes
Beta2-macroglobulin	Serum	90th %ile	6.3	2.1	3.1	No
Ferritin	Serum	90th %ile	14.6	2.1	8.0	No
Interstitial cell adhesion molecule-1	Serum	90th %ile	23.4	6.4	4.5	Yes
Interleukin-6	Serum	90th %ile	10.4	8.3	1.3	No
C-reactive protein	Serum	90th %ile	10.4	6.3	1.7	No
Cortisol	Serum	90th %ile	10.4	2.1	5.5	No
Lactoferrin	Serum	90th %ile	11.6	9.3	1.3	No
Defensins	Serum	90th %ile	20.9	4.7	5.4	Yes
Relaxin	Serum	90th %ile	10.9	10.9	1.0	No
Interleukin-10	Serum	90th %ile	6.4	12.8	0.5	No
Granulocyte colony stimulating factor	Serum	90th %ile	8.5	10.6	0.8	No
Activan	Serum	Pos	8.5	10.6	0.8	No
Interleukin-6	Cervix	90th %ile	20.4	6.1	3.9	Yes
Lactoferrin	Cervix	90th %ile	4.3	0.0	Inf	No
Defensins	Cervix	90th %ile	10.5	18.4	0.5	No
Sialidase	Cervix	90th %ile	8.2	6.1	1.4	No
Short cervix	Ultrasound	<25mm	44.9	12.2	5.8	Yes
Fetal fibronectin	Cervix/ Vagina	≥50 ng/mL	40.0	2.0	32.7	Yes
Gram stain score	Vagina	≥9	30.0	24.0	1.4	No
PH	Vagina	≥5.0	42.9	18.4	3.3	Yes
Chlamydia	Vagina	Pos	15.2	6.5	2.6	No
Previous SPTB	History	Pos	42.0	14.0	4.5	Yes
Uterine Contractions	History	Pos	24.0	32.0	0.7	No
Bleeding	History	Pos	36.0	24.0	1.8	No
Body mass index	Measured	<19.8	29.2	14.6	2.4	No

The data shown in this table are reproduced (with modification) from Goldenberg et al. with the permission of the publisher (Reference 220).

6.0.1 Fetal Fibronectin

In the study of NICHD MFMU the measurement of a positive vaginal fetal fibronectin (>50 ng/ml) at 24 weeks of gestation was associated with a sensitivity of 63% and an odds ratio of 60 for a subsequent preterm birth occurring between 24–28 weeks of gestation. The authors reached the following conclusion: (1) a positive fetal fibronectin test was associated with a relative risk of 14.1 (95% CI 9.3–21.4) for delivery <32 weeks and a relative risk of 6.7 (95% CI 4.9–9.2) for delivery <35 weeks of gestation; (2) vaginal fetal fibronectin is most sensitive when measured in asymptomatic patients near to the occurrence of the preterm delivery; and (3) the predictive value of fetal fibronectin before 22 weeks of gestation was much poorer [28,220]. Additionally, the NICHD MFMU found that repeated measurements of fetal fibronectin increase its sensitivity for the detection of preterm birth [28,220]. This finding was in accord with the results of a meta-analysis of 40 studies (10,000 patients), in which repeated measurements of fetal fibronectin in women at risk for preterm birth increases the sensitivity for the detection of preterm delivery <34 weeks [221].

Table VII. Risk factors and tests for spontaneous preterm birth <35 weeks obtained or available at 24 weeks' gestational age in cases and controls.

Factor	Source of Data or Fluid	Test Cutoff	%Positive Cases n= 107	% Positive Controls n= 107	OR Cases vs. Controls	Significant (P< .05)
Corticotropin releasing factor	Serum	90th %ile	11.7	8.3	1.5	No
Alpha fetoprotein	Serum	90th %ile	35.3	13.5	3.5	Yes
Alkaline phosphatase	Serum	90th %ile	14.9	3.3	5.1	Yes
Beta2-macroglobulin	Serum	90th %ile	5.1	6.8	0.7	No
Ferritin	Serum	90th %ile	9.9	7.4	1.4	No
Interstitial cell adhesion molecule-1	Serum	90th %ile	16.4	9.1	2.0	No
Interleukin-6	Serum	90th %ile	10.0	9.2	1.1	No
C-reactive protein	Serum	90th %ile	8.3	6.7	1.3	No
Cortisol	Serum	90th %ile	12.6	7.6	1.8	No
Lactoferrin	Serum	90th %ile	8.8	11.4	0.8	No
Defensins	Serum	90th %ile	18.4	10.5	1.9	No
Relaxin	Serum	90th %ile	13.6	8.2	1.8	No
Interleukin-10	Serum	90th %ile	4.3	10.3	0.4	No
Granulocyte colony stimulating factor	Serum	90th %ile	7.7	7.7	1.0	No
Activan	Serum	Pos	14.2	11.7	1.3	No
Interleukin-6	Cervix	90th %ile	20.0	9.6	2.4	No
Lactoferrin	Cervix	90th %ile	5.0	0.0	Inf	Yes
Defensins	Cervix	90th %ile	16.7	10.0	1.8	No
Sialidase	Cervix	90th %ile	9.6	9.6	1.0	No
Short cervix	Ultrasound	≤25 mm	36.8	9.6	5.5	Yes
Fetal fibronectin	Cervix/vagina	≥50 ng/mL	22.8	3.2	9.1	Yes
Gram stain score	Vagina	≥9	22.8	15.0	1.7	No
PH	Vagina	>5	38.1	21.4	2.3	Yes
Chlamydia	Vagina	Pos	12.8	5.1	2.7	Yes
Previous SPB	History	Pos	43.3	15.0	4.3	Yes
Contractions	History	Pos	31.5	31.5	1.0	No
Bleeding	History	Pos	35.4	20.5	2.1	Yes
Body mass index	Measured	<19.8	30.9	17.9	2.1	Yes

*The data shown in this table are reproduced (with modification) from Goldenberg et al. with the permission of the publisher (Reference 220).

Table VIII. Odds ratios for preterm delivery stratified according to gestational age at delivery and cervical length

	10 mm	15 mm	20 mm	25 mm	30 mm
28 wk					
Cervical length					
OR (95% CI)	27.15 (9.85-27.86)	33.12 (17.09-64.20)	27.01 (15.35-47.53)	17.36 (10.69-28.20)	4.34 (2.94-6.40)
Previous preterm delivery					
OR (95% CI)	1.41 (1.11-1.80)	1.34 (1.03-1.74)	1.30 (0.99-1.71)	1.32 (1.01-1.73)	1.34 (1.05-1.71)
African American					
OR (95% CI)	3.59 (1.75-7.38)	3.50 (1.70-7.22)	3.40 (1.65-6.94)	3.37 (1.64-6.94)	3.35 (1.63-6.88)
30 wk					
Cervical length					
OR (95% CI)	26.39 (9.86-70.63)	29.26 (15.30-55.96)	21.89 (12.65-37.87)	14.23 (8.97-22.58)	3.90 (2.75-5.34)
Previous preterm delivery					
OR (95% CI)	1.69 (1.40-2.04)	1.64 (1.35-1.99)	1.62 (1.33-1.96)	1.63 (1.34-1.98)	1.62 (1.33-1.95)
African American					
OR (95% CI)	3.85 (2.02-7.34)	3.79 (1.98-7.26)	3.70 (1.93-7.08)	3.66 (1.19-6.98)	3.60 (1.89-6.86)
32 wk					
Cervical length					
OR (95% CI)	29.28 (11.32-75.75)	24.32 (12.88-45.90)	18.25 (10.75-30.99)	13.42 (8.75-20.58)	3.24 (2.37-4.44)
Previous preterm delivery					
OR (95% CI)	1.90 (1.61-2.23)	1.85 (1.57-2.18)	1.83 (1.55-2.16)	1.84 (1.56-2.17)	1.84 (1.55-2.17)
African American					
OR (95% CI)	2.36 (1.51-3.70)	2.31 (1.48-3.64)	2.27 (1.45-3.57)	2.25 (1.43-3.53)	2.24 (1.43-3.50)
34 wk					
Cervical length					
OR (95% CI)	22.54 (8.76-57.99)	25.06 (13.25-47.36)	20.79 (12.44-34.76)	12.40 (8.33-18.45)	2.94 (2.25-3.85)
Previous preterm delivery					
OR (95% CI)	1.93 (1.67-2.24)	1.89 (1.63-2.19)	1.87 (1.61-2.17)	1.88 (1.62-2.18)	1.89 (1.63-2.20)
African American					
OR (95% CI)	1.39 (1.03-1.88)	1.36 (1.00-1.85)	1.34 (0.98-1.84)	1.33 (0.98-1.81)	1.34 (0.99-1.81)

36 wk

Cervical length					
OR (95% CI)	14.29 (5.47-37.36)	15.21 (7.96-29.10)	13.20 (7.86-22.19)	9.01 (6.14-13.23)	2.24 (1.79-2.80)
Previous preterm delivery					
OR (95% CI)	2.08 (1.83-2.37)	2.05 (1.80-2.33)	2.03 (1.78-2.31)	2.03 (1.79-2.32)	2.06 (1.81-2.35)
African American					
OR (95% CI)	1.26 (1.01-1.57)	1.24 (0.99-1.56)	1.23 (0.98-1.54)	1.23 (0.98-1.53)	1.23 (0.99-1.53)

OR, Odds ratio; 95% CI, 95% confidence interval

Cervical length in each column dichotomized as less than the noted value versus greater than the noted value. Outcomes for designated gestational ages at delivery are further subdivided by the covariates associated with each gestational age. The odds ratio for a cervical length of 10 mm at a gestational age of 32 weeks, for example, reflects the risk of preterm delivery at δ32 weeks' gestation for cervical lengths δ10 mm versus >10 mm. The odds ratios for history of preterm delivery and maternal race are also provided. *The data shown in this table are reproduced (with modification) from Hassan et al. with the permission of the publisher (Reference 225).

6.0.2 Sonographic Cervical Length

Cervical sonography is the most objective and reliable method to assess cervical length [222-226] and sonographic cervical length is the single most powerful predictor for preterm birth in the index pregnancy [227], and it is far more informative than a history of previous preterm delivery [228-232]. The shorter the sonographic cervical length in the mid-trimester, the higher the risk of spontaneous preterm labor/delivery [226]. However, there is no agreement on the definition of a sonographic short cervix. Iams et al. [226] proposed that a cervix of 26 mm or shorter at 24 weeks of gestation increases the risk for spontaneous preterm delivery (RR 6.19, 95% CI 3.84–9.97); however, others have proposed a cutoff of 15 mm [224,225,233-241] because it is associated with nearly 50% risk of spontaneous preterm delivery at ≤32 weeks of gestation (Table VIII) [242]. Vaisbuch et al. [243] reported that asymptomatic women with a sonographic cervical length ≤15 mm diagnosed before 20 weeks of gestation have a higher risk of very early preterm delivery (<28 weeks) than women diagnosed with this condition between 20-24 weeks (77% vs. 31%, respectively, p<0.001).

An individualized risk assessment for preterm birth by using sonographic cervical length and other maternal risk factors such as maternal age, ethnic group, body mass index, cigarette smoking and previous cervical surgery was developed by To et al. [242]. However, sonographic cervical length is not a good screening test for the identification of patients at risk for spontaneous preterm delivery because only some of the patients who will have a spontaneous preterm birth have a short cervix in the mid-trimester. Rather, it is a method for risk assessment for spontaneous preterm delivery. The importance of sonographic measurement of cervical length derives from the observation that some of the patients with a history of previous preterm birth who shorten their cervix during the index pregnancy may benefit from therapeutic cervical cerclage [48,244,245] and patients with a short cervix may benefit from vaginal progesterone administration to reduce the rate of spontaneous preterm birth [246].

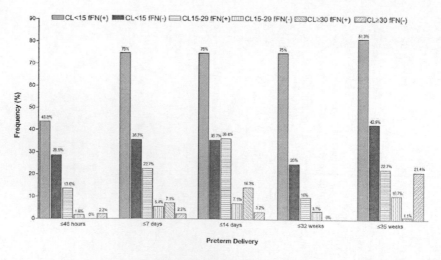

Figure 5. Frequency of spontaneous preterm delivery according to cervical length (CL) results (categorized as <15 mm, 15–29 mm, and ≥30 mm) and vaginal fetal fibronectin (fFN) determination. Adopted from Gomez et al. [241] with permission.

The effect of the combination of a short sonographic cervical length (<15 mm) and fetal fibronectin test in the risk assessment of patients with preterm labor was studied by Gomez et al. [241]. Of patients with a sonographic short cervix and a positive fetal fibronectin test, 43% delivered within 48 hours and 75% delivered <32 weeks of gestation (Figure 5). Moreover, this group had a shorter examination-to-delivery interval in comparison to patients with a cervical length > 15 mm or negative fetal fibronectin test (Figure 6). The results of this study and others support the approach of a combined assessment of cervical length and fetal fibronectin especially among patients at risk.

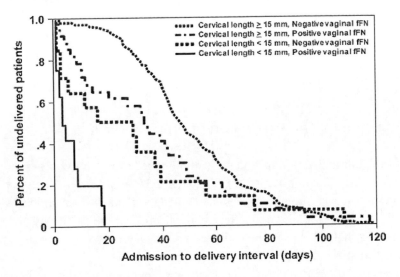

Figure 6. Survival curve of the admission-to-delivery interval (days) according to cervical length and vaginal fetal fibronectin (fFN) results (Kaplan Meier with log rank test, P <0.0001). Adopted from Gomez et al. [241] with permission.

7. Prevention of Preterm Birth

The prevention of preterm birth is one of the major objectives of modern obstetrics. In the US there is an initiative to reduce the rate of preterm birth to 6.1% by 2010, and the March of Dimes has made this topic its main field of interest. In spite of all efforts, at present there is no specific treatment for spontaneous preterm birth and this is attributed to the syndromic nature of preterm delivery that cannot be resolved by a single medication or intervention.

Currently there is wide agreement regarding the beneficial effect of two treatments: (1) the administration of corticosteroids for patients at risk for preterm birth to reduced acute neonatal morbidity; and (2) prophylactic antibiotic treatment for patients with preterm PROM that has occurred from 24 to 32 weeks of gestation [247,248] but not for preterm labor with intact membranes [249]. This treatment has been proven to prolong pregnancy and reduce the rate of acute neonatal morbidity [247,248]. However, the results of the follow up of children after 7 years were as follows: (1) In children who were born after preterm PROM, neither antibiotic regime was associated with a significant effect on the overall level of behavioral, medical status and academics achievements [250]. (2) In contrast, prophylactic antibiotic treatment of patients with preterm labor had a negative effect on the children's outcome at the age of 7. Treatment with erythromycin was associated with increased functional impairment of children of mother with preterm labor and intact membranes [250]. The more worrisome outcome was the higher rate of cerebral palsy among children whose mothers were treated with erythromycin (OR 1.93, 95% CI 1.21–3.09) as well as in those treated with co-amoxicalve (OR 1.69, 95% CI 1.07–2.67) [251]. Thus, prophylactic antibiotic treatment should not be administrated to patients with preterm labor with intact membranes.

Yet, these treatments are targeted to reduce the rate of complications rather than to prevent the "disease". In the recent years, attempts to prevent spontaneous preterm birth are mainly by two approaches: (1) the administration of progesterone to patients with a history of preterm birth or with a short sonographic cervix; and (2) placement of cerclage for cervical os insufficiency.

7.1 Progesterone for the Prevention of Preterm Birth

Progestogens administration for the prevention of recurrent abortion or preterm birth has been a subject of investigation [229,230,252-257,257-261] and meta-analyses [262-264] for several decades. However, progesterone gained a wide acceptance as a valid treatment for the prevention of preterm birth [265] only after the publication of the studies by da Fonseca [232] and the NICHD MFMU [231] who investigated its efficacy in the prevention of preterm birth in women with a history of preterm delivery.

Da Fonseca et al. [232] reported the results of a randomized, double-blinded, placebo-controlled study including 142 high-risk singleton pregnancies including patients with: (1) at least one previous spontaneous preterm birth; (2) prophylactic cervical cerclage; or (3) a uterine malformation. The patients were randomized to receive either daily vaginal suppository of micronized progesterone (100 mg) or placebo, from 24 to 34 weeks of gestation. The rate of preterm delivery <37 weeks and <34 weeks was lower in the progesterone group than in the placebo group (<37 weeks, progesterone: 13.8% vs. placebo: 28.5%, p=0.03; and < 34 weeks, progesterone: 2.8% vs. 18.6%, p=0.002) [232]. The authors concluded that prophylactic vaginal progesterone appeared to reduce the rate of preterm delivery in women at high risk for preterm birth [232].

The NICHD-MFMU network [231] reported the results of a multicenter double-blind, placebo-controlled clinical trial testing whether 17-hydroxy progesterone caproate (OHPC) administration can reduce the rate of preterm delivery in patients with a history of spontaneous preterm birth. The patients were enrolled at 16 to 20 weeks of gestation and randomly assigned in a 2:1 ratio to receive either a weekly injection of 250 mg of 17-OHPC or a weekly injection of placebo until delivery or 36 weeks of gestation. Treatment with 17-OHPC significantly reduced the rate of preterm delivery at less than 37 weeks, less than 35 weeks, and less than 32 weeks of gestation (<37 weeks, RR 0.66; 95% CI 0.54–0.81; <35 weeks, RR 0.67; 95% CI 0.48–0.93; and <32 weeks, RR 0.58; 95% CI 0.37–0.91]. Moreover, neonates born to women treated with 17-OHPC had significantly lower rates of NEC, IVH and need for supplemental oxygen [231]. Thus, among women at high risk for preterm delivery, a weekly injection of 17-OHPC resulted in a reduction in the rate of recurrent preterm birth and several neonatal complications [231]. Although the results of this study appear promising, some have raised concerns about the high rate of preterm delivery (54.9% [84/153]) in the control group [266,267], suggesting that this may be due to the effect of castor oil that was used as the placebo and as a carrier for the synthetic progestin [266]. However, the beneficial effect of 17-OHPC and vaginal progesterone in the reduction of preterm birth and of 17-OHPC in the reduction of the rate of neonates with low birth weight were further supported by systematic reviews meta-analyses and a Cochrane review [268-272].

In 2007, three new randomized clinical trials on the efficacy of progestogens in preventing preterm birth were reported [228,246,273]. The recent randomized clinical trials [228,231,232,246,273] yielded conflicting results. O'Brien et al. [228] reported the results of a multinational, randomized, double-blind, placebo-controlled trial of progesterone vaginal gel administration to patients with a history of spontaneous preterm birth between 20 to 35 weeks of gestation. Women were randomized, between 18 to 22 completed weeks of gestation, to receive daily treatment of progesterone vaginal polycarbophil-based gel (Crinone®, 8%, 90 mg) or placebo (Replens®) [228] that were self-administered either until delivery, 37 weeks of gestation, or the occurrence of PROM. Vaginal progesterone did not reduce the rate of preterm birth at ≤32, ≤35, or ≤37 weeks of gestation. Moreover, there were no differences in the neonatal and maternal outcomes [228].

The beneficial effect of progesterone in patients with a sonographic short cervix has been recently reported [58,246,274]. A randomized prospective clinical trial [58] in which women with preterm labor and intact membranes (25 to 33 6/7 weeks) were allocated to either observation or IM administration of 341 mg of 17-OHPC twice a week until 36 weeks of gestation or delivery was performed. Patients allocated to receive 17-OHPC had a longer sonographic cervical length than those in the observation group [58]; suggesting that progesterone may have major effects on the uterine cervix.

Fonseca et al. [246] reported the results of a randomized clinical trial evaluating the efficacy of vaginal progesterone in reducing the rate of preterm birth in women with a sonographic short cervix (≤15 mm by transvaginal ultrasound between 20 to 25 weeks of gestation). Women were allocated to daily vaginal administration of 200 mg of micronized progesterone or placebo (safflower oil) from 24 to 34 weeks. The frequency of spontaneous preterm delivery <34 weeks was significantly lower in the progesterone group than that in patients allocated to placebo (19.2% vs. 34.4%; $p=0.007$). A secondary analysis of this trial indicated that among women without a history of delivery <34 weeks, the incidence of preterm birth was significantly lower in women receiving progesterone than in those allocated to placebo (RR 0.57, 95% CI 0.35–0.93) suggesting that progesterone may be beneficial to patients with a sonographic short cervix even without a history of preterm birth.

The secondary retrospective analysis [274] of the study of O'Brien et al. [228] supports the findings of Fonseca et al. [246]—that patients with a short cervix may benefit from vaginal progesterone administration. However, the authors [274] reported that vaginal progesterone gel may have a beneficial effect in reducing preterm delivery <32 weeks of gestation at a sonographic cervical length of <28 mm [274]. These findings imply that the cutoff of 15 mm may be too stringent and progesterone may also work in women with a longer cervix. As the frequency of a cervix of ≤15 mm is 1.7% but that of <28 mm is about 10% [226,274], this could expand the therapeutic range of progesterone.

The study of De Franco et al. [274] provides the first hint that vaginal progesterone administration may improve infant outcome in properly selected patients. The frequency of NICU admission was lower in women with a cervical length of ≤30 mm and <28 mm and who had received progesterone treatment than in those allocated to placebo. The same was the case for the duration of NICU length of stay [274]. However, these conclusions must be considered tentative because they derive from a secondary analysis which is intended to be hypothesis-generating [275].

In contrast to the results in singleton gestations, the administration of progesterone for the prevention of preterm birth in twin gestation had no beneficial effect. Hartikainen-Sorri et al. [260] more than twenty-five years ago, and recently Rouse et al. [273] reported the results of a multicenter, placebo-controlled, double-blind, randomized clinical trials of 17-OHPC for prevention of preterm birth in twin pregnancies. Both studies concluded that there was no beneficial effect of 17-OHPC administration for the prevention of preterm birth in twin gestation.

7.2 Cerclage

Keeping with the view that cervical insufficiency is a mechanical disorder of the cervix, placement of a cervical stitch (cerclage) has been proposed as a treatment for this disorder. The clinical value of cervical cerclage has been subject of many observational and randomized clinical trials [239,240,244,276-298] and systematic reviews [299-301]. Yet controversies still exist regarding the subset of patients who will benefit from cerclage.

The current evidence suggests the following: (1) Women who are at low risk for preterm delivery (by history) and have a sonographic short cervix (≤15 mm) will not benefit from cerclage [240]. (2) The benefit of cerclage in women who have a high risk for preterm birth, both by history and a sonographic short cervix observed during the current pregnancy, is controversial [278,296,297,302,303]. However, a recent randomize clinical trial conducted by the NICHD MFM network among patients with a prior preterm birth <34 weeks of gestation. Patients with a cervical length <25 mm randomly assigned to cerclage reported a beneficial effect of cerclage. This benefit was highly concentrated in women with very short cervical length (<15 mm) [304]. (3) Among patients at risk for preterm delivery, serial sonographic examinations of the cervix followed by cerclage in those who shortened the cervix is a reasonable alternative to prophylactic placement of cerclage based upon uncontrolled studies [240,295,305]. (4) The role of prophylactic cerclage in high-risk patients without a sonographic short cervix for the prevention of preterm delivery/midtrimester abortion (by history) is unclear [276-278,294,306]. (5) In one trial, emergency cerclage combined with indomethacin administration appeared to reduce the rate of preterm delivery in patients with the clinical presentation of "cervical insufficiency" [298]. This evidence indicates that only patients with the clinical presentation of "acute cervical insufficiency" and those with a previous history consistent with "cervical insufficiency" and progressive shortening of the cervix demonstrated by ultrasound may benefit from cerclage placement.

The inflammatory status of the endocervix may be an additional criterion to identify those patients that could benefit from cerclage placement and those for whom this intervention may be harmful [245].

8. Summary

Preterm birth is a syndrome and a clinical end point of many underlying pathologies. The recent years have shown changes in the epidemiology of preterm birth with more emphasis on late preterm birth after 34 weeks, indicated preterm birth and increased contribution of pregnancies conceived by assisted reproduction. The available tools to predict and prevent preterm birth are limited, yet they may be suitable for a specific subset of patients. A better understanding of the underlying mechanism leading to preterm birth will facilitate tailoring future diagnostic and prediction modalities as well as more successful treatments.

References

[1]   Goldenberg RL, Culhane JF, Iams JD, Romero R. Epidemiology and causes of preterm birth. *Lancet* 2008; 371(9606):75-84.

[2]   Nardi O, Zureik M, Courbon D, Ducimetiere P, Clavel-Chapelon F. Preterm delivery of a first child and subsequent mothers' risk of ischaemic heart disease: a nested case-control study. *Eur J Cardiovasc Prev Rehabil* 2006; 13(2):281-283.

[3]   Smith GC, Pell JP, Walsh D. Pregnancy complications and maternal risk of ischaemic heart disease: a retrospective cohort study of 129,290 births. *Lancet* 2001; 357(9273):2002-2006.

[4]   Moster D, Lie RT, Markestad T. Long-term medical and social consequences of preterm birth. *N Engl J Med* 2008; 359(3):262-273.

[5]   Mazaki-Tovi S, Romero R, Kusanovic JP, Erez O, Pineles BL, Gotsch F et al. Recurrent preterm birth. *Semin Perinatol* 2007; 31(3):142-158.

[6]   Romero R, Mazor M, Munoz H, Gomez R, Galasso M, Sherer DM. The preterm labor syndrome. *Ann N Y Acad Sci* 1994; 734:414-429.

[7]   Martin JA, Hamilton BE, Sutton PD, Ventura SJ, Menacker F, Kirmeyer S et al. Births: Final Data for 2006. *Natl Vital Stat Rep* 2009; 57(7):1-121.

[8]   Slattery MM, Morrison JJ. Preterm delivery. *Lancet* 2002; 360(9344):1489-1497.

[9]   Martin JA, Hamilton BE, Sutton PD, Ventura SJ, Menacker F, Kirmeyer S et al. Births: Final Data for 2005. *Natl Vital Stat Rep* 2007; 56(6):1-104.

[10]   Martin JA, Hamilton BE, Sutton PD, Ventura SJ, Menacker F, Munson ML. Births: Final Data for 2003. *Natl Vital Stat Rep* 2005; 54(2):1-116.

[11]   PRAMS and Preterm Delivery Fact Sheet. http://www.cdc.gov/reproductivehealth/ products&pubs/PDFs/Preterm%20Delivery%20FS pdf [2006

[12]   Mercer BM. Preterm premature rupture of the membranes. *Obstet Gynecol* 2003; 101(1):178-193.

[13] Meis P, Ernest J, Moore M, Michielutte R, Sharp P, Buescher PA. Regional program for prevention of premature birth in northwestern North Carolina. *American Journal of Obstetrics & Gynecology* 1987; 157(3):550-556.

[14] Meis PJ, Michielutte R, Peters TJ, Wells HB, Sands RE, Coles EC et al. Factors associated with preterm birth in Cardiff, Wales. II. Indicated and spontaneous preterm birth. *Am J Obstet Gynecol* 1995; 173(2):597-602.

[15] Meis PJ, Goldenberg RL, Mercer BM, Iams JD, Moawad AH, Miodovnik M et al. The preterm prediction study: risk factors for indicated preterm births. Maternal-Fetal Medicine Units Network of the National Institute of Child Health and Human Development. *Am J Obstet Gynecol* 1998; 178(3):562-567.

[16] McElrath TF, Hecht JL, Dammann O, Boggess K, Onderdonk A, Markenson G et al. Pregnancy disorders that lead to delivery before the 28th week of gestation: an epidemiologic approach to classification. *Am J Epidemiol* 2008; 168(9):980-989.

[17] Ananth CV, Getahun D, Peltier MR, Salihu HM, Vintzileos AM. Recurrence of spontaneous versus medically indicated preterm birth. *Am J Obstet Gynecol* 2006; 195(3):643-650.

[18] Ananth CV, Vintzileos AM. Maternal-fetal conditions necessitating a medical intervention resulting in preterm birth. *Am J Obstet Gynecol* 2006; 195(6):1557-1563.

[19] Ananth CV, Vintzileos AM. Epidemiology of preterm birth and its clinical subtypes. *J Matern Fetal Neonatal Med* 2006; 19(12):773-782.

[20] Preterm singleton births—United States, 1989–1996. *MMWR Morb Mortal Wkly Rep* 1999; 48(9):185-189.

[21] Joseph KS, Kramer MS, Marcoux S, Ohlsson A, Wen SW, Allen A et al. Determinants of preterm birth rates in Canada from 1981 through 1983 and from 1992 through 1994. *N Engl J Med* 1998; 339(20):1434-1439.

[22] Vintzileos AM, Ananth CV, Smulian JC, Scorza WE, Knuppel RA. The impact of prenatal care in the United States on preterm births in the presence and absence of antenatal high-risk conditions. *Am J Obstet Gynecol* 2002; 187(5):1254-1257.

[23] Romero R, Espinoza J, Mazor M, Chaiworapongsa T. The preterm parturition syndrome. In: Critchely H, Bennett P, Thornton S, editors. *Preterm Birth*. London: RCOG Press; 2004. 28-60.

[24] Romero R, Sepulveda W, Baumann P, Yoon BH, Brandt F, Gomez R et al. The preterm labor syndrome: Biochemical, cytologic, immunologic, pathologic, microbiologic, and clinical evidence that preterm labor is a heterogeneous disease. *Am J.Obstet.Gynecol.* 168, 288. 1993. Ref Type: Abstract

[25] Romero R. The child is the father of the man. *Prenat Neonat Med* 1996; 1:8-11.

[26] Romero R, Athayde N, Maymon E, Pacora P, Bahado-Singh R. Premature rupture of the membranes. In: Reece A, Hobbins J, editors. *Medicine of the Fetus and Mother*. Philadelphia: JB Lippincott; 1998. 1581-1625.

[27] Mercer BM, Goldenberg RL, Das A, Moawad AH, Iams JD, MPJ et al. The Preterm Prediction Study: A clinical risk assessment system. *American Journal of Obstetrics & Gynecology* 1996; 174(6):1885-1895.

[28] Goldenberg RL, Iams JD, Mercer BM, Meis PJ, Moawad AH, Copper RL et al. The preterm prediction study: the value of new vs standard risk factors in predicting early

and all spontaneous preterm births. NICHD MFMU Network. *Am J Public Health* 1998; 88(2):233-238.

[29] Mercer BM, Goldenberg RL, Moawad AH, Meis PJ, Iams JD, Das AF et al. The preterm prediction study: effect of gestational age and cause of preterm birth on subsequent obstetric outcome. National Institute of Child Health and Human Development Maternal-Fetal Medicine Units Network. *Am J Obstet Gynecol* 1999; 181(5 Pt 1):1216-1221.

[30] Ananth CV, Joseph KS, Oyelese Y, Demissie K, Vintzileos AM. Trends in preterm birth and perinatal mortality among singletons: United States, 1989 through 2000. *Obstet Gynecol* 2005; 105(5 Pt 1):1084-1091.

[31] Ladfors L, Mattsson LA, Eriksson M, Milsom I. Prevalence and risk factors for prelabor rupture of the membranes (PROM) at or near-term in an urban Swedish population. *J Perinat Med* 2000; 28(6):491-496.

[32] Harger JH, Hsing AW, Tuomala RE, Gibbs RS, Mead PB, Eschenbach DA et al. Risk factors for preterm premature rupture of fetal membranes: a multicenter case-control study. *Am J Obstet Gynecol* 1990; 163(1 Pt 1):130-137.

[33] Spinillo A, Nicola S, Piazzi G, Ghazal K, Colonna L, Baltaro F. Epidemiological correlates of preterm premature rupture of membranes. *Int J Gynaecol Obstet* 1994; 47(1):7-15.

[34] Mercer BM, Goldenberg RL, Meis PJ, Moawad AH, Shellhaas C, Das A et al. The Preterm Prediction Study: prediction of preterm premature rupture of membranes through clinical findings and ancillary testing. The National Institute of Child Health and Human Development Maternal-Fetal Medicine Units Network. *Am J Obstet Gynecol* 2000; 183(3):738-745.

[35] Shiono P, Klebanoff M, Nugent R, Cotch M, Wilkins D, Rollins D et al. The impact of cocaine and marijuana use on low birth weight and preterm birth: A multicenter study. *American Journal of Obstetrics & Gynecology* 1995; 172(1):19-27.

[36] Iams JD, Goldenberg RL, Mercer BM, Moawad A, Thom E, Meis PJ et al. The Preterm Prediction Study: recurrence risk of spontaneous preterm birth. National Institute of Child Health and Human Development Maternal-Fetal Medicine Units Network. *Am J Obstet Gynecol* 1998; 178(5):1035-1040.

[37] Menard MK, Newman RB, Keenan A, Ebeling M. Prognostic significance of prior preterm twin delivery on subsequent singleton pregnancy. *Am J Obstet Gynecol* 1996; 174(5):1429-1432.

[38] Bloom SL, Yost NP, McIntire DD, Leveno KJ. Recurrence of preterm birth in singleton and twin pregnancies. *Obstet Gynecol* 2001; 98(3):379-385.

[39] Rydhstroem H. Gestational duration in the pregnancy after a preterm twin delivery. *Am J Obstet Gynecol* 1998; 178(1 Pt 1):136-139.

[40] Lee SE, Romero R, Park CW, Jun JK, Yoon BH. The frequency and significance of intraamniotic inflammation in patients with cervical insufficiency. *Am J Obstet Gynecol* 2008; 198(6):633-638.

[41] Kiwi R, Neuman MR, Merkatz IR, Selim MA, Lysikiewicz A. Determination of the elastic properties of the cervix. *Obstet Gynecol* 1988; 71(4):568-574.

[42] PAGE EW. Incompetent internal os of the cervix causing late abortion and premature labor; technic for surgical repair. *Obstet Gynecol* 1958; 12(5):509-515.

[43] Toaff R, Toaff ME, Ballas S, Ophir A. Cervical incompetence: diagnostic and therapeutic aspects. *Isr J Med Sci* 1977; 13(1):39-49.

[44] Zlatnik FJ, Burmeister LF, Feddersen DA, Brown RC. Radiologic appearance of the upper cervical canal in women with a history of premature delivery. II. Relationship to clinical presentation and to tests of cervical compliance. *J Reprod Med* 1989; 34(8):525-530.

[45] ACOG Practice Bulletin. Cervical insufficiency. *Obstet Gynecol* 2003; 102(5 Pt 1):1091-1099.

[46] Fliegner JR. Can anything be done about mid-trimester fetal wastage? *Aust N Z J Obstet Gynaecol* 1987; 27(3):205-209.

[47] Lidegaard O. Cervical incompetence and cerclage in Denmark 1980-1990. A register based epidemiological survey. *Acta Obstet Gynecol Scand* 1994; 73(1):35-38.

[48] Romero R, Espinoza J, Erez O, Hassan S. The role of cervical cerclage in obstetric practice: can the patient who could benefit from this procedure be identified? *Am J Obstet Gynecol* 2006; 194(1):1-9.

[49] Craig CJ. Congenital abnormalities of the uterus and foetal wastage. *S Afr Med J* 1973; 47(42):2000-2005.

[50] Levine RU, Berkowitz KM. Conservative management and pregnancy outcome in diethylstilbestrol-exposed women with and without gross genital tract abnormalities. *Am J Obstet Gynecol* 1993; 169(5):1125-1129.

[51] Ludmir J, Landon MB, Gabbe SG, Samuels P, Mennuti MT. Management of the diethylstilbestrol-exposed pregnant patient: a prospective study. *Am J Obstet Gynecol* 1987; 157(3):665-669.

[52] Mangan CE, Borow L, Burtnett-Rubin MM, Egan V, Giuntoli RL, Mikuta JJ. Pregnancy outcome in 98 women exposed to diethylstilbestrol in utero, their mothers, and unexposed siblings. *Obstet Gynecol* 1982; 59(3):315-319.

[53] Kristensen J, Langhoff-Roos J, Wittrup M, Bock JE. Cervical conization and preterm delivery/low birth weight. A systematic review of the literature. *Acta Obstet Gynecol Scand* 1993; 72(8):640-644.

[54] Moinian M, Andersch B. Does cervix conization increase the risk of complications in subsequent pregnancies? *Acta Obstet Gynecol Scand* 1982; 61(2):101-103.

[55] Raio L, Ghezzi F, Di NE, Gomez R, Luscher KP. Duration of pregnancy after carbon dioxide laser conization of the cervix: influence of cone height. *Obstet Gynecol* 1997; 90(6):978-982.

[56] Mays JK, Figueroa R, Shah J, Khakoo H, Kaminsky S, Tejani N. Amniocentesis for selection before rescue cerclage. *Obstet Gynecol* 2000; 95(5):652-655.

[57] Romero R, Gonzalez R, Sepulveda W, Brandt F, Ramirez M, Sorokin Y et al. Infection and labor. VIII. Microbial invasion of the amniotic cavity in patients with suspected cervical incompetence: prevalence and clinical significance. *Am J Obstet Gynecol* 1992; 167(4 Pt 1):1086-1091.

[58] Facchinetti F, Paganelli S, Comitini G, Dante G, Volpe A. Cervical length changes during preterm cervical ripening: effects of 17-alpha-hydroxyprogesterone caproate. *Am J Obstet Gynecol* 2007; 196(5):453-454.

[59] Sherman AI. Hormonal therapy for control of the incompetent os of pregnancy. *Obstet Gynecol* 1966; 28(2):198-205.

[60] Harger JH. Cervical cerclage: patient selection, morbidity, and success rates. *Clin Perinatol* 1983; 10(2):321-341.

[61] Iams JD, Johnson FF, Sonek J, Sachs L, Gebauer C, Samuels P. Cervical competence as a continuum: a study of ultrasonographic cervical length and obstetric performance. *Am J Obstet Gynecol* 1995; 172(4 Pt 1):1097-1103.

[62] Guzman ER, Mellon R, Vintzileos AM, Ananth CV, Walters C, Gipson K. Relationship between endocervical canal length between 15-24 weeks gestation and obstetric history. *J Matern Fetal Med* 1998; 7(6):269-272.

[63] Benedetti TJ, Valle R, Ledger WJ. Antepartum pneumonia in pregnancy. *Am J Obstet Gynecol* 1982; 144(4):413-417.

[64] Cunningham FG, Morris GB, Mickal A. Acute pyelonephritis of pregnancy: A clinical review. *Obstet Gynecol* 1973; 42(1):112-117.

[65] Fan YD, Pastorek JG, Miller JM, Jr., Mulvey J. Acute pyelonephritis in pregnancy. *Am J Perinatol* 1987; 4(4):324-326.

[66] Finland M, Dublin T.D. Pneumococcic pneumonia complicating pregnancy and the puerperium. *JAMA* 1939; 112:1027-1032.

[67] Gilles HM, Lawson JB, Sibelas M, Voller A, Allan N. Malaria, anaemia and pregnancy. *Ann Trop Med Parasitol* 1969; 63(2):245-263.

[68] Herd N, Jordan T. An investigtion of malaria during pregnancy in Zimbabwe. *Afr J Med* 1981; 27:62.

[69] Hibbard L, Thrupp L, Summeril S, Smale M, Adams R. Treatment of pyelonephritis in pregnancy. *Am J Obstet Gynecol* 1967; 98(5):609-615.

[70] Kass E. Maternal urinary tract infection. *NY State J Med* 1962; 1:2822-2826.

[71] Madinger NE, Greenspoon JS, Ellrodt AG. Pneumonia during pregnancy: has modern technology improved maternal and fetal outcome? *Am J Obstet Gynecol* 1989; 161(3):657-662.

[72] McLane CM. Pyelitis of pregnancy: a five-year study. *Am J Obstet Gynecol* 1939; 38:117.

[73] Oxhorn H. The changing aspects of pneumonia complicating pregnancy. *Am J Obstet Gynecol* 1955; 70:1057.

[74] Stevenson CS, Glasko A.J., Gillespie EC. Treatment of typhoid in pregnancy with chloramphenicol (chloromycetin). *JAMA* 1951; 146:1190.

[75] Wing ES, Troppoli D.V. The intrauterine transmission of typhoid. *JAMA* 1930; 95:405.

[76] Goncalves LF, Chaiworapongsa T, Romero R. Intrauterine infection and prematurity. *Ment Retard Dev Disabil Res Rev* 2002; 8(1):3-13.

[77] Minkoff H. Prematurity: infection as an etiologic factor. *Obstet Gynecol* 1983; 62(2):137-144.

[78] Romero R, Mazor M, Wu Y, Sirtori M, Oyarzun E, Mitchell M et al. Infection in the pathogenesis of preterm labor. *Seminars in Perinatology* 1988; 12(4):262-279.

[79] Romero R, Sirtori M, Oyarzun E, Avila C, Mazor M, Callahan R et al. Infection and labor. V. Prevalence, microbiology, and clinical significance of intraamniotic infection in women with preterm labor and intact membranes. *Am J Obstet Gynecol* 1989; 161(3):817-824.

[80] Bang B. The etiology of epizootic abortion. *J Comp Anthol Ther* 1987; 10:125.

[81] Fidel PL, Jr., Romero R, Wolf N, Cutright J, Ramirez M, Araneda H et al. Systemic and local cytokine profiles in endotoxin-induced preterm parturition in mice. *Am J Obstet Gynecol* 1994; 170(5 Pt 1):1467-1475.

[82] Kullander S. Fever and parturition. An experimental study in rabbits. *Acta Obstet Gynecol Scand Suppl* 1977;(66):77-85.

[83] McDuffie RS, Jr., Sherman MP, Gibbs RS. Amniotic fluid tumor necrosis factor-alpha and interleukin-1 in a rabbit model of bacterially induced preterm pregnancy loss. *Am J Obstet Gynecol* 1992; 167(6):1583-1588.

[84] McKay DG, Wong TC. The effect of bacterial endotoxin on the placenta of the rat. *Am J Pathol* 1963; 42:357-377.

[85] Rieder RF, Thomas L. Studies on the mechanisms involved in the production of abortion by endotoxin. *J Immunol* 1960; 84:189-193.

[86] Romero R, Munoz H, Gomez R, Ramirez M, Araneda H, Cutright J et al. Antibiotic therapy reduces the rate of infection-induced preterm delivery and perinatal mortality. *Am J.Obstet.Gynecol.* 170, 390. 1994. Ref Type: Abstract

[87] Skarnes RC, Harper MJ. Relationship between endotoxin-induced abortion and the synthesis of prostaglandin F. *Prostaglandins* 1972; 1(3):191-203.

[88] Takeda Y, Tsuchiya I. Studies on the pathological changes caused by the injection of the Shwartzman filtrate and the endotoxin into pregnant rabbits. *Jap J Exper Med* 1953; 21:9-16.

[89] Zahl PA, Bjerknes C. Induction of decidua-placental hemorrhage in mice by the endotoxins of certain gram-negative bacteria. *Proc Soc Exper Biol Med* 1943; 54:329-332.

[90] Gomez R, Ghezzi F, Romero R, Munoz H, Tolosa JE, Rojas I. Premature labor and intra-amniotic infection. Clinical aspects and role of the cytokines in diagnosis and pathophysiology. *Clin Perinatol* 1995; 22(2):281-342.

[91] Romero R, Salafia CM, Athanassiadis AP, Hanaoka S, Mazor M, Sepulveda W et al. The relationship between acute inflammatory lesions of the preterm placenta and amniotic fluid microbiology. *Am J Obstet Gynecol* 1992; 166(5):1382-1388.

[92] Romero R, Espinoza J, Chaiworapongsa T, Kalache K. Infection and prematurity and the role of preventive strategies. *Semin Neonatol* 2002; 7(4):259-274.

[93] Romero R, Mazor M. Infection and preterm labor. *Clin Obstet Gynecol* 1988; 31(3):553-584.

[94] Alanen A. Polymerase chain reaction in the detection of microbes in amniotic fluid. *Ann Med* 1998; 30(3):288-295.

[95] Hitti J, Riley DE, Krohn MA, Hillier SL, Agnew KJ, Krieger JN et al. Broad-spectrum bacterial rDNA polymerase chain reaction assay for detecting amniotic fluid infection among women in premature labor. *Clin Infect Dis* 1997; 24(6):1228-1232.

[96] Watts DH, Krohn MA, Hillier SL, Eschenbach DA. The association of occult amniotic fluid infection with gestational age and neonatal outcome among women in preterm labor. *Obstet Gynecol* 1992; 79(3):351-357.

[97] Romero R, Quintero R, Oyarzun E, Wu YK, Sabo V, Mazor M et al. Intraamniotic infection and the onset of labor in preterm premature rupture of the membranes. *Am J Obstet Gynecol* 1988; 159(3):661-666.

[98] Averbuch B, Mazor M, Shoham-Vardi I, Chaim W, Vardi H, Horowitz S et al. Intra-uterine infection in women with preterm premature rupture of membranes: maternal and neonatal characteristics. *Eur J Obstet Gynecol Reprod Biol* 1995; 62(1):25-29.

[99] Carroll SG, Papaioannou S, Ntumazah IL, Philpott-Howard J, Nicolaides KH. Lower genital tract swabs in the prediction of intrauterine infection in preterm prelabour rupture of the membranes. *Br J Obstet Gynaecol* 1996; 103(1):54-59.

[100] Cotton DB, Hill LM, Strassner HT, Platt LD, Ledger WJ. Use of amniocentesis in preterm gestation with ruptured membranes. *Obstet Gynecol* 1984; 63(1):38-43.

[101] Coultrip LL, Grossman JH. Evaluation of rapid diagnostic tests in the detection of microbial invasion of the amniotic cavity. *Am J Obstet Gynecol* 1992; 167(5):1231-1242.

[102] Garite TJ, Freeman RK, Linzey EM, Braly P. The use of amniocentesis in patients with premature rupture of membranes. *Obstet Gynecol* 1979; 54(2):226-230.

[103] Zlatnik FJ, Cruikshank DP, Petzold CR, Galask RP. Amniocentesis in the identification of inapparent infection in preterm patients with premature rupture of the membranes. *J Reprod Med* 1984; 29(9):656-660.

[104] Bujold E, Morency AM, Rallu F, Ferland S, Tetu A, Duperron L et al. Bacteriology of amniotic fluid in women with suspected cervical insufficiency. *J Obstet Gynaecol Can* 2008; 30(10):882-887.

[105] Romero R, Shamma F, Avila C, Jimenez C, Callahan R, Nores J et al. Infection and labor. VI. Prevalence, microbiology, and clinical significance of intraamniotic infection in twin gestations with preterm labor. *Am J Obstet Gynecol* 1990; 163(3):757-761.

[106] Romero R, Nores J, Mazor M, Sepulveda W, Oyarzun E, Parra M et al. Microbial invasion of the amniotic cavity during term labor. Prevalence and clinical significance. J Reprod Med 1993; 38(7):543-548.

[107] Leitich H, Bodner-Adler B, Brunbauer M, Kaider A, Egarter C, Husslein P. Bacterial vaginosis as a risk factor for preterm delivery: a meta-analysis. *Am J Obstet Gynecol* 2003; 189(1):139-147.

[108] Vidaeff AC, Ramin SM. From concept to practice: the recent history of preterm delivery prevention. Part II: Subclinical infection and hormonal effects. *Am J Perinatol* 2006; 23(2):75-84.

[109] Newton ER, Piper J, Peairs W. Bacterial vaginosis and intraamniotic infection. *Am J Obstet Gynecol* 1997; 176(3):672-677.

[110] Ralph SG, Rutherford AJ, Wilson JD. Influence of bacterial vaginosis on conception and miscarriage in the first trimester: cohort study. *BMJ* 1999; 319(7204):220-223.

[111] Llahi-Camp JM, Rai R, Ison C, Regan L, Taylor-Robinson D. Association of bacterial vaginosis with a history of second trimester miscarriage. *Hum Reprod* 1996; 11(7):1575-1578.

[112] Watts DH, Krohn MA, Hillier SL, Eschenbach DA. Bacterial vaginosis as a risk factor for post-cesarean endometritis. *Obstet Gynecol* 1990; 75(1):52-58.

[113] Watts DH, Eschenbach DA, Kenny GE. Early postpartum endometritis: the role of bacteria, genital mycoplasmas, and Chlamydia trachomatis. *Obstet Gynecol* 1989; 73(1):52-60.

[114] Chaim W, Mazor M, Leiberman JR. The relationship between bacterial vaginosis and preterm birth. A review. *Arch Gynecol Obstet* 1997; 259(2):51-58.

[115] McDonald HM, O'Loughlin JA, Vigneswaran R, Jolley PT, Harvey JA, Bof A et al. Impact of metronidazole therapy on preterm birth in women with bacterial vaginosis flora (Gardnerella vaginalis): a randomised, placebo controlled trial. *Br J Obstet Gynaecol* 1997; 104(12):1391-1397.

[116] Carey JC, Klebanoff MA, Hauth JC, Hillier SL, Thom EA, Ernest JM et al. Metronidazole to prevent preterm delivery in pregnant women with asymptomatic bacterial vaginosis. National Institute of Child Health and Human Development Network of Maternal-Fetal Medicine Units. *N Engl J Med* 2000; 342(8):534-540.

[117] Kekki M, Kurki T, Pelkonen J, Kurkinen-Raty M, Cacciatore B, Paavonen J. Vaginal clindamycin in preventing preterm birth and peripartal infections in asymptomatic women with bacterial vaginosis: a randomized, controlled trial. *Obstet Gynecol* 2001; 97(5 Pt 1):643-648.

[118] Ugwumadu A, Manyonda I, Reid F, Hay P. Effect of early oral clindamycin on late miscarriage and preterm delivery in asymptomatic women with abnormal vaginal flora and bacterial vaginosis: a randomised controlled trial. *Lancet* 2003; 361(9362):983-988.

[119] McDonald H, Brocklehurst P, Parsons J, Vigneswaran R. Antibiotics for treating bacterial vaginosis in pregnancy. *Cochrane Database Syst Rev* 2003;(2):CD000262.

[120] Guaschino S, Ricci E, Franchi M, Frate GD, Tibaldi C, Santo DD et al. Treatment of asymptomatic bacterial vaginosis to prevent pre-term delivery: a randomised trial. *Eur J Obstet Gynecol Reprod Biol* 2003; 110(2):149-152.

[121] Okun N, Gronau KA, Hannah ME. Antibiotics for bacterial vaginosis or Trichomonas vaginalis in pregnancy: a systematic review. *Obstet Gynecol* 2005; 105(4):857-868.

[122] Shennan A, Crawshaw S, Briley A, Hawken J, Seed P, Jones G et al. A randomised controlled trial of metronidazole for the prevention of preterm birth in women positive for cervicovaginal fetal fibronectin: the PREMET Study. *BJOG* 2006; 113(1):65-74.

[123] McDonald H, Brocklehurst P, Parsons J. Antibiotics for treating bacterial vaginosis in pregnancy. *Cochrane Database Syst Rev* 2005;(1):CD000262.

[124] McDonald HM, Brocklehurst P, Gordon A. Antibiotics for treating bacterial vaginosis in pregnancy. *Cochrane Database Syst Rev* 2007;(1):CD000262.

[125] Hoffman HJ, Bakketeig LS. Risk factors associated with the occurrence of preterm birth. *Clin Obstet Gynecol* 1984; 27(3):539-552.

[126] Roberts WE, Morrison JC, Hamer C, Wiser WL. The incidence of preterm labor and specific risk factors. *Obstet Gynecol* 1990; 76(1 Suppl):85S-89S.

[127] Heinonen KM, Jokela V. Multiple fetuses, growth deviations and mortality in a very preterm birth cohort. *J Perinat Med* 1994; 22(1):5-11.

[128] Imseis HM, Albert TA, Iams JD. Identifying twin gestations at low risk for preterm birth with a transvaginal ultrasonographic cervical measurement at 24 to 26 weeks' gestation. *Am J Obstet Gynecol* 1997; 177(5):1149-1155.

[129] Wennerholm UB, Holm B, Mattsby-Baltzer I, Nielsen T, Platz-Christensen J, Sundell G et al. Fetal fibronectin, endotoxin, bacterial vaginosis and cervical length as predictors of preterm birth and neonatal morbidity in twin pregnancies. *Br J Obstet Gynaecol* 1997; 104(12):1398-1404.

[130] Wright SP, Mitchell EA, Thompson JM, Clements MS, Ford RP, Stewart AW. Risk factors for preterm birth: a New Zealand study. *N Z Med J* 1998; 111(1058):14-16.

[131] Kiely JL. What is the population-based risk of preterm birth among twins and other multiples? *Clin Obstet Gynecol* 1998; 41(1):3-11.

[132] Newman RB. Obstetric management of high-order multiple pregnancies. *Baillieres Clin Obstet Gynaecol* 1998; 12(1):109-129.

[133] oseph KS, Allen AC, Dodds L, Vincer MJ, Armson BA. Causes and consequences of recent increases in preterm birth among twins. *Obstet Gynecol* 2001; 98(1):57-64.

[134] Ananth CV, Demissie K, Hanley ML. Birth weight discordancy and adverse perinatal outcomes among twin gestations in the United States: the effect of placental abruption. *Am J Obstet Gynecol* 2003; 188(4):954-960.

[135] Vintzileos AM, Ananth CV, Smulian JC, Scorza WE. The impact of prenatal care on preterm births among twin gestations in the United States, 1989-2000. Am J Obstet Gynecol 2003; 189(3):818-823.

[136] Blickstein I. Do multiple gestations raise the risk of cerebral palsy? *Clin Perinatol* 2004; 31(3):395-408.

[137] Elliott JP, Istwan NB, Collins A, Rhea D, Stanziano G. Indicated and non-indicated preterm delivery in twin gestations: impact on neonatal outcome and cost. *J Perinatol* 2005; 25(1):4-7.

[138] Ananth CV, Joseph KS, Demissie K, Vintzileos AM. Trends in twin preterm birth subtypes in the United States, 1989 through 2000: impact on perinatal mortality. *Am J Obstet Gynecol* 2005; 193(3 Pt 2):1076-1082.

[139] Gardner MO, Goldenberg RL, Cliver SP, Tucker JM, Nelson KG, Copper RL. The origin and outcome of preterm twin pregnancies. *Obstet Gynecol* 1995; 85(4):553-557.

[140] Wilcox L, Kiely J, Melvin C, Martin M. Assisted reproductive technologies: estimates of their contribution to multiple births and newborn hospital days in the United States. *Fertility and Sterility* 1996; 65(2):361-366.

[141] Martin JA, Hamilton BE, Ventura SJ, Menacker F, Park MM, SPD. Births: Final data for 2001. 51[2], 1-103. 2002. Hyattsville, Maryland: National Center for Health Statistics. Ref Type: Report

[142] Green NS. Risks of Birth Defects and Other Adverse Outcomes Associated With Assisted Reproductive Technology. *Pediatrics* 2004; 114(1):256-259.

[143] Jain T, Missmer SA, Hornstein MD. Trends in Embryo-Transfer Practice and in Outcomes of the Use of Assisted Reproductive Technology in the United States. *N Engl J Med* 2004; 350(16):1639-1645.

[144] Meis P, Michielutte R, Peters T, Wells H, Sands R, Coles E et al. Factors associated with preterm birth in Cardiff, Wales. *American Journal of Obstetrics and Gynecology* 1995; 173(2):597-602.

[145] Yang J, Hartmann KE, Savitz DA, Herring AH, Dole N, Olshan AF et al. Vaginal bleeding during pregnancy and preterm birth. *Am J Epidemiol* 2004; 160(2):118-125.

[146] Ekwo EE, Gosselink CA, Moawad A. Unfavorable outcome in penultimate pregnancy and premature rupture of membranes in successive pregnancy. *Obstet Gynecol* 1992; 80(2):166-172.

[147] Combs CA, Katz MA, Kitzmiller JL, Brescia RJ. Experimental preeclampsia produced by chronic constriction of the lower aorta: validation with longitudinal blood pressure measurements in conscious rhesus monkeys. *Am J Obstet Gynecol* 1993; 169(1):215-223.

[148] Kim YM, Bujold E, Chaiworapongsa T, Gomez R, Yoon BH, Thaler HT et al. Failure of physiologic transformation of the spiral arteries in patients with preterm labor and intact membranes. *Am J Obstet Gynecol* 2003; 189(4):1063-1069.

[149] Kim YM, Chaiworapongsa T, Gomez R, Bujold E, Yoon BH, Rotmensch S et al. Failure of physiologic transformation of the spiral arteries in the placental bed in preterm premature rupture of membranes. *Am J Obstet Gynecol* 2002; 187(5):1137-1142.

[150] Gomez R, Romero R, Nien JK, Medina L, Carstens M, Kim YM et al. Idiopathic vaginal bleeding during pregnancy as the only clinical manifestation of intrauterine infection. *J Matern Fetal Neonatal Med* 2005; 18(1):31-37.

[151] Chaiworapongsa T, Espinoza J, Yoshimatsu J, Kim YM, Bujold E, Edwin S et al. Activation of coagulation system in preterm labor and preterm premature rupture of membranes. *J Matern Fetal Neonatal Med* 2002; 11(6):368-373.

[152] Elovitz MA, Saunders T, Ascher-Landsberg J, Phillippe M. Effects of thrombin on myometrial contractions in vitro and in vivo. *Am J Obstet Gynecol* 2000; 183(4):799-804.

[153] Elovitz MA, Ascher-Landsberg J, Saunders T, Phillippe M. The mechanisms underlying the stimulatory effects of thrombin on myometrial smooth muscle. *Am J Obstet Gynecol* 2000; 183(3):674-681.

[154] Elovitz MA, Baron J, Phillippe M. The role of thrombin in preterm parturition. *Am J Obstet Gynecol* 2001; 185(5):1059-1063.

[155] Gomez R, Athayde N, Pacora P, Mazor M, Yoon BH, Romero R. Increased Thrombin in Intrauterine Inflammation. *Am J Obstet Gynecol* 1998; 178(1):S62.

[156] Ananth CV, Misra DP, Demissie K, Smulian JC. Rates of preterm delivery among Black women and White women in the United States over two decades: an age-period-cohort analysis. *Am J Epidemiol* 2001; 154(7):657-665.

[157] Kistka ZA, Palomar L, Lee KA, Boslaugh SE, Wangler MF, Cole FS et al. Racial disparity in the frequency of recurrence of preterm birth. *Am J Obstet Gynecol* 2007; 196(2):131-136.

[158] Palomar L, DeFranco EA, Lee KA, Allsworth JE, Muglia LJ. Paternal race is a risk factor for preterm birth. *Am J Obstet Gynecol* 2007; 197(2):152-157.

[159] Brady E. Hamilton, PhD, Joyce A. Martin, MPH, and Stephanie J. Ventura, MA. Birth: Preliminary Data for 2006. 12-5-2007. CDC. National Vital Statistic Reports. Ref Type: Report

[160] Adams MM, Read JA, Rawlings JS, Harlass FB, Sarno AP, Rhodes PH. Preterm delivery among black and white enlisted women in the United States Army. *Obstet Gynecol* 1993; 81(1):65-71.

[161] Meis PJ, Ernest JM, Moore ML. Causes of low birth weight births in public and private patients. *Am J Obstet Gynecol* 1987; 156(5):1165-1168.

[162] Brown HL, Chireau MV, Jallah Y, Howard D. The "Hispanic paradox": an investigation of racial disparity in pregnancy outcomes at a tertiary care medical center. *Am J Obstet Gynecol* 2007; 197(2):197.

[163] Wong LF, Caughey AB, Nakagawa S, Kaimal AJ, Tran SH, Cheng YW. Perinatal outcomes among different Asian-American subgroups. *Am J Obstet Gynecol* 2008; 199(4):382-386.

[164] Zeitlin J, Bucourt M, Rivera L, Topuz B, Papiernik E. Preterm birth and maternal country of birth in a French district with a multiethnic population. *BJOG* 2004; 111(8):849-855.

[165] Aveyard P, Cheng KK, Manaseki S, Gardosi J. The risk of preterm delivery in women from different ethnic groups. *BJOG* 2002; 109(8):894-899.

[166] Craig ED, Mantell CD, Ekeroma AJ, Stewart AW, Mitchell EA. Ethnicity and birth outcome: New Zealand trends 1980-2001. Part 1. Introduction, methods, results and overview. *Aust N Z J Obstet Gynaecol* 2004; 44(6):530-536.

[167] Leung TN, Roach VJ, Lau TK. Incidence of preterm delivery in Hong Kong Chinese. *Aust N Z J Obstet Gynaecol* 1998; 38(2):138-141.

[168] Melamed Y, Bashiri A, Shoham-Vardi I, Furman B, Hackmon-Ram R, Mazor M. Differences in preterm delivery rates and outcomes in Jews and Bedouins in Southern Israel. *Eur J Obstet Gynecol Reprod Biol* 2000; 93(1):41-46.

[169] Segal S, Gemer O, Yaniv M. The outcome of pregnancy in an immigrant Ethiopian population in Israel. *Arch Gynecol Obstet* 1996; 258(1):43-46.

[170] Simhan HN, Krohn MA. Paternal race and preterm birth. *Am J Obstet Gynecol* 2008; 198(6):644-646.

[171] Lu MC, Chen B. Racial and ethnic disparities in preterm birth: the role of stressful life events. *Am J Obstet Gynecol* 2004; 191(3):691-699.

[172] Dole N, Savitz DA, Siega-Riz AM, Hertz-Picciotto I, McMahon MJ, Buekens P. Psychosocial factors and preterm birth among African American and White women in central North Carolina. *Am J Public Health* 2004; 94(8):1358-1365.

[173] Stein AL, March CM. Pregnancy outcome in women with mullerian duct anomalies. *J Reprod Med* 1990; 35(4):411-414.

[174] Rackow BW, Arici A. Reproductive performance of women with mullerian anomalies. *Curr Opin Obstet Gynecol* 2007; 19(3):229-237.

[175] Erez O, Dukler D, Novack L, Rozen A, Zolotnik L, Bashiri A et al. Trial of labor and vaginal birth after cesarean section in patients with uterine Mullerian anomalies: a population-based study. *Am J Obstet Gynecol* 2007; 196(6):537-11.

[176] Raga F, Bauset C, Remohi J, Bonilla-Musoles F, Simon C, Pellicer A. Reproductive impact of congenital Mullerian anomalies. *Hum Reprod* 1997; 12(10):2277-2281.

[177] Barnes DL, Adair LS, Popkin BM. Women's physical activity and pregnancy outcome: a longitudinal analysis from the Philippines. *Int J Epidemiol* 1991; 20(1):162-172.

[178] Croteau A, Marcoux S, Brisson C. Work activity in pregnancy, preventive measures, and the risk of preterm delivery. *Am J Epidemiol* 2007; 166(8):951-965.

[179] Saurel-Cubizolles MJ, Subtil D, Kaminski M. Is preterm delivery still related to physical working conditions in pregnancy? *J Epidemiol Community Health* 1991; 45(1):29-34.

[180] Klebanoff MA, Shiono PH, Carey JC. The effect of physical activity during pregnancy on preterm delivery and birth weight. *Am J Obstet Gynecol* 1990; 163(5 Pt 1):1450-1456.

[181] Ortayli N, Ozugurlu M, Gokcay G. Female health workers: an obstetric risk group. *Int J Gynaecol Obstet* 1996; 54(3):263-270.

[182] Meyer JD, Warren N, Reisine S. Job control, substantive complexity, and risk for low birth weight and preterm delivery: an analysis from a state birth registry. *Am J Ind Med* 2007; 50(9):664-675.

[183] Reagan PB, Salsberry PJ. Race and ethnic differences in determinants of preterm birth in the USA: broadening the social context. *Soc Sci Med* 2005; 60(10):2217-2228.

[184] Hourani L, Hilton S. Occupational and environmental exposure correlates of adverse live-birth outcomes among 1032 US Navy women. *J Occup Environ Med* 2000; 42(12):1156-1165.

[185] Auger N, Luo ZC, Platt RW, Daniel M. Do mother's education and foreign born status interact to influence birth outcomes? Clarifying the epidemiological paradox and the healthy migrant effect. *J Epidemiol Community Health* 2008; 62(5):402-409.

[186] Grjibovski A, Bygren LO, Svartbo B. Socio-demographic determinants of poor infant outcome in north-west Russia. *Paediatr Perinat Epidemiol* 2002; 16(3):255-262.

[187] Parker JD, Schoendorf KC, Kiely JL. Associations between measures of socioeconomic status and low birth weight, small for gestational age, and premature delivery in the United States. *Ann Epidemiol* 1994; 4(4):271-278.

[188] Savitz DA, Kaufman JS, Dole N, Siega-Riz AM, Thorp JM, Jr., Kaczor DT. Poverty, education, race, and pregnancy outcome. *Ethn Dis* 2004; 14(3):322-329.

[189] Morgen CS, Bjork C, Andersen PK, Mortensen LH, Nybo Andersen AM. Socioeconomic position and the risk of preterm birth--a study within the Danish National Birth Cohort. *Int J Epidemiol* 2008; 37(5):1109-1120.

[190] Neonatal and perinatal mortality: Country, Regional, and Global Estimate. WHO Press; 2006.

[191] Health, United States, 2004 with Chartbook on Trends in the Health of Americans. 12-2-2004. Hyattsville, Maryland, National Center for Health Statistics. Ref Type: Report

[192] Fanaroff AA, Hack M, Walsh MC. The NICHD neonatal research network: changes in practice and outcomes during the first 15 years. *Seminars in Perinatology* 2003; 27(4):281-287.

[193]   (193)   Draper ES, Manktelow B, Field DJ, James D. Prediction of survival for preterm births by weight and gestational age: retrospective population based study. *BMJ* 1999; 319(7217):1093-1097.

[194] Gibson AT. Outcome following preterm birth. *Best Pract Res Clin Obstet Gynaecol* 2007; 21(5):869-882.

[195] Cartlidge PH, Stewart JH. Survival of very low birthweight and very preterm infants in a geographically defined population. *Acta Paediatr* 1997; 86(1):105-110.

[196] Bohin S, Draper ES, Field DJ. Impact of extremely immature infants on neonatal services. *Arch Dis Child Fetal Neonatal Ed* 1996; 74(2):F110-F113.

[197] Hagan R, Benninger H, Chiffings D, Evans S, French N. Very preterm birth—a regional study. Part 2: The very preterm infant. *Br J Obstet Gynaecol* 1996; 103(3):239-245.

[198] Tyson J, Younes N, Verter J, et al. Viability, morbidity, and resource use among newborns of 501- to 800-g birth weight. *JAMA* 1996; 276:1645-1651.

[199] Barton L, Hodgman J, Pavlova Z. Causes of death in the extremely low birth weight infant. *Pediatrics* 1999; 102:446-451.

[200] Effer SB, Moutquin JM, Farine D, Saigal S, Nimrod C, Kelly E et al. Neonatal survival rates in 860 singleton live births at 24 and 25 weeks gestational age. A Canadian multicentre study. *BJOG* 2002; 109(7):740-745.

[201] Bottoms SF, Paul RH, Iams JD, Mercer BM, Thom EA, Roberts JM et al. Obstetric determinants of neonatal survival: influence of willingness to perform cesarean delivery on survival of extremely low-birth-weight infants. National Institute of Child Health and Human Development Network of Maternal-Fetal Medicine Units. *Am J Obstet Gynecol* 1997; 176(5):960-966.

[202] Shankaran S, Fanaroff A, Wright L, Stevenson D, Donovan E, Ehrenkranz R et al. Risk factors for early death among extremely low-birth-weight infants. *American Journal of Obstetrics and Gynecology* 2002; 186(4):796-802.

[203] Vohr BR, Wright LL, Dusick AM, Perritt R, Poole WK, Tyson JE et al. Center Differences and Outcomes of Extremely Low Birth Weight Infants. *Pediatrics* 2004; 113(4):781-789.

[204] Villar J, Abalos E, Carroli G, Giordano D, Wojdyla D, Piaggio G et al. Heterogeneity of Perinatal Outcomes in the Preterm Delivery Syndrome. *Obstet Gynecol* 2004; 104(1):78-87.

[205] Yoon BH, Kim CJ, Romero R, Jun JK, Park KH, Choi ST et al. Experimentally induced intrauterine infection causes fetal brain white matter lesions in rabbits. *Am J Obstet Gynecol* 1997; 177(4):797-802.

[206] Yoon BH, Jun JK, Romero R, Park KH, Gomez R, Choi JH et al. Amniotic fluid inflammatory cytokines (interleukin-6, interleukin-1beta, and tumor necrosis factor-alpha), neonatal brain white matter lesions, and cerebral palsy. *Am J Obstet Gynecol* 1997; 177(1):19-26.

[207] Yoon BH, Romero R, Kim CJ, Koo JN, Choe G, Syn HC et al. High expression of tumor necrosis factor-alpha and interleukin-6 in periventricular leukomalacia. *Am J Obstet Gynecol* 1997; 177(2):406-411.

[208] Yoon BH, Romero R, Park JS, Kim CJ, Kim SH, Choi JH et al. Fetal exposure to an intra-amniotic inflammation and the development of cerebral palsy at the age of three years. *Am J Obstet Gynecol* 2000; 182(3):675-681.

[209] Bozynski ME, Nelson MN, Genaze D, Rosati-Skertich C, Matalon TA, Vasan U et al. Cranial ultrasonography and the prediction of cerebral palsy in infants weighing less than or equal to 1200 grams at birth. *Dev Med Child Neurol* 1988; 30(3):342-348.

[210] Pinto-Martin JA, Riolo S, Cnaan A, Holzman C, Susser MW, Paneth N. Cranial ultrasound prediction of disabling and nondisabling cerebral palsy at age two in a low birth weight population. *Pediatrics* 1995; 95(2):249-254.

[211] Ment LR, Vohr B, Oh W, Scott DT, Allan WC, Westerveld M et al. Neurodevelopmental outcome at 36 months' corrected age of preterm infants in the Multicenter Indomethacin Intraventricular Hemorrhage Prevention Trial. *Pediatrics* 1996; 98(4 Pt 1):714-718.

[212] de Vries LS, Rademaker KJ, Groenendaal F, Eken P, van H, I, Vandertop WP et al. Correlation between neonatal cranial ultrasound, MRI in infancy and neurodevelopmental outcome in infants with a large intraventricular haemorrhage with or without unilateral parenchymal involvement. *Neuropediatrics* 1998; 29(4):180-188.

[213] Chiang MF, Arons RR, Flynn JT, Starren JB. Incidence of retinopathy of prematurity from 1996 to 2000: analysis of a comprehensive New York state patient database. *Ophthalmology* 2004; 111(7):1317-1325.

[214] Marlow N, Wolke D, Bracewell MA, Samara M, the EPICure Study Group. Neurologic and Developmental Disability at Six Years of Age after Extremely Preterm Birth. *N Engl J Med* 2005; 352(1):9-19.

[215] Cooke RW. Perinatal and postnatal factors in very preterm infants and subsequent cognitive and motor abilities. *Arch Dis Child Fetal Neonatal Ed* 2005; 90(1):F60-F63.

[216] Huddy CL, Johnson A, Hope PL. Educational and behavioural problems in babies of 32-35 weeks gestation. *Arch Dis Child Fetal Neonatal Ed* 2001; 85(1):F23-F28.

[217] Saigal S, Lambert M, Russ C, Hoult L. Self-esteem of adolescents who were born prematurely. *Pediatrics* 2002; 109(3):429-433.

[218] Khashu M, Narayanan M, Bhargava S, Osiovich H. Perinatal outcomes associated with preterm birth at 33 to 36 weeks' gestation: a population-based cohort study. *Pediatrics* 2009; 123(1):109-113.

[219] Shapiro-Mendoza CK, Tomashek KM, Kotelchuck M, Barfield W, Nannini A, Weiss J et al. Effect of late-preterm birth and maternal medical conditions on newborn morbidity risk. *Pediatrics* 2008; 121(2):e223-e232.

[220] Goldenberg RL, Iams JD, Mercer BM, Meis P, Moawad A, Das A et al. What we have learned about the predictors of preterm birth. Semin Perinatol 2003; 27(3):185-193.

[221] Leitich H, Kaider A. Fetal fibronectin--how useful is it in the prediction of preterm birth? *BJOG* 2003; 110 Suppl;%20:66-70.:66-70.

[222] Andersen HF, Nugent CE, Wanty SD, Hayashi RH. Prediction of risk for preterm delivery by ultrasonographic measurement of cervical length. *Am J Obstet Gynecol* 1990; 163(3):859-867.

[223] Taipale P, Hiilesmaa V. Sonographic measurement of uterine cervix at 18-22 weeks' gestation and the risk of preterm delivery. *Obstet Gynecol* 1998; 92(6):902-907.

[224] Heath VC, Southall TR, Souka AP, Elisseou A, Nicolaides KH. Cervical length at 23 weeks of gestation: prediction of spontaneous preterm delivery. *Ultrasound Obstet Gynecol* 1998; 12(5):312-317.

[225] Hassan SS, Romero R, Berry SM, Dang K, Blackwell SC, Treadwell MC et al. Patients with an ultrasonographic cervical length < or =15 mm have nearly a 50% risk of early spontaneous preterm delivery. *Am J Obstet Gynecol* 2000; 182(6):1458-1467.

[226] Iams JD, Goldenberg RL, Meis PJ, Mercer BM, Moawad A, Das A et al. The length of the cervix and the risk of spontaneous premature delivery. National Institute of Child Health and Human Development Maternal Fetal Medicine Unit Network. *N Engl J Med* 1996; 334(9):567-572.

[227] Owen J, Yost N, Berghella V, Thom E, Swain M, Dildy GA, III et al. Mid-trimester endovaginal sonography in women at high risk for spontaneous preterm birth. *JAMA* 2001; 19;286(11):1340-1348.

[228] O'Brien JM, Adair CD, Lewis DF, Hall DR, DeFranco EA, Fusey S et al. Progesterone vaginal gel for the reduction of recurrent preterm birth: primary results from a randomized, double-blind, placebo-controlled trial. *Ultrasound Obstet Gynecol* 2007; 30(5):687-696.

[229] Yemini M, Borenstein R, Dreazen E, Apelman Z, Mogilner BM, Kessler I et al. Prevention of premature labor by 17 alpha-hydroxyprogesterone caproate. *Am J Obstet Gynecol* 1985; 151(5):574-577.

[230] Johnson JW, Austin KL, Jones GS, Davis GH, King TM. Efficacy of 17alpha-hydroxyprogesterone caproate in the prevention of premature labor. N Engl J Med 1975; 293(14):675-680.

[231] Meis PJ, Klebanoff M, Thom E, Dombrowski MP, Sibai B, Moawad AII et al. Prevention of recurrent preterm delivery by 17 alpha-hydroxyprogesterone caproate. *N Engl J Med* 2003; 348(24):2379-2385.

[232] da Fonseca EB, Bittar RE, Carvalho MH, Zugaib M. Prophylactic administration of progesterone by vaginal suppository to reduce the incidence of spontaneous preterm birth in women at increased risk: a randomized placebo-controlled double-blind study. *Am J Obstet Gynecol* 2003; 188(2):419-424.

[233] Heath VC, Daskalakis G, Zagaliki A, Carvalho M, Nicolaides KH. Cervicovaginal fibronectin and cervical length at 23 weeks of gestation: relative risk of early preterm delivery. *BJOG* 2000; 107(10):1276-1281.

[234] Palma-Dias RS, Fonseca MM, Stein NR, Schmidt AP, Magalhaes JA. Relation of cervical length at 22-24 weeks of gestation to demographic characteristics and obstetric history. *Braz J Med Biol Res* 2004; 37(5):737-744.

[235] Gomez R, Romero R, Nien JK, Chaiworapongsa T, Medina L, Kim YM et al. A short cervix in women with preterm labor and intact membranes: a risk factor for microbial invasion of the amniotic cavity. *Am J Obstet Gynecol* 2005; 192(3):678-689.

[236] Hassan S, Romero R, Hendler I, Gomez R, Khalek N, Espinoza J et al. A sonographic short cervix as the only clinical manifestation of intra-amniotic infection. *J Perinat Med* 2006; 34(1):13-19.

[237] Alfirevic Z, len-Coward H, Molina F, Vinuesa CP, Nicolaides K. Targeted therapy for threatened preterm labor based on sonographic measurement of the cervical length: a randomized controlled trial. *Ultrasound Obstet Gynecol* 2007; 29(1):47-50.

[238] Kusanovic JP, Espinoza J, Romero R, Goncalves L, Nien JK, Soto E et al. Clinical significance of the presence of amniotic fluid 'sludge' in asymptomatic patients at high risk for spontaneous preterm delivery. Ultrasound Obstet Gynecol 2007.

[239] To MS, Palaniappan V, Skentou C, Gibb D, Nicolaides KH. Elective cerclage vs. ultrasound-indicated cerclage in high-risk pregnancies. *Ultrasound Obstet Gynecol* 2002; 19(5):475-477.

[240] To MS, Alfirevic Z, Heath VC, Cicero S, Cacho AM, Williamson PR et al. Cervical cerclage for prevention of preterm delivery in women with short cervix: randomised controlled trial. *Lancet* 2004; 363(9424):1849-1853.

[241] Gomez R, Romero R, Medina L, Nien JK, Chaiworapongsa T, Carstens M et al. Cervicovaginal fibronectin improves the prediction of preterm delivery based on sonographic cervical length in patients with preterm uterine contractions and intact membranes. *Am J Obstet Gynecol* 2005; 192(2):350-359.

[242] To MS, Skentou CA, Royston P, Yu CK, Nicolaides KH. Prediction of patient-specific risk of early preterm delivery using maternal history and sonographic measurement of cervical length: a population-based prospective study. *Ultrasound Obstet Gynecol* 2006; 27(4):362-367.

[243] Vaisbuch E, Romero R, Erez O, Kusanovic JP, Gotsch F, Mazaki-Tovi S et al. The clinical significance of early (< 20 weeks) versus late (20-24 weeks) detection of a sonographic short cervix in asymptomatic women. *Ultrasound Obstet Gynecol*. 32[3], 276. 2008. Ref Type: Abstract

[244] Althuisius S, Dekker G, Hummel P, Bekedam D, Kuik D, van GH. Cervical Incompetence Prevention Randomized Cerclage Trial (CIPRACT): effect of therapeutic cerclage with bed rest vs. bed rest only on cervical length. *Ultrasound Obstet Gynecol* 2002; 20(2):163-167.

[245] Sakai M, Shiozaki A, Tabata M, Sasaki Y, Yoneda S, Arai T et al. Evaluation of effectiveness of prophylactic cerclage of a short cervix according to interleukin-8 in cervical mucus. *Am J Obstet Gynecol* 2006; 194(1):14-19.

[246] Fonseca EB, Celik E, Parra M, Singh M, Nicolaides KH. Progesterone and the risk of preterm birth among women with a short cervix. *N Engl J Med* 2007; 357(5):462-469.

[247] Mercer BM, Miodovnik M, Thurnau GR, Goldenberg RL, Das AF, Ramsey RD et al. Antibiotic therapy for reduction of infant morbidity after preterm premature rupture of the membranes. A randomized controlled trial. National Institute of Child Health and Human Development Maternal-Fetal Medicine Units Network. *JAMA* 1997; 278(12):989-995.

[248] Kenyon SL, Taylor DJ, Tarnow-Mordi W. Broad-spectrum antibiotics for preterm, prelabour rupture of fetal membranes: the ORACLE I randomised trial. ORACLE Collaborative Group. *Lancet* 2001; 357(9261):979-988.

[249] Kenyon SL, Taylor DJ, Tarnow-Mordi W. Broad-spectrum antibiotics for spontaneous preterm labour: the ORACLE II randomised trial. ORACLE Collaborative Group. *Lancet* 2001; 357(9261):989-994.

[250] Kenyon S, Brocklehurst P, Jones D, Marlow N, Salt A, Taylor D. MRC ORACLE Children Study. Long term outcomes following prescription of antibiotics to pregnant women with either spontaneous preterm labour or preterm rupture of the membranes. *BMC Pregnancy Childbirth* 2008; 8:14.:14.

[251] Kenyon S, Pike K, Jones DR, Brocklehurst P, Marlow N, Salt A et al. Childhood outcomes after prescription of antibiotics to pregnant women with spontaneous preterm labour: 7-year follow-up of the Oracle II trial. *Lancet* 2008; 372(9646):1319-1327.

[252] Papiernik-Berkhauer E. Etude en double aveugle d'un medicament prevenant la survenue prematurée de l'accouchement chez des femmes 'a risque eleve' d'accouchement premature. Edition Schering, Serie IV, fiche 3. 1970. 65-68.

[253] Levine L. Habitual Abortion. A controlled Study of Progestational Therapy. *West J Surg Obstet Gynecol* 1964; 72:30-6.:30-36.

[254] Bishop PM, Richards NA, Doll R. Habitual abortion; prophylactic value of progesterone pellet implantation. *Br Med J* 1950; 2(4671):130-133.

[255] Bishop PM, Richards NA. Habitual abortion; further observations on the prophylactic value of progesterone pellet implantation. *Br Med J* 1952; 1(4752):244-246.

[256] Check JH, Chase JS, Nowroozi K, Wu CH, Adelson HG. Progesterone therapy to decrease first-trimester spontaneous abortions in previous aborters. *Int J Fertil* 1987; 32(3):192-193.

[257] Breart G, Lanfranchi M, Chavigny C, Rumeau-Rouquette C, Sureau C. A comparative study of the efficiency of hydroxyprogesterone caproate and of chlormadinone acetate in the prevention of premature labor. *Int J Gynaecol Obstet* 1979; 16(5):381-384.

[258] Tognoni G, Ferrario L, Inzalaco M, Crosignani PG. Progestagens in threatened abortion. *Lancet* 1980; 2(8206):1242-1243.

[259] Gerhard I, Gwinner B, Eggert-Kruse W, Runnebaum B. Double-blind controlled trial of progesterone substitution in threatened abortion. *Biol Res Pregnancy Perinatol* 1987; 8(1 1ST Half):26-34.

[260] Hartikainen-Sorri AL, Kauppila A, Tuimala R. Inefficacy of 17 alpha-hydroxyprogesterone caproate in the prevention of prematurity in twin pregnancy. *Obstet Gynecol* 1980; 56(6):692-695.

[261] Hauth JC, Gilstrap LC, III, Brekken AL, Hauth JM. The effect of 17 alpha-hydroxyprogesterone caproate on pregnancy outcome in an active-duty military population. *Am J Obstet Gynecol* 1983; 146(2):187-190.

[262] Daya S. Efficacy of progesterone support for pregnancy in women with recurrent miscarriage. A meta-analysis of controlled trials. *Br J Obstet Gynaecol* 1989; 96:275-280.

[263] Goldstein P, Berrier J, Rosen S, Sacks HS, Chalmers TC. A meta-analysis of randomized control trials of progestational agents in pregnancy. *Br J Obstet Gynaecol* 1989; 96(3):265-274.

[264] Keirse MJ. Progestogen administration in pregnancy may prevent preterm delivery. *Br J Obstet Gynaecol* 1990; 97(2):149-154.

[265] ACOG Committee Opinion. Use of progesterone to reduce preterm birth. *Obstet Gynecol* 2003; 102(5 Pt 1):1115-1116.

[266] Brancazio LR, Murtha AP, Heine RP. Prevention of recurrent preterm delivery by 17 alpha-hydroxyprogesterone caproate. *N Engl J Med* 2003; 349(11):1087-1088.

[267] Greene MF. Progesterone and preterm delivery--deja vu all over again. *N Engl J Med* 2003; 348(24):2453-2455.

[268] Sanchez-Ramos L, Kaunitz AM, Delke I. Progestational agents to prevent preterm birth: a meta-analysis of randomized controlled trials. *Obstet Gynecol* 2005; 105(2):273-279.

[269] Dodd JM, Crowther CA, Cincotta R, Flenady V, Robinson JS. Progesterone supplementation for preventing preterm birth: a systematic review and meta-analysis. *Acta Obstet Gynecol Scand* 2005; 84(6):526-533.

[270] Coomarasamy A, Thangaratinam S, Gee H, Khan KS. Progesterone for the prevention of preterm birth: a critical evaluation of evidence. *Eur J Obstet Gynecol Reprod Biol* 2006; 129(2):111-118.

[271] Mackenzie R, Walker M, Armson A, Hannah ME. Progesterone for the prevention of preterm birth among women at increased risk: a systematic review and meta-analysis of randomized controlled trials. *Am J Obstet Gynecol* 2006; 194(5):1234-1242.

[272] Dodd JM, Flenady V, Cincotta R, Crowther CA. Prenatal administration of progesterone for preventing preterm birth. *Cochrane Database Syst Rev* 2006;(1):CD004947.

[273] Rouse DJ, Caritis SN, Peaceman AM, Sciscione A, Thom EA, Spong CY et al. A trial of 17 alpha-hydroxyprogesterone caproate to prevent prematurity in twins. *N Engl J Med* 2007; 357(5):454-461.

[274] De Franco EA, O'Brien JM, Adair CD, Lewis DF, Hall DR, Fusey S et al. Vaginal progesterone is associated with a decrease in risk for early preterm birth and improved neonatal outcome in women with a short cervix: a secondary analysis from a randomized, double-blind, placebo-controlled trial. *Ultrasound Obstet Gynecol* 2007; 30(5):697-705.

[275] Klebanoff MA. Subgroup analysis in obstetrics clinical trials. *Am J Obstet Gynecol* 2007; 197(2):119-122.

[276] Lazar P, Gueguen S, Dreyfus J, Renaud R, Pontonnier G, Papiernik E. Multicentred controlled trial of cervical cerclage in women at moderate risk of preterm delivery. *Br J Obstet Gynaecol* 1984; 91(8):731-735.

[277] Final report of the Medical Research Council/Royal College of Obstetricians and Gynaecologists multicentre randomised trial of cervical cerclage. MRC/RCOG Working Party on Cervical Cerclage. *Br J Obstet Gynaecol* 1993; 100(6):516-523.

[278] Althuisius SM, Dekker GA, Hummel P, Bekedam DJ, van Geijn HP. Final results of the Cervical Incompetence Prevention Randomized Cerclage Trial (CIPRACT): therapeutic cerclage with bed rest versus bed rest alone. *Am J Obstet Gynecol* 2001; 185(5):1106-1112.

[279] Briggs RM, Thompson WB, Jr. Treatment of the incompetent cervix. *Obstet Gynecol* 1960; 16(4):414-418.

[280] Seppala M, Vara P. Cervical cerclage in the treatment of incompetent cervix. A retrospective analysis of the indications and results of 164 operations. *Acta Obstet Gynecol Scand* 1970; 49(4):343-346.

[281] Robboy MS. The management of cervical incompetence. UCLA experience with cerclage procedures. *Obstet Gynecol* 1973; 41(1):108-112.

[282] Crombleholme WR, Minkoff HL, Delke I, Schwarz RH. Cervical cerclage: an aggressive approach to threatened or recurrent pregnancy wastage. *Am J Obstet Gynecol* 1983; 146(2):168-174.

[283] Ayhan A, Mercan R, Tuncer ZS, Tuncer R, Kisnisci HA. Postconceptional cervical cerclage. *Int J Gynaecol Obstet* 1993; 42(3):243-246.

[284] Golan A, Wolman I, Arieli S, Barnan R, Sagi J, David MP. Cervical cerclage for the incompetent cervical os. Improving the fetal salvage rate. *J Reprod Med* 1995; 40(5):367-370.

[285] Olatunbosun OA, al Nuaim L, Turnell RW. Emergency cerclage compared with bed rest for advanced cervical dilatation in pregnancy. *Int Surg* 1995; 80(2):170-174.

[286] Guzman ER, Houlihan C, Vintzileos A, Ivan J, Benito C, Kappy K. The significance of transvaginal ultrasonographic evaluation of the cervix in women treated with emergency cerclage. *Am J Obstet Gynecol* 1996; 175(2):471-476.

[287] Berghella V, Daly SF, Tolosa JE, DiVito MM, Chalmers R, Garg N et al. Prediction of preterm delivery with transvaginal ultrasonography of the cervix in patients with high-risk pregnancies: does cerclage prevent prematurity? *Am J Obstet Gynecol* 1999; 181(4):809-815.

[288] Kurup M, Goldkrand JW. Cervical incompetence: elective, emergent, or urgent cerclage. *Am J Obstet Gynecol* 1999; 181(2):240-246.

[289] Novy MJ, Gupta A, Wothe DD, Gupta S, Kennedy KA, Gravett MG. Cervical cerclage in the second trimester of pregnancy: a historical cohort study. *Am J Obstet Gynecol* 2001; 184(7):1447-1454.

[290] Hassan SS, Romero R, Maymon E, Berry SM, Blackwell SC, Treadwell MC et al. Does cervical cerclage prevent preterm delivery in patients with a short cervix? *Am J Obstet Gynecol* 2001; 184(7):1325-1329.

[291] Guzman ER, Ananth CV. Cervical length and spontaneous prematurity: laying the foundation for future interventional randomized trials for the short cervix. *Ultrasound Obstet Gynecol* 2001; 18(3):195-199.

[292] Berghella V, Haas S, Chervoneva I, Hyslop T. Patients with prior second-trimester loss: prophylactic cerclage or serial transvaginal sonograms? *Am J Obstet Gynecol* 2002; 187(3):747-751.

[293] Odibo AO, Farrell C, Macones GA, Berghella V. Development of a scoring system for predicting the risk of preterm birth in women receiving cervical cerclage. *J Perinatol* 2003; 23(8):664-667.

[294] Rush RW, Isaacs S, McPherson K, Jones L, Chalmers I, Grant A. A randomized controlled trial of cervical cerclage in women at high risk of spontaneous preterm delivery. *Br J Obstet Gynaecol* 1984; 91(8):724-730.

[295] Guzman ER, Forster JK, Vintzileos AM, Ananth CV, Walters C, Gipson K. Pregnancy outcomes in women treated with elective versus ultrasound-indicated cervical cerclage. *Ultrasound Obstet Gynecol* 1998; 12(5):323-327.

[296] Berghella V, Odibo AO, Tolosa JE. Cerclage for prevention of preterm birth in women with a short cervix found on transvaginal ultrasound examination: a randomized trial. *Am J Obstet Gynecol* 2004; 191(4):1311-1317.

[297] Althuisius SM, Dekker GA, van Geijn HP, Bekedam DJ, Hummel P. Cervical incompetence prevention randomized cerclage trial (CIPRACT): study design and preliminary results. *Am J Obstet Gynecol* 2000; 183(4):823-829.

[298] Althuisius SM, Dekker GA, Hummel P, van Geijn HP. Cervical incompetence prevention randomized cerclage trial: emergency cerclage with bed rest versus bed rest alone. *Am J Obstet Gynecol* 2003; 189(4):907-910.

[299] Belej-Rak T, Okun N, Windrim R, Ross S, Hannah ME. Effectiveness of cervical cerclage for a sonographically shortened cervix: a systematic review and meta-analysis. *Am J Obstet Gynecol* 2003; 189(6):1679-1687.

[300] Drakeley AJ, Roberts D, Alfirevic Z. Cervical cerclage for prevention of preterm delivery: meta-analysis of randomized trials. *Obstet Gynecol* 2003; 102(3):621-627.

[301] Drakeley AJ, Roberts D, Alfirevic Z. Cervical stitch (cerclage) for preventing pregnancy loss in women. *Cochrane Database Syst Rev* 2003;(1):CD003253.

[302] Rust OA, Atlas RO, Reed J, van Gaalen J, Balducci J. Revisiting the short cervix detected by transvaginal ultrasound in the second trimester: why cerclage therapy may not help. *Am J Obstet Gynecol* 2001; 185(5):1098-1105.

[303] Rust OA, Atlas RO, Jones KJ, Benham BN, Balducci J. A randomized trial of cerclage versus no cerclage among patients with ultrasonographically detected second-trimester preterm dilatation of the internal os. *Am J Obstet Gynecol* 2000; 183(4):830-835.

[304] Owen J. Multicenter randomized trial of cerclage for preterm birth prevention in high-risk women with shorten mid-trimester cervical length. *Am.J.Obstet Gynecol* (199), s3. 2008. Ref Type: Abstract

[305] Higgins SP, Kornman LH, Bell RJ, Brennecke SP. Cervical surveillance as an alternative to elective cervical cerclage for pregnancy management of suspected cervical incompetence. *Aust N Z J Obstet Gynaecol* 2004; 44(3):228-232.

[306] Odibo AO, Elkousy M, Ural SH, Macones GA. Prevention of preterm birth by cervical cerclage compared with expectant management: a systematic review. *Obstet Gynecol Surv* 2003; 58(2):130-136.

In: Textbook of Perinatal Epidemiology
Editor: Eyal Sheiner, pp. 593-618

ISBN: 978-1-60741-648-7
© 2010 Nova Science Publishers, Inc.

Chapter XXVII

Genetic Epidemiology of Preterm Birth

Ramkumar Menon[*1-2] *and Digna R. Velez Edwards*[3]

Department of Epidemiology, Rollins School of Public Health, and the Department of
Obstetrics and Gynecology, Emory University, Atlanta, GA,[1] The Perinatal Research
Center, Nashville, TN, USA[2]
Deparment of Obstetrics and Gynecology, Vanderbilt Epidemiology Center, Vanderbilt
University Medical Center, Nashville, TN[3]

Definitions

- Epistasis: Gene-gene interactions or epistasis is the interaction of multiple genetic variants (usually at different loci) such that the net phenotypic effect of carrying more than one variant is different than would be predicted by simply combining the effects of each individual variant.
- Genome-wide association study (GWAS): GWAS is involves scanning genetic risk markers across the complete set of DNA or entire genome to find genetic variations associated with a particular disease.
- HapMap: Haplotypes are regions of DNA inherited together and HapMap is a consortium that describes the common patterns of human DNA sequence variation in four populations of the world (Chinese, Japanese, Yorubans and Caucasians of European ancestry).
- Linkage disequilibrium (LD): LD is a correlation between close by genetic variations such that the alleles at neighboring markers are associated within a

* For Correspondence: Ramkumar Menon, Ph.D., Associate Professor (Research), Department of Epidemiology, Rollins School of Public Health of Emory University, , 1518 Clifton Rd NE, Atlanta, GA 30322, rmenon3@emory.edu; Research Director, The Perinatal Research Center, Centennial Women's Hospital, 2300 Patterson Street, Nashville, TN 37203; Phone - 615 342 3917(Office) ; Fax-615 342 6541; Cell - 615 335 5564, E- Mail - fortunat@edge.net,

population more often than if they were unlinked. LD is normally seen between variants within the same chromosome.

- Single nucleotide polymorphisms: Single nucleotide polymorphisms (SNPs) are DNA variations that occur throughout the human genome and their frequency is expected to be >1% in the population. If they are more frequent in a specific disease phenotype than normal control population, they are likely associated with that disease.

Introduction

Preterm birth (below 37 weeks of gestation) is an important cause of perinatal mortality and morbidity with long-term adverse consequences for child health.[1-3] Children who were born preterm and with low birth weight (LBW, below 2500 grams) have higher rates of cerebral palsy, sensory deficits, learning disabilities, and respiratory illnesses compared to children born at term. The morbidity associated with preterm birth often extends to later life, resulting in enormous physical, psychological and economic costs.[4;5] The National Institute of Medicine report on prematurity (July 2006) indicates that 12.5% of babies are born preterm in the USA, totaling approximately half a million babies each year and care of these infants costs ~$26 billion/year in medical and social expenses.[6;7] Preterm birth rate continues to rise, increasing by as much as 30% during the last twenty-five years, despite advances in medical care.[8] There are two major classes of preterm birth; namely spontaneous (mostly unknown etiology) and indicated (known risk factors such as preeclampsia, multiple gestations, gestational diabetes etc). This chapter is focused on **spontaneous preterm birth (PTB)**.

Tremendous knowledge has been gained in the past decade regarding various etiological factors, pathophysiologic pathways, genetic and bio-markers associated with preterm birth. Studies have identified multiple risk factors associated with preterm birth that include but are not limited to socio-economic factors, psycho-social stressors, behavioral factors, maternal infection, prior history, race and genetics.[9-17] Nonetheless, the knowledge gained has not been translated into proper screening and effective intervention reflected by the non-decreasing rate of preterm birth.

Understanding of PTB is further complicated by racial disparity observed in PTB rate among various ethnic groups. In 2003, the rate for African Americans (AA) was 17.8 percent, while the rates were 10.5 percent for Asian and Pacific Islanders and 11.5 percent for Caucasians[18]. LBW remains twice as high for AA women as for Caucasian women. High rates of PTB among AA and LBW are the leading cause of excess infant mortality among AA compared to other ethnic groups in the US. These disparities cannot be fully explained by differences in socioeconomic conditions, access to care, or maternal behaviors, such as smoking or drug use.[7;8] Studies over the last 15 years have focused on elucidating individual risk factors associated with adverse birth outcomes and assessing their importance across racial subgroups, but have not led to elimination of the disparity.[19-25]

Factors Affecting Understanding of PTB

Spontaneous preterm birth (PTB) is a complex disease resulting from a biological response from multiple pathophysiologic pathways. The trigger that initiates each of these pathways is still unclear making intervention and prevention extremely difficult. This complexity is due in part to etiologic and pathophysiologic heterogeneity.[15] A generalized assessment of etiology and pathophysiology without considering individual's own risk factors such as genetic, epigenetics, socio-environmental, behavioral and combinations of risk factors (gene and environmental) has led to ambiguity in understanding and therefore providing proper intervention to prevent PTB.

Why Genetics?

Advances in the understanding of complex diseases have progressed greatly over the last decade due to recent progress in studies focused on genetic variations (polymorphisms) in the human genome.[25-27] These studies have been motivated by growing evidence indicating that familial or intergenerational factors influence PTB. This influence may reflect shared environmental factors or genetic factors, or both. The evidence for a genetic predisposition to PTB includes: 1) Twin studies supporting a genetic predisposition to PTB give heritability estimates ranging from almost 20% to almost 40%.[28;29] This estimated heritability is approximately the same as that traditionally reported for hypertension, a condition generally accepted to have a clear genetic component. 2) History of previous preterm delivery is one of the best outcome predictors for future PTB[26;28] 3) Observations that mothers who were preterm themselves or who have a sister who had a PTB have an increased risk of giving birth preterm.[30-33] 4) Data showing that ethnic disparity exists in the PTB rates in the US, regardless of the socio-economic status of mothers also supports a genetic component to PTB.[20;21] Although these data are individually inconclusive, taken together they strongly support a role for genetic variation in the etiology of PTB. Additional data suggesting a significant genetic component are the data collected on over 120,000 live births in the United Kingdom, where there is evidence of differential gestational periods among ethnic groups[34]. These data suggest that there is some innate difference among ethnic groups with respect to normal gestational age. In addition there is evidence that PTB is higher in Asians than Caucasians with an odds ratio (OR) of ~1.5, supporting previous studies.

How to Design and Conduct Genetic Association Studies

Technological revolution and development of sophisticated analytical methods and advances in the genomic research field such as the International HapMap consortium (http://www.hapmap.org)[35] make it possible to understand the genetic complexities in preterm birth. However, the success of any such research depends on how the studies are being designed and conducted, source and processing of samples etc. Feasibility of the study and necessary sample size and statistical power depend critically on the study design. It is important that all the available information about the disease/trait be used fully when decisions are made about the sampling schemes, sampling units, and analytical methods. Before detailing the analytical aspects we describe some fundamental aspects of study designs. This starts with the definition of the phenotype.

Phenotype Definition is the Key for a Successful Outcome of any Study

Definition by World Health Organization states preterm birth as birth before less than 37 completed weeks gestation.[1;36] This standard definition has been misinterpreted and misquoted in the literature. A review of literature documented the following terminologies used to describe this condition include; preterm birth, premature birth, preterm labor and delivery, prematurity, preterm premature labor, unexplained preterm labor, unexplained early delivery, unexplained spontaneous preterm labor, spontaneous preterm labor and delivery, spontaneous preterm birth, preterm premature rupture of the membranes and preterm birth, preterm prelabor rupture of the membranes, indicated preterm birth, and iatrogenic preterm birth. It is very hard to understand the phenotype studied in many of the published literature due this ambiguity in phenotype definition. Different definitions of the phenotype do lead to different results. Heterogeneities in complex disease such as preterm birth arise due to different clinical manifestations, differences in biological pathways leading to disease diagnosis and differences in severity of symptoms. Appropriate definition and description of the phenotype studied can avoid this dilemma. Preterm birth can be classified into three major groups namely; medically indicated (iatrogenic) preterm birth, spontaneous or idiopathic preterm birth (PTB) and preterm premature rupture of membranes (pPROM) leading to preterm birth. PTB can also be classified into 3 groups based on the gestational age at delivery, namely; mild preterm (32–37 weeks), moderate preterm (28–31 weeks) and very preterm (<28 weeks). We suggest that defining the phenotype is the key component before designing the studies.

Study Design

Genetic studies can employ classical epidemiological study designs such as cohort studies, case-control studies or cross sectional studies.[61]

Cohort studies: A genetic cohort study design to detect genetic markers of PTB will involve a group of pregnant women followed throughout their pregnancies. The risk factor characteristics of their pregnancies is monitored throughout the pregnancy and the outcome (preterm vs. term delivery) can be recorded.[37] Cohort studies can be conducted prospectively, although classical epidemiological studies use both prospective and retrospective models. Prospective studies allow the investigator to follow the natural case history through preclinical and clinical visits. Multiple disease outcomes such as pPROM, preeclampsia, gestational diabetes, placental insufficiency, fetal anomalies can be monitored during the course of study. Inclusion and exclusion criteria can be developed to create variables and confounders to be considered during analysis, providing homogeneity in studied subjects. In many cases putative risk factors can also be monitored before the onset of disease (e.g., bacterial vaginosis (BV) during first trimester). However, the state of biological specimens (e.g., amniotic fluid and blood samples) collected for genotype-phenotype comparisons may be affected by clinical treatment of the subjects.[38;39] Prospective cohort studies also reduce both the bias and confounding encountered in other study designs where status is assigned and data is collected retrospectively. Additional limitations include both the time and cost required to complete the study. The prevalence rate of PTB can greatly affect the amount of time it takes to collect enough subjects for analysis; as a result it can take several years to recruit enough subjects to provide sufficient power for PTB genetic associations given its incidence. Hence these studies can be very expensive.

Case-control studies: These are observational studies where cases are selected on the basis of an outcome variable and controls are normal or non-diseased individuals.[40-42] To date, most of the PTB genetic studies use a case-control design, often consisting of unrelated cases and controls although family trios may be used. In this retrospective study, cases and controls are well defined and all cases that validate the inclusion criteria by the investigating team can be included. Similarly, controls will be selected based on stringent inclusion criteria. Case-control studies are mostly retrospective and hence the time required for recruitment is relatively short (proper review of the subjects medical history is often sufficient).[42] It is important that the cases and controls are recruited from the same population as population stratification can produce spurious results.[43;44] Although only one outcome is typically considered in a case-control study, multiple risk factors can be ascertained based on the inclusion criteria. However, some of the advantages of cohort studies can be disadvantages for case-control design. Risk factors such as level of stress, dietary information, smoking and other behavioral changes, subclinical infections and BV during pregnancy provide some of the confounding variables that cannot always be known with a great deal of reliability, as determining risk factors retrospectively can suffer because of recall bias. In addition, biological specimens may be affected by environmental exposures for which data are impossible to collect as the critical variables occur prior to entry into the study. If confounders are identified and stratified properly for analysis, genetic associations and their effects on PTB phenotype can still be made with case-control designs. In those cases, where a larger cohort is available for multiple studies a nested case-control study can be created; this may be the ideal study, as it has most advantages of the cohort study (follow-up) design and those from the case-control study design.[45]

Cross-sectional studies: In this design study subjects are assessed at a single time during the study period.[37;42] Cross-sectional study subjects can be recruited from an ongoing cohort study. This will shorten recruitment time and cost of the study, i.e. the major limitations of cohort studies. However, this design is not popular in genetic epidemiological studies as it rarely identifies risk factors during selection and if these factors are identified, they may or may not be associated with disease.[37] For example, in PTB of unknown etiology, this design may not allow an investigator to perform an amniocentesis to identify intraamniotic infection (IAI). Signs of subclinical infection may not accurately identify IAI. It is unlikely that this design will associate disease and selected single nucleotide polymorphisms (SNP); however, carefully designed cross-sectional studies can provide pilot data by screening the population, giving ample information to design future cohort or case-control studies.

Family-based studies: Although a family-based study design is not considered to be a classical epidemiological ascertainment scheme (as family-based genetic study can technically be collected with a cohort or a cross-sectional design) in the field of genetics this is an important study design to consider given the heritability of the traits examined. The majority of PTB studies are performed on unrelated cases and controls. However, there are studies that look at family trios, multiplex families with more than one affected offspring, extended pedigrees with multiple generations, or sib-pairs. Statistical methods that measure association in pedigree data generally evaluate the relationship between the trait of interest and transmissions from parents to offspring. Thereby two possible designs are to ascertain parents and offspring from PTB events, scoring the offspring as cases, or to ascertain the mothers who deliver preterm and the maternal grandparents of the preterm offspring, scoring the mothers as cases. With the first approach, the effect is assumed to arise in the offspring of a PTB event, and is an early-onset trait. With the second, the effect is assumed to arise in the mother of a PTB event and is a late-onset trait. Ascertainment for late-onset traits might encounter higher rates of missing parents, which contribute substantially to power in pedigree-based association studies. As previously noted, these studies can follow many of the above mentioned epidemiological ascertainment schemes; therefore, in addition to considering the issue pertaining to family structure the previously described ascertainment schemes must also be applied to make it a sound genetic and epidemiological study.

We have not discussed some other designs (case only studies, cohort-case studies, etc.) as these are not likely to be as effective for genetic association studies in PTB.

Population stratification: Regardless of the study design, population stratification is another important factor to consider in the design of an association study, particularly with regard to the classification of individuals within subgroups and status groups. Population stratification is the differences in allele frequencies between cases and controls due to factors such as ancestry between individuals classified into a group. This can result in invalid associations of genes with disease. It can arise because of population admixture a sample consists of a mixture of subpopulations and/or distinct ancestral groups. This can greatly compromise the interpretability of one's results (e.g. analyzing data consisting of a combination of African-American and Caucasian samples can remove or add association signals from either population)[46]. This is a major source of spurious association even in the most well designed studies. For this reason care must be taken in grouping individuals into racial groups. If self-reported ethnicity is used, it is advisable to only include individuals within a given group if they can trace their ethnicity back two generations to their parents. An alternative approach is to use ancestry-informative markers, markers that have established allele frequency differences between different geographic populations. Using a group of these highly differentiated ancestry informative markers across the genome will help to estimate an individual's geographic origin. This, however, will come at additional costs given that these additional markers will need to be genotyped in addition to the markers being examined for association with disease.

Genetic Association Studies in Preterm Birth

Sample size and power: An appropriately designed genetic association study requires sample size and power calculations prior to beginning both ascertainment and genotyping to understand if there is enough data available or if more data must be obtained to allow for the detection of the trait of interest. Determining the appropriate sample size and power ensures that the study is powered to detect the subtle genetic effects expected for a complex disease such as PTB. Power analysis can be used to determine the sample size, marker allele frequencies, and density of markers that are required to detect an association with the trait of interest. This information should be obtained prior to sample collection to aid in developing strategies for sample ascertainment and collection and to determine the cost for an optimal study design. Software commonly used for determining power are based on the ascertainment schemes, outcome measurement, and the statistical test used to detect association (e.g. OR, relative risk, or slope of a regression line). The majority of PTB genetic association studies have been performed with a case-control study design and power can easily be computed using freely available software. Commonly, software to calculate power assumes the most simplistic genetic model of a single diallelic disease mutation that is tested for association. This may not be the ideal model for association every genetic study and other software is available that can allow for modeling of more complex disease phenotypes including the power to detect association in the presence of linkage disequilibrium (LD) between markers, the power to detect gene x gene or gene x environment interactions, and more complex study designs (e.g. trios or sib-pairs).

Calculating power: In a case-control PTB study, if samples are collected for both mother and fetus, they are treated as independent samples. For a case-control study design power can easily be calculated using several methods. One freely available software is Power and Sample Size Calculation (PS), developed by Dupont and Plummer.[47] For a retrospective case-control study power is parameterized in terms of the 1) type I error rate, 2) number of case patients, 3) the minimum minor allele frequency acceptable for any given marker, 4) the ratio of control to case patients, and 5) OR of exposure in cases relative to exposure in controls. For example, given a type I error rate of 0.05, 100 cases, a minimum minor allele frequency of 0.20, and a 1:1 ratio of cases to controls, power would be 57%; however, if power is plotted (Figure 1), it can be seen that increasing sample size to 150 cases and controls provide 80% power. This software can also be used if the study outcome is a normally distributed continuous measure, e.g. gestational age in weeks or amniotic fluid concentration cytokine levels.

Power studies for family data utilize a combination of simulations and analytical methods to determine power[48;49]. Often Monte Carlo simulations are used and power is calculated by simulating pedigrees under different genetic models and recombination rates between markers and disease loci; this, however, can be time consuming and other analytical approaches. Quanto, the method developed by Gauderman and Morrison (2006)[50], can be used to calculate power for case-siblings (each case is matched to one unaffected sibling) and family trios. Quanto can be used for power calculations for both binary and quantitative and gene x gene or gene x environment interactions. Quanto, in contrast to PS, computes the power for a given number of sampling units, where a sampling unit can be a sibling pair or a case-parent trio. For a simple log-additive genetic model, power to calculate a main effect for trio data is measured from the following parameter 1) outcome (disease or continuous), 2) hypothesis (gene only, gene x environment interaction, environment only, or gene x gene interaction), 3) allele frequency, 4) inheritance mode, 5) susceptibility frequency, 6) disease risk parameters (baseline/population risk, genetic effect), 7) sample size, and 8) type I error rate.

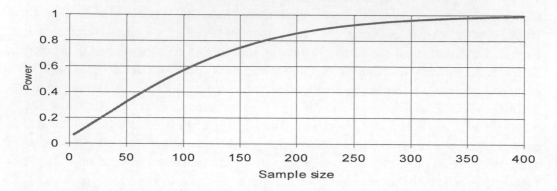

Figure 1. Power to detect association given a type I error rate of 0.05, 100 cases, a minimum minor allele frequency of 0.20, and a 1:1 ratio of cases to controls. Power is located on the y-axis and case sample size is located on the x-axis. This figure was created using PS software created by Dupont and Plummer.

Single Locus Associations and Analytical Strategies

Studies designed to identify genetic risk factors in PTB encounter all of the same problems faced by studies of any complex disease.[51] PTB does not follow a simple Mendelian mode of inheritance; this poses analytical challenges, since maternal, fetal, or both maternal and fetal genetic information may be related to PTB. For this reason, the birth event is treated as the outcome for all analyses performed (born less than <37 weeks gestation is preterm or >37 week gestation is full term) and the same status is assigned to both mother and baby. Treating the birth event as the outcome, rather than designating an affected individual, allows for more analytical approaches to be used to evaluate genetic risks.

Studies examining PTB have predominantly been performed using a case-control dyad study design where maternal and fetal genetic information are both collected, but analyzed as independent samples. Studies utilizing this approach are performed by comparing allele and/or genotype frequency between term and PTB, in both maternal and fetal data. The dyad case-control design has the advantage that it is not necessary to recruit fathers into the study. Ascertaining and recruiting fathers would increase expense substantially and thus reduce sample size, either due to financial constraints or unavailable fathers.

Trio and family-based study designs have also been performed, but analytical methods are more limited due to the ambiguous affection scoring of mothers and babies.

Single Locus Analysis on Case-Control Studies

Case-control studies on PTB are performed on maternal and fetal genetic data separately. Subjects are selected based on their status, where status can be defined as binary (preterm case or term control) or continuous (gestational age in weeks). Despite the increase in power gained by using a continuous outcome, gestational age is more commonly measured as a binary variable, as this simplifies interpretation of results and there is clinical evidence supporting these thresholds. Cases and controls must be appropriately matched for age and race as well as selected from the same inclusion and exclusion criteria; otherwise, these variables should be adjusted for in a linear model, which decreases statistical power.

Prior to performing single locus tests of association deviations from Hardy-Weinberg equilibrium (HWE) are examined in cases and controls for each marker examined. Tests for deviations from HWE tell you if a population adheres to expected distribution for a randomly mating population. HWE assumes: diploid organisms, equal allele frequencies in the sexes, no migration, no mutation, no selection, sexual reproduction, no overlapping generations, random mating, and a large population size.[52] The test looks for deviations from the following equation $1 = p^2 + 2pq + q^2$, where p and q are the frequencies of the major and minor allele, respectively. p^2 is the frequency of the homozygous major allele, 2pq is the frequency of the heterozygote, and q^2 is the frequency of the homozygous minor allele and the frequencies of all of the genotypes sum to 1. It is assumed that the control population adheres to HWE, but not cases as a deviation from HWE in cases can indicate the presence of an association. A significant deviation from HWE in controls for a given SNP most commonly can indicate the presence of genotyping error and as a result the marker is either dropped from the analysis or regenotyped.

Single marker analyses using a binary outcome are performed by comparing cases to controls with respect to the presence or absence of a particular allele or genotype using a chi-squared test. In this case the presence or absence of an allele or genotype is considered the exposure. The minor allele is usually assumed to be the risk allele. Analyses are stratified by both race and whether the samples are from mothers or babies. For single marker analyses of case-control binary outcome data the most common tests are chi-square, Fisher's exact test, Cochran Armitage trend test, and logistic regression. These tests can be used to assess association with alleles, genotypes, and genetic models, such as dominant, additive and recessive modes of inheritance. Alleles are usually coded for in a genetic model based on the presence or absence of the minor allele (e.g. the data would be coded 0 (homozygous major allele), 1 (heterozygous), 2 (homozygous minor allele) for an additive model in a logistic regression analysis). If single marker analyses are adjusted for potential confounding factors, (e.g. smoking, alcohol consumption, or other known risk factors) Mantel Haenzel chi-square analyses and logistic regression can be used.

There are two common ways to interpret an association in a genetic study. The association can be interpreted as a direct or indirect association (Figure 2). A direct association is observed if the marker analyzed directly leads to disease phenotype (Figure 2a). An indirect association results if an association is observed at a locus due to a more complex relationship between the marker and the phenotype (Figure 2b). Commonly when associations are observed at a marker, rather than indicating a direct casual relationship, the association is observed because the marker is in LD with the causal locus or environmental factor that directly cause the disease. LD is the nonrandom association of alleles at nearby loci (correlation). The human genome contains many areas of strong LD, which vary by ethnicity and local recombination rates, and these patterns should be considered when evaluating association results. Under these circumstances the locus of interest is in close proximity to the disease locus. For a large majority of studies the most common approach is to select markers that are in strong LD with several other markers in a gene. These markers are generally termed tag SNPs. A tag SNP approach allows for a few SNPs to provide coverage for a larger genetic area through strong correlations between the genotypes and ungenotyped markers. Understanding the LD structure of the data being examined is an important step in the analytical process for both case-control and family-based association studies. These patterns should be examined for differences between cases and controls and regions of low haplotype diversity, where a single direct association might result in several indirect significant test results. Causal relationships can be complicated and may involve interactions with other genes or environmental variables. A linear model is the most straightforward and interpretable statistical method to evaluate interactions; however, for searches without specific testable hypotheses, a data reduction method or machine learning algorithm may be more optimal.

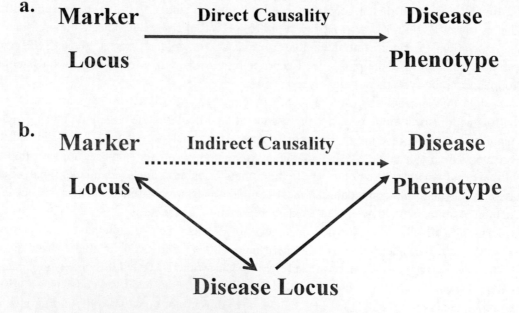

Figure 2. Direct and indirect associations. Dotted lines indicate indirect causality and solid lines indicate direct causality. A is an example of a direction association while b is an example of an indirect association (e.g. LD between the marker and the disease locus).

SNPs and their association with PTB have been studied extensively. A comprehensive list of case control studies done to understand genetic association can be found in review published by Plunkett and Muglia.[53]

Multilocus Interactions or Genetic Epistasis

Due to locus and allelic heterogeneities, researchers in the field have started to explore gene-gene interaction or genetic epistasis. Model free approaches have been developed due to the reality that complex diseases derive from multiple genetic and nongenetic determinants, including interactions between them. Genetic epistasis studies involve analysis of SNPs from multiple candidate genes selected from multitudes of pathophysiologic pathways and using statistical methods interaction between various SNPs are determined.

Multilocus Interaction Methodologies

Gene x gene (GXG) and gene x environmental (GXE) interactions have been proposed as potential factors contributing towards PTB risk, but development of analytical methods has been limited. These methods use a variety of approaches to analyze both maternal and fetal genetic data. The majority have been developed for case-control rather than trio study designs, where the child is termed the affected and both parents are collected, for the same statistical reasons that case-control study designs are preferred for single locus analyses. A discussion of these analytical approaches has been previously reviewed by Hoh and Ott (2003)[54]. These approaches to test for GXG and GXE interactions in case-control data include: 1) logistic regression; 2) Monte Carlo logic regression[55] ; 3) classification and regression trees; 4) classification and regression trees (CART) [56]; 5) the focused interaction testing framework (FITF)[57]; 6) patterning and recursive partitioning (PRP) [58]; 7) neural networks[59]; and 7) multifactor dimensionality reduction (MDR).[60] Extensions to the log-linear approach described by Wilcox et al[61] and Weinberg et al[40], an approach that tests for the overrepresentation of the inheritance of specific alleles, has been proposed, but has not been explored extensively for use with PTB data.

Multifactor Dimensionality Reduction (MDR)

MDR has been used recently in PTB and other traits, including psychiatric diseases, physiological conditions, and pathogen susceptibilities. Multilocus associations contributing to PTB can be searched for and detected using MDR.[60,62] MDR is a nonparametric approach, developed to detect epistatic interactions in the absence of main effects, that accepts case-control categorical and binary data.[60;62] Since MDR does not account for familial relationships, maternal and fetal data are analyzed separately to detect effects associated with either the maternal or fetal genome. It is also possible to use MDR for analysis of maternal-fetal interaction by searching through the maternal and fetal loci as if they represented different genomic sites. Thereby, interactions within mothers, within fetuses, and between mothers and fetus could be evaluated simultaneously, at the expense of some increased computation time and decreased statistical power due to multiple comparisons. Analysis of maternal-fetal interactions would involve the doubling of the dimensions of the MDR model. For example, if 27 loci were genotyped 54 dimensions would be assessed (27 from mother and 27 from fetus). Simulation studies, however, have not been performed examining the efficiency and validity of this approach.

The MDR algorithm functions as follows (Figure 3):

In the first step of MDR, the dataset is divided into multiple partitions for K-fold cross validation (CV)[60] and an exhaustive list of multilocus models is generated. CV mitigates the effect of overfitting models to the data. Overfitting is when a model fits a sample very well, but does not generalize to other independent samples. This is often the result of large searches when no procedure such as CV or bootstrapping is used. Five-fold CV rather than ten-fold CV is more commonly used as studies suggest that this is a powerful and computationally efficient approach to find multilocus associations [59]. In five-fold CV, the training set is comprised of 4/5 of the data, while the testing set is comprised of the remaining 1/5 of the data.

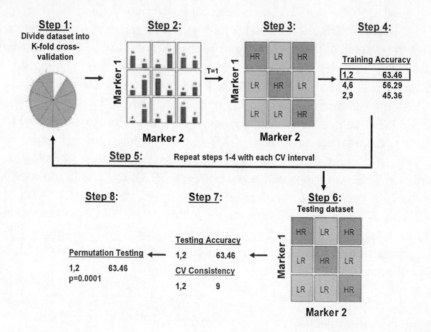

Figure 3. The Multifactor Dimensionality Reduction algorithm adapted from MDR algorithm Figure 1 published in Ritchie et al. 2001 *Am J Hum Genet*.

In step 2, MDR considers a multilocus combination of SNPs and calculates the ratio of cases to controls and genotypes or levels of variables are collapsed on the basis of the ratio of cases to controls in each genotype in step 3. In step 4 all models are summarized in the training set with a classification accuracy statistic, which measures the relationship between loci in a model and the outcome. Step 5 iterates over all models using steps 1-4. Step 6 uses the test set data to evaluate the locus combinations of each order (2-locus, 3-locus, etc.) with the highest classification accuracy. This provides a measure of the accuracy of the model in an unobserved sample. Repeating the process of steps 1-4 using each CV fold as a test set, and taking the average of classification accuracy estimates from each test set provides an unbiased estimate of a model's ability to predict an outcome in an independent sample. In step 7, MDR evaluates the CV consistency, or the number of times a model of some order is the best in the training set, and the average testing accuracy. The final model is chosen from this set of models based upon maximization of testing accuracy and CV consistency. When prediction accuracy and CV consistency indicate different models, parsimony is used to choose the simplest model (the model with the fewest loci). Step 8 is a permutation test, where case and control status is randomly shuffled and the analysis is performed many times. This procedure will correctly estimate the distribution of the test statistics under the null hypothesis, given the correlation structure in the data, the number of comparisons performed, and the presence of non-independent multilocus models in the search space.

If the data consists of an unbalanced ratio of cases to controls (high risk cells; a higher ratio of cases to controls) are labeled in dark grey and low risk cells (a higher ratio of controls to cases) are labeled in light grey in Figure 3), balanced accuracy is used for the analyses in place of the default fitness function, accuracy.[63] Balanced accuracy is statistically equivalent to accuracy when datasets are completely balanced and is calculated from the average of sensitivity (the ability of a test to correctly identify those who have the disease) and specificity (the ability of a test to correctly identify those who do not have the disease) of the MDR model. Open-source MDR software is available at MDR (available at www.epistasis.org). Our laboratory has explored this approach with a small set of candidate genes.[64-66]

Haplotype Associations and Analytical Strategies

Single locus association studies are rarely restricted to the analysis of the effect of a single SNP even with a well established candidate. The examination of multiple SNPs, comprising a haplotype, within a gene can provide additional information that cannot be gained from a SNP alone. A haplotype is a specific set of alleles on a chromosome. Individuals without chromosomal abnormalities have a single paternal and a maternal haplotype, which was assembled with recombination and transmitted to the gamete during meiosis. There are several benefits from performing haplotype association. Principally, they provide more biologically relevant information than single SNP analysis. For example, if you observe that several mutations are in a haplotype in *cis* (mutations that are on the same chromosome), a different biological effect may occur, relative to *trans* (mutations that are on different chromosomes), because they might interact to cause changes in protein-protein interactions *in vivo*. Mutations that are *cis* can have a very different impact on phenotype than *trans*. In addition to this, simulation and analytical studies have shown that haplotype analyses can have greater power to detect indirect association than single SNP association analyses. Haplotypes also provide information regarding population history. For example, if the mutation that leads to disease was introduced into the population at some point in the population's genetic history, on a single haplotype of an individual, knowledge of the haplotype information can provide some additional information regarding the disease. The structure of haplotypes can provide some insight into the recombination rates, genetic drift, mutations, natural selection, and population migrations that lead to the current state of the disease. As a result, analytical approaches have been developed to examine the role of haplotypes and disease.

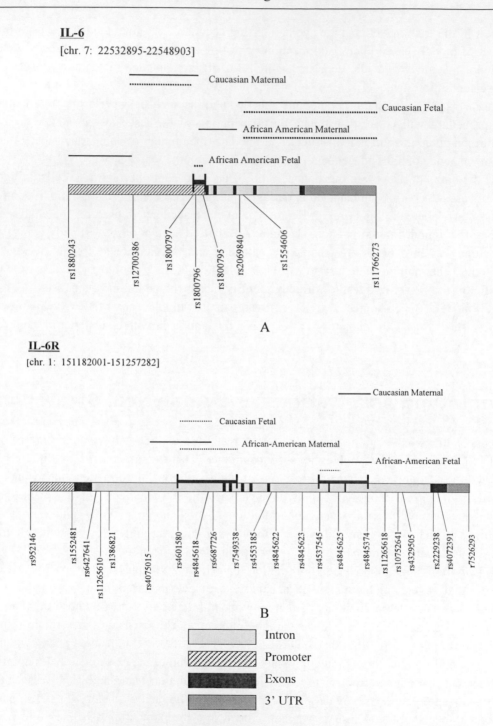

Figure 4. Interleukin 6 and Interleukin 6 Receptor haplotype associations across African-American and Caucasian samples. Dark lines with bounded vertical lines indicate haplotypes that were associated with dichotomous outcome and dashed lines indicate haplotype that were associated with continuous outcome, dark bounded lines on the x-axis indicate regions of overlapping haplotype associations. Introns are labeled with light grey, promoter with dashed lines, exons with solid black rectangles, and 3'UTR with dark grey. a) Results for haplotype analyses for IL-6; b) results for haplotype analyses for IL-6R. (Velez et al 2008).

Haplotypes cannot be directly observed in genotype data, and as a result methods have been developed to reconstruct haplotypes and to estimate haplotype frequencies. When using family data haplotypes are more directly reconstructed from family pedigrees by following genetic information from parent to offspring. These methods do not resolve haplotypes unambiguously and as a result methods were developed to reconstruct diplotypes in pedigree data. The Lander-Green algorithm is used to reconstruct haplotypes in family data and is implemented in MERLIN software.[67] The Lander-Green algorithm uses the conditional independence along a chromosome (assuming no interference) considering all individuals jointly for every chromosome position. It utilizes inheritance vectors that summarize the inheritance of an individual at a specific location in the genome and from this the pedigree likelihoods can be computed that allows for the enumeration of the complete multilocus diplotype. In unrelated case-control data haplotype reconstruction is less straightforward and commonly the Clark[68] algorithm utilizing maximum parsimony is used so that diplotypes are resolved with the minimum number of distinct possible haplotypes. Using this approach unambiguous multilocus genotypes are resolved first forming the set of known haplotypes and the remaining are resolved based on the patterns observed at those resolved haplotypes. In both unrelated case-control and family-based haplotype methods, haplotypes are reconstructed by the use of an expectation maximization (EM) algorithm[69;70], where the maximum-likelihood estimates of the population haplotype frequencies are determined.

The approaches commonly used to test for haplotype association have been previously reviewed by Schaid et al.[71;72] Commonly the haplotype trend regression test (available in commonly used genetic analysis software PLINK[73], JMP Genomics software from SAS[74], POWERMARKER software[75]) or generalized linear models (available in R package HAPLO.STAT)[76;77] are used to test for haplotype association. The majority of these software packages allow for the analysis of both categorical and continuously distributed outcomes. For PTB haplotype analyses, determining which haplotype methods to use is based on whether a categorical or continuous outcome is going to be examined, as well as whether covariates are going to be analyzed.

Studies by our group have successfully performed haplotype analyses using both continuous phenotype and categorical PTB data (Figure 4).[78] We examined Interleukin (IL)-6 and IL-6 receptor (IL-6R) for haplotype associations with outcome considered as dichotomous (preterm vs. term) and continuous (IL-6 cytokine concentration (pg/ml)) using haplotype trend regression tests of association. African-American, Caucasian, maternal and fetal samples were analyzed separately. Significant associations from both dichotomous and continuous haplotype analyses and across geographic populations converged on three regions in both IL-6 and Il-6R: in IL-6 markers (rs1800797, rs1800796, and rs1800795); in IL-6R markers (rs4601580, rs4645618, rs6687726, and rs7549338) and IL-6R markers (rs4537545, rs4845625, and rs4845374). These results allowed us to narrow down common regions of the IL-6 and IL-6R genes that seem to have significant associations across populations, illustrating how haplotype analyses might be successfully implemented in an analysis of PTB given status, phenotype data, and genotypic information.

Reproducibility and Reliability of Data

Unfortunately, many of these single locus association studies have failed to replicate in subsequent studies. One possible explanation for this failure to replicate is the potential for genetic heterogeneity. One approach to address this potential heterogeneity is through meta-analysis. In one case, meta-analysis has shown no significant association between the risk of PTB and a SNP in the tumor necrosis factor $-\alpha$ gene (TNF) promoter at -308 previously reported to be associated with pregnancy outcome.[79] Recently, authors of this chapter and others , as a part of preterm birth international collaborative (PREBIC) with support from World Health Organization and March of Dimes, USA conducted a systematic review of genetic association studies in preterm birth to document true associations.[80] Until 2007 December, 88 manuscripts documented genetic associations in spontaneous preterm birth and data were extracted from only 48 of them as most other studies did not fit the inclusion criteria due to various reasons such as improper study designs, reporting issues etc. In summary, the analysis included data on 144 polymorphisms in 76 genes and 19 meta-analyses were performed. Three gene variants (two in the maternal [beta-2 adrenergic receptor (rs1042713) and interferon gamma (rs2430561)) and one in the neonatal genome (coagulation factor 2 [rs1799963] have shown nominally significant associations, but all three have weak epidemiological credibility.

Heterogeneity of Association Studies

Significant differences in study designs, definitions of phenotype, and analytical approaches have the potential to contribute to inconsistent findings. False positive or false negative results can also arise due to population stratification. This issue of stratification is particularly important in studies where the sample is pooled from a population such as the United States, which has the potential for significant ethnic heterogeneity.[81;82] However, some recent analytical methods have been developed to address the issue of stratification. Due to complex etiology of preterm birth multiple gene variants may be involved in the disease process. This creates locus heterogeneity. Alternatively, different variants in the same gene may cause different phenotypes. This is referred to as allelic heterogeneity. In either case, the array of predisposing variants can be large, making the study of PTB difficult.[27;83]

Complex patterns of association caused by allelic heterogeneity and locus heterogeneity can often result from the presence of multiple rare variants (MRV).[84] The primary models used for association studies on disease variants are based on the concept of common disease common variant (CDCV,[85;86]) and MRV[84]. Briefly, CDCV models of association assume that the mutation has different recombination histories that are common to specific populations and these populations have common genetic variants/alleles that have a large effect on common disease.[86] This is in contrast to the concept of MRV which assumes that diseases result from multiple minor and modest effects that increase risk caused by the summation of a number of low frequency variants on several different genes. MRV is relatively difficult to detect because of the lack of adequate methods to differentiate these effects from other sources of heterogeneity. The truth is likely that diseases result from a combination of

CDCV and MRV. Despite the numerous concerns involved with many studies to date, we are beginning to elucidate the genetic predispositions and pathophysiologic mechanisms of PTB.

Genome Wide Association Studies (GWAS) in Spontaneous Preterm Birth

At the time of writing of this chapter, no GWAS have been reported in PTB although many are underway.[87] GWAS studies are gaining popularity due to several reasons; 1) Single locus analyses have literally littered the field with errors and misunderstandings regarding the true causal variant 2) Due to complexity of causation of PTB, candidate gene selections are incomplete or uneven as many of the underlying pathways are either ignored or not yet understood. This bias during the candidate gene selection stage in fact may miss some causal variant. 3) The candidate gene studies reported so far are not adequately powered and the associations that are found to be significant may be just an artifact due to genetic differences introduced due to population admixture. 4) Etiologic, pathophysiologic, genetic (allelic and locus) heterogeneities makes even large scale candidate gene associations less reliable. GWAS studies genetic variation across the entire human genome in which many genetic variations contribute to a person's risk. Information obtained from GWAS in combination with environmental and other clinical and demographic data can better predict the risk and also help to understand the basic biological processes affecting the disease outcome. A catalog of all reported GWAS can be seen at http://www.genome.gov/gwastudies/

The rest of this chapter will discuss different platforms and analytical methods for GWAS that can potentially be applied to preterm birth research.

GWAS Methodologies

GWAS methodologies have only recently been made possible with advances in genotyping technologies and the success of the HapMap project.[35] GWAS systematically search through the entire human genome without *a priori* hypotheses about the biology of the disease examined or the location of potential susceptibility genes. In contrast to a candidate gene-based approach which uses known biology to guide selection of genes and markers for analysis, a GWAS might provide novel insight into the biology of a disease. GWAS have been applied to several diseases (http://www.genome.gov/gwastudies/). Recent studies examining PTB have been small-scale candidate gene association studies based on hypothesized PTB pathways, along with a few larger-scale high-throughput candidate studies that have been published in the literature. GWAS methodologies can be very useful for a complex disease such as PTB where the biology is not completely understood and candidate genes, as a result, might miss important sources of genetic risk.

GWAS have advantages over the candidate gene-based approaches that have been more commonly used in PTB genetic association studies. The cost of GWAS genotyping platforms are decreasing and the prices for performing a GWAS over a candidate gene study may be comparable, depending on the number of SNPs in the candidate gene study. The advantages in genomic coverage; however, may not necessarily outweigh the limitations of a GWAS today. Principally due to stringent significance thresholds due to multiple testing corrections, GWAS have less power than a more confined study to detect genes with small effects that may localize disease genes more tightly. It is therefore very important to consider the sample size available to the study when deciding whether to proceed with a GWAS or a smaller genotyping platform. For example, if a study featured a small sample, and the candidate gene and GWAS genotyping were the same cost, then the candidate gene study would be more likely to succeed due to power after multiple testing corrections were applied. However, for a sufficiently large sample, the GWAS methodology might be more likely to succeed due to increased genomic coverage. These questions can be answered using the power software packages described above.

Due to current analytical methods and computational limitations, data sample structures can be prohibitive, e.g. studies may be limited to unrelated cases and controls or family trios rather than extended pedigrees or more complicated family structures. Type I error (the false positive rate) is also a considerable problem in GWAS studies, as analyzing hundreds of thousands of markers across the human genome can limit the interpretability of the results. This is compounded by the fact that the markers being tested are not independent due to LD, which makes a straight forward analytical correction approach (such as Bonferroni correction) highly conservative. Analytic methods to deal with the large multiple testing corrections associated with testing hundreds of thousands of markers across the genome have been under development.[88] Finally, the volume of genotypic data that is generated creates large computational demands, both in terms of data storage and analysis. This means that, although financially available, GWAS are limited to those with access to high-performance computing.

Genotyping for GWAS are currently performed under two genotyping platforms, Affymetrix and Illumina.

Affymetrix: Affymetrix is currently being used to analyze over 1.8 million SNPs on one chip; of the two platforms, Affymetrix is the more cost-effective of the genotyping platforms using ~250 nanograms of DNA per genotype (http://affymetrix.com/index.affx). Affymetrix uses DNA microarrays for high-throughput SNP detection using photolithography to create site-specific primers that are attached to a silicon chip. Primers attach to specifically amplified DNA that is equivalent to a site-specific complement probe. For detection a reporter (e.g. fluorescent molecule) attaches to either a photolithographic probe or an amplified DNA probe, and is chemically released upon hybridization of the two oligo chains. The current Affymetrix Genome-wide Human SNP array 6.0 allows for the selection of more than 906,600 SNPs from a combination of 482,000 unbiased "historical SNPs" selected by Affymetrix and a combination of 424,000 additional SNPs that consist of tags, mitochondrial SNPs, SNPs in recombination hotspots, SNPs on chromosomes X and Y, and new SNPs added to the dbSNP database. The remaining 946,000 markers consist of copy number variant (CNV) probes.

Illumina: The Illumina genotyping platform is currently able to analyze 1.1 million SNPs on an Illumina Human1M-duo beadchip array. The Illumina system consists of a complex bead array that allows all SNPs to be detected at once. Much like Affymetrix, this system also relies on a fluorescence reporting mechanism, but with a locus specification step at the beginning of the process that creates a specifically addressed oligonucleotide chain that is then amplified by a process that is similar to whole genome amplification (http://www.illumina.com). SNPs for the Illumina platform are selected based on being tag SNPs in the populations from the International HapMap Project dataset.[35] Additional SNPs are selected based on SNP coverage Reference Sequence (RefSeq) genes (within 10 kilo bases) (http://www.ncbi.nlm.nih.gov/RefSeq/), non-synonymous SNPs, ADME SNPs, and SNPs found in the major histocompatibility complex (MHC) region. With regard to genomic coverage Affymetrix and Illumina are comparable[89].

GWAS Data Analysis

GWAS data analysis, following implementation of genotype-calling algorithms (genotype-calling algorithms are available in Bead Studio software for Illumina and Birdsuite software for Affymetrix) and laboratory quality control (QC), is comprised of four distinct parts: QC analysis, data summary statistics, association analysis, and detailed follow-up analysis. Today the method most commonly used to perform GWAS analysis is PLINK software available for Window and UNIX operating systems including Linux, Solaris, and Mac OS (http://pngu.mgh.harvard.edu/purcell/plink/).[73] PLINK is a software that merges the majority of GWAS data analysis into one package. PLINK can analyze both case-control and family trio data. For the purposes of PTB GWAS data analysis, PLINK is most useful for the analysis of case-control data. Several quality control steps can be performed using PLINK. Some of the primary ways it can be used for QC is to identify and remove duplicated individuals, SNPs that have low minor allele frequencies, SNPs with departures from HWE, and SNPs and individuals with excess missing data.

There are regions of the human chromosome with considerable allele frequency differences between both geographic and racial populations.[90] As a result, PLINK has implemented approaches to help both group individuals appropriately and evaluate population stratification. PLINK has implemented a method based on principal component analysis (PCA) and multidimensional scaling (MDS). A detailed description of the method is available in the PLINK user's manual (http://pngu.mgh.harvard.edu/purcell/plink/). This approach can either be used as a QC step to remove outlier individuals who appear not be to belong to a particular population or as a follow-up analysis approach to understand the reason for an association (e.g. whether most of the association signals are coming from a subgroup of the data).

Single marker, haplotype, and gene x gene association analyses can all be performed using PLINK with adjustments for multiple testing. PLINK is designed to handle large quantities of data, which is not the case for more commonly used genetic analysis software. The first step in a GWAS analysis involves single SNP analyses. Single SNP analyses can involve five tests of association including, allelic, genotypic, Cochran-Armitage trend, dominant association, and recessive association. Some investigators prefer one test over another depending on the hypotheses being pursued. As a result, rather than having to keep track of the number of tests performed, PLINK will determine this and make an adjustment for multiple comparisons from a selection of several commonly used approaches (Bonferroni,

False Discovery Rate, Holm, and Sidak corrections). The most interesting/significant associations can be followed-up with haplotype analyses within genes. Haplotype analyses are performed as previously described for non-GWAS studies. The haplotype tests implemented in PLINK are trend tests of association.

As a final step, more complex analyses may be performed with PLINK. For example, PLINK also allows gene x environment interactions and gene x gene interactions to be modeled with the logistic regression option. PLINK can test gene x gene epistasis for case/control population-based samples using either linear or logistic regression, depending on whether the phenotype is a quantitative or binary trait with models based on allele dosage for each SNP (additive effects) and no covariates. Currently, in case-only analysis, only SNPs that are more than 1 Mb apart, or on different chromosomes, are included in case-only tests due to a strict assumption of independent SNPs. Eventually the option for gene-based tests of epistasis will be implemented in PLNK.

For family trio data, the transmission disequilibrium test can be used for analyses.[91] The transmission disequilibrium test, however, is not useful for PTB analyses given the ambiguity of the maternal and fetus status; therefore, PLINK is primarily useful for the case-control analyses. Although PLINK is a commonly preferred method for GWAS analysis, other techniques and software are available to analyze GWAS software.

Summary

Lack of understanding of risk factors and pathophysiologic events leading to PTB has made prevention of PTB a major clinical dilemma and a major public health concern. Many studies have linked genetic variations in maternal and fetal genes as risk factors of PTB; however, conclusive evidence still does not exist to use as a 'high risk pregnancy' screening tool. Proper identification of genetic risk factors is essential because genetic risk factors are static markers and association of these markers may provide an early screening strategy. As GWAS methodologies are becoming easily available and commercially feasible, successful outcome of a study will dependent on many of the factors described in this chapter starting with phenotype definition, appropriate study design, power and analytical methods. Replication of data in multiple cohorts using similar strategies is one of the major and essential aspects of any genetic association study. This chapter did not detail the dynamic changes that can influence the pathophysiology of pregnancy outcome due to gene-environmental interactions. It is unlikely that statistical associations established through genetic association studies have any direct impact in the outcome of the phenotype. Biological associations need to be established through gene x environmental interaction studies in order to design proper biomarker screening and develop intervention methods.

References

[1]   International Classification of Diseases and Related Health Problems - 10th revision. Geneva, Switzerland: *World Health Organization,* 1992.

[2]   Huddy CL, Johnson A, Hope PL. Educational and behavioral problems in babies of 32-35 weeks gestation. *Arch Dis Child Fetal Neonatal Ed* 2001;85:F23-F28.

[3]   Wang ML, Dorer DJ, Fleming MP, Catlin EA. Clinical outcomes of near-term infants. *Pediatrics* 2004;114:372-76.

[4]   Petrou S. The economic consequences of preterm birth during the first 10 years of life. *BJOG* 2005;112 Suppl 1:10-15.

[5]   Petrou S, Mehta Z, Hockley C, Cook-Mozaffari P, Henderson J, Goldacre M. The impact of preterm birth on hospital inpatient admissions and costs during the first 5 years of life. *Pediatrics* 2003;112:1290-97.

[6]   Preterm births: U.S. 1992-2002. *National Center for Health Statistics* 2006.

[7]   Preterm birth: causes, consequences, and prevention. *Institute of Medicine* 2006.

[8]   Raju TN, Higgins RD, Stark AR, Leveno KJ. Optimizing care and outcome for late-preterm (near-term) infants: a summary of the workshop sponsored by the National Institute of Child Health and Human Development. *Pediatrics* 2006;118:1207-14.

[9]   Brooke OG, Anderson HR, Bland JM, Peacock JL, Stewart CM. Effects on birth weight of smoking, alcohol, caffeine, socioeconomic factors, and psychosocial stress. *BMJ* 1989;298:795-801.

[10] Dominguez TP. Race, racism, and racial disparities in adverse birth outcomes. *Clin.Obstet.Gynecol.* 2008;51:360-70.

[11] Fiscella K. Race, genes and preterm delivery. *J.Natl.Med.Assoc.* 2005;97:1516-26.

[12] Goldenberg RL, Andrews WW. Intrauterine infection and why preterm prevention programs have failed. *Am.J.Public Health* 1996;86:781-83.

[13] Jesse DE, Reed PG. Effects of spirituality and psychosocial well-being on health risk behaviors in Appalachian pregnant women. *J.Obstet.Gynecol.Neonatal Nurs.* 2004;33:739-47.

[14] McCormick MC, Brooks-Gunn J, Shorter T, Holmes JH, Wallace CY, Heagarty MC. Factors associated with smoking in low-income pregnant women: relationship to birth weight, stressful life events, social support, health behaviors and mental distress. *J.Clin.Epidemiol.* 1990;43:441-48.

[15] Menon R. Spontaneous preterm birth, a clinical dilemma: etiologic, pathophysiologic, and genetic heterogeneities and racial disparity. *Acta. Obstet. Gynecol. Scand.* 2008; 87:590-600. Swamy GK, Ostbye T, Skjaerven R. Association of preterm birth with long-term survival, reproduction, and next-generation preterm birth. *JAMA* 2008;299:1429-36.

[16] Wadhwa PD, Culhane JF, Rauh V, Barve SS, Hogan V, Sandman CA et al. Stress, infection and preterm birth: a biobehavioural perspective. *Paediatr.Perinat.Epidemiol.* 2001;15 Suppl 2:17-29.

[17] Martin JA, Kung HC, Mathews TJ, Hoyert DL, Strobino DM, Guyer B et al. Annual summary of vital statistics: 2006. *Pediatrics* 2008;121:788-801.

[18] Cockey CD. Premature births hit record high. *AWHONN.Lifelines.* 2005;9:365-70.

[19] Foster HW, Wu L, Bracken MB, Semenya K, Thomas J, Thomas J. Intergenerational effects of high socioeconomic status on low birthweight and preterm birth in African Americans. *J Natl Med Assoc* 2000;92:213-21.

[20] Lu MC, Halfon N. Racial and ethnic disparities in birth outcomes: a life-course perspective. *Matern.Child Health J* 2003;7:13-30.

[21] MacDorman MF, Martin JA, Mathews TJ, Hoyert DL, Ventura SJ. Explaining the 2001-02 infant mortality increase: data from the linked birth/infant death data set. *Natl Vital Stat Rep*. 2005;53:1-22.

[22] Martin JA, Kochanek KD, Strobino DM, Guyer B, MacDorman MF. Annual summary of vital statistics--2003. *Pediatrics* 2005;115:619-34.

[23] Minino AM, Arias E, Kochanek KD, Murphy SL, Smith BL. Deaths: final data for 2000. *Natl Vital Stat Rep*. 2002;50:1-119.

[24] Ward R. Familial aggregation and genetic epidemiology of blood pressure. In: Brenner JMLaBM, editor. *Hypertension: pathophysiology, diagnosis and management.* New York: Raven Press; 1990.

[25] Romero R, Chaiworapongsa T, Kuivaniemi H, Tromp G. Bacterial vaginosis, the inflammatory response and the risk of preterm birth: a role for genetic epidemiology in the prevention of preterm birth. *Am J.Obstet.Gynecol.* 2004;190:1509-19.

[26] Varner MW, Esplin MS. Current understanding of genetic factors in preterm birth. *BJOG.* 2005;112 Suppl 1:28-31.

[27] Clausson B, Lichtenstein P, Cnattingius S. Genetic influence on birthweight and gestational length determined by studies in offspring of twins. *BJOG.* 2000;107:375-81.

[28] Treloar SA, Macones GA, Mitchell LE, Martin NG. Genetic influences on premature parturition in an Australian twin sample. *Twin.Res.* 2000;3:80-82.

[29] Bakketeig LS, Hoffman HJ, Harley EE. The tendency to repeat gestational age and birth weight in successive births. *Am J.Obstet.Gynecol.* 1979;135:1086-103.

[30] Carr-Hill RA, Hall MH. The repetition of spontaneous preterm labour. *Br.J.Obstet.Gynaecol.* 1985;92:921-28.

[31] Rotimi CN, Cooper RS, Cao G, Ogunbiyi O, Ladipo M, Owoaje E et al. Maximum-likelihood generalized heritability estimate for blood pressure in Nigerian families. *Hypertension* 1999;33:874-78.

[32] Winkvist A, Mogren I, Hogberg U. Familial patterns in birth characteristics: impact on individual and population risks. *Int.J.Epidemiol.* 1998;27:248-54.

[33] Patel RR, Steer P, Doyle P, Little MP, Elliott P. Does gestation vary by ethnic group? A London-based study of over 122,000 pregnancies with spontaneous onset of labour. *Int J Epidemiol.* 2004;33:107-13.

[34] The International HapMap Consortium. The International HapMap Project. *Nature* 2003;426:789-96.

[35] Births: preliminary data for 2005. *National Center for Health Statistics* 2006.

[36] *Fundamentals of Epidemiology*. New York: Oxford University Press, 1993.

[37] Adams MM, Finley S, Hansen H, Jahiel RI, Oakley GP, Jr., Sanger W et al. Utilization of prenatal genetic diagnosis in women 35 years of age and older in the United States, 1977 to 1978. *Am J.Obstet.Gynecol*. 1981;139:673-77.

[38] Heinonen OP, Slone D, Monson RR, Hook EB, Shapiro S. Cardiovascular birth defects and antenatal exposure to female sex hormones. *N.Engl.J.Med*. 1977;296:67-70.

[39] Weinberg CR, Wilcox AJ, Lie RT. A log-linear approach to case-parent-triad data: assessing effects of disease genes that act either directly or through maternal effects and that may be subject to parental imprinting. *Am J.Hum.Genet.* 1998;62:969-78.

[40] Zheng G, Tian X. Robust trend tests for genetic association using matched case-control design. *Stat.Med.* 2006;25:3160-73.

[41] *Modern Epidemiology.* Boston: Little, Brown & Co., 1986.

[42] Heiman GA, Hodge SE, Gorroochurn P, Zhang J, Greenberg DA. Effect of population stratification on case-control association studies. I. Elevation in false positive rates and comparison to confounding risk ratios (a simulation study). *Hum.Hered.* 2004;58:30-39.

[43] Voight BF, Pritchard JK. Confounding from cryptic relatedness in case-control association studies. *PLoS.Genet.* 2005;1:e32.

[44] Thorsen P, Schendel DE, Deshpande AD, Vogel I, Dudley DJ, Olsen J. Identification of biological/biochemical marker(s) for preterm delivery. *Paediatr.Perinat.Epidemiol.* 2001;15 Suppl 2:90-103.

[45] Sullivan PF, Eaves LJ, Kendler KS, Neale MC. Genetic case-control association studies in neuropsychiatry. *Arch.Gen.Psychiatry* 2001;58:1015-24.

[46] Dupont WD, Plummer WD, Jr. Power and sample size calculations for studies involving linear regression. *Control Clin.Trials* 1998;19:589-601.

[47] Kaplan NL, Martin ER, Weir BS. Power studies for the transmission/disequilibrium tests with multiple alleles. *Am J.Hum.Genet.* 1997;60:691-702.

[48] Kaplan NL, Martin ER. Power calculations for a general class of tests of linkage and association that use nuclear families with affected and unaffected sibs. *Theor.Popul.Biol.* 2001;60:193-201.

[49] Gauderman , W. J. and Morrison, J. M. QUANTO 1.2: A computer program for power and sample size calculations for genetic-epidemiology studies. 2007. *Ref Type: Computer Program*

[50] Hirschhorn JN, Daly MJ. Genome-wide association studies for common diseases and complex traits. *Nat.Rev Genet.* 2005;6:95-108.

[51] Hartl DL. Genetic variation. *In: Sinauer AD, editor. A Primer of Population Genetics.* Sunderland, Massachusetts: Sinauer Associates, Inc; 2000. p. 26-29.

[52] Plunkett J, Muglia LJ. Genetic contributions to preterm birth: implications from epidemiological and genetic association studies. *Ann Med.* 2008;40:167-95.

[53] Hoh J, Ott J. Mathematical multi-locus approaches to localizing complex human trait genes. *Nat.Rev Genet.* 2003;4:701-09.

[54] Kooperberg C, Ruczinski I. Identifying interacting SNPs using Monte Carlo logic regression. *Genet Epidemiol* 2005;28:157-70.

[55] Brelman L, Friedman JH, Olshen RA, Stone CJ. *Classification and regression trees.* New York, NY: Chapman & Hall, 1984.

[56] Millstein J, Conti DV, Gilliland FD, Gauderman WJ. A testing framework for identifying susceptibility genes in the presence of epistasis. *Am.J.Hum.Genet.* 2006;78:15-27.

[57] Bastone L, Reilly M, Rader DJ, Foulkes AS. MDR and PRP: a comparison of methods for high-order genotype-phenotype associations. *Hum Hered.* 2004;58:82-92.

[58] Motsinger AA, Ritchie MD. The effect of reduction in cross-validation intervals on the performance of multifactor dimensionality reduction. *Genet Epidemiol* 2006;30:546-55.

[59] Ritchie MD, Hahn LW, Roodi N, Bailey LR, Dupont WD, Parl FF et al. Multifactor-dimensionality reduction reveals high-order interactions among estrogen-metabolism genes in sporadic breast cancer. *Am J Hum Genet* 2001;69:138-47.

[60] Wilcox AJ, Weinberg CR, Lie RT. Distinguishing the effects of maternal and offspring genes through studies of "case-parent triads". *Am J.Epidemiol.* 1998;148:893-901.

[61] Hahn LW, Ritchie MD, Moore JH. Multifactor dimensionality reduction software for detecting gene-gene and gene-environment interactions. *Bioinformatics* 2003;19:376-82.

[62] Velez DR, White BC, Motsinger AA, Bush WS, Ritchie MD, Williams SM et al. A balanced accuracy function for epistasis modeling in imbalanced datasets using multifactor dimensionality reduction. *Genet Epidemiol* 2007;31:306-15.

[63] Fortunato SJ, Menon R, Velez DR, Thorsen P, Williams SM. Racial disparity in maternal-fetal genetic epistasis in spontaneous preterm birth. *Am J.Obstet.Gynecol.* 2008;198:666-69.

[64] Menon R, Velez DR, Simhan H, Ryckman K, Jiang L, Thorsen P et al. Multilocus interactions at maternal tumor necrosis factor-alpha, tumor necrosis factor receptors, interleukin-6 and interleukin-6 receptor genes predict spontaneous preterm labor in European-American women. *Am J.Obstet.Gynecol.* 2006;194:1616-24.

[65] Velez DR, Fortunato SJ, Thorsen P, Lombardi SJ, Williams SM, Menon R. Preterm birth in Caucasians is associated with coagulation and inflammation pathway gene variants. *PLoS.ONE.* 2008;3:e3283.

[66] Abecasis GR, Cherny SS, Cookson WO, Cardon LR. Merlin--rapid analysis of dense genetic maps using sparse gene flow trees. *Nat.Genet.* 2002;30:97-101.

[67] Clark AG. Inference of haplotypes from PCR-amplified samples of diploid populations. *Mol.Biol.Evol.* 1990;7:111-22.

[68] Excoffier L, Slatkin M. Maximum-likelihood estimation of molecular haplotype frequencies in a diploid population. *Mol.Biol.Evol.* 1995;12:921-27.

[69] Hawley ME, Kidd KK. HAPLO: a program using the EM algorithm to estimate the frequencies of multi-site haplotypes. *J.Hered.* 1995;86:409-11.

[70] Schaid DJ. Genetic epidemiology and haplotypes. *Genet.Epidemiol.* 2004;27:317-20.

[71] Schaid DJ. Linkage disequilibrium testing when linkage phase is unknown. *Genetics* 2004;166:505-12.

[72] Purcell S, Neale B, Todd-Brown K, Thomas L, Ferreira MA, Bender D et al. PLINK: a tool set for whole-genome association and population-based linkage analyses. *Am J.Hum.Genet.* 2007;81:559-75.

[73] JMP Genomics. (3.2). 2008. NC, SAS Institute Inc. *Ref Type: Computer Program*

[74] Liu K, Muse SV. PowerMarker: an integrated analysis environment for genetic marker analysis. *Bioinformatics*. 2005;21:2128-29.

[75] Schaid DJ, Rowland CM, Tines DE, Jacobson RM, Poland GA. Score tests for association between traits and haplotypes when linkage phase is ambiguous. *Am J.Hum.Genet.* 2002;70:425-34.

[76] Sinwell, J. P. and Schaid, D. J. haplo.stats: statistical analysis of haplotypes with traits and covariates when linkage phase in ambiguous. (R package version 1.3.8). 2005. *Ref Type: Computer Program*

[77] Velez DR, Fortunato SJ, Williams SM, Menon R. Interleukin-6 (IL-6) and receptor (IL6-R) gene haplotypes associate with amniotic fluid protein concentrations in preterm birth. *Hum.Mol.Genet.* 2008;17:1619-30.

[78] Menon R, Merialdi M, Betran AP, Dolan S, Jiang L, Fortunator SJ et al. Lack of association between tumor necrosis factor-alpha promoter polymorphism (-208), TNF concentration, and preterm birth. *Am J.Obstet.Gynecol.* 2008.

[79] Dolan, S. M., Hollegaard, M. V., Merialdi, M., Betran, A. P, Allen, T., Abelow, C., Eckardt, J., Lin, B. K., Khoury, M. J., Ioannidis, J. P. A., Bertram, L., Zheng, X., Dubin, R. A., Velez, D. R., and Menon, R. *Synopsis of preterm birth genetic association studies: the preterm birth genomics knowledge base (PTBGene).* Public Health genomics 2010. In Press

[80] Colhoun HM, McKeigue PM, Davey SG. Problems of reporting genetic associations with complex outcomes. *Lancet* 2003;361:865-72.

[81] Pfaff CL, Parra EJ, Bonilla C, Hiester K, McKeigue PM, Kamboh MI et al. Population structure in admixed populations: effect of admixture dynamics on the pattern of linkage disequilibrium. *Am J.Hum.Genet.* 2001;68:198-207.

[82] Esplin MS, Varner MW. Genetic factors in preterm birth--the future. *BJOG.* 2005;112 Suppl 1:97-102.

[83] Neale BM, Sham PC. The future of association studies: gene-based analysis and replication. *Am J.Hum.Genet.* 2004;75:353-62.

[84] Chakravarti A. Population genetics--making sense out of sequence. *Nat.Genet.* 1999;21:56-60.

[85] Weiss KM, Clark AG. Linkage disequilibrium and the mapping of complex human traits. *Trends Genet.* 2002;18:19-24.

[86] Biggio J, Christiaens I, Katz M, Menon R, Merialdi M, Morken NH et al. A call for an international consortium on the genetics of preterm birth. *Am J.Obstet.Gynecol.* 2008;199:95-97.

[87] Cardon LR, Bell JI. Association study designs for complex diseases. *Nat.Rev Genet.* 2001;2:91-99.

[88] Barrett JC, Cardon LR. Evaluating coverage of genome-wide association studies. *Nat.Genet.* 2006;38:659-62.

[89] A haplotype map of the human genome. *Nature* 2005;437:1299-320.

[90] Spielman RS, McGinnis RE, Ewens WJ. Transmission test for linkage disequilibrium: the insulin gene region and insulin-dependent diabetes mellitus (IDDM). *Am J.Hum.Genet.* 1993;52:506-16.

In: Textbook of Perinatal Epidemiology
Editor: Eyal Sheiner, pp. 619-637

ISBN: 978-1-60741-648-7
© 2010 Nova Science Publishers, Inc.

Chapter XXVIII

Epidemiology of Placental Abruption

*Cande V. Ananth**

Definitions

- Placental abruption: Premature separation of the normally implanted placenta prior to delivery of the fetus.

Introduction

Uterine bleeding, especially in the second-half of pregnancy, is a major cause for concern. While up to a third of all bleeding episodes is attributable to placental abruption and about 20% to placental previa, roughly half of bleeding episodes are undetermined.[1-3] In normal pregnancies, the placenta detaches after birth, whereas in cases of placental abruption the placental detachment occurs earlier. The premature placental separation may be partial or complete, with varied consequences on both the mother and the ensuing fetus. Placental abruption is also termed ablatio placentae and accidental hemorrhage. Despite its clinical significance, there are no reliable diagnostic tests or biomarkers to predict or prevent the occurrence of abruption. In fact, the condition even lacks a universal and standardized definition. However, the clinical hallmarks of abruption include painful vaginal bleeding accompanied by tetanic uterine contractions, uterine hypertonicity, and a nonreassuring fetal heart rate patterns.

Placental abruption is associated with excessively high rates of perinatal mortality and morbidity, preterm birth, and restricted fetal growth. The condition also portends increased

* For Correspondence: Cande V. Ananth , Professor and Director, Division of Epidemiology and Biostatistics, Department of Obstetrics, Gynecology, and Reproductive Sciences, UMDNJ-Robert Wood Johnson Medical School, New Brunswick NJ 08901,USA, Tel: (732) 235-7940 / Fax: (732) 235-6627, Email: cande.ananth@umdnj.edu

risks of an array of outcomes in the mother, including hemorrhage requiring blood transfusions, hemorrhagic shock, disseminated intravascular coagulation, need for hysterectomy, renal failure and involvement of other organ systems including the liver and kidneys. Maternal death as a consequence of placental abruption is, however, very rare.

The etiology of placental abruption remains elusive. Rupture of defective maternal vessels in the decidua basalis is known to be the leading initiating cause for the placental separation.[4, 5] In a few other instances, the bleeding may also emanate from the fetal-placental vessels. The accumulating blood entrapped between the placenta and the decidua subsequently splits the decidua from the site of placental attachment in the uterine wall. The entrapped blood (hematoma) is often severe enough to result in a complete or near-complete placental separation. In such scenarios, there is often loss of gas exchange and nutrients to the fetus, potentially leading to in utero fetal demise or fetal growth restriction. In a majority of instances, placental abruption is "revealed" in that blood tracks between the membranes and the decidua, and escapes through the cervix into the vagina (Fig 1, panel A). In other less common instances the placental abruption is said to be "concealed" when blood accumulates behind the placenta, with no obvious external bleeding (Fig 1, panel B).[5]

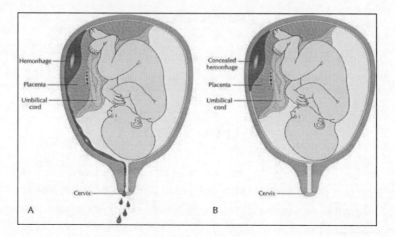

Figure 1. Types of placental abruption. A. Revealed placental abruption, where blood tracks between the membranes, and escapes through the vagina and cervix. B. Concealed placental abruption where blood collects behind the placenta, with no evidence of vaginal bleeding. Figure reproduced, with permission from Oyelese and Ananth5 Placental abruption. Obstetrics and Gynecology 2006;108:1005-1016.

Incidence and Temporal Trends

Placental abruption complicates roughly 1 in 100 to 120 (0.8% to 1%) pregnancies,[6, 7] but estimates vary considerably between countries and regions. The rate is reported to be as low as 1 in 300 (0.3%) in Norway[8] and 1 in 250 (0.4%) in Sweden[9] and Finland[10] to as high as 1 in 50 pregnancies in the United States Collaborative Perinatal Project [11, 12] and other hospital-based studies.[13] Placental abruption severe enough to result in a stillbirth complicated roughly 1 in 420 deliveries in a large hospital-based study.[14] In fact, the rate of placental abruption varies dramatically by gestational age at delivery (Fig 2), with the rate being 10-

fold higher at very preterm gestations and sharply declining and pregnancy progresses toward term. Sheiner and colleagues reported a rate of abruption of 5.4% and 0.3% at preterm and term gestations, respectively.[15, 16]

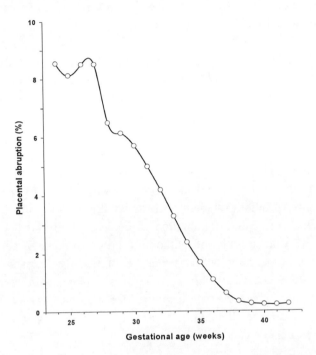

Figure 2. Risk of placental abruption by gestational age at delivery in the United States, 2003-04.

The incidence of placental abruption had increased by 23% between 1979-81 (0.81%) and 1999-01 (1.00%) in the United States, and that increase was evident among more black women than among white women.[17] In fact, the rate almost doubled among blacks (relative risk 1.97, 95% confidence interval 1.88-1.96) and increased by 15% among whites (relative risk 1.15, 95% confidence interval 1.14-1.16). These trends were also observed in studies from Norway, where Rasmussen and colleagues[8, 18] showed that the frequency of placental abruption increased by 72% between 1971 (0.53%) and 1990 (0.91%). Although causes for such temporal increases in placental abruption could be varied and numerous, it is likely that diagnostic criterion for abruption, among other clinical and socio-behavioral risk factors, may have contributed much to these trends.[17]

Maternal Mortality and Complications

Placental abruption is associated with a variety of maternal complications, but maternal deaths from pregnancies complicated by abruption, although rare, have also been documented.[19-23] Maternal risks associated with placental abruption include disseminated intravascular coagulation, hemorrhagic shock, uterine rupture, hysterectomy, and acute renal failure.[19, 24]

Etiology and Pathophysiology

Placental abruption can be the end-result of an acute process/event or the final culmination of long-standing chronic processes.[25, 26] Mechanical forces to the abdomen, including blunt trauma and sudden uterine decompression, can lead to premature placental separation suggesting an acute process. In the latter, thrombosis, inflammation, infection, decidual vasculopathy of the uteroplacental vasculature are suggestive of chronic processes that can lead to premature placental separation. Epidemiologic evidence suggesting that placental abruption is largely a chronic disease condition was recently demonstrated using population-based data of singleton births in the United States.[26] Rates of 1) acute-inflammation–associated clinical conditions (premature rupture of membranes and intrauterine infection); 2) chronic processes associated with vascular dysfunction or chronic inflammation (chronic and pregnancy-induced hypertension, preexisting or gestational diabetes, small for gestational age, and maternal smoking); and 3) both acute and chronic processes, were examined among women with and without abruption (Fig 3). These data show that the frequency of acute-inflammation associated conditions declined steadily with gestational age in both women with and without an abruption (Fig 3, panel A). In contrast, rates of chronic processes increased with advancing gestation (Fig 2, panel B); among women with abruption, the rate increased steadily up to term, and plateaued thereafter, in contrast to women without abruption where the rate began to decline much earlier (around 28 weeks.) Rates of both acute and chronic clinical processes (Fig 3, panel C) were similar to those with acute-inflammation-associated conditions.[26]

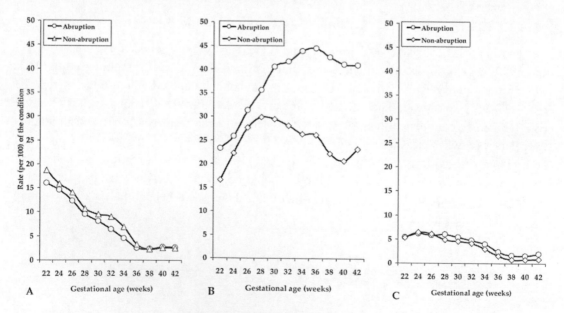

Figure 3. Rates (per 100 births) of acute-inflammation–associated conditions (A), chronic clinical processes (B), and acute-inflammation– associated conditions and chronic clinical processes combined (C) among women with and without placental abruption (Figure reproduced, with permission, from Ananth *et al.*[26] Placental abruption in term and preterm gestations: evidence for heterogeneity in clinical pathways. Obstet Gynecol 2006;107:785-92.).

Epidemiology and Risk Factors

Despite extensive research, the cause of the majority of placental abruption cases remain unknown.[27] A number of epidemiologic and clinical studies have identified several predisposing risk factors for this condition. Risk factors that trigger acute-onset placental abruption include abdominal trauma/injury, short umbilical cord, and sudden uterine decompression.[28-35] In their study of women in California that gave birth while being hospitalized for trauma, El-Kady et al.[36] noted a 9.2-fold (95% confidence interval 7.8-11.0) increased odds of placental abruption in comparison to women without any traumatic experience. In the same study, the authors found a 1.6-fold (95% confidence interval 1.3-1.9) increased odds of abruption in women that sustained trauma prenatally, but who delivered later.[36] More recently, Schiff[37] reported data from Washington State that the risk of placental abruption was 8-fold higher (95% confidence interval 4.3-15.0) among women hospitalized for falls.

Maternal Age and Parity

Young and advanced maternal age and multiparity have been implicated as predisposing risk factors for a variety of obstetrical complications, including placental abruption. However, these associations have been strongly disputed. Some studies showed evidence of an association between maternal age and abruption risk[38-40] while others demonstrated associations between parity and placental abruption.[1, 20, 41]

With concerns attributable to inadequate study designs and inadequate adjustments for confounding factors aside, the chief reason for such wide-spread disparity in previous findings is that maternal age and parity are tightly correlated. Therefore, efforts to disentangle the associations amongst age, parity and abruption, in principle, must examine the associations jointly. A large, cohort study from Nova Scotia, Canada showed that teenaged women and women with repeated pregnancies are at particularly increased risk of abruption,[42] observations that corroborates several previous studies.[10, 23, 38, 43-48] More importantly, Ananth and colleagues[42] reported a strong interaction between maternal age and parity on the risk of abruption, with increased risk among multiparous women that were young (<30 years). These observations suggest a joint influence of aging effects of the uterus (repeated pregnancies) and a natural biologic aging process on abruption risk.

Preterm Premature Rupture of Membranes and Intrauterine Infection

The occurrence of placental abruption has a strong infectious underpinning, but the pathophysiologic mechanisms for such purported associations remain poorly understood. Intrauterine infections, notably chorioamnionitis, are associated with increased risk of placental abruption. Several studies have shown that inflammatory lesions of the placenta, both at preterm and term gestations are associated with abruption.[17, 43, 49-52] Darby and colleagues[50] showed that the frequency of chorioamnionitis was 10-fold greater in preterm abruption cases than controls (41% versus 4%, P<0.001). Importantly, the association between chorioamnionitis and abruption risk was stronger at preterm (odds ratio 3.6, 95% confidence interval 1.7-10.5) than at term (odds ratio 2.8, 95% confidence interval 1.3-6.1) gestations.[53] However, this association was largely driven by severe chorioamnionitis. Since abruption is associated with a thrombin-enhanced expression of a potent neutrophil chemoattractant — interleukin-8, it is speculated that that the association may be the consequence of marked infiltration of decidual neutrophils.[54, 55]

Mechanisms that support increased risk of placental abruption in relation to prolonged rupture of membranes is speculative, but likely many. Vintzileos *et al.*[13] concluded that infections do not seem to be implicated in the pathway through which preterm premature rupture of membranes (PROM) predisposes to abruption. Nelson *et al.*[56] fuelled speculations that the mechanism was similar to placental separation in the third stages of labor, and perhaps a sudden reduction in uterine volume was the cause of placental abruption. As more studies began to report the associations amongst preterm PROM,[13, 27, 43, 44, 46, 52, 56, 57] intra-uterine infections[43, 46, 50, 52, 53] and abruption, it became apparent that both these conditions were independently associated with increased risk of abruption.

Despite speculations regarding the temporal association between preterm PROM and abruption, the evidence of a dose-effect in the increasing latency between preterm PROM and risk of abruption suggests that preterm PROM is likely a predisposing risk factor for abruption. It has been estimated that roughly 6% of placental abruption cases are attributable to pregnancies complicated by both preterm PROM and intrauterine infections.[52]

Hypertensive Disorders Complicating Pregnancy

The first documented anecdotal observation regarding an association between toxemia of pregnancy and placental abruption by a noted obstetrician Chantrueil dates back to the early 19th century. Subsequent to these initial observations, scores of studies either have validated the association between hypertensive disorders complicating pregnancy, notably, preeclampsia and risk of abruption[7, 40, 44, 46, 58-60] or have refuted it.[20, 61] A meta-analysis reported that women diagnosed with preexisting or chronic hypertension are over 3-fold (odds ratio 3.1, 95% confidence interval 2.0-4.8) likely to develop placental abruption,[6] and this association has been confirmed in subsequent studies.[7, 12, 15, 16, 46, 48, 60, 62] Preeclampsia and preeclampsia superimposed on chronic hypertension are two other hypertensive complications that are established risk factors for abruption, with odds ratios of 2-5 to 4-fold for preeclampsia[7, 12, 42] and even higher estimates for superimposed hypertension.[7]

The initial reports that did not detect an association between hypertension and abruption speculated that hypertension was the result of vasoconstriction caused by hemorrhage or release of vaso-constrictive substances.[1] As more and more data began to accrue, these initial findings were challenged, and it remains fairly well-established now that both chronic hypertension and preeclampsia are strong risk factors for placental abruption. Unfortunately, anti-hypertensive therapy does not appear to be beneficial in reducing the risk of placental abruption in women diagnosed with preexisting (chronic) hypertension.[63]

Tobacco, Cocaine, Marijuana, and Drug Use

Smoking during pregnancy has to be one of the most consistently reported risk factors for most obstetrical complications and perinatal outcomes.[64] One notable exception to this association is preeclampsia (discussed below). Smoking is associated with roughly a doubling of risk of abruption,[62] although evidence for a dose-response effect with number of cigarettes smoked per day appears modest.[40, 44, 45, 65-67] In fact, based on a study in Nova Scotia, Canada, we[66] demonstrated a threshold effect of number of cigarettes smoked per day and risk of abruption. These data indicated a linear increase in risk of abruption with increasing number of cigarettes smoked up to 10, and plateaued thereafter. Naeye and colleagues[11] reported that not only was there a linear increase in the risk of abruption in relation to increasing number of cigarettes smoked, but that the risk was also dependent on the number of years smoked.

Cocaine, an alkaloid in its free form, is a strong risk factor for placental abruption. Women that ingest cocaine are generally at 2- to 3-fold increased risk of abruption.[68-71] Similarly, marijuana use during pregnancy has been shown to be associated with increased risk of placental abruptio, but this association was found only when women reported using marijuana continuously during pregnancy.[40]

Both maternal smoking and hypertensive disorders complicating pregnancy are established risk factors for placental abruption, but smoking is also protective for preeclampsia.[72-75] However, despite the paradoxical association between smoking and preeclampsia, when women smoke and develop preeclampsia, their risk of abruption appears elevated to an extent greater than the sum of the individual effects, suggesting a strong interaction. This joint effect between chronic hypertension and maternal smoking on the risk of abruption was first reported by Williams et al.[58] Subsequently, Ananth and colleagues[7] confirmed this association, and additionally reported a 5.9-fold (95% confidence interval 3.4-10.3) and 7.8-fold (95% confidence interval 2.4-25.9) increased risks of abruption among smokers that developed severe preeclampsia and chronic hypertension with superimposed preeclampsia, respectively.

Other Putative Risk Factors

Recent studies suggest that surgical disruption of the uterine cavity, including prior cesarean delivery[76-78] and a short inter-pregnancy interval are risk factors of abruption.[78] Exposure to snakebite[79] and excessive stimulation of the nipple during antepartum electronic fetal heart rate surveillance[80] have been associated with increased risks of placental abruption, but these findings remain anecdotal and unconfirmed. Other studies suggest that maternal uterine fibroids may also predispose women to an increased risk of placental abruption,[81] although this association remains uncorroborated. Maternal iron deficiency anemia has been suggested as a potential risk factor for placental abruption,[82] but the evidence remains weak. Epidemiologic studies have also observed a slight excess of male fetuses in women diagnosed with abruption.[27, 44, 46]

Poor maternal diet and inadequate nutrition during pregnancy, especially during the early stages of pregnancy, is suggested to be associated with increased risk of placental abruption. It is generally thought that inadequate nutrition, including folate deficiency is associated with abruption[1, 83-86], but these findings have also been challenged.[87, 88] More recently, Nilsen *et al.*[89] reported a 32% reduction in the incidence of placental abruption in women that took both folate and multivitamin during pregnancy, suggesting some benefit of dietary and supplementation folate on abruption risk.

Recurrence of Placental Abruption

Among all known risk factors for placental abruption, perhaps the strongest predictor of risk is prior abruption.[6, 10, 12, 90-95] The recurrence risk for placental abruption has been estimated to range between 6% and 15%, suggesting that a vast majority of abruption cases likely bear an underlying chronic process.[25, 26] Data from a large hospital-based cohort study suggested that up to 7% of women diagnosed with abruption that was severe enough to result in stillbirths would encounter the same outcome in the subsequent pregnancy.[14] Evidence suggesting a dose-response increase in risk based on the number of prior abruptions is, however, weak. Hibbard and Jeffcoate[1] reported that women with two previous abruptions carried a 25% likelihood of developing abruption in the next pregnancy and, in a more serious form.[96]

Despite the increased recurrence and importance of placental abruption as a determinant of adverse pregnancy outcomes (discussed later), there are no reliable methods for risk assessment or biologic markers for predicting risk.[97] This leaves the undesired consequence of uncertain obstetrical management of patients that have experienced placental abruption in a previous pregnancy or those at impending risk. Perhaps the most complicating factor to this conundrum is the lack of a universal and acceptable diagnosis of this devastating obstetrical complication.

Ischemic Placental Disease

Numerous attempts to understand and characterize the etiology of placental abruption and related obstetrical complications have been disappointing. Rasmussen *et al.*[98] reported data from the Medical Birth Registry of Norway that showed that women with a previous small for gestational age birth, chronic hypertension or diabetes mellitus were at 2 to 4-fold increased risk of placental abruption in the subsequent pregnancy.[98] They speculated that small for gestational age, hypertension and diabetes were conditions that involved some dysfunction of the placenta. Subsequently, in an effort to better understand the etiology of abruption, Ananth and Vintzileos[99, 100] proposed that preeclampsia, intrauterine growth restriction and placental abruption were obstetrical complications that involved the placenta, and conditions with variable clinical manifestations on an underlying disorder – ischemic placental disease. This concept of a unified pathophysiologic mechanism was subsequently supported through epidemiologic patterns of cross-recurrence of each of the 3 conditions. Specifically, they showed that women that had preeclampsia in the first pregnancy were not only at increased risk of preeclampsia in the second pregnancy, by also carried increased risk of placental abruption.[95, 101]

Familial Predisposition

Studies have recently shown that placental abruption tends to aggregate more in families of women with that have experienced an abruption. This was first demonstrated by Toivonen et al.[102] in a Finnish study, who compared rates of abruption in first-degree female relatives (mothers and sisters) to that of 29,605 women in a general obstetrical population. The risk of abruption in first-degree relatives of abruption probands (0.4%) was similar to that in the general population (0.6%). However, when these data were restricted to probands with recurrent placental abruption, the odds ratio for familial aggregation of abruption in mothers and sisters combined was 5.6 (95% confidence interval 1.4-23.2). These observations suggest a role for a genetic predisposition for placental abruption,[103-113] although the evidence needs further corroboration.

Placental Abruption and Adverse Perinatal Outcomes

Placental abruption is fairly rare and complicates about 1 in 100 pregnancies, yet it contributed disproportionately to excessively high rates of preterm birth, fetal growth restriction and perinatal mortality. It has been estimated that up to a quarter of all preterm births can be attributed to placental abruption, and especially preterm births that are medically indicated.[114]

Placental abruption is strongly associated with increased risk of low birthweight (<2,500 g). Several studies have demonstrated that the association between abruption and low birthweight[30, 115-117] is chiefly mediated through the strong associations with preterm births and, to a lesser extent, through intrauterine growth restriction.[44, 114, 118-120] Babies born to women diagnosed with abruption are delivered early (Fig 4, left panel), and these babies weigh, on average, 400 g lower in comparison to babies of women without abruption (Fig 4, right panel). The consistently lower birthweight-for-gestational age among abruption births strongly suggest that such babies are likely growth restricted. Ananth and Wilcox[121] showed that in the United States, babies in the lowest centile of weight (<1% adjusted for gestational age) were nearly nine times as likely to be born with placenta abruption than those babies in the heaviest (≥90%) birthweight centiles, with progressively declining risk with increasing birthweight centiles (Table 1.) To isolate effects of early (preterm) delivery from growth restriction, the association between abruption and growth restriction at term was indeed strong, suggesting that placental abruption is strongly associated with early delivery and affects fetal growth. These observations led them to speculate that the origins of placental abruption lie at least in mid-pregnancy and may perhaps even extend earlier the stages of placental implantation.[121]

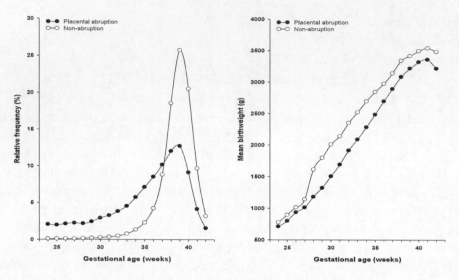

Figure 4. Distribution of gestational age (panel A) and mean birthweight-for-gestational age in singleton live births from pregnancies with and without placental abruption in the United States, 2003-04.

Table 1. Relative risk for placental abruption in relation to gestational age-specific centiles of birthweight: United States singleton live births, 1995-96.

Gestational age-specific birthweight centile (%)	Adjusted relative risk (95% confidence interval)	
	All births	Term births
<1	8.8 (8.2-9.5)	9.8 (9.0-10.5)
1-2	5.1 (4.8-5.4)	4.6 (4.3-5.0)
3-4	4.2 (4.0-4.5)	3.5 (3.2-3.8)
5-9	3.6 (3.4-3.8)	2.7 (2.5-2.9)
10-19	3.1 (3.0-3.3)	2.0 (1.9-2.1)
20-19	2.8 (2.7-2.9)	1.7 (1.6-1.8)
30-39	2.5 (2.4-2.7)	1.5 (1.3-1.5)
40-49	2.3 (2.2-2.5)	1.4 (1.3-1.5)
50-59	2.1 (2.0-2.3)	1.4 (1.3-1.5)
60-69	1.8 (1.7-1.9)	1.2 (1.1-1.3)
70-79	1.5 (1.4-1.6)	1.2 (1.2-1.3)
80-89	1.3 (1.2-1.3)	1.1 (1.0-1.2)
≥90	1.0 (Reference)	1.0 (Reference)

Reproduced, with permission, from Ananth and Wilcox[121] (American Journal of Epidemiology 2001;153: 332-337)

Placental abruption has potentially disastrous effects to the fetus, with perinatal mortality as high as 60%.[18, 20, 39, 114] Karegard and Gennser[9] reported a perinatal mortality rate of 202 per 1000 births complicated by abruption in Sweden, in contrast to a rate of 10.4 per 1000 births not complicated by abruption. Using data from the Medical Birth Registry of Norway, Rasmussen and colleagues[18] reported a perinatal mortality rate of 124 per 1000 births complicated by abruption – a rate that was roughly 60-fold higher in comparison to births not complicated by abruption.

Overall risks of stillbirth in singleton births in the United States among abruption and non-abruption births were 71.4 and 3.5 per 1000 births, respectively (relative risk 22.0, 95% confidence interval 21.1-22.9). Even among babies that were live-born, the risk of neonatal mortality was 27.4 and 2.2 per 1000 live births, respectively (relative risk 13.0, 95% confidence interval 12.2-13.9). The gestational age-specific stillbirth (Fig 5, left panel) and neonatal mortality (Fig 5, right panel) among abruption and non-abruption births show marked increase in mortality rates among abruption births. In fact, the excessively high perinatal mortality with placental abruption was due, in part, to its strong association with preterm delivery; 55% of the excess perinatal deaths associated with abruption were due to early delivery, and an additional 9% to fetal growth restriction.[121]

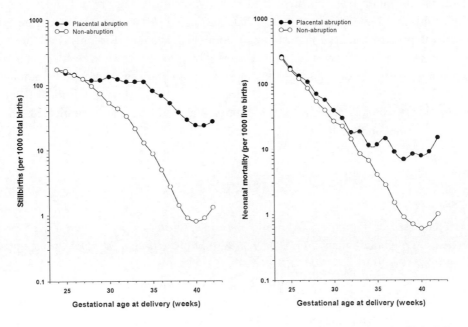

Figure 5. Risks of stillbirth and neonatal mortality in relation to placental abruption in the United States, 2003-04.

Using population-based data of all singleton, twin and triplet births in the United States (1995-98), Salihu and colleagues[122] reported that the frequency of placental abruption were 6.2, 12.2 and 15.6 per 1,000 singleton, twin, and triplet gestations respectively. In contrast to the increasing rate by plurality, these authors showed that the (adjusted) odds ratio for perinatal mortality in relation to abruption were 14.3 (95% confidence interval 13.2-15.4) among singletons, 4.4 (95% confidence interval 3.9-4.9) among twins and 3.0 (95% confidence interval 2.0-4.6) among triplet gestations.[122]

Other Adverse Perinatal Outcomes

Placental abruption has also been associated with other adverse perinatal outcomes. Several studies have reported increased risk of cerebral palsy.[65, 123-126] A recent study from Sweden[127] reported an odds ratio of 8.6 (95% confidence interval 5.6-13.3) for cerebral palsy in infants born of pregnancies complicated by placental abruption. Other newborn complications resulting from placental abruption include intraventricular hemorrhage and periventricular leukomalacia.[128] Placental abruption is also associated with a variety of major congenital malformations (relative risk 2.6, 95% confidence interval 1.5-4.4), and importantly, congenital heart defects in the newborn (relative risk 4.6, 95% confidence interval 2.5-8.6).[44]

Conclusion

Placental abruption was first described over two centuries ago by a famous obstetrician Edward Rigby in 1775.[61] It is estimated that both acute-inflammatory process and chronic processes (at preterm and term gestations) combined account for only half of placental abruption cases.[26] This observation alone underscores how little we understand the etiologic underpinnings of this serious obstetrical complication. In addition, there are no biomarkers or clinical tests to predict the condition, and efforts leading to such biomarker identification may prove beneficial to understand placental abruption – a condition that is implicated in a variety of adverse maternal and fetal outcomes.

References

[1]   Hibbard BM, Jeffcoate TN. Abruptio placentae. *Obstet Gynecol* 1966;27:155-67.

[2]   Lowe TW, Cunningham FG. Placental abruption. *Clinical obstetrics and gynecology* 1990;33:406-13.

[3]   Nielson EC, Varner MW, Scott JR. The outcome of pregnancies complicated by bleeding during the second trimester. *Surg Gynecol Obstet* 1991;173:371-4.

[4]   Clark SL. Placenta previa and abruptio placentae. In: Creasy RK, Resnik R, eds. *Maternal Fetal Medicine*. 5th edition. Philadelphia, PA: WB Saunders Company; 2004:715-7.

[5]   Oyelese Y, Ananth CV. Placental abruption. *Obstet Gynecol* 2006;108:1005-16.

[6]   Ananth CV, Savitz DA, Williams MA. Placental abruption and its association with hypertension and prolonged rupture of membranes: A methodologic review and meta-analysis. *Obstet Gynecol* 1996;88:309-18.

[7]   Ananth CV, Savitz DA, Bowes WA, Jr., Luther ER. Influence of hypertensive disorders and cigarette smoking on placental abruption and uterine bleeding during pregnancy. *Br J Obstet Gynaecol* 1997;104:572-8.

[8]   Rasmussen S, Irgens LM, Bergsjo P, Dalaker K. The occurrence of placental abruption in Norway 1967-1991. *Acta Obstet Gynecol Scand* 1996;75:222-8.

[9]   Karegard M, Gennser G. Incidence and recurrence rate of abruptio placentae in Sweden. *Obstet Gynecol* 1986;67:523-8.

[10] Tikkanen M, Nuutila M, Hiilesmaa V, Paavonen J, Ylikorkala O. Clinical presentation and risk factors of placental abruption. *Acta Obstet Gynecol Scand* 2006;85:700-5.

[11] Naeye RL. Abruptio placentae and placenta previa: Frequency, perinatal mortality, and cigarette smoking. *Obstet Gynecol* 1980;55:701-4.

[12] Misra DP, Ananth CV. Risk factor profiles of placental abruption in first and second pregnancies: Heterogeneous etiologies. *J Clin Epidemiol* 1999;52:453-61.

[13] Vintzileos AM, Campbell WA, Nochimson DJ, Weinbaum PJ. Preterm premature rupture of the membranes: A risk factor for the development of abruptio placentae. *Am J Obstet Gynecol* 1987;156:1235-8.

[14] Pritchard JA, Mason R, Corley M, Pritchard S. Genesis of severe placental abruption. *Am J Obstet Gynecol* 1970;108:22-7.

[15] Sheiner E, Shoham-Vardi I, Hadar A, Hallak M, Hackmon R, Mazor M. Incidence, obstetric risk factors and pregnancy outcome of preterm placental abruption: a retrospective analysis. *J Matern Fetal Neonatal Med* 2002;11:34-9.

[16] Sheiner E, Shoham-Vardi I, Hallak M, et al. Placental abruption in term pregnancies: Clinical significance and obstetric risk factors. *J Matern Fetal Neonatal Med* 2003;13:45-9.

[17] Ananth CV, Oyelese Y, Yeo L, Pradhan A, Vintzileos AM. Placental abruption in the United States, 1979 through 2001: Temporal trends and potential determinants. *Am J Obstet Gynecol* 2005;192:191-8.

[18] Rasmussen S, Irgens LM, Bergsjo P, Dalaker K. Perinatal mortality and case fatality after placental abruption in Norway 1967-1991. *Acta Obstet Gynecol Scand* 1996;75:229-34.

[19] Brame RG, Harbert GM, Jr., McGaughey HS, Jr., Thornton WN, Jr. Maternal risk in abruption. *Obstet Gynecol* 1968;31:224-7.

[20] Paterson ME. The aetiology and outcome of abruptio placentae. *Acta Obstet Gynecol Scand* 1979;58:31-5.

[21] Rai L, Duvvi H, Rao UR, Vaidehi, Nalinii V. Severe abruptio placentae--still unpreventable. *Int J Gynaecol Obstet* 1989;29:117-20.

[22] Sibai BM, Ramadan MK, Usta I, Salama M, Mercer BM, Friedman SA. Maternal morbidity and mortality in 442 pregnancies with hemolysis, elevated liver enzymes, and low platelets (HELLP syndrome). *Am J Obstet Gynecol* 1993;169:1000-6.

[23] Yla-Outinen A, Palander M, Heinonen PK. Abruptio placentae--risk factors and outcome of the newborn. *Eur J Obstet Gynecol Reprod Biol* 1987;25:23-8.

[24] Leunen K, Hall DR, Odendaal HJ, Grove D. The profile and complications of women with placental abruption and intrauterine death. *J Trop Pediatr* 2003;49:231-4.

[25] Ananth CV, Oyelese Y, Prasad V, Getahun D, Smulian JC. Evidence of placental abruption as a chronic process: Associations with vaginal bleeding early in pregnancy and placental lesions. *Eur J Obstet Gynecol Reprod Biol* 2006;128:15-21.

[26] Ananth CV, Getahun D, Peltier MR, Smulian JC. Placental abruption in term and preterm gestations: evidence for heterogeneity in clinical pathways. *Obstet Gynecol* 2006;107: 785-92.

[27] Ananth CV, Smulian JC, Demissie K, Vintzileos AM, Knuppel RA. Placental abruption among singleton and twin births in the United States: risk factor profiles. *Am J Epidemiol* 2001; 153:771-8.

[28] Lavin JP, Jr., Miodovnik M. Delayed abruption after maternal trauma as a result of an automobile accident. *J Reprod Med* 1981;26:621-4.

[29] Higgins SD, Garite TJ. Late abruptio placenta in trauma patients: implications for monitoring. *Obstet Gynecol* 1984;63:10S-2S.

[30] Brink AL, Odendaal HJ. Risk factors for abruptio placentae. *S Afr Med J* 1987;72:250-2.

[31] Kettel LM, Branch DW, Scott JR. Occult placental abruption after maternal trauma. *Obstet Gynecol* 1988;71:449-53.

[32] Pearlman MD, Tintinallli JE, Lorenz RP. A prospective controlled study of outcome after trauma during pregnancy. *Am J Obstet Gynecol* 1990;162:1502-7.

[33] Pritchard JA, Cunningham FG, Pritchard SA, Mason RA. On reducing the frequency of severe abruptio placentae. *Am J Obstet Gynecol* 1991;165:1345-51.

[34] Cook KE, Jenkins SM. Pathologic uterine torsion associated with placental abruption, maternal shock, and intrauterine fetal demise. *Am J Obstet Gynecol* 2005;192:2082-3.

[35] Munro KI, Horne AW, Martin CW, Calder AA. Uterine torsion with placental abruption. *J Obstet Gynaecol* 2006;26:167-9.

[36] El-Kady D, Gilbert WM, Anderson J, Danielsen B, Towner D, Smith LH. Trauma during pregnancy: an analysis of maternal and fetal outcomes in a large population. *Am J Obstet Gynecol* 2004;190:1661-8.

[37] Schiff MA. Pregnancy outcomes following hospitalisation for a fall in Washington State from 1987 to 2004. *BJOG* 2008;115:1648-54.

[38] Eriksen G, Wohlert M, Ersbak V, Hvidman L, Hedegaard M, Skajaa K. Placental abruption. A case-control investigation. *Br J Obstet Gynaecol* 1991;98:448-52.

[39] Naeye RL, Harkness WL, Utts J. Abruptio placentae and perinatal death: A prospective study. *Am J Obstet Gynecol* 1977;128:740-6.

[40] Williams MA, Lieberman E, Mittendorf R, Monson RR, Schoenbaum SC. Risk factors for abruptio placentae. *Am J Epidemiol* 1991;134:965-72.

[41] Abu-Heija A, al-Chalabi H, el-Iloubani N. Abruptio placentae: risk factors and perinatal outcome. *J Obstet Gynaecol Res* 1998;24:141-4.

[42] Ananth CV, Wilcox AJ, Savitz DA, Bowes WA, Jr., Luther ER. Effect of maternal age and parity on the risk of uteroplacental bleeding disorders in pregnancy. *Obstet Gynecol* 1996;88: 511-6.

[43] Saftlas AF, Olson DR, Atrash HK, Rochat R, Rowley D. National trends in the incidence of abruptio placentae, 1979-1987. *Obstet Gynecol* 1991;78:1081-6.

[44] Raymond EG, Mills JL. Placental abruption. Maternal risk factors and associated fetal conditions. *Acta Obstet Gynecol Scand* 1993;72:633-9.

[45] Cnattingius S. Maternal age modifies the effect of maternal smoking on intrauterine growth retardation but not on late fetal death and placental abruption. *Am J Epidemiol* 1997; 145:319-23.

[46] Kramer MS, Usher RH, Pollack R, Boyd M, Usher S. Etiologic determinants of abruptio placentae. *Obstet Gynecol* 1997;89:221-6.

[47] Sanchez SE, Pacora PN, Farfan JH, et al. Risk factors of abruptio placentae among Peruvian women. *Am J Obstet Gynecol* 2006;194:225-30.

[48] Shen TT, DeFranco EA, Stamilio DM, Chang JJ, Muglia LJ. A population-based study of race-specific risk for placental abruption. *BMC Pregnancy Childbirth* 2008;8:43.

[49] Naeye RL. Coitus and antepartum haemorrhage. *Br J Obstet Gynaecol* 1981;88:765-70.

[50] Darby MJ, Caritis SN, Shen-Schwarz S. Placental abruption in the preterm gestation: An association with chorioamnionitis. *Obstet Gynecol* 1989;74:88-92.

[51] Holmgren PA, Olofsson JI. Preterm premature rupture of membranes and the associated risk for placental abruption. Inverse correlation to gestational length. *Acta Obstet Gynecol Scand* 1997;76:743-7.

[52] Ananth CV, Oyelese Y, Srinivas N, Yeo L, Vintzileos AM. Preterm premature rupture of membranes, intrauterine infection, and oligohydramnios: risk factors for placental abruption. *Obstet Gynecol* 2004;104:71-7.

[53] Nath CA, Ananth CV, Smulian JC, Shen-Schwarz S, Kaminsky L. Histologic evidence of inflammation and risk of placental abruption. *Am J Obstet Gynecol* 2007;197:319 e1-6.

[54] Lockwood CJ, Toti P, Arcuri F, et al. Mechanisms of abruption-induced premature rupture of the fetal membranes: thrombin-enhanced interleukin-8 expression in term decidua. *Am J Pathol* 2005;167:1443-9.

[55] Rosen T, Schatz F, Kuczynski E, Lam H, Koo AB, Lockwood CJ. Thrombin-enhanced matrix metalloproteinase-1 expression: a mechanism linking placental abruption with premature rupture of the membranes. *J Matern Fetal Neonatal Med* 2002;11:11-7.

[56] Nelson DM, Stempel LE, Zuspan FP. Association of prolonged, preterm premature rupture of the membranes and abruptio placentae. *J Reprod Med* 1986;31:249 53.

[57] Major CA, de Veciana M, Lewis DF, Morgan MA. Preterm premature rupture of membranes and abruptio placentae: is there an association between these pregnancy complications? *Am J Obstet Gynecol* 1995;172:672-6.

[58] Williams MA, Mittendorf R, Monson RR. Chronic hypertension, cigarette smoking, and abruptio placentae. *Epidemiology* 1991;2:450-3.

[59] Zetterstrom K, Lindeberg SN, Haglund B, Hanson U. Maternal complications in women with chronic hypertension: A population-based cohort study. *Acta Obstet Gynecol Scand* 2005; 84:419-24.

[60] Ananth CV, Peltier MR, Kinzler WL, Smulian JC, Vintzileos AM. Chronic hypertension and risk of placental abruption: Is the association modified by ischemic placental disease? *Am J Obstet Gynecol* 2007;197:273 e1-7.

[61] Hibbard BM, Hibbard ED. Aetiological factors in abruptio placentae. *British Medical Journal* 1963;2:1430-6.

[62] Ananth CV, Smulian JC, Vintzileos AM. Incidence of placental abruption in relation to cigarette smoking and hypertensive disorders during pregnancy: A meta-analysis of observational studies. *Obstet Gynecol* 1999;93:622-8.

[63] Sibai BM, Mabie WC, Shamsa F, Villar MA, Anderson GD. A comparison of no medication versus methyldopa or labetalol in chronic hypertension during pregnancy. *Am J Obstet Gynecol* 1990;162:960-6; discussion 6-7.

[64] Cnattingius S. The epidemiology of smoking during pregnancy: smoking prevalence, maternal characteristics, and pregnancy outcomes. *Nicotine Tob Res* 2004;6 Suppl 2:S125-40.

[65] Spinillo A, Fazzi E, Stronati M, Ometto A, Capuzzo E, Guaschino S. Early morbidity and neurodevelopmental outcome in low-birthweight infants born after third trimester bleeding. *Am J Perinatol* 1994;11:85-90.

[66] Ananth CV, Savitz DA, Luther ER. Maternal cigarette smoking as a risk factor for placental abruption, placenta previa, and uterine bleeding in pregnancy. *Am J Epidemiol* 1996; 144:881-9.

[67] Cnattingius S, Mills JL, Yuen J, Eriksson O, Salonen H. The paradoxical effect of smoking in preeclamptic pregnancies: Smoking reduces the incidence but increases the rates of perinatal mortality, abruptio placentae, and intrauterine growth restriction. *Am J Obstet Gynecol* 1997; 177:156-61.

[68] Siegel RK. Cocaine smoking. *N Engl J Med* 1979;300:373.

[69] Acker D, Sachs BP, Tracey KJ, Wise WE. Abruptio placentae associated with cocaine use. *Am J Obstet Gynecol* 1983;146:220-1.

[70] Townsend RR, Laing FC, Jeffrey RB, Jr. Placental abruption associated with cocaine abuse. *Am J Roentgenol* 1988;150:1339-40.

[71] Flowers D, Clark JF, Westney LS. Cocaine intoxication associated with abruptio placentae. *J Natl Med Assoc* 1991;83:230-2.

[72] Zhang J, Klebanoff MA, Levine RJ, Puri M, Moyer P. The puzzling association between smoking and hypertension during pregnancy. *Am J Obstet Gynecol* 1999;181:1407-13.

[73] England L, Zhang J. Smoking and risk of preeclampsia: a systematic review. *Front Biosci* 2007;12:2471-83.

[74] Peltier MR, Ananth CV. Is the association of maternal smoking and pregnancy-induced hypertension dependent on fetal growth? *Am J Obstet Gynecol* 2007;196:532 e1-6.

[75] Ness RB, Zhang J, Bass D, Klebanoff MA. Interactions between smoking and weight in pregnancies complicated by preeclampsia and small-for-gestational-age birth. *Am J Epidemiol* 2008;168:427-33.

[76] Hemminki E, Merilainen J. Long-term effects of cesarean sections: Ectopic pregnancies and placental problems. *Am J Obstet Gynecol* 1996;174:1569-74.

[77] Lydon-Rochelle M, Holt VL, Easterling TR, Martin DP. First-birth cesarean and placental abruption or previa at second birth. *Obstet Gynecol* 2001;97:765-9.

[78] Getahun D, Oyelese Y, Salihu HM, Ananth CV. Previous cesarean delivery and risks of placenta previa and placental abruption. *Obstet Gynecol* 2006;107:771-8.

[79] Zugaib M, de Barros AC, Bittar RE, Burdmann EA, Neme B. Abruptio placentae following snake bite. *Am J Obstet Gynecol* 1985;151:754-5.

[80] Taylor RN, Green JR. Abruptio placentae following nipple stimulation. *Am J Perinatol* 1987;4:94-7.

[81] Rice JP, Kay HH, Mahony BS. The clinical significance of uterine leiomyomas in pregnancy. *Am J Obstet Gynecol* 1989;160:1212-6.

[82] Duthie SJ, King PA, To WK, Lopes A, Ma HK. A case controlled study of pregnancy complicated by severe maternal anaemia. *Aust NZ J Obstet Gynaecol* 1991;31:125-7.

[83] Hibbard BM. The role of folic acid in pregnancy; with particular reference to anaemia, abruption and abortion. *J Obstet Gynaecol Br Commonw* 1964;71:529-42.

[84] Stone ML, Luhby AL, Feldman R, Gordon M, Cooperman JM. Folic acid metabolism in pregnancy. *Am J Obstet Gynecol* 1967;99:638-48.

[85] Hibbard BM. Folates and the fetus. *S Afr Med J* 1975;49:1223-6.

[86] Ray JG, Laskin CA. Folic acid and homocyst(e)ine metabolic defects and the risk of placental abruption, pre-eclampsia and spontaneous pregnancy loss: A systematic review. *Placenta* 1999;20:519-29.

[87] Alperin JB, Haggard ME, McGanity WJ. Folic acid, pregnancy, and abruptio placentae. *Am J Clin Nutr* 1969;22:1354-61.

[88] Whalley PJ, Scott DE, Pritchard JA. Maternal folate deficiency and pregnancy wastage. I. Placental abruption. *Am J Obstet Gynecol* 1969;105:670-8.

[89] Nilsen RM, Vollset SE, Rasmussen SA, Ueland PM, Daltveit AK. Folic acid and multivitamin supplement use and risk of placental abruption: A population-based registry study. *Am J Epidemiol* 2008;167:867-74.

[90] Rasmussen S, Irgens LM, Dalaker K. The effect on the likelihood of further pregnancy of placental abruption and the rate of its recurrence. *Br J Obstet Gynaecol* 1997;104:1292-5.

[91] Rasmussen S, Irgens LM, Dalaker K. Outcome of pregnancies subsequent to placental abruption: a risk assessment. *Acta Obstet Gynecol Scand* 2000;79:496-501.

[92] Furuhashi M, Kurauchi O, Suganuma N. Pregnancy following placental abruption. *Arch Gynecol Obstet* 2002;267:11-3.

[93] Karri K, Dwarakanath L. Recurrent preterm abruption--case report. *Med Gen Med* 2005; 7:63.

[94] Ananth CV, Cnattingius S. Influence of maternal smoking on placental abruption in successive pregnancies: A population-based prospective cohort study in Sweden. *Am J Epidemiol* 2007;166:289-95.

[95] Ananth CV, Peltier MR, Chavez MR, Kirby RS, Getahun D, Vintzileos AM. Recurrence of ischemic placental disease. *Obstet Gynecol* 2007;110:128-33.

[96] Knab DR. Abruptio placentae. An assessment of the time and method of delivery. *Obstet Gynecol* 1978;52:625-9.

[97] Neilson JP. Interventions for treating placental abruption. *Cochrane Database Syst Rev* 2003:CD003247.

[98] Rasmussen S, Irgens LM, Dalaker K. A history of placental dysfunction and risk of placental abruption. *Paediatr Perinat Epidemiol* 1999;13:9-21.

[99] Ananth CV, Vintzileos AM. Maternal-fetal conditions necessitating a medical intervention resulting in preterm birth. *Am J Obstet Gynecol* 2006;195:1557-63.

[100] Ananth CV, Vintzileos AM. Epidemiology of preterm birth and its clinical subtypes. *J Matern Fetal Neonatal Med* 2006;19:773-82.

[101] Ananth CV, Vintzileos AM. Medically indicated preterm birth: Recognizing the importance of the problem. *Clin Perinatol* 2008;35:53-67.

[102] Toivonen S, Keski-Nisula L, Saarikoski S, Heinonen S. Risk of placental abruption in first-degree relatives of index patients. *Clin Genet* 2004;66:244-6.

[103] Dizon-Townson DS, Meline L, Nelson LM, Varner M, Ward K. Fetal carriers of the factor V Leiden mutation are prone to miscarriage and placental infarction. *Am J Obstet Gynecol* 1997;177:402-5.

[104] El-Khairy L, Vollset SE, Refsum H, Ueland PM. Plasma total cysteine, pregnancy complications, and adverse pregnancy outcomes: the Hordaland Homocysteine Study. *Am J Clin Nutr* 2003;77:467-72.

[105] Facchinetti F, Marozio L, Grandone E, Pizzi C, Volpe A, Benedetto C. Thrombophilic mutations are a main risk factor for placental abruption. *Haematologica* 2003;88:785-8.

[106] Jaaskelainen E, Toivonen S, Romppanen EL, et al. M385T polymorphism in the factor V gene, but not Leiden mutation, is associated with placental abruption in Finnish women. *Placenta* 2004;25:730-4.

[107] Jaaskelainen E, Keski-Nisula L, Toivonen S, et al. MTHFR C677T polymorphism is not associated with placental abruption or preeclampsia in Finnish women. *Hypertens Pregnancy* 2006;25:73-80.

[108] Jarvenpaa J, Pakkila M, Savolainen ER, Perheentupa A, Jarvela I, Ryynanen M. Evaluation of Factor V Leiden, Prothrombin and Methylenetetrahydrofolate Reductase gene mutations in patients with severe pregnancy complications in Northern Finland. *Gynecol Obstet Invest* 2006;62:28-32.

[109] Mousa HA, Alfirevic Z. Do placental lesions reflect thrombophilia state in women with adverse pregnancy outcome? *Hum Reprod* 2000;15:1830-3.

[110] Mousa HA, Alfirevic Z. Thrombophilia and adverse pregnancy outcome. *Croat Med J* 2001;42:135-45.

[111] Ananth CV, Elsasser DA, Kinzler WL, et al. Polymorphisms in methionine synthase reductase and betaine-homocysteine S-methyltransferase genes: Risk of placental abruption. *Mol Genet Metab* 2007;91:104-10.

[112] Ananth CV, Peltier MR, De Marco C, et al. Associations between 2 polymorphisms in the methylenetetrahydrofolate reductase gene and placental abruption. *Am J Obstet Gynecol* 2007; 197:385 e1-7.

[113] Ananth CV, Peltier MR, Moore DF, Kinzler WL, Leclerc D, Rozen RR. Reduced folate carrier 80A-->G polymorphism, plasma folate, and risk of placental abruption. *Hum Genet* 2008;124:137-45.

[114] Ananth CV, Berkowitz GS, Savitz DA, Lapinski RH. Placental abruption and adverse perinatal outcomes. *JAMA* 1999;282:1646-51.

[115] Niswander KR, Friedman EA, Hoover DB, Pietrowski H, Westphal MC. Fetal morbidity following potentially anoxigenic obstetric conditions. I. Abruptio placentae. *Am J Obstet Gynecol* 1966;95:838-45.

[116] Krohn M, Voigt L, McKnight B, Daling JR, Starzyk P, Benedetti TJ. Correlates of placental abruption. *Br J Obstet Gynaecol* 1987;94:333-40.

[117] Aiken CG. The causes of perinatal mortality in Bulawayo, Zimbabwe. Cent *Afr J Med* 1992;38:263-81.

[118] Voigt LF, Hollenbach KA, Krohn MA, Daling JR, Hickok DE. The relationship of abruptio placentae with maternal smoking and small for gestational age infants. *Obstet Gynecol* 1990;75:771-4.

[119] Kyrklund-Blomberg NB, Gennser G, Cnattingius S. Placental abruption and perinatal death. *Paediatr Perinat Epidemiol* 2001;15:290-7.

[120] Hung TH, Hsieh CC, Hsu JJ, Lo LM, Chiu TH, Hsieh TT. Risk factors for placental abruption in an Asian population. *Reprod Sci* 2007;14:59-65.

[121] Ananth CV, Wilcox AJ. Placental abruption and perinatal mortality in the United States. *Am J Epidemiol* 2001;153:332-7.

[122] Salihu HM, Bekan B, Aliyu MH, Rouse DJ, Kirby RS, Alexander GR. Perinatal mortality associated with abruptio placenta in singletons and multiples. *Am J Obstet Gynecol* 2005;193: 198-203.

[123] Spinillo A, Fazzi E, Stronati M, Ometto A, Iasci A, Guaschino S. Severity of abruptio placentae and neurodevelopmental outcome in low birth weight infants. *Early Hum Dev* 1993; 35:45-54.

[124] Kayani SI, Walkinshaw SA, Preston C. Pregnancy outcome in severe placental abruption. *BJOG* 2003;110:679-83.

[125] Matsuda Y, Maeda T, Kouno S. Comparison of neonatal outcome including cerebral palsy between abruptio placentae and placenta previa. *Eur J Obstet Gynecol Reprod Biol* 2003; 106:125-9.

[126] Matsuda Y, Maeda T, Kouno S. Fetal/neonatal outcome in abruptio placentae during preterm gestation. *Semin Thromb Hemost* 2005;31:327-33.

[127] Thorngren-Jerneck K, Herbst A. Perinatal factors associated with cerebral palsy in children born in Sweden. *Obstet Gynecol* 2006;108:1499-505.

[128] Gibbs JM, Weindling AM. Neonatal intracranial lesions following placental abruption. *Eur J Pediatr* 1994;153:195-7.

In: Textbook of Perinatal Epidemiology
Editor: Eyal Sheiner, pp. 639-662

ISBN: 978-1-60741-648-7
© 2010 Nova Science Publishers, Inc.

Chapter XXIX

Epidemiology of Placenta Previa

Yinka Oyelese[*] and Cande V. Ananth[2]

Professor and Director, Division of Epidemiology and Biostatistics, Department of
Obstetrics, Gynecology, and Reproductive Sciences, UMDNJ-Robert Wood Johnson
Medical School, New Brunswick NJ 08901, USA[2]

Definitions

- Placenta previa: A placenta that is situated partially or completely in the lower uterine segment of the uterus, and either overlies, or is in close proximity to, the internal os of the cervix.
- Placenta accreta: The placenta is abnormally adherent to the myometrium.
- Placenta increta: The placenta invades the myometrium.
- Placenta percreta: The placenta invades through the entire myometrium and uterine serosa, and often into surrounding structures such as the bladder and ureters.
- Vasa previa: A condition in which fetal vessels run, unprotected by placental tissue or umbilical cord, over the cervix and under the presenting part.

Introduction

Approximately one-third of cases of second- and third-trimester bleeding are due to placenta previa, making it one of the leading causes of bleeding in the second half of

[*]For Correspondence: Yinka Oyelese, Associate Professor, Division of Maternal Fetal Medicine, Department of Obstetrics & Gynecology, Tennessee Institute of Fetal Maternal and Infant Health, University of Tennessee Health Sciences Center, Memphis, TN, USA Tel: (732) 236-6307/ Fax: (732) 235-6627, Email: yinkamd@aol.com

pregnancy.[1, 2] It is also an important cause of maternal and perinatal mortality and morbidity. In 1869, Gay wrote "Of the danger to the female, in unavoidable hemorrhage, from presentation of the placenta, Professor Simpson says that "the peril of life is as great as though the patient were seized with yellow fever or malignant cholera".[3] Meigs went further, stating that "he believed the peril of placenta previa to be greater to the woman than if a pistol ball were fired at her head from the distance of a few paces."[3] While the mortality from this condition has dropped drastically in modern medicine, primarily as a result of blood transfusions, improved surgical and anesthetic techniques, asepsis and antibiotics, it continues to be associated with significant maternal and perinatal mortality, especially in the developing world.

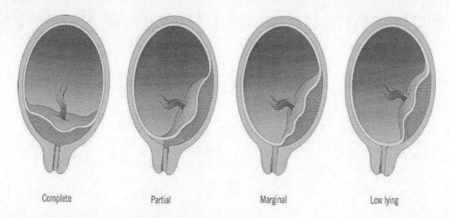

Complete   Partial   Marginal   Low lying

Figure 1. Types of placenta previa: (i) Complete placenta previa: the placenta completely overlies the internal cervical os; (ii) Partial placenta previa: the placenta partially covers the internal os, which is slightly dilated; (iii) Marginal placenta previa: the lower placental edge just reaches the internal cervical os, but does not cover it; (iv) Low-lying placenta: part of the placenta lies within the lower uterine segment. The lower placental edge does not reach the internal cervical os, but reaches within 5 cm of it. (From: Oyelese Y. Smulian JC. Placenta previa, placenta accreta, and vasa previa. (Obstet Gynecol 2006;107:927–41) ©2006 by The American College of Obstetricians and Gynecologists. Published by Lippincott Williams & Wilkins. Used by permission.).

The term "placenta previa" is derived from the word "placenta" and the Latin words "pre" meaning "before", and "via", which comes from the same origin as "viaduct" and "avenue", describing a passageway. Thus, "placenta previa" means that the placenta lies before the fetus and in the passageway, which in this case is the area over the cervix. Placenta previa is defined as a placenta that is situated partially or completely in the lower uterine segment of the uterus, and either overlies, or is in close proximity to, the internal os of the cervix. The placenta normally implants in the fundus, or the upper part of the uterus (Fig 1). In pregnancies complicated by placenta previa, when labor starts, and the cervix begins dilating, the placenta separates from the uterine wall, and bleeding is inevitable. This bleeding may be severe and life-threatening, and therefore placenta previa is one of the most important obstetric complications. There are four types of placenta previa, categorized by the relationship between the placenta and the internal cervical os.[1] When the placenta completely overlies the cervix, attempts at vaginal birth invariably lead to serious bleeding. To prevent maternal death or serious morbidity, these women need to be delivered by cesarean. In cases where the lower placental edge lies greater than 2 centimeters away from the cervix, in the absence of other contraindications to labor, vaginal birth may be safely attempted.[4, 5]

Placenta previa was historically diagnosed early in the third trimester, when the woman experienced painless vaginal bleeding.[6] The episodes of bleeding were usually recurrent and typically consisted of small volumes of blood. An unstable lie or fetal malpresentation also often led to a suspicion of placenta previa.[1, 7] These resulted from the placenta occupying the area over the cervix, a position that is usually occupied by the fetal head. More recently, the almost universal use of second trimester antenatal ultrasound has resulted in most cases being diagnosed early in pregnancy on routine sonographic examination. However, approximately 90% of women who have an apparent placenta previa in the mid-trimester will no longer have one at term.[8, 9] This phenomenon is attributed to "placental migration" in which the placenta appears to move away from the cervix as gestation advances.[9, 10] Transvaginal sonography for the diagnosis of placenta previa has been shown to be more accurate than transabdominal ultrasound.[11, 12] Abdominal sonography is associated with 12.5% false positive and false negative rates.[12]

The management of placenta previa includes hospitalization when the patient experiences bleeding, and cesarean delivery at about 36-37 weeks of gestation or if severe bleeding occurs earlier.[1] Women diagnosed with placenta previa may be put on bed rest for prolonged periods during the pregnancy. Steroids should be administered to promote fetal lung maturation in pregnancies less than 34 weeks of gestation.[1]

It is preferable to schedule delivery before the onset of labor, or before the patient experiences a massive bleed.[1] This allows surgery to proceed in a controlled environment, rather than as an emergency in a woman who has suffered continuing massive blood loss.[1] Often, an amniocentesis is performed to document fetal lung maturation prior to delivery. The greatest risk with placenta previa is of maternal hemorrhage, which may be massive. In addition, cesarean delivery may be associated with maternal mortality or morbidity, including surgical and anesthetic complications, blood transfusions, and need for hysterectomy. Placenta previa is also associated with increased rates of preterm birth, perinatal mortality, and neonatal morbidity.

Etiology

Placenta previa is caused by an abnormal location of implantation of the blastocyst in the lower segment of the uterine cavity. Damage to the endometrium or myometrium, delayed ovulation, or disorders of endometrial vascularization appear to predispose to this low implantation. Although several risk factors have been identified, the etiology of placenta previa remains elusive.[13]

Incidence

Placenta previa complicates about 0.4% of births,[14] although reported incidences have ranged up to 1.9%. The true incidence of placenta previa will vary according to how placenta previa is defined, at what gestational age the diagnosis is made, and how accurate the diagnosis is. Crenshaw and colleagues[15] reviewed all women treated for placenta previa at the Duke University Medical Center between 1950 and 1969. During that 20-year time span, in which 28,837 patients were delivered, they found that 1 in 271 pregnancies (0.37%) were affected with placenta previa.[15] A similar incidence of placenta previa had previously been reported by Davidson et al.,[16] and Reich.[17] Hibbard[18] in 1968, in a review of 102,670 deliveries at the University of Southern California Medical Center in Los Angeles over the years 1948-1953, found a rate of placenta previa of 1 per 214 deliveries, a rate of 0.46%. More recent studies continue to find a similar incidence. Monica and Lilja[19] analyzed data from 1,825,998 deliveries from 1973-90 in the Swedish Birth Registry, and found 5,683 cases of placenta previa, a rate of 0.3%. Iyasu and colleagues[20] performed a population-based study of the epidemiology of placenta previa, using data from the National Hospital Discharge Survey in the United States. They found an average incidence of placenta previa of 0.48%. They also found that the rates increased among black and other minority women, while rates among white women remained stable. This incidence has been fairly common across populations, with a rate of 0.4% reported in Croatia.[14] Wang and co-workers[21] found 126 cases of placenta previa in Malaysia, giving a rate of 0.49%. Interestingly, Hemminki and colleagues,[22] using discharge data from New York State from 1976 to 1982 found 9.9 hospital discharges for placenta previa per 1,000 live births.

The proportion of placenta previa among all pregnancies varies across gestation. This is the consequence of two separate factors; the diagnosis and ascertainment of cases of placenta previa in the second trimester, and the deliveries of cases of placenta previa as gestational age advances (Fig 2).

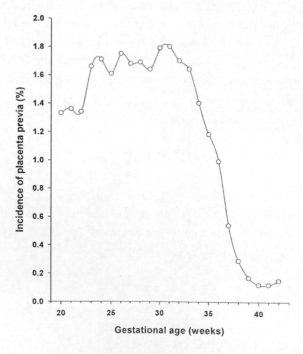

Figure 2. Rates of live births and stillbirths from placenta previa across gestation in the United States, 2003-04.

Recurrence Risk

Women with placenta previa have an increased risk of placenta previa in a subsequent pregnancy.[23, 24] Williams in 1967 described a case of a woman with placenta previa in 4 consecutive pregnancies.[25] Gorodeski and colleagues[23] studied 33,135 women who delivered from 1968-78 at the Beilinson Medical Center in Israel, and found that women who had a prior placenta previa had a rate of 3.2% of placenta previa in a subsequent pregnancy, a 6-fold increased risk.[23] Rasmussen and co-workers,[24] in a cohort study using the Medical Birth Registry of Norway, found a recurrence rate of 2.3%. Monica and Lilja[19] found a 7.2 fold increased rate of placenta previa among women who had a prior placenta previa. Endometrial or decidual damage from cesarean delivery, uterine curettage, myomectomy, or other uterine surgery appears to be implicated in the etiology of placenta previa, making it reasonable to expect that a woman with placenta previa in one pregnancy would be at increased risk in another pregnancy.

Epidemiology of Placenta Previa

Maternal Age and Parity

Increased maternal age is associated with an elevated risk for placenta previa.[14, 24, 26, 27] Sheiner and colleagues,[26] in a population-based study, found that maternal age greater than 40 years had a 3-fold higher risk of placenta previa (odds ratio 3.1, 95% confidence interval 2.0-4.9). Zhang and Savitz,[27] in a population-based, case-control study, using Vital Records from North Carolina (1986-88), observed a dose-response pattern in risk for placenta previa with increasing maternal age. Women aged ≥34 years old had a two to three times higher risk of placenta previa compared to women <20 years old. In particular, women aged greater than 45 years appear to be at increased risk of placenta previa.[14] However, women who are older tend to have increased parity. Nonetheless, this increased incidence with maternal age remains in most studies that have corrected for parity.[27] Tuzovic and colleagues,[14] in a retrospective case control study over 10 years in Croatia found maternal age ≥35 years to be a risk factor for placenta previa, even after controlling for parity. Both Babinszki and colleagues[28] and Abu-Heija and associates[29] observed that the rate of placenta previa was higher in women of higher parity. Thus, placenta previa is more common in older women, both because of age and increased parity.

Ananth and colleagues[30], using data from a population-based prospective cohort study in Nova Scotia, Canada (1980-93), reported that the risk of placenta previa increased dramatically with advancing maternal age after adjustment for potential confounders, including parity. In fact, they also reported strong interactions between maternal age and parity no the risk of developing previa.[30] They speculated that the natural ageing and aging of the uterine environment (i.e., parity effect) both play important roles in the epidemiology of placenta previa.

Maternal Race and Ethnicity

Few studies have evaluated the association of maternal race with placenta previa. Iyasu and co-workers,[20] in a U.S. study found that the risk of placenta previa was higher in black women than in white women (rate ratio 1.3, 95% confidence interval 1.0-1.7). These authors also observed that the rate of placenta previa in the US had increased among black women, while remaining stable in white women. An increased risk of placenta previa has been shown among women of Asian origin. Taylor and associates conducted a population based case-control study of 810 women using data from the Washington State birth certificates from 1984-1987.[31] They found that women of Asian origin had an 86% increased likelihood of placenta previa than were white women (odds ratio 1.86, 95% confidence interval 1.38-2.51)

Maternal Smoking

Several studies have demonstrated that smoking in pregnancy is associated with an increased risk for placenta previa.[32] Naeye,[33, 34] using data from the Collaborative Perinatal Project in the U.S., found an increased risk of placenta previa among women who smoked, and found that the frequency of placenta previa was strongly associated with the number of years the mothers had smoked, rather than how much they smoked during pregnancy. In fact, this author was of the opinion that at least half of the excessive perinatal deaths associated with maternal smoking during pregnancy were the consequence of placenta previa and placental abruption. Women who stopped smoking in pregnancy had a third fewer losses from placenta previa compared to those who continued smoking. Williams and associates performed a case-control analysis of 69 pregnancies with placenta previa and 12,351 controls, using interview and medical record data from the Boston Hospital for women (1977-80).[35] These investigators found that the relative risk for placenta previa in mothers that "ever smoked" during pregnancy was 1.9 (95% confidence interval 1.2-3.0). After adjusting for confounders, this risk rose (odds ratio 2.6, 95% confidence interval 1.3-5.5). Kramer and colleagues, using the Washington State birth certificate data from 1984 to 1987, conducted a case-control study of the relationship between smoking and placenta previa. They compared 598 pregnancies complicated by placenta previa and compared them with 2,422 randomly selected controls -pregnancies from the same time period without placenta previa. They found that smoking doubled the risk of placenta previa after adjustment for confounders (odds ratio 2.1, 95% confidence interval 1.7-2.5). Monica and Lilja examined 5,683 cases of placenta previa, and determined that smoking had a 53% increased risk for developing placenta previa.[19] These authors also found a dose-response relationship between the number of cigarettes smoked and the risk of placenta previa. Chelmlow and colleagues[36] found that smoking in pregnancy carried a 2.6 to 4.4 fold increased risk of placenta previa. Others have found such an increased risk of placenta previa among smoking women. Conversely, Zhang and Fried[37] examined the North Carolina vital records for 1988 and 1989, and found that the prevalence of placenta previa increased according to the number of cigarettes smoked per day during pregnancy, but found that after correcting for potential confounders, the odds ratio for placenta previa among smokers was only 1.3 (95% confidence interval 1.1-1.6). Thus, in Zhang and Fried's study, the magnitude of the impact of smoking on the risk of placenta previa was very modest. Ananth and associates[38] also observed such a modest risk increase when they carried out a prospective cohort study of 87,184 pregnancies from Nova Scotia, and found that smoking carried a 1.4 relative risk (95% confidence interval 1.0-1.8) of placenta previa when compared to non-smokers. These authors did not find a dose-response increased risk based on the number of cigarettes smoked per day.[38] Meyer and colleagues[39] found that smoking in pregnancy carried an increased risk of placenta previa that followed a dose-response pattern. Women who smoked more than a pack per day had a doubling of their risk of placenta previa, while those who smoked less than 1 pack per day had an increased risk of 25%. In a case-control study of 304 cases of placenta previa, Handler and colleagues[32] found a dose-response relationship between smoking cigarettes and placenta previa. Pregnant women who smoked ≥20 cigarettes per day were over two times as likely to experience a placenta previa as nonsmokers (odds ratio 2.3, 95% confidence interval 1.5-3.5).[32] Kramer and colleagues[40] proposed that the increased risk of placenta previa in smokers may be due to an increased placental size in these women.

Nicotine has been shown to cause vasoconstriction in the placenta, and impaired utero-placental blood flow, resulting in a state of placental hypoxia. Smokers, as well as women who live at high altitudes, both conditions associated with chronic oxygen deprivation, both have larger placentas.

Cocaine Use

Cocaine use has been associated with an increased risk of placenta previa. In a case-control study, Handler and associates[32] found that women who used cocaine were more 1.4 (95% confidence interval 0.8-2.4) times likely to have a placenta previa than women who did not. Maccones and colleagues[41] found, in a case-control study, that cocaine use was associated with a 4-fold increased risk of placenta previa after controlling for other variables (odds ratio 4.4, 95% confidence interval 1.2-16.4).

Infertility Treatment

Infertility treatment has been associated with an increased risk for placenta previa. Romundstadt and colleagues, examining 845,384 pregnancies from the Norway Medical Births Registry compared the risk of placenta previa in 7568 pregnancies conceived by assisted reproductive technologies (ART) with pregnancies conceived naturally.[42] They found a 6-fold higher risk of placenta previa among those singleton pregnancies conceived by ART (odds ratio 5.6, 95% confidence interval 4.4-7.0). Shevell and associates[43] similarly found that in vitro fertilization increased the risk for placenta previa. Sheiner and co-workers,[26] in a case-control study of over 78,000 births, including 298 cases of placenta previa, observed that infertility treatments were associated with a 3-fold increased risk of placenta previa (odds ratio 3.1, 95% confidence interval 1.8-5.6). Allen and co-workers[44] evaluated outcomes in pregnancies conceived by ART and also found that ART was associated with an increased risk of placenta previa. A meta-analysis by Jackson and associates[45] of complications resulting from ART also found an increased risk of placenta previa in pregnancies conceived by IVF.

It is thought that uterine contractions, possibly due to prostaglandin release, may occur following intrauterine placement of the embryos using a catheter.[46] It is possible that these contractions result in more embryos implanting in the lower uterine segment. It has also been shown that lower implantation within the uterus is associated with higher rates of successful implantation, and that some may choose to deliberately replace the embryos lower in the uterus.[47] These two mechanisms may, to some extent, explain why ART may be associated with increased risk of placenta previa.

Prior Cesarean Delivery

Perhaps the strongest risk factor for development of placenta previa is a history of a cesarean delivery in a prior pregnancy.[14, 48, 49] One of the earliest to suggest that a uterine scar predisposed to placenta previa in a subsequent pregnancy was Bender.[50] In a study of 41,206 consecutive pregnancies from Saudi Arabia, that included 222 cases of placenta previa, Chattopadhay and colleagues found that there was a five-fold increased rate of placenta previa in women with a prior cesarean scar (2.54% versus 0.44%).[51] Ananth and colleagues[48] published a meta-analysis examining the association of placenta previa with a history of prior cesarean delivery and abortion. This meta-analysis combined 36 studies and included 3.7 million women, out of which 13,992 were diagnosed with placenta previa. These authors found a strong association between these risk factors and the subsequent development of placenta previa.[48] The odds ratio for developing a placenta previa among women with a prior cesarean was 2.6 (95% confidence interval 2.3, 3.0). Further analysis of two studies showed that there was a dose-response pattern for the risk of placenta previa based on the number of prior cesarean deliveries (Fig 3). Subsequent to Ananth's meta-analysis,[48] Hendricks et al.[52] in a retrospective cohort study of all single gestations at the National University Hospital of Singapore between 1993 and 1997 found that the increased risk of developing placenta previa among women with 1,2, and 3 prior cesareans were 2.2 (95% confidence interval 1.4-3.4), 4.1 (95% confidence interval 1.9-8.8), and 22.4 (95% confidence interval 6.4-78.3) respectively.

To and colleagues reviewed patients with placenta previa over 10 years and found that a prior cesarean carried an increased risk of placenta previa (1.31%) compared with those with an unscarred uterus (0.75%; relative risk 1.6). These investigators found that this risk increased as the number of previous cesarean sections increased (relative risk 1.5 for one previous section and 2.6 for two or more).[53]

Lydon-Rochelle and colleagues[54] in a retrospective population-based, cohort analysis using data from the Washington State Birth Events Record database, found that a cesarean in a first pregnancy carried an increased risk of placenta previa (odds ratio 1.4, 95% confidence interval 1.1-1.6) in the subsequent pregnancy when compared with women who had a vaginal delivery in their first pregnancy. We studied women in their first two singleton pregnancies using the Missouri longitudinally linked data 1989-1997 and calculated the relative risk for associations between cesarean delivery and risk of previa in subsequent pregnancies, after adjusting for several confounders. We found that the pregnancy after a cesarean delivery was associated with increased risk of placenta previa compared with a vaginal delivery (relative risk 1.5, 95% confidence interval confidence interval 1.3-1.8).[55]

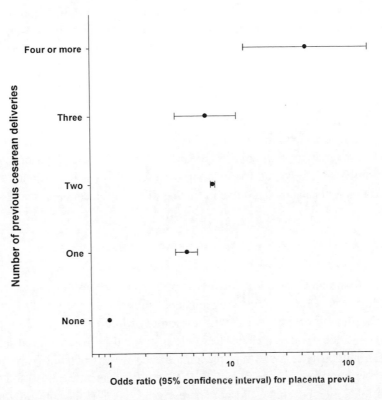

Figure 3. Odds ratios for placenta previa depending on number of prior cesarean deliveries. Data from Ananth et al.[48]

Interestingly, cesarean delivery in the first and second births conferred a two-fold increased risk of previa in the third pregnancy (relative risk 2.0, 95% confidence interval 1.3-3.0) compared with first two vaginal deliveries, suggesting a dose-response relationship between the number of cesareans and risk of placenta previa in a subsequent pregnancy. Yang and colleagues,[56] in a retrospective cohort study of 5,146,762 births in the US, found that a cesarean birth in a first pregnancy carried an odds ratio of 1.47 (95% confidence interval 1.41, 1.52) for a placenta previa in the subsequent pregnancy. Similarly, Kennare et al.,[57] in a an Australian study of over 35,000 pregnancies, found an odds ratio of 1.7 (95% confidence interval 1.3-2.1) for placenta previa in women who had a prior cesarean delivery, when compared with those who had a prior vaginal birth. The risk increased with the number of prior cesarean deliveries.[57]

Based on these data, one can infer that women with a prior cesarean have approximately double the risk of placenta previa in a subsequent pregnancy, with the risks increasing thereafter in a dose-response relationship with the number of prior cesareans. However, not all investigators have found this dose-response relationship. Hershkowitz and colleagues[58] reviewed 284 women with placenta previa. These authors found no difference in the frequency of placenta previa among women with one (1.54%), two (1.39%) and three (10.37/1,000; 1.04%) prior cesarean deliveries.[58] However, the frequency of placenta previa was significantly lower (0.79%) in women with no prior cesarean delivery.[58] It is thought that the increased risk of placenta previa results from scarring or disruption of the endometrium, which, in turn, forces implantation of the placenta in the scarred lower uterine segment. In fact, the National Institutes of Health recognizes this and states in their consensus statement that maternal cesarean on request should be discouraged in women desiring several children partly because of the risk of placenta previa in subsequent pregnancies.[59]

The cesarean delivery rate has risen dramatically in developed countries in recent years, with the most recent cesarean rate in the US in 2006 being 31.1%, up from 20.7% in 1996. Even more importantly, fewer women are attempting a vaginal birth after cesarean. This proportion dropped from 28.3% in 1996 to 9.2% in 2004.[60] Women who have had two prior cesareans almost invariably will have a cesarean for all subsequent births. Thus, the proportion of women who have had two or more cesarean scars will continue to rise. It is to be expected that this will cause a steep rise in the incidence of placenta previa.

Prior Abortion

Studies have found an association between a prior spontaneous or induced abortion. In a case-control study from Croatia, reviewing placenta previa over 10 years, Tuzovic et al.[14] found a prior abortion to be associated with an almost triple risk of placenta previa (odds ratio 2.8, 95% confidence interval 2.04-3.83). Johnson and colleagues,[61] in a case-control study from Washington State, found that placenta previa was associated with the number of prior sharp uterine curettages (odds ratio 2.9, 95% confidence interval 1.0-8.5 for ≥3 prior curettages), while suction curettage did not increase the risk for placenta previa (odds ratio 0.9, 95% confidence interval 0.6-1.5).[61] A population-based study by Taylor et al.,[62] also from Washington State, of 486 women with placenta previa and 1598 controls found that after adjusting for confounders, women with one or more prior induced abortions had a 28% increased risk for placenta previa (odds ratio 1.3, 95% confidence interval 1.0-1.6). For women with one or more spontaneous abortions, the odds ratio was 1.30 (95% confidence interval 1.01-1.66). A meta-analysis by Ananth and colleagues[48] found that there was an increased risk of placenta previa following spontaneous (relative risk 1.6, 95% confidence interval 1.0-2.6) and induced abortion (relative risk 1.7, 95% confidence interval 1.0-2.9). Others have not found this association. Grimes and co-workers[63] found that after correcting for the effects of age and gravidity, legal abortion did not increase the risk for placenta previa in a subsequent pregnancy. These data collectively suggest that there is an association between abortion and development of placenta previa in a subsequent pregnancy, but that this association is weak.

Gestational Hypertension

The risk of pregnancy-induced hypertension appears to be reduced in pregnancies complicated by placenta previa. This observation was first reported by Bieniarz in 1958, who stated "there is no eclampsia in placenta previa cases and, on the other hand, in severe toxemia of pregnancy, low implantation of the placenta is met only exceptionally".[64] Ananth and colleagues[65] carried out a population based study of 121,082 pregnancies from Nova Scotia, of which 416 had placenta previa. The risk of pregnancy-induced hypertension in women with placenta previa was 0.5 (95% confidence interval 0.4-3.7).[65] This risk reduction was still present when these investigators adjusted for length of gestation, suggesting that the reduced risk for gestational hypertension was not mediated by the earlier delivery of women with placenta previa. Wang and co-workers[21] carried out retrospective study of 25,844 singleton primigravid pregnancies in Malaysia, and assessed the relationship between pregnancy induced hypertension and placenta previa. These authors found a slight inverse association between the two, with an odds ratio of 0.93 (95% confidence interval 0.89-0.97). Nicolaides et al.[66] had similar findings in Nottingham, England. They found a 3.0% incidence of pregnancy-induced hypertension (PIH) among women with placenta previa compared with an incidence of 15.3% of PIH among women without placenta previa. Leiberman and associates[67] in Israel compared 491 women with placenta previa with 106,866 without placenta previa. These investigators found a relative risk of 0.4 (95% confidence interval 0.3-0.8) for PIH among women with placenta previa compared with women with normal placental location. This reduction persisted even when parity and gestational age were accounted for. Multivariate logistic regression analysis determined that patients with placenta previa had a third of the risk of PIH regardless of gestational age at delivery and parity.

While the exact mechanism by which placenta previa is protective against PIH is uncertain, it has been suggested that the arteries supplying a placenta previa do not undergo pressure from the myometrium and broad ligament that can occur in those supplying a fundally implanted placenta. They proposed that narrowing in the distal segment of the uterine artery ascending branch that supplies a normally implanted placenta predisposes to placental ischemia and preeclampsia. However, since this does not occur in the vessels supplying a placenta previa, the blood flow to the placenta is improved, preventing trophoblastic hypoxia, which in turn lowers the risk for pregnancy-induced hypertension.

Multiple Gestations

The rate of placenta previa is higher among twins than in singleton pregnancies. Strong and Brar reviewed the incidence of placenta previa over a 10 year period at the Women's Hospital, Los Angeles County/University of Southern California Medical Center and found that placenta previa occurred in 0.55% of twin births, compared with in 0.31% of singleton births.[68] Ananth and colleagues,[69] in a population-based study using US natality files (1989-98) comprised of 37,956,020 singleton births and 961,578 twin births, found that placenta previa was 40% higher in twin births (3.9 per 1,000 live births, n=3,793 births) than in singleton pregnancies (2.8 per 1,000 live births, n=104,754 births). Conversely, a retrospective cohort study by Francois and colleagues[70] from Arizona found that placenta previa complicated 0.18% of singleton pregnancies and 0.46% of twin pregnancies (P=0.09), and concluded that there was no significant difference in the rate of placenta previa between singleton and twin pregnancies.

Multiple gestations are associated with increased placental mass. Hence, it is reasonable to expect the placenta to extend into the lower uterine segment more frequently than in singleton pregnancies.

Fetal Gender

Retrospective studies have found an association between male fetal gender and risk of placenta previa, even though reasons for this association are unclear. MacGillivray and colleagues found an increased male-female sex ratio of 1.273 among women with placenta previa, compared with 1.050 in women without placenta previa in Cape Town, South Africa.[71] These authors proposed that the increased proportion of male fetuses in pregnancies complicated by placenta previa might be the result of delayed development of the blastocyst, which in turn leads to the low implantation. Jakobovits and Zubek[72] also, in a case-control study, found a male fetus preponderance in pregnancies with placenta previa. Demissie and colleagues[73] conducted both a historical cohort analysis of singleton live births in New Jersey and a meta-analysis to assess the association between placenta previa and male gender at birth. In the cohort study, the male-to-female ratio among newborns in pregnancies with placenta previa was 1.19 to 1, compared to 1.05 to 1 among those pregnancies that did not have a placenta previa.[73] Their meta-analysis showed an increased rate of placenta previa of 14% among pregnancies with male fetuses when compared with those with female fetuses.[73] While a male fetus appears to be associated with an increased risk for placenta previa, no biologically plausible reason for this association has been suggested.

Maternal Mortality and Morbidity

While placenta previa was formerly a leading cause of maternal mortality, the death of a mother from placenta previa in the developed world is becoming increasingly rare. However, placenta previa continues to be a cause of significant maternal morbidity, especially when it is associated with placenta accreta. Crane and colleagues[74] found that placenta previa was associated with increased risks for hysterectomy (relative risk 33.3), antepartum bleeding (relative risk 9.8), and intrapartum (relative risk 2.5) and postpartum (relative risk 1.9) hemorrhages, blood transfusion (relative risk 10.1), septicemia (relative risk 5.6), and thrombophlebitis (relative risk 4.9). McShane and colleagues[75] in a review of 147 cases of placenta previa found similar maternal risks. Takayama and colleagues[76] found that cesarean section in women with placenta previa was associated with increased blood loss when compared with cesareans in women without placenta previa (1,154 ml ± 924 ml versus 632 ml ± 357 ml; P <0.001). In that study, a hysterectomy was performed in 4/88 women with placenta previa, while none were performed in the 176 controls. There was a 6.5 fold higher blood transfusion rate among women with placenta previa compared with controls.

Sheiner and colleagues[77] found a relative risk of 8 for obstetric hysterectomy in patients who had a placenta previa (odds ratio 8.2, 95% confidence interval 2.2-31.0). Grobman and colleagues[78] found that adverse maternal outcomes (a composite of transfusion, hysterectomy, operative injury, coagulopathy, venous thromboembolism, pulmonary edema, or death) increased in women with placenta previa as the number of prior cesareans increased (odds ratio 1.9, 95% confidence interval 1.2-2.9). However, these authors did not correct for the number of cesareans the patient had previously had. Thus, it is not possible to say whether this increased maternal morbidity was the consequence of placenta previa with an increasing number of prior cesareans, or the consequence of an increasing number of cesareans alone (independent of placenta previa). Likewise, Crane and colleagues[74] found an increased risk for hysterectomy (relative risk 33.3), antepartum, intrapartum, and postpartum bleeding among patients with placenta previa.

Perinatal Mortality and Morbidity

Placenta previa has long been recognized to be associated with increased perinatal mortality and morbidity. In the early 20th century, the condition was resulted in a fetal mortality as high as 70%. This was primarily because at the time cesarean was not a safe operation, and most efforts were geared toward preserving the life of the mother rather than the fetus. Labor was induced or hastened, and high forceps deliveries or breech extractions were performed in an attempt to empty the uterus expeditiously. Later in the century, it was recommended that women with suspected placenta previa should be immediately delivered by cesarean at the time of the first bleed, which typically occurred early in the third trimester. This invariably led to a high perinatal mortality from prematurity. It was Macafee[79] and Johnson,[80] who, in separate publications in 1945 changed the outcome of the fetus in cases of placenta previa, when they advocated that delivery should be delayed until greater fetal maturity was achieved. Nesbitt and colleagues in 1962 reported that the perinatal mortality from placenta previa decreased from 44.3% in 1942 to 33.2% in 1951, coinciding with the advent of expectant management of placenta previa.[81] Similarly, Hibrd[18] in 1968 reported the perinatal mortality rate for pregnancies complicated by placenta previa as 24.7% from 1962-66.

More contemporaneous data show a marked reduction in perinatal deaths from placenta previa.[75, 77] However, placenta previa is still associated with increased perinatal mortality and morbidity. Sheiner and colleagues[26] reported a perinatal mortality rate of 2.3% among infants born to women with pregnancies complicated by placenta previa, compared with 0.9% among controls, giving odds ratio for perinatal mortality of 2.6 (95% confidence interval 1.1-5.6). These authors determined that early gestational age at delivery and the presence of congenital malformations were the significant risk factors for perinatal mortality. They also found that placenta previa carried a four-fold increased risk of Apgar scores less than 7 at 5 minutes (odds ratio 4.4, 95% confidence interval 2.3-8.3). Iyasu and colleagues,[20] in a US study, assessed placenta previa to carry a 5.5 fold increase in stillbirth compared to women without placenta previa. Ananth and co-workers,[82] in a US population-based study from 1989 to 1997, found that there was an increased neonatal mortality of 10.7 per 1,000 live births, compared with 2.5 per 1,000 for infants born to women with placenta previa compared with those born to women without placenta previa (relative risk 4.3, 95% confidence interval 4.0-4.8). These investigators also found, rather interestingly, that the perinatal mortality in pregnancies with placenta previa was lower than those without placenta previa up to a gestational age of 37 weeks. However, after 37 weeks of gestation, there was a higher perinatal mortality in pregnancies with placenta previa. They proposed that the reason for the reduced mortality below 37 weeks of gestation in pregnancies complicated by placenta previa was primarily due to aggressive use of steroids to promote fetal lung maturation in those pregnancies complicated by previa. Based on their findings, they recommended 36 to 37 weeks as an ideal gestational age for delivery of fetuses in pregnancies with placenta previa.

Using data from the US vital records (2003-04), we examined the distributions of gestational age and gestational age-specific birthweight (i.e., birthweight-for-gestational age) in those with and without placenta previa. These data indicated that women with placenta previa were delivered earlier than those without previa, suggesting an increased preterm birth rate in women with previa (Fig 4). Babies born to women placenta previa had, on average, 250g lower birthweight at early gestations in comparison to those born to women without previa (Fig 5). Although rates of stillbirth were similar in women with and without placenta previa (Fig 6), an analysis restricted to live births indicated lower neonatal mortality rates in pregnancies diagnosed with placenta previa at prior to 37 weeks, and higher thereafter, when compared with those pregnancies without placenta previa (Fig 7).

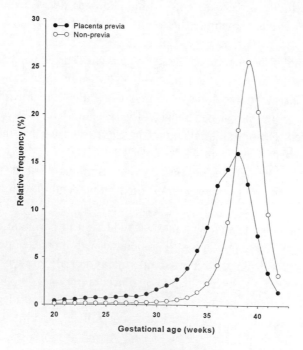

Figure 4. Distribution of gestational ages in pregnancies diagnosed with (filled circles) and without (open circles) placenta previa in the United States, 2003-04.

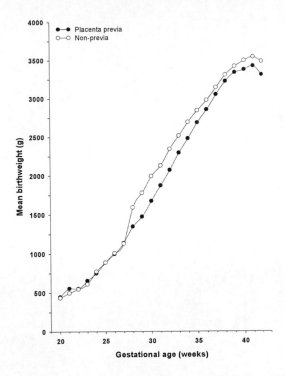

Figure 5. Distribution of mean birthweights in pregnancies with (filled circles) and without (open circles) placenta previa across gestation in the United States 2003-04.

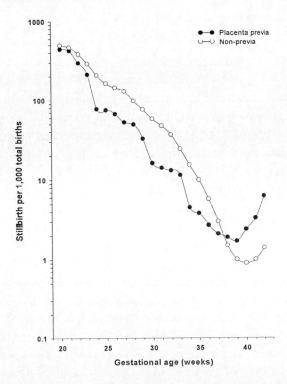

Figure 6. Rates of stillbirth compared across gestation between pregnancies complicated by placenta previa (filled circles) and those without placenta previa (open circles) in the United States 2003-04.

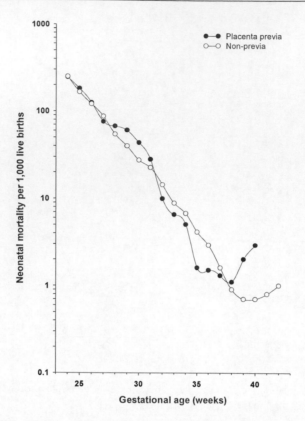

Figure 7. Rates of neonatal death compared across gestation between pregnancies complicated by placenta previa (filled circles) and those without placenta previa (open circles) in the United States 2003-04.

Salihu and colleagues[83] found that placenta previa tripled the risk of neonatal death after live birth (hazard ratio 3.1, 95% confidence interval 2.4-3.9), and attributed this increased risk to preterm delivery. Crane and colleagues,[84] examining births in Nova Scotia found an association between placenta previa and preterm birth, congenital anomalies (odds ratio 2.5), respiratory distress syndrome (odds ratio 4.9) and neonatal anemia (odds ratio 2.7). Khashoggi,[85] using data from Saudi Arabia, found a perinatal mortality rate for cases of placenta previa of 41.6 per 1,000 births, compared to 12.4 per 1,000 for women without placenta previa. These authors also reported the rate of respiratory distress syndrome to be 18.7% among neonates born in pregnancies complicated by placenta previa. McShane and colleagues[75] reviewed 147 cases of placenta previa from the Boston Hospital for Women and the Brigham and Women's Hospital in Boston from 1975 to 1982. These authors found a crude perinatal mortality rate of 81 per 1,000 births. Four of the 12 perinatal deaths were stillbirths. All the neonatal deaths were the consequence of respiratory distress or other complication of preterm birth. Interestingly, these authors found that apart from preterm birth, the gestational age at first bleed and the gestational age at major bleed correlated with perinatal mortality. Twenty percent of the newborns were anemic. Fetal anemia is a complication of placenta previa; bleeding from either the placental separation or the incision into the placenta at the time of cesarean may cause fetal blood loss. Thus, infants born to mothers with placenta previa have a high rate of blood transfusions.

Zlatnik and associates[86] carried out a retrospective cohort study of women with placenta previa and observed that women with placenta previa were 5 times as likely to be delivered before 34 weeks as women without placenta previa. The majority of deliveries in cases of placenta previa are delivered before 37 weeks, and therefore the infants are likely to suffer the increased mortality and morbidity associated with preterm birth. McShane and colleagues[75] found that two-thirds of patients with placenta previa were delivered prior to 36 weeks. Placenta previa is also associated with an increased risk of respiratory distress syndrome in the newborn, again primarily the consequence of preterm birth.[75, 87]

In summary, the data show that placenta previa is associated with increased perinatal mortality and morbidity and for the most part these adverse outcomes are the consequence of preterm birth.

Related Conditions

Placenta previa is closely associated with 2 other conditions that cause significant perinatal and maternal mortality and morbidity. Thus, a discussion of placenta previa would be incomplete without a brief discussion of these two conditions namely, placenta accreta and vasa previa.

Placenta Accreta

Placenta accreta is said to occur when the placenta is abnormally adherent to the myometrium.[1] Placenta accreta rarely occurs in the absence of a prior cesarean delivery. Normally, there is a clear plane of cleavage between the placenta and the myometrium (Nitabuch's layer). Absence or deficiency of this layer leads to placental invasion of the myometrium. It is now felt that placenta accreta results from implantation of the pregnancy in the prior cesarean scar. Attempts to remove the placenta at the time of delivery are unsuccessful and lead to severe life-threatening hemorrhage. There are three types of placenta accreta, based on degree of placental invasion *Placenta accreta* is attached to the myometrium, *placenta increta* actually invades the myometrium, while *placenta percreta* invades through the entire myometrium and uterine serosa, and often into surrounding structures such as the bladder and ureters.[1] The average blood loss at delivery is in excess of 5,000 ml. Thus, placenta accreta is associated with significant maternal morbidity and mortality.

Placenta accreta complicates approximately 1 in 2,500 pregnancies.[88] It is considered that this is a 10-fold increase over the past 50 years.[89] The main risk factors for placenta accreta are a prior cesarean and placenta previa. Clark and colleagues[90] found that the risk of placenta accreta for women with a placenta previa who also had a prior uterine incision was 24%, 47%, 40%, and 67%, depending on whether they had had one, two, three and four prior cesareans, respectively. These authors also found increasing age and parity to be associated with an increased risk of placenta accreta. Placenta accreta is ideally treated with hysterectomy after delivery of the fetus.[1] In fact, placenta accreta has become the leading indication for peripartum hysterectomy.[91] Several recent reports have documented conservative management of placenta accreta, leaving the placenta *in situ* after delivery, sometimes administering methotrexate to destroy the remaining placental tissue.[92] Embolization of the uterine arteries has also been used as in cases where the placenta has been left in place.[93]

Vasa Previa

Vasa previa is a condition in which fetal vessels run, unprotected by placental tissue or umbilical cord, over the cervix and under the presenting part.[1, 94] This is a consequence of either velamentous insertion, in which the cord inserts into the membranes rather than the placenta, or vessels running between lobes of a bi-lobate placenta.[94] The condition is of utmost importance because when the membranes break, either spontaneously or iatrogenically, these vessels often rupture, resulting in rapid fetal exsanguination and death.[94]

Vasa previa is rare, and the exact incidence remains unknown. However, data suggest that it occurs in about 1 in 2,500 births.[94] Risk factors for vasa previa include a placenta previa in the mid-trimester, even if the placenta is no longer previa at term,[95, 96] in-vitro fertilization,[95, 97, 98] multifetal gestations,[98] and bi-lobed placentas.[98]

Good perinatal outcomes with vasa previa depend on prenatal diagnosis and delivery by cesarean prior to rupture of the membranes.[99] In a multi-center cohort study of 155 pregnancies affected by vasa previa, we found that the perinatal survival was 97% in cases diagnosed prenatally compared with 44% in cases not diagnosed prenatally (P <0.001).[99] In addition, among survivors in cases not diagnosed prenatally, median 1- and 5-minute Apgar scores were only 1 and 4, compared with 8 and 9, respectively, in cases diagnosed prenatally (P <0.001). Over 50% (24 of 41) of surviving neonates born to women without prenatal diagnosis required blood transfusions compared with 2 of 59 diagnosed prenatally (P <0.001). Multivariable logistic regression analysis showed that the only significant predictors of neonatal survival were prenatal diagnosis (P <0.001) and gestational age at delivery (P=0.01)

Conclusions

Placenta previa complicates approximately 1 in 250 births. The most important risk factor for placenta previa is a prior cesarean delivery. Other risk factors include maternal smoking, multiparity, prior abortion, increasing maternal age, and male fetal gender. Placenta previa is associated with significant maternal morbidity, and, more rarely, mortality. The increased perinatal mortality associated with placenta previa is mainly the consequence of preterm birth. Because of the increasing cesarean rate in developed countries, it is to be anticipated that the rate of placenta previa will continue to rise. Reduction of the escalating cesarean delivery rate should be a focus of health care planning.

References

[1]   Oyelese Y, Smulian JC. Placenta previa, placenta accreta, and vasa previa. *Obstet Gynecol* 2006;107:927-41.

[2]   Koifman A, Levy A, Zaulan Y, Harlev A, Mazor M, Wiznitzer A, Sheiner E. The clinical significance of bleeding during the second trimester of pregnancy. *Arch Gynecol Obstet* 2008;278:47-51.

[3]   Gay C. Placenta praevia. *Trans NY State Med Soc* 1869:219-28.

[4]   Oppenheimer LW, Farine D, Ritchie JW, Lewinsky RM, Telford J, Fairbanks LA. What is a low-lying placenta? *Am J Obstet Gynecol* 1991;165:1036-8.

[5]   Bhide A, Prefumo F, Moore J, Hollis B, Thilaganathan B. Placental edge to internal os distance in the late third trimester and mode of delivery in placenta praevia. *BJOG* 2003;110:860-4.

[6]   Percival R. The management of placenta praevia. *Br J Clin Pract* 1957;11:193-202.

[7]   Gemer O, Segal S. Incidence and contribution of predisposing factors to transverse lie presentation. *Int J Gynaecol Obstet* 1994;44:219-21.

[8]   McClure N, Dornal JC. Early identification of placenta praevia. *Br J Obstet Gynaecol* 1990;97:959-61.

[9]   Becker RH, Vonk R, Mende BC, Ragosch V, Entezami M. The relevance of placental location at 20-23 gestational weeks for prediction of placenta previa at delivery: evaluation of 8650 cases. *Ultrasound Obstet Gynecol* 2001;17:496-501.

[10]   Oppenheimer L, Holmes P, Simpson N, Dabrowski A. Diagnosis of low-lying placenta: can migration in the third trimester predict outcome? *Ultrasound Obstet Gynecol* 2001;18:100-2.

[11]   Farine D, Peisner DB, Timor-Tritsch IE. Placenta previa--is the traditional diagnostic approach satisfactory? *J Clin Ultrasound* 1990;18:328-30.

[12]   Oyelese Y. Placenta previa and vasa previa: time to leave the Dark Ages. *Ultrasound Obstet Gynecol* 2001;18:96-9.

[13]   Faiz AS, Ananth CV. Etiology and risk factors for placenta previa: an overview and meta-analysis of observational studies. *J Matern Fetal Neonatal Med* 2003;13:175-90.

[14]   Tuzovic L, Djelmis J, Ilijic M. Obstetric risk factors associated with placenta previa development: case-control study. *Croat Med J* 2003;44:728-33.

[15]   Crenshaw C, Jr., Jones DE, Parker RT. Placenta previa: a survey of twenty years experience with improved perinatal survival by expectant therapy and cesarean delivery. *Obstet Gynecol Surv* 1973;28:461-70.

[16]   Davidson VA, Brunken R. Placenta praevia: its incidence, diagnosis and treatment. *J Int Coll Surg* 1957;27:466-70.

[17]   Reich AM. Placenta previa; a critical appraisal based on a thirty-five-year study at Bellevue Hospital; 1919-1954. *Am J Obstet Gynecol* 1956;72:277-89.

[18]   Hibrd LT. Placenta previa. *Trans Pac Coast Obstet Gynecol Soc* 1968;36:14-26.

[19]   Monica G, Lilja C. Placenta previa, maternal smoking and recurrence risk. *Acta Obstet Gynecol Scand* 1995;74:341-5.

[20] Iyasu S, Saftlas AK, Rowley DL, Koonin LM, Lawson HW, Atrash HK. The epidemiology of placenta previa in the United States, 1979 through 1987. *Am J Obstet Gynecol* 1993;168:1424-9.

[21] Wang JC, Hin LY, Ng KB. Pregnancy-induced hypertension and placenta previa: a racial and geographical perspective. *Int J Gynaecol Obstet* 1999;67:177-8.

[22] Hemminki E, Glebatis DM, Therriault GD, Janerich DT. Incidence of placenta previa and abruptio placentae in New York State. *N Y State J Med* 1987;87:594-8.

[23] Gorodeski IG, Bahari CM, Schachter A, Neri A. Recurrent placenta previa. *Eur J Obstet Gynecol Reprod Biol* 1981;12:7-11.

[24] Rasmussen S, Albrechtsen S, Dalaker K. Obstetric history and the risk of placenta previa. *Acta Obstet Gynecol Scand* 2000;79:502-7.

[25] Williams GL. Recurrence of placenta praevia in four consecutive pregnancies. *J Obstet Gynaecol Br Commonw* 1967;74:609-10.

[26] Sheiner E, Shoham-Vardi I, Hallak M, Hershkowitz R, Katz M, Mazor M. Placenta previa: obstetric risk factors and pregnancy outcome. *J Matern Fetal Med* 2001;10:414-9.

[27] Zhang J, Savitz DA. Maternal age and placenta previa: a population-based, case-control study. *Am J Obstet Gynecol* 1993;168:641-5.

[28] Babinszki A, Kerenyi T, Torok O, Grazi V, Lapinski RH, Berkowitz RL. Perinatal outcome in grand and great-grand multiparity: effects of parity on obstetric risk factors. *Am J Obstet Gynecol* 1999;181:669-74.

[29] Abu-Heija AT, El-Jallad F, Ziadeh S. Placenta previa: effect of age, gravidity, parity and previous caesarean section. *Gynecol Obstet Invest* 1999;47:6-8.

[30] Ananth CV, Wilcox AJ, Savitz DA, Bowes WA, Jr., Luther ER. Effect of maternal age and parity on the risk of uteroplacental bleeding disorders in pregnancy. *Obstet Gynecol* 1996;88:511-6.

[31] Taylor VM, Peacock S, Kramer MD, Vaughan TL. Increased risk of placenta previa among women of Asian origin. *Obstet Gynecol* 1995;86:805-8.

[32] Handler AS, Mason ED, Rosenberg DL, Davis FG. The relationship between exposure during pregnancy to cigarette smoking and cocaine use and placenta previa. *Am J Obstet Gynecol* 1994;170:884-9.

[33] Naeye RL. The duration of maternal cigarette smoking, fetal and placental disorders. *Early Hum Dev* 1979;3:229-37.

[34] Naeye RL. Abruptio placentae and placenta previa: frequency, perinatal mortality, and cigarette smoking. *Obstet Gynecol* 1980;55:701-4.

[35] Williams MA, Mittendorf R, Lieberman E, Monson RR, Schoenbaum SC, Genest DR. Cigarette smoking during pregnancy in relation to placenta previa. *Am J Obstet Gynecol* 1991;165:28-32.

[36] Chelmow D, Andrew DE, Baker ER. Maternal cigarette smoking and placenta previa. *Obstet Gynecol* 1996;87:703-6.

[37] Zhang J, Fried DB. Relationship of maternal smoking during pregnancy to placenta previa. *Am J Prev Med* 1992;8:278-82.

[38] Ananth CV, Savitz DA, Luther ER. Maternal cigarette smoking as a risk factor for placental abruption, placenta previa, and uterine bleeding in pregnancy. *Am J Epidemiol* 1996;144:881-9.

[39] Meyer MB, Tonascia JA. Maternal smoking, pregnancy complications, and perinatal mortality. *Am J Obstet Gynecol* 1977;128:494-502.

[40] Kramer MD, Taylor V, Hickok DE, Daling JR, Vaughan TL, Hollenbach KA. Maternal smoking and placenta previa. *Epidemiology* 1991;2:221-3.

[41] Macones GA, Sehdev HM, Parry S, Morgan MA, Berlin JA. The association between maternal cocaine use and placenta previa. *Am J Obstet Gynecol* 1997;177:1097-100.

[42] Romundstad LB, Romundstad PR, Sunde A, von During V, Skjaerven R, Vatten LJ. Increased risk of placenta previa in pregnancies following IVF/ICSI; a comparison of ART and non-ART pregnancies in the same mother. *Hum Reprod* 2006;21:2353-8.

[43] Shevell T, Malone FD, Vidaver J, et al. Assisted reproductive technology and pregnancy outcome. *Obstet Gynecol* 2005;106:1039-45.

[44] Allen C, Bowdin S, Harrison RF, et al. Pregnancy and perinatal outcomes after assisted reproduction: a comparative study. *Ir J Med Sci* 2008;177:233-41.

[45] Jackson RA, Gibson KA, Wu YW, Croughan MS. Perinatal outcomes in singletons following in vitro fertilization: a meta-analysis. *Obstet Gynecol* 2004;103:551-63.

[46] Fanchin R, Righini C, Olivennes F, Taylor S, de Ziegler D, Frydman R. Uterine contractions at the time of embryo transfer alter pregnancy rates after in-vitro fertilization. *Hum Reprod* 1998;13:1968-74.

[47] Waterstone J, Curson R, Parsons J. Embryo transfer to low uterine cavity. Lancet 1991;337:1413.

[48] Ananth CV, Smulian JC, Vintzileos AM. The association of placenta previa with history of cesarean delivery and abortion: a metaanalysis. *Am J Obstet Gynecol* 1997;177:1071-8.

[49] McMahon MJ, Li R, Schenck AP, Olshan AF, Royce RA. Previous cesarean birth. A risk factor for placenta previa? *J Reprod Med* 1997;42:409-12.

[50] Bender S. Placenta previa and previous lower segment cesarean section. *Surg Gynecol Obstet* 1954;98:625-8.

[51] Chattopadhyay SK, Kharif H, Sherbeeni MM. Placenta praevia and accreta after previous caesarean section. *Eur J Obstet Gynecol Reprod Biol* 1993;52:151-6.

[52] Hendricks MS, Chow YH, Bhagavath B, Singh K. Previous cesarean section and abortion as risk factors for developing placenta previa. *J Obstet Gynaecol Res* 1999;25:137-42.

[53] To WW, Leung WC. Placenta previa and previous cesarean section. *Int J Gynaecol Obstet* 1995;51:25-31.

[54] Lydon Rochelle M, Holt VL, Easterling TR, Martin DP. First-birth cesarean and placental abruption or previa at second birth(1). *Obstet Gynecol* 2001;97:765-9.

[55] Getahun D, Oyelese Y, Salihu HM, Ananth CV. Previous cesarean delivery and risks of placenta previa and placental abruption. *Obstet Gynecol* 2006;107:771-8.

[56] Yang Q, Wen SW, Oppenheimer L, Chen XK, Black D, Gao J, Walker MC.. Association of caesarean delivery for first birth with placenta praevia and placental abruption in second pregnancy. *BJOG* 2007;114:609-13.

[57] Kennare R, Tucker G, Heard A, Chan A. Risks of adverse outcomes in the next birth after a first cesarean delivery. *Obstet Gynecol* 2007;109:270-6.

[58] Hershkowitz R, Fraser D, Mazor M, Leiberman JR. One or multiple previous cesarean sections are associated with similar increased frequency of placenta previa. *Eur J Obstet Gynecol Reprod Biol* 1995;62:185-8.

[59] NIH State-of-the-Science Conference Statement on cesarean delivery on maternal request. *NIH Consens State Sci Statements* 2006;23:1-29.

[60] Menacker F, Declercq E, Macdorman MF. Cesarean delivery: background, trends, and epidemiology. *Semin Perinatol* 2006;30:235-41.

[61] Johnson LG, Mueller BA, Daling JR. The relationship of placenta previa and history of induced abortion. *Int J Gynaecol Obstet* 2003;81:191-8.

[62] Taylor VM, Kramer MD, Vaughan TL, Peacock S. Placental previa in relation to induced and spontaneous abortion: a population-based study. *Obstet Gynecol* 1993;82:88-91.

[63] Grimes DA, Techman T. Legal abortion and placenta previa. *Am J Obstet Gynecol* 1984;149:501-4.

[64] Bieniarz J. The patho-mechanism of late pregnancy toxemia and obstetrical hemorrhages. I. Contradiction in the clinical pictures of eclampsia and placenta previa depending upon the placental site. *Am J Obstet Gynecol* 1958;75:444-53.

[65] Ananth CV, Bowes WA, Jr., Savitz DA, Luther ER. Relationship between pregnancy-induced hypertension and placenta previa: a population-based study. *Am J Obstet Gynecol* 1997;177:997-1002.

[66] Nicolaides KH, Faratian B, Symonds EM. Effect on low implantation of the placenta on maternal blood pressure and placental function. *Br J Obstet Gynaecol* 1982;89:806-10.

[67] Leiberman JR, Fraser D, Kasis A, Mazor M. Reduced frequency of hypertensive disorders in placenta previa. *Obstet Gynecol* 1991;77:83-6.

[68] Strong TH, Jr., Brar HS. Placenta previa in twin gestations. *J Reprod Med* 1989;34:415-6.

[69] Ananth CV, Demissie K, Smulian JC, Vintzileos AM. Placenta previa in singleton and twin births in the United States, 1989 through 1998: a comparison of risk factor profiles and associated conditions. *Am J Obstet Gynecol* 2003;188:275-81.

[70] Francois K, Johnson JM, Harris C. Is placenta previa more common in multiple gestations? *Am J Obstet Gynecol* 2003;188:1226-7.

[71] MacGillivray I, Davey D, Isaacs S. Placenta praevia and sex ratio at birth. *Br Med J (Clin Res Ed)* 1986;292:371-2.

[72] Jakobovits AA, Zubek L. Sex ratio and placenta praevia. *Acta Obstet Gynecol Scand* 1989;68:503-5.

[73] Demissie K, Breckenridge MB, Joseph L, Rhoads GG. Placenta previa: preponderance of male sex at birth. *Am J Epidemiol* 1999;149:824-30.

[74] Crane JM, Van den Hof MC, Dodds L, Armson BA, Liston R. Maternal complications with placenta previa. *Am J Perinatol* 2000;17:101-5.

[75] McShane PM, Heyl PS, Epstein MF. Maternal and perinatal morbidity resulting from placenta previa. *Obstet Gynecol* 1985;65:176-82.

[76] Takayama T, Minakami H, Koike T, Watanabe T, Sato I. Risks associated with cesarean sections in women with placenta previa. *J Obstet Gynaecol Res* 1997;23:375-9.

[77] Sheiner E, Levy A, Katz M, Mazor M. Identifying risk factors for peripartum cesarean hysterectomy. A population-based study. *J Reprod Med* 2003;48:622-6.

[78] Grobman WA, Gersnoviez R, Landon MB, et al. Pregnancy outcomes for women with placenta previa in relation to the number of prior cesarean deliveries. *Obstet Gynecol* 2007;110:1249-55.

[79] MacAfee C. Placenta previa: study of 174 cases. *J Obstet Gynecol Br Emp* 1945;52:313-24.

[80] Johnson H. The conservative management of some varieties of placenta previa. *Am J Obstet Gynecol* 1945;50:248.

[81] Nesbitt JR, Yankauer A , Schlesinger ER , Allaway N. Investigation of perinatal mortality rates associated with placenta previa in upstate New York, 1942-1958. *N Engl J Med* 1962;267:381-6.

[82] Ananth CV, Smulian JC, Vintzileos AM. The effect of placenta previa on neonatal mortality: a population-based study in the United States, 1989 through 1997. *Am J Obstet Gynecol* 2003;188:1299-304.

[83] Salihu HM, Li Q, Rouse DJ, Alexander GR. Placenta previa: neonatal death after live births in the United States. *Am J Obstet Gynecol* 2003;188:1305-9.

[84] Crane JM, van den Hof MC, Dodds L, Armson BA, Liston R. Neonatal outcomes with placenta previa. *Obstet Gynecol* 1999;93:541-4.

[85] Khashoggi T. Maternal and neonatal outcome in major placenta previa. *Ann Saudi Med* 1995;15:313-6.

[86] Zlatnik MG, Cheng YW, Norton ME, Thiet MP, Caughey AB. Placenta previa and the risk of preterm delivery. *J Matern Fetal Neonatal Med* 2007;20:719-23.

[87] Bekku S, Mitsuda N, Ogita K, Suehara N, Fujimura M, Aono T. High incidence of respiratory distress syndrome (RDS) in infants born to mothers with placenta previa. *J Matern Fetal Med* 2000;9:110-3.

[88] Miller DA, Chollet JA, Goodwin TM. Clinical risk factors for placenta previa-placenta accreta. *Am J Obstet Gynecol* 1997;177:210-4.

[89] ACOG Committee opinion. Number 266, January 2002 : placenta accreta. *Obstet Gynecol* 2002;99:169-70.

[90] Clark SL, Koonings PP, Phelan JP. Placenta previa/accreta and prior cesarean section. *Obstet Gynecol* 1985;66:89-92.

[91] Kastner ES, Figueroa R, Garry D, Maulik D. Emergency peripartum hysterectomy: experience at a community teaching hospital. *Obstet Gynecol* 2002;99:971-5.

[92] Nijman RG, Mantingh A, Aarnoudse JG. Persistent retained placenta percreta: methotrexate treatment and Doppler flow characteristics. *BJOG* 2002;109:587-8.

[93] Clement D, Kayem G, Cabrol D. Conservative treatment of placenta percreta: a safe alternative. *Eur J Obstet Gynecol Reprod Biol* 2004;114:108-9.

[94] Oyelese KO, Turner M, Lees C, Campbell S. Vasa previa: an avoidable obstetric tragedy. *Obstet Gynecol Surv* 1999;54:138-45.

[95] Oyelese Y, Spong C, Fernandez MA, McLaren RA. Second trimester low-lying placenta and in-vitro fertilization? Exclude vasa previa. *J Matern Fetal Med* 2000;9:370-2.

[96] Oyelese KO, Schwarzler P, Coates S, Sanusi FA, Hamid R, Campbell S. A strategy for reducing the mortality rate from vasa previa using transvaginal sonography with color Doppler. *Ultrasound Obstet Gynecol* 1998;12:434-8.

[97] Schachter M, Tovbin Y, Arieli S, Friedler S, Ron-El R, Sherman D. In vitro fertilization is a risk factor for vasa previa. *Fertil Steril* 2002;78:642-3.

[98] Gandhi M, Cleary-Goldman J, Ferrara L, Ciorica D, Saltzman D, Rebarber A. The association between vasa previa, multiple gestations, and assisted reproductive technology. *Am J Perinatol* 2008;25:587-9.

[99] Oyelese Y, Catanzarite V, Prefumo F, Lashley S, Schachter M, Tovbin Y, Goldstein V, Smulian JC. Vasa previa: the impact of prenatal diagnosis on outcomes. *Obstet Gynecol* 2004;103:937-42.

In: Textbook of Perinatal Epidemiology
Editor: Eyal Sheiner, pp. 663-677

ISBN: 978-1-60741-648-7
© 2010 Nova Science Publishers, Inc.

Chapter XXX

Epidemiology of Breech Delivery

Henry Chong Lee [*] *and Jeffrey B. Gould* [2]

MD, MPH, Robert L. Hess Professor of Pediatrics, Department of Pediatrics, Division of Neonatal and Developmental Medicine, Director, Perinatal Epidemiology and Health Outcomes Research Unit, Stanford University School of Medicine, 750 Welch Rd., #315, Stanford, CA 94305, email: jbgould@stanford.edu [2]

Definitions

- Breech presentation: The fetus's bottom presents downward toward the cervix.
- Frank breech: The hips are flexed and knees extended with buttocks presenting and feet near the head.
- Complete breech: The hips and knees are flexed with buttocks and feet presenting in a crosslegged position.
- Footling or incomplete breech: One or both feet present first, before the breech.

Introduction

Breech presentation, in which the fetus's bottom presents downward toward the cervix, was described as early as about 400 – 600 A.D. in the Moschion manuscript with figures of the fetus, which were adopted by obstetric texts of the 16 to 18th centuries.[1, 2] Leonardo di Vinci described a fetus in complete breech presentation in his notebook.[1] There are three types of breech presentation: frank breech which is the most common in which hips are flexed and knees extended with buttocks presenting and feet near the head, complete breech

---

[*] For Correspondence: Henry Chong Lee, MD, MS, Assistant Clinical Professor of Pediatrics, University of California, San Francisco, 533 Parnassus Avenue, Room U503, San Francisco, CA 94143-0734, (415) 476-1888 (phone), (415) 476-9976 (fax), email: LeeHC@peds.ucsf.edu

when hips and knees are flexed with buttocks and feet presenting in a crosslegged position, and footling or incomplete breech, when one or both feet present first.

Incidence

A precise incidence of breech presentation at birth is difficult to ascertain. The reported incidence of breech is usually 3-4%, ranging from 2.7% to 5.2%.[3-7] This variability may be due to demographic differences in the composition of the population under study and in the operational definition of breech delivery. When considering the reported rates of breech presentation, one should note the inclusion criteria, as incidence can be significantly influenced by the composition of the population under study. For example, preterm infants and multiple gestation births are more likely to have higher incidence of breech as are infants with congenital anomalies. When reporting rates, it should be noted whether these groups were excluded from analysis.

For example, using the Netherlands Perinatal Registry which included more than 1.3 million singleton births, the breech incidence in an 8 year period was 5.2% for all singletons, but only 3% for term singletons.[8] However these may be higher estimates then what might be expected in a general population in that the Netherlands registry captures data at higher proportions (95-99%) for births at higher risk centers than at low risk hospitals (90%). Because data is biased towards centers where breech presentation would be expected to be higher, the rate reported could be an overestimate of actual country-wide incidence.

A second difficulty in estimating the incidence of breech is ascertainment. The best estimate of the true incidence of breech would presumably be from data collection from a large population. When using administrative datasets, it is important to see how variables are defined and recorded. Large population data such as a country's vital records dataset may not differentiate between breech presentation and other malpresentations. In our study of United States birth certificate data, we found a breech incidence in the whole U.S. population of 3.8% over a 7 year period, which included more than 28 million births.[6] The coding for U.S. birth certificate data has included "malpresentation" as part of the breech variable. Therefore, the validity of this measure, while commonly used as an estimate of breech presentation rates, is dependent on the diagnosis of other malpresentations. In our analysis, we also saw a variation of breech incidence by state ranging from an incidence of 1.5 to 4.1%. While the ascertainment of breech or transverse lie should be uniform, it is possible that there may be variability in the diagnosis of other malpresentations.

Etiology / Associations, Congenital Malformations

In some infants, breech presentation may occur as a result of disorders in which there is decreased movement in utero. Infants with congenital malformations and / or neuromuscular disorders have been found with higher incidence of breech than expected and conversely, breech infants have been found with higher rates of malformations.[4, 9, 10] A study of cases from dysmorphology clinics found that the proportion of breech presentation for various congenital disorders, such as Trisomy 18 and Zelleweger syndrome, was higher than expected.[11] Breech incidence was as high as 50% for Prader-Willi syndrome, a well known cause of hypotonia. Fetal alcohol syndrome and Smith-Lemli-Opitz syndrome had breech incidence of 40%. When considering studies of developmental outcome in breech infants, it would be important to consider the potential impact of these associations.

Prematurity and Size

The incidence of breech declines as a function of increasing gestational age, as more fetuses engage in the vertex position as pregnancy ensues. In a study of the Netherlands Perinatal Registry, the incidence of breech decreased linearly with gestation from 40% at 24 weeks to 3% at term. In our analysis of the United States birth certificates, we found a similar decline for singletons, however starting at 25% incidence at 24 weeks and declining to 3% at 39 weeks and 2% at 40 weeks (figure 1). Another study of singletons born in Washington State reported similar rates – 20.6% at 25 – 26 weeks gestation, declining to 2.6% at 40 weeks.[12] These differences at earlier gestations between the U.S. data and the Netherlands may be due to differences in reporting or management of preterm births. The steeper drop from 39 to 40 weeks (which is seen at 37 weeks in the Netherlands Registry) may be due to elective cesarean deliveries occurring prior to those gestational age weeks.

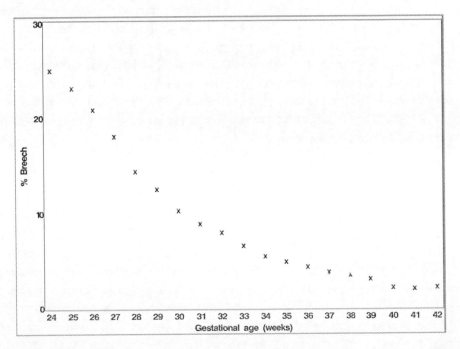

Figure 1. Incidence of breech presentation at birth by gestational age. Data source: National Center for Health Statistics.

Small size independent of gestational age has also been shown as a risk factor for breech presentation. After controlling for gestational age, parity, and maternal age, a 500 gram decrease in birth weight was associated with an increased risk of breech presentation in singletons (OR 1.32, 95% CI 1.26, 1.38).[10] In a similar study of Australian term newborns, small for gestational age (< 10th percentile for birth weight) was associated with breech presentation (OR 1.33, 95% CI 1.28, 1.38).[13]

Gender

In a study of the Netherlands Perinatal Registry, for infants born after 32 weeks gestation, there were significantly more singleton girls than boys in breech position at delivery.[8] The study included more than 70,000 breech births. At 40 weeks, 43.4% of breech infants were boys, with 3.6% of girls and 2.8% of boys being born in breech position. This difference in breech presentation with females having higher incidence has also been shown in other cohorts.[3, 13, 14] In our investigation of the United States birth certificate dataset from 2003, we also found a higher incidence of breech in singleton females (3.3%) than males (3.0%).[15] The reason for this gender difference may be due to the smaller size of girls or differences in body proportion.

Multiple Births

Breech presentation is more common in multiple births. In twin pregnancies, the incidence of breech in the first presenting or lower twin has been reported to be 17.7% to 27.0%.[16] For the second presenting twin, the incidence was higher, from 30.7% to 40.8%.[16] The incidence of breech in higher order multiples has been less well reported, although it would presumably be higher than for singletons. In a series of 41 triplet pregnancies, the incidence of breech in the first presenting triplet was 17.6%, the second triplet 28.5%, and the third triplet 29.1%.[17] It is notable that almost all of those pregnancies were preterm, which is also associated with breech presentation.

Developmental Dysplasia of the Hip

Breech presentation has been noted as a risk factor for developmental dysplasia of the hip (DDH). The etiology of DDH is multi-factorial including genetic predisposition and hormonal. However, intra-uterine mechanical factors would likely play an important role in the forces which cause hip instability and dysplasia, and would explain the higher risk of DDH seen in breech born infants. The risk of DDH from breech presentation is probably a result of some period of time spent in that position, and has been shown to remain higher for infants who were in breech position at 36 weeks, but then subsequently delivered in vertex position after version.[18]

The incidence of DDH is difficult to pinpoint for several reasons: the condition encompasses a spectrum of hip instability from subluxation to dislocation, there is no gold standard for diagnosis, and the condition may be present or absent at varying times in an infant's life.[19] Earlier studies describing risk factors for DDH were based on registries of patients with that condition. As the incidence of breech is relatively stable across populations, knowing the proportion of breech in a cohort of DDH can give an idea of the increased risk conferred by the abnormal position in utero. Reported incidence of breech in such studies range from 11% to 25% in patients with DDH.[20-22]

A population based approach may allow for a clearer indication of the risk of a breech infant for DDH. In an Australian cohort, breech presentation was found to be the most significant factor associated with DDH.[23] Vaginally delivered breech infants (OR 17.2, 95% CI 12.8, 23.0) and cesarean delivered breech infants (OR 10.0, 95% CI 8.6 11.7) were more likely to have DDH compared to non-breech presentation.

In a population based study of the Norwegian birth registry of more than 1 million births, the breech rate of neonatal hip instability was 4.4% compared to the overall prevalence of 0.9%.[24] In that study, neonatal hip instability was defined as positive Ortolani sign or congenital dislocation of the hip. There was a slight increase in prevalence for vaginally delivered breech infants (4.54%) compared to cesarean born breech infants (4.25%).

Mortality and Morbidity

The process of labor and delivery present several risks to the fetus presenting in breech position, including cord prolapse, head entrapment, and other birth traumas.[25-27] Other associated morbidities include potential brain injury, spinal cord injury, brachial plexus injury, skull fracture, fracture of long bones or clavicle, and genital injury; such injuries may be more prevalent in vaginal breech births.[28-36]

Determining the risk contribution of breech presentation to various morbidities is not always straightforward. The presence of various obstetric conditions and injuries may partly be a result of the factors which led to breech presentation, and not the breech presentation per se. Breech presentation would also influence the mode of delivery, which could potentially contribute to or attenuate certain morbidities. For example, cord prolapse is more common in preterm infants and the preterm state could have contributed to the prolapse as well as breech presentation.

Cord prolapse is a rare obstetric complication which often requires emergent cesarean delivery, with an incidence of 0.1% to 0.6% in the general population, and ensuing cord compression can lead to asphyxia and encephalopathy.[27] The reported incidence of cord prolapse is 2% to 6% in breech presentation with a decreasing trend in more recent reports.[27] This may be partly due to the increase in elective cesarean delivery for breech infants. In a large case-control study examining risk factors of cord prolapse, breech presentation conferred a significantly higher risk of prolapse (OR 2.5, 95% CI 1.7, 3.9) after controlling for other factors.[37]

Infants born in breech position are at generally higher risk of asphyxia and encephalopathy, conferring a 4 to 20-fold risk compared to vertex births.[38-42] This risk is present for both preterm and term infants, but is more of a factor for term births.[39]

Neonatal mortality is higher for infants born in breech position, this risk likely related to the above morbidities, conferring a 1.5 to 2-fold risk compared to vertex births.[29, 43-45] When considering mortality, there is the possibility of risk factors for breech presentation also being risks for mortality. During a 9 year period in California amongst term births, there were 0.6 deaths per 1,000 breech deliveries compared to 0.3 per 1000 vertex deliveries.[29] Neonatal mortality was higher for breech babies born vaginally (1.8 per 1000).

Version

External version of breech fetuses can be attempted in order to reduce the potential for complications and cesarean delivery. The procedure has been shown to reduce the incidence of breech presentation at term.[46, 47] At 36 weeks gestation, the success rate is about 65%.[25] Complications such as placental separation or umbilical cord compression can lead to the need for emergent cesarean delivery. However, the current literature has not shown a significantly high rate of ultimate adverse outcomes for infant or mother.[48] Although cesarean delivery may be necessary due to a complication or failure of version, the overall cesarean rate could be reduced by attempts at version.[25, 46]

Cesarean and Breech

The suggestion that cesarean delivery may be of routine benefit for breech presentation surfaced in the 1950's.[25, 49, 50] Prior to that time, vaginal breech delivery was the standard. The cesarean rate for breech steadily increased in the United States in the 1970's. At one university center in the 1970's, the cesarean rate for singleton breech infants with birth weight greater than 2,500 grams increased from 13% to 54%, and from 5% to 55% in smaller infants.[51]

Retrospective Studies

Most past studies on the potential benefit of cesarean delivery for term infants have been retrospective cohort studies and have had relatively low power to detect significant differences in both neonatal and maternal outcomes.[52-54] Some investigators have found no significant impact from the mode of delivery when considering other factors, both short and long term.[55-58] Others have found reduction in mortality and morbidity.[5, 7, 29] Conclusions from such studies have been difficult to make due to their retrospective nature and issues of selection bias and confounding. The framework for when to have a trial of labor for certain patients have not been uniform, nor the reasons for switching to cesarean delivery.

Larger population-based studies have also been performed which have tended to show some benefit to cesarean in regard to mortality. In a study of 3,447 term breech births in the North West Thames region, there was a relative risk of 20 (95% CI, 2.5, 163) of mortality for vaginal vs. cesarean delivery. However, this study did not incorporate potential confounders in the analysis. A study of term breech births (n = 100,667) in California from 1991 to 1999 found higher mortality (OR 9.2, 95% CI 3.3, 25.6) for singleton breech vaginal vs. cesarean delivery, but no difference in mortality by mode of delivery when the mother had a prior vaginal delivery.[29] However, morbidities such as asphyxia and brachial plexus injury were increased for vaginal delivery in both nulliparous mothers and those with prior vaginal delivery.

Other large observational studies have also shown that cesarean delivery for breech presentation is associated with lower incidence of acidemia, low Apgar score, and neurologic injury.[7, 59, 60] Although such studies may have power to detect differences in outcome, they often have less clinical detail, particularly regarding the decisions surrounding the mode of delivery. This limits the practical application of these studies, due to the potential that the factors which influenced the mode of delivery could ultimately have impacted outcome, more so than the mode of delivery itself. In an era where the benefit of cesarean is at least contemplated by many obstetricians, could there have been extenuating circumstances which led to a vaginal delivery, which could have been the cause of the adverse outcome, and not the mode of delivery per se? Presumably, a study with more clinical details could be beneficial in answering such questions. However, with more detail, one generally compromises on sample size and power.

Randomized Trials

There have been three randomized trials examining this question. Two were published more than 20 years ago and had relatively small sample size. In a randomized trial of 208 term frank breech infants, the ultimate decision for vaginal delivery was based on x-ray pelvimetry. Of 112 women assigned to the vaginal group, 52 had inadequate pelvic measurements and were scheduled for cesarean delivery. Of the 60 planned vaginal deliveries, 49 had successful vaginal births and 11 ultimately underwent cesarean delivery for difficulties during labor. Their conclusion was that in selected cases, vaginal delivery could be performed in term frank breech presentation.[61] A randomized trial of 105 term nonfrank breech infants also found that 59% of those assigned to the planned vaginal group had inadequate dimensions on x-ray pelvimetry.[62] Although they concluded that selective vaginal delivery was a potential option, their numbers were small, with 31 patients ultimately delivering vaginally, one of which ended in neonatal death due to "inadequate resuscitation".

The largest randomized trial conducted by Hannah et al., the Term Breech Trial, was a multicenter trial involving 2083 women in 121 hospitals in 26 countries.[63] The initial results were published in October 2000 and demonstrated improved outcome for selective cesarean delivery.[63] They found a lower rate of neonatal mortality and serious morbidity in the planned cesarean group (1.6% vs. 5.0%) without significant maternal morbidity or mortality. However, follow-up data from this trial did not demonstrate improvement in outcomes for cesarean delivery neither for infants at 2 years, nor for mothers, although there was also no harm seen for mothers.[64, 65] The number of patients followed up to 2 years was reduced from the original group to 923 children.

Several studies have found increased morbidity for mothers undergoing cesarean compared to vaginal delivery.[7, 58, 66] However, the Term Breech Trial found similar outcomes and no significant increase in morbidity for mothers in the planned cesarean group compared to selective delivery.[64]

If there is a select group of singleton breech infants that can be delivered safely by skilled practitioners, the potential for training and maintaining the skill level of obstetricians may be limited. Even in Sweden, where breech vaginal deliveries were relatively high, the average number of estimated vaginal deliveries by each obstetrician would be less than one per year.[7]

Recent Trends

Largely in response to the Term Breech Trial, the American College of Obstetricians and Gynecologists Committee on Obstetric Practice published an opinion statement in 2001 which recommended cesarean delivery for singleton term breech presentation.[67] The opinion statement was modified in 2006 to allow for the possibility of vaginal delivery in specific situations with skilled physicians and appropriate counseling of mothers.[68] Although there has been some controversy surrounding the implications of the Term Breech Trial, it appears to have had implications for practice as seen by increased cesarean rates in various countries. In Sweden, the cesarean section rate for term breech infants increased from 75.3% to 86.0% from 1999 to 2001.[69] In the Netherlands, the cesarean section rate increased from 50% to 80% within two months after publication of the Term Breech Trial.[70] In the United States, cesarean rates had already been high at 83.8% in 1997. There was a modest increase up to 85.1% in 2003 after the recommendations surrounding the Term Breech Trial.[6]

It is worth noting that there is somewhat wide variability of cesarean delivery rates for breech across different states, ranging from 62 to 96% within the same year.[6] We found that those states having higher reporting of breech incidence tended to have lower rates of cesarean delivery for breech.(figure 2).

It is possible that lowered rates in those states may be secondary to an overestimate of breech incidence rather than a true decrease in cesearean delivery for breech presentation due to inclusion of infants who were in "malpresentation" and not truly in breech presentation. This would be the case if cases labeled as "malpresentation" represented relatively benign situations in which cesarean delivery would not usually be required.

There still remain researchers in the obstetric community who believe that in the care of a skilled provider and in selected circumstances, delivery of a breech infant by vaginal route can be a safe practice.[66, 71, 72]

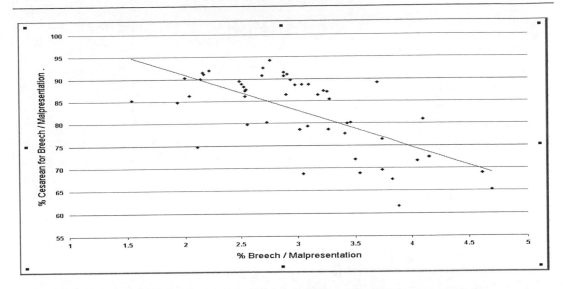

Figure 2. Cesarean rates for breech presentation by breech incidence for individual states. Data source: National Center for Health Statistics.

Preterm Breech and Cesarean

The potential benefit of cesarean delivery for preterm breech infants has also been debated. Although there have been a few randomized trials attempted for preterm breech and mode of delivery, they have suffered from poor enrollment, possibly due to both a lack of enthusiasm in both practitioners and patients.[73-75] One study which involved 26 centers was only able to recruit 13 patients from 6 of those centers over a period of 17 months, despite many more patients having been eligible for the study.[74] The largest study was able to recruit 38 patients over a five year period.[75] Although there was a trend toward higher Apgar scores in the immediate cesarean group, there were not enough numbers to draw conclusions about the optimal mode of delivery in this population.

There have been multiple retrospective studies on preterm breech mode of delivery. These have shown a potential benefit of cesarean compared to vaginal delivery in regard to mortality.[45, 76, 77] Other outcomes such as intraventricular hemorrhage and adverse neurologic sequelae have been associated with vaginal delivery compared to cesarean delivery in breech infants with birth weights 750 to 1,500 grams.[78-80] However, the conclusions of such studies are limited due to their retrospective design. The decisions regarding mode of delivery would be influenced by the circumstances surrounding viability of preterm infants and the mother's health. It is also possible that the medical management of an infant could also be influenced by the mode of delivery, with a stronger push for survival after a mother has undergone a surgical delivery.

Despite this uncertainty, the majority of preterm infants are delivered by cesarean, with greater than 80% cesarean rates for most gestational age groups and often exceeding 90% in the US.[81]

Conclusion

Breech presentation occurs at approximately 3-4% at birth. Although the majority of infants born in breech position will be healthy "well babies", there is increased risk of adverse outcome, which may in part be due to the "cause" of breech presentation, and in some situations, the circumstances of the breech delivery. There has been an increasing trend in cesarean delivery of breech due to various studies which have shown an advantage to planned cesarean delivery, most notably the Term Breech Trial.[63] However, there is still debate about the necessity of cesarean delivery for all breech births.[82, 83] As another randomized clinical trial of large magnitude seems unlikely, epidemiologic studies may continue to play an important role in furthering this debate.

References

[1] Confino E, Gleicher N, Elrad H, Ismajovich B, David MP. The breech dilemma. A review. *Obstet Gynecol Surv* 1985;40(6):330-7.

[2] Barbour AHF. Early Contributions of Anatomy to Obstetrics. *Edinburgh Medical Journal* 1888;34(4):328-35.

[3] Hall MH, Carr-Hill R. Impact of sex ratio on onset and management of labour. *Br Med J (Clin Res Ed)* 1982;285(6339):401-3.

[4] Ho NK. Neonatal outcome of breech babies in Toa Payoh Hospital 1984-1989. *Singapore Med J* 1992;33(4):333-6.

[5] Thorpe-Beeston JG, Banfield PJ, Saunders NJ. Outcome of breech delivery at term. *Bmj* 1992;305(6856):746-7.

[6] Lee HC, El-Sayed YY, Gould JB. Population trends in cesarean delivery for breech presentation in the United States, 1997-2003. *Am J Obstet Gynecol* 2008;199(1):59 e1-8.

[7] Roman J, Bakos O, Cnattingius S. Pregnancy outcomes by mode of delivery among term breech births: Swedish experience 1987-1993. *Obstet Gynecol* 1998;92(6):945-50.

[8] Rietberg CC, Elferink-Stinkens PM, Visser GH. Term breech delivery in *The Netherlands:* Utrecht University; 2006.

[9] Axelrod FB, Leistner HL, Porges RF. Breech presentation among infants with familial dysautonomia. *J Pediatr* 1974;84(1):107-9.

[10] Rayl J, Gibson PJ, Hickok DE. A population-based case-control study of risk factors for breech presentation. *Am J Obstet Gynecol* 1996;174(1 Pt 1):28-32.

[11] Braun FH, Jones KL, Smith DW. Breech presentation as an indicator of fetal abnormality. *J Pediatr* 1975;86(3):419-21.

[12] Hickok DE, Gordon DC, Milberg JA, Williams MA, Daling JR. The frequency of breech presentation by gestational age at birth: a large population-based study. *Am J Obstet Gynecol* 1992;166(3):851-2.

[13] Roberts CL, Algert CS, Peat B, Henderson-Smart D. Small fetal size: a risk factor for breech birth at term. *Int J Gynaecol Obstet* 1999;67(1):1-8.

[14] Jonas O, Roder D. Breech presentation in South Australia, 1987-1989. *Aust N Z J Obstet Gynaecol* 1993;33(1):17-21.

[15] National Center for Health Statistics. 2003 Natality public-use tape and CD-ROM. . Hyattsville, MD: *National Center for Health Statistics.*

[16] Sekulic SR, Petrovic DS, Runic R, Williams M, Vejnovic TR. Does a probability of breech presentation of more than 50% exist among diseases and medical conditions? *Twin Res Hum Genet* 2007;10(4):649-54.

[17] Ziadeh SM. Perinatal outcome in 41 sets of triplets in Jordan. *Birth* 2000;27(3):185-8.

[18] Andersson JE, Oden A. The breech presentation and the vertex presentation following an external version represent risk factors for neonatal hip instability. *Acta Paediatr* 2001;90(8):895-8.

[19] Clinical practice guideline: early detection of developmental dysplasia of the hip. Committee on Quality Improvement, Subcommittee on Developmental Dysplasia of the Hip. American Academy of Pediatrics. *Pediatrics* 2000;105(4 Pt 1):896-905.

[20] Woolf CM, Koehn JH, Coleman SS. Congenital hip disease in Utah: the influence of genetic and nongenetic factors. *Am J Hum Genet* 1968;20(5):430-9.

[21] Carter CO, Wilkinson JA. Genetic and environmental factors in the etiology of congenital dislocation of the hip. *Clin Orthop Relat Res* 1964;33:119-28.

[22] Record RG, Edwards JH. Environmental influences related to the aetiology of congenital dislocation of the hip. *Br J Prev Soc Med* 1958;12(1):8-22.

[23] Chan A, McCaul KA, Cundy PJ, Haan EA, Byron-Scott R. Perinatal risk factors for developmental dysplasia of the hip. *Arch Dis Child Fetal Neonatal Ed* 1997;76(2):F94-100.

[24] Hinderaker T, Daltveit AK, Irgens LM, Uden A, Reikeras O. The impact of intra-uterine factors on neonatal hip instability. An analysis of 1,059,479 children in Norway. *Acta Orthop Scand* 1994;65(3):239-42.

[25] Bowes Jr. WA, Thorp Jr. JM. Clinical Aspects of Normal and Abnormal Labor. *In: Creasy RK, Resnik R, eds. Maternal-Fetal Medicine. 5th ed.* Philadelphia: Saunders; 2004:671-706.

[26] Dilbaz B, Ozturkoglu E, Dilbaz S, Ozturk N, Sivaslioglu AA, Haberal A. Risk factors and perinatal outcomes associated with umbilical cord prolapse. *Arch Gynecol Obstet* 2006;274(2):104-7.

[27] Lin MG. Umbilical cord prolapse. *Obstet Gynecol Surv* 2006;61(4):269-77.

[28] Bassaw B, Rampersad N, Roopnarinesingh S, Sirjusingh A. Correlation of fetal outcome with mode of delivery for breech presentation. *J Obstet Gynaecol* 2004;24(3):254-8.

[29] Gilbert WM, Hicks SM, Boe NM, Danielsen B. Vaginal versus cesarean delivery for breech presentation in California: a population-based study. *Obstet Gynecol* 2003;102(5 Pt 1):911-7.

[30] Tiwary CM. Testicular injury in breech delivery: possible implications. *Urology* 1989;34(4):210-2.

[31] Erkaya S, Tuncer RA, Kutlar I, Onat N, Ercakmak S. Outcome of 1040 consecutive breech deliveries: clinical experience of a maternity hospital in Turkey. *Int J Gynaecol Obstet* 1997;59(2):115-8.

[32] Nadas S, Gudinchet F, Capasso P, Reinberg O. Predisposing factors in obstetrical fractures. *Skeletal Radiol* 1993;22(3):195-8.

[33] Vialle R, Pietin-Vialle C, Ilharreborde B, Dauger S, Vinchon M, Glorion C. Spinal cord injuries at birth: a multicenter review of nine cases. *J Matern Fetal Neonatal Med* 2007;20(6):435-40.

[34] Franken EA, Jr. Spinal cord injury in the newborn infant. *Pediatr Radiol* 1975;3(2):101-4.

[35] van Ouwerkerk WJ, van der Sluijs JA, Nollet F, Barkhof F, Slooff AC. Management of obstetric brachial plexus lesions: state of the art and future developments. *Childs Nerv Syst* 2000;16(10-11):638-44.

[36] Geutjens G, Gilbert A, Helsen K. Obstetric brachial plexus palsy associated with breech delivery. A different pattern of injury. *J Bone Joint Surg Br* 1996;78(2):303-6.

[37] Critchlow CW, Leet TL, Benedetti TJ, Daling JR. Risk factors and infant outcomes associated with umbilical cord prolapse: a population-based case-control study among births in Washington State. *Am J Obstet Gynecol* 1994;170(2):613-8.

[38] Lindstrom K, Hallberg B, Blennow M, Wolff K, Fernell E, Westgren M. Moderate neonatal encephalopathy: pre- and perinatal risk factors and long-term outcome. *Acta Obstet Gynecol Scand* 2008;87(5):503-9.

[39] MacDonald HM, Mulligan JC, Allen AC, Taylor PM. Neonatal asphyxia. I. Relationship of obstetric and neonatal complications to neonatal mortality in 38,405 consecutive deliveries. *J Pediatr* 1980;96(5):898-902.

[40] Milsom I, Ladfors L, Thiringer K, Niklasson A, Odeback A, Thornberg E. Influence of maternal, obstetric and fetal risk factors on the prevalence of birth asphyxia at term in a Swedish urban population. *Acta Obstet Gynecol Scand* 2002;81(10):909-17.

[41] Mbweza E. Risk factors for perinatal asphyxia at Queen Elizabeth Central Hospital, Malawi. *Clin Excell Nurse Pract* 2000;4(3):158-62.

[42] Chandra S, Ramji S, Thirupuram S. Perinatal asphyxia: multivariate analysis of risk factors in hospital births. *Indian Pediatr* 1997;34(3):206-12.

[43] Kambarami RA. Levels and risk factors for mortality in infants with birth weights between 500 and 1,800 grams in a developing country: a hospital based study. *Cent Afr J Med* 2002;48(11-12):133-6.

[44] Evans N, Hutchinson J, Simpson JM, Donoghue D, Darlow B, Henderson-Smart D. Prenatal predictors of mortality in very preterm infants cared for in the Australian and New Zealand Neonatal Network. *Arch Dis Child Fetal Neonatal Ed* 2007;92(1):F34-40.

[45] Demol S, Bashiri A, Furman B, Maymon E, Shoham-Vardi I, Mazor M. Breech presentation is a risk factor for intrapartum and neonatal death in preterm delivery. *Eur J Obstet Gynecol Reprod Biol* 2000;93(1):47-51.

[46] Hofmeyr GJ, Kulier R. External cephalic version for breech presentation at term. *Cochrane Database Syst Rev* 2000(2):CD000083.

[47] Zhang J, Bowes WA, Jr., Fortney JA. Efficacy of external cephalic version: a review. *Obstet Gynecol* 1993;82(2):306-12.

[48] Nassar N, Roberts CL, Barratt A, Bell JC, Olive EC, Peat B. Systematic review of adverse outcomes of external cephalic version and persisting breech presentation at term. *Paediatr Perinat Epidemiol* 2006;20(2):163-71.

[49] Goethals TR. Cesarean section as the method of choice in management of breech delivery. *Am J Obstet Gynecol* 1956;71(3):536-52.

[50] Wright RC. Reduction of perinatal mortality and morbidity in breech delivery through routine use of cesarean section. *Obstet Gynecol* 1959;14:758-63.

[51] Bowes WA, Jr., Taylor ES, O'Brien M, Bowes C. Breech delivery: evaluation of the method of delivery on perinatal results and maternal morbidity. A*m J Obstet Gynecol* 1979;135(7):965-73.

[52] Bingham P, Hird V, Lilford RJ. Management of the mature selected breech presentation: an analysis based on the intended method of delivery. *Br J Obstet Gynaecol* 1987;94(8):746-52.

[53] Cheng M, Hannah M. Breech delivery at term: a critical review of the literature. *Obstet Gynecol* 1993;82(4 Pt 1):605-18.

[54] Hannah M, Hannah W. Caesarean section or vaginal birth for breech presentation at term. *Bmj* 1996;312(7044):1433-4.

[55] Munstedt K, von Georgi R, Reucher S, Zygmunt M, Lang U. Term breech and long-term morbidity -- cesarean section versus vaginal breech delivery. *Eur J Obstet Gynecol Reprod Biol* 2001;96(2):163-7.

[56] Danielian PJ, Wang J, Hall MH. Long-term outcome by method of delivery of fetuses in breech presentation at term: population based follow up. *Bmj* 1996;312(7044):1451-3.

[57] McBride WG, Black BP, Brown CJ, Dolby RM, Murray AD, Thomas DB. Method of delivery and developmental outcome at five years of age. *Med J Aust* 1979;1(8):301-4.

[58] Sanchez-Ramos L, Wells TL, Adair CD, Arcelin G, Kaunitz AM, Wells DS. Route of breech delivery and maternal and neonatal outcomes. *Int J Gynaecol Obstet* 2001;73(1):7-14.

[59] Herbst A, Thorngren-Jerneck K. Mode of delivery in breech presentation at term: increased neonatal morbidity with vaginal delivery. *Acta Obstet Gynecol Scand* 2001;80(8):731-7.

[60] Ulander VM, Gissler M, Nuutila M, Ylikorkala O. Are health expectations of term breech infants unrealistically high? *Acta Obstet Gynecol Scand* 2004;83(2):180-6.

[61] Collea JV, Chein C, Quilligan EJ. The randomized management of term frank breech presentation: a study of 208 cases. *Am J Obstet Gynecol* 1980;137(2):235-44.

[62] Gimovsky ML, Wallace RL, Schifrin BS, Paul RH. Randomized management of the nonfrank breech presentation at term: a preliminary report. *Am J Obstet Gynecol* 1983;146(1):34-40.

[63] Hannah ME, Hannah WJ, Hewson SA, Hodnett ED, Saigal S, Willan AR. Planned caesarean section versus planned vaginal birth for breech presentation at term: a randomised multicentre trial. Term Breech Trial Collaborative Group. *Lancet* 2000;356(9239):1375-83.

[64] Hannah ME, Whyte H, Hannah WJ, et al. Maternal outcomes at 2 years after planned cesarean section versus planned vaginal birth for breech presentation at term: the

international randomized Term Breech Trial. *Am J Obstet Gynecol* 2004;191(3):917-27.

[65]   Whyte H, Hannah ME, Saigal S, et al. Outcomes of children at 2 years after planned cesarean birth versus planned vaginal birth for breech presentation at term: the International Randomized Term Breech Trial. *Am J Obstet Gynecol* 2004;191(3):864-71.

[66]   Irion O, Hirsbrunner Almagbaly P, Morabia A. Planned vaginal delivery versus elective caesarean section: a study of 705 singleton term breech presentations. *Br J Obstet Gynaecol* 1998;105(7):710-7.

[67]   ACOG committee opinion: number 265, December 2001. Mode of term single breech delivery. *Obstet Gynecol* 2001;98(6):1189-90.

[68]   ACOG Committee Opinion No. 340. Mode of term singleton breech delivery. *Obstet Gynecol* 2006;108(1):235-7.

[69]   Alexandersson O, Bixo M, Hogberg U. Evidence-based changes in term breech delivery practice in Sweden. *Acta Obstet Gynecol Scand* 2005;84(6):584-7.

[70]   Rietberg CC, Elferink-Stinkens PM, Visser GH. The effect of the Term Breech Trial on Medical Intervention Behavior and Neonatal Outcome in The Netherlands: An Analysis of 35,453 Term Breech Infants. *Obstet Gynecol Surv* 2005;60(5):289-90.

[71]   Kayem G, Goffinet F, Clement D, Hessabi M, Cabrol D. Breech presentation at term: morbidity and mortality according to the type of delivery at Port Royal Maternity hospital from 1993 through 1999. *Eur J Obstet Gynecol Reprod Biol* 2002;102(2):137-42.

[72]   Hauth JC, Cunningham FG. Vaginal breech delivery is still justified. *Obstet Gynecol* 2002;99(6):1115-6.

[73]   Lumley J, Lester A, Renou P, Wood C. A failed RCT to determine the best method of delivery for very low birth weight infants. *Control Clin Trials* 1985;6(2):120-7.

[74]   Penn ZJ, Steer PJ, Grant A. A multicentre randomised controlled trial comparing elective and selective caesarean section for the delivery of the preterm breech infant. *Br J Obstet Gynaecol* 1996;103(7):684-9.

[75]   Zlatnik FJ. The Iowa premature breech trial. *Am J Perinatol* 1993;10(1):60-3.

[76]   Lee KS, Khoshnood B, Sriram S, Hsieh HL, Singh J, Mittendorf R. Relationship of cesarean delivery to lower birth weight-specific neonatal mortality in singleton breech infants in the United States. *Obstet Gynecol* 1998;92(5):769-74.

[77]   Main DM, Main EK, Maurer MM. Cesarean section versus vaginal delivery for the breech fetus weighing less than 1,500 grams. *Am J Obstet Gynecol* 1983;146(5):580-4.

[78]   Gorbe E, Chasen S, Harmath A, Patkos P, Papp Z. Very-low-birthweight breech infants: short-term outcome by method of delivery. *J Matern Fetal Med* 1997;6(3):155-8.

[79]   Granati B, Rondinelli M, Capoti C, Carnielli V, Bottos M, Rubaltelli FF. The premature breech presentation: outcome of newborn infants born by vaginal or abdominal delivery. *Am J Perinatol* 1984;1(2):145-7.

[80]   Weissman A, Blazer S, Zimmer EZ, Jakobi P, Paldi E. Low birthweight breech infant: short-term and long-term outcome by method of delivery. *Am J Perinatol* 1988;5(3):289-92.

[81] Lee HC, El-Sayed YY, Gould JB. Delivery mode by race for breech presentation in the US. *J Perinatol* 2007;27(3):147-53.

[82] Yamamura Y, Ramin KD, Ramin SM. Trial of vaginal breech delivery: current role. *Clin Obstet Gynecol* 2007;50(2):526-36.

[83] Turner MJ. The Term Breech Trial: are the clinical guidelines justified by the evidence? *J Obstet Gynaecol* 2006;26(6):491-4.

In: Textbook of Perinatal Epidemiology
Editor: Eyal Sheiner, pp. 679-688

ISBN: 978-1-60741-648-7
© 2010 Nova Science Publishers, Inc.

Chapter XXXI

Epidemiology of Postpartum Hemorrhage

Iris Ohel, Gershone Holcberg and Eyal Sheiner[*]

Departments of Obstetrics and Gynecology, Soroka University Medical Center, Ben-Gurion University of the Negev, Beer-Sheva, Israel

Definitions

- Postpartum hemorrhage (PPH): blood loss of more than 500 ml after vaginal delivery or above 1000 ml after cesarean delivery.
- Early postpartum hemorrhage: PPH that occurs within 24 hours after delivery.
- Late postpartum hemorrhage: PPH that occurs between 24 hours and 6 weeks after delivery.

Introduction

Postpartum hemorrhage (PPH) is excessive bleeding after childbirth. It is considered to be one of the treatable emergency situations in obstetrics, and if not treated in time could cause significant morbidity and mortality. In most parts of the world, postpartum hemorrhage accounts for 35–55% of maternal deaths. In rural regions and developing countries, where access to quick medical attendance is limited, this could be a major health problem. It is usually agreed that objective evaluation and estimation of the amount of bleeding after labor may be difficult, especially when bleeding is slow and steady, or in the presence of concomitant intra-abdominal bleeding or concealed bleeding. Also, the clinical signs of blood loss such as decrease in blood pressure and increased heart rate tend to appear late, only when the quantity of blood loss reaches 1500 ml, mainly due to the high blood volume in pregnant

[*] For Correspondence: Eyal Sheiner, M.D, PhD, Department of Obstetrics and Gynecology, Soroka University Medical Center, P.O. Box 151, Beer-Sheva, Israel. Tel 972-8-6403551, Fax 972-8-6403294, E-mail sheiner@bgu.ac.il

women. Practitioners tend to underestimate the amount of blood loss surrounding labor and delivery. Still, some use a rough estimation of blood loss of more than 500 ml to define PPH, and above 1000 ml for severe PPH or for PPH after cesarean delivery. Perhaps a more precise description would be afforded by evaluating the decrease in hematocrit. A drop of 10% volume would be defined as PPH, or a need for blood transfusion.

Incidence

The attempts to define PPH still leave us with vague definitions; this is obvious in a retrospective review of charts of women after delivery. Clinicians use different definitions, and the estimation of the exact amount of bleeding is imprecise and sometimes even missing, making the evaluation of incidence difficult. Each article or review dealing with the incidence of PPH around the world addresses this issue. The variations of PPH incidence are enormous because of inconsistencies in definition and lack of reporting, especially in developing countries [1] and rural areas where out-of-hospital deliveries, with their associated increased risk for adverse maternal outcomes, specifically hemorrhage, are more frequent [2].

Maternal Mortality and PPH

The problem becomes an epidemiologic one once the significance of maternal mortality related to PPH is understood. Maternal death might occur within a short period of time due to irreversible shock. A comprehensive summary of the magnitude and distribution of the causes of maternal deaths is critical to conducting programs for treatment. This was done by the World Health Organization (WHO) analysis of causes of maternal death [3,4]. For developing countries without routine registration of cause of death, measuring who dies and why is almost impossible. To emphasize this, roughly two-thirds of countries do not even have the means to count their populations [5]. In the analysis done by the WHO of joint causes of death, hemorrhage was the leading cause of maternal death in Africa and Asia, causing >30% of deaths. Hypertensive disorders represent the highest cause of maternal mortality in Latin America and the Caribbean with 25% of the total, followed by hemorrhage with 21%. As expected, this systematic analysis of the causes of maternal deaths showed a rate of reported PPH of between 1.4–49.6%, both across and within geographical regions. The data confirm the prominent role of hemorrhage as a cause of maternal death in developing countries. This systematic review highlights the need for increased emphasis on programs relevant to specific settings, such as the prevention and treatment of hemorrhage both prepartum and postpartum. The authors emphasize that "at the very least, most postpartum hemorrhage deaths should be avoidable by appropriate diagnosis and management" [5].

Efforts are being made around the world to collect data, and as a result some figures do exist. An example from Nigeria is a 5-year (1996–2000) review of the causes of maternal mortality in a centrally located mission hospital in Benin City.[6] A total of 7055 women gave birth during the 5-year period, with 32 maternal deaths, which gives a Maternal Mortality Ratio (MMR) of 454/100,000 live births. Eclampsia (34.4%), hemorrhage (25.0%), infections (18.8%), and abortions (12.5%) were the four leading causes of death. In a study from Malawi, East Africa, MMR reached 1027/100,000 live births [7]. Obstetric hemorrhage comprised 10.6% of total deaths and was the fourth leading cause of maternal mortality after puerperal sepsis, post-abortion complications, and other infectious conditions.

The maternal mortality rates emphasize one of the most striking differences between well-resourced and under-resourced countries (see the next chapter). The average overall maternal mortality ratio (MMR) per 100,000 live births is 13 in industrialized countries and reported to be 2 in Sweden [8]. The importance of this point is to understand that mothers suffer complications of pregnancy even when they live in an environment of national prosperity. The reduction of mortality rates over the years is the result of specific improvements in pregnancy care including confidential enquiries into maternal death cases. For example, in the UK there were 17 deaths from obstetric hemorrhage in 2000–2002, out of a total of almost two million births [9]. Of some 6000 cases of major obstetric hemorrhage, over 99% of cases of life-threatening bleeding were treated successfully. In all countries, the way to reduce maternal mortality is to ensure that high quality care is accessible, particularly by those most at risk.

Trends in Rates of PPH over Time

There are reports of increasing rates of PPH in developed countries. The data from Soroka University Medical Center, Beer-Sheva, Israel, show that from 1988 until 2006 there was a gradual overall rise in the incidence of reported PPH from all births, rising from 2.37% up to 10.32% (Figure 1).

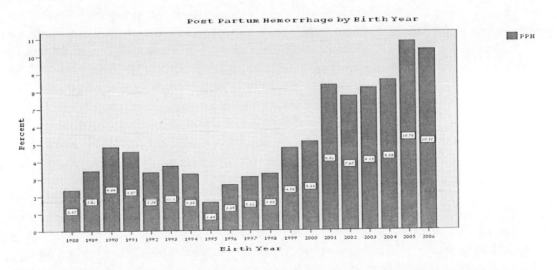

Figure 1. Reported PPH from all births 1988–2006; data from Soroka University Medical Center, Beer-Sheva, Israel

Soroka University Medical Center serves as a referral and sole hospital for the entire population of the Negev region in Israel. The maternity ward and delivery room are busy with more than 12,000 births a year; all data are collected and computerized in a large perinatal database. Trying to understand this trend toward higher rates of PPH over the years and whether this is a reflection of only a reporting bias, we looked at the rates of PPH by mode of delivery. Of the total cesarean deliveries (CDs) and vaginal births, there were 0.33% and 0.55% cases of PPH, respectively. Nevertheless, while we could not collect exact data regarding recurrent CD, it seems that multiple operations increase the risk for PPH. These figures imply that perhaps the rising rates of CDs with its consequences of repeat CDs and the known accompanying complications, such as adherent placenta, may be one of the causes for the general rise in PPH over the years. The rise in risk factors for PPH (such as multiple gestations) [2] might be another contributor to the gradual rise in the incidence of PPH.

A study from Australia aimed at determining whether changes in risk factors for PPH over time are associated with a rise in postpartum hemorrhage rates [10]. This was a population-based study of 752,374 women giving birth in 1994–2002. It was evident that there was an increased proportion of women aged 35 years or older and more nulliparous and cesarean deliveries. Observed PPH rates increased from 4.7 to 6.0, but this increase was not explained by the changing risk profile of the women but rather by a rise in reporting of PPH. Another study from Canada investigated a recent observation of an increase in hysterectomies for PPH [11]. They concluded that there has been an unexplained increase in the frequency, and possibly the severity, of atonic PPH in Canada, leading to higher rates of hysterectomy.

Recurrent PPH

It is well recognized from daily clinical practice that parturients who experienced PPH in their previous delivery are at greater risk of PPH in the index delivery. The medical staff should be prepared to act immediately and use measures of prevention and quick management in the face of recurrent PPH. This finding was proved in a study examining the risk of recurrence of PPH in subsequent pregnancies as determined using record linkage of women's singleton pregnancies over the years 1994 through 2002 [12]. Among the 125,295 women with consecutive pregnancies, the rate of PPH in their first pregnancy was 5.8%. The risk of having PPH in the third pregnancy rose from 4.4% when there was no PPH in the first two pregnancies, to 10.2% when there was PPH in the first pregnancy but not in the second, 14.3% when the PPH event occurred in the second delivery only, and 21.7% for women who had had two prior PPHs. These data represent a risk of recurrent PPH 3.3 times greater than for women with no history of PPH (RR, 3.3; 95% CI, 3.1–3.5) and a relative risk of 5 (RR, 5.0; 95% CI, 3.8–6.5) for women who had had two prior PPHs. The increased risk of recurrence was also evident when mode of delivery was taken into account. This study shows that the risk of a first PPH in any pregnancy is one in 20 (risk of about 5%), while the risk of recurrent PPHs increases to one in seven for a second pregnancy and one in five for a third.

Etiologies and Risk Factors

Predisposing factors and causes for PPH may be grouped by the site of bleeding:

Uterus
1) Uterine atony: This is a general description of a hypotonic myometrium. Predisposing factors include:

- Problems in the perfusion of the uterine muscle
  - Hemorrhage resulting in hypotensive shock
  - Some anesthetics used in conduction analgesia

- Over-distended uterus having trouble contracting after it is emptied
  - large fetus
  - multifetal pregnancy
  - polyhydramnion
  - high parity

- Prolonged or precipitate labor
- Chorioamnionitis

2) Retained placental fragments or pathological adherence like placenta accreta.
3) Uterine rupture

Genital tract
Lacerations of the cervix, vagina, or perineum

Coagulation abnormalities which may be revealed for the first time in the woman's life during labor and could intensify all of the above.

A population-based study of risk factors for early PPH characterized 154,311 women with singleton gestations [13]. Early PPH complicated 0.43% of all singleton deliveries included in this study (n=66/154,311). Independent risk factors for early PPH using multivariate analysis included retained placenta (OR 3.5, 95% CI 2.1–5.8), failure to progress during the second stage of labor (OR 3.4, 95% CI 2.4–4.7), placenta accreta (OR 3.3, 95% CI 1.7–6.4), lacerations (OR 2.4, 95% CI 2.0–2.8), instrumental delivery (OR 2.3, 95% CI 1.6–3.4), large for gestational age (LGA) newborn (OR 1.9, 95% CI 1.6–2.4), hypertensive disorders (OR 1.7, 95% CI 1.2–2.1), induction of labor (OR 1.4, 95% CI 1.1–1.7) and augmentation of labor with oxytocin (OR 1.4, 95% CI 1.2–1.7). Women were than assigned into three different groups according to the assessed severity of PPH, assuming that the severe cases were handled by revision of the birth canal under anesthesia, and the most severe cases required in addition treatment with blood products. A significant linear association was found between the severity of bleeding and the following factors: vacuum extraction (P<0.001), oxytocin augmentation (P<0.001), hypertensive disorders (P<0.001), as well as perinatal mortality (P<0.001), uterine rupture (P<0.001), peripartum hysterectomy (P<0.001), and uterine or internal iliac artery ligation (P<0.001).

At the same institute—Soroka University Medical Center—we have also shown that most cases of PPH recorded occurred around term, obviously since most deliveries take place during this period. While there are almost no cases of PPH at delivery of up to 34 weeks gestation, most cases occur in term deliveries between 37–42 weeks' gestation, with a peak at 40 weeks (Figure 2).

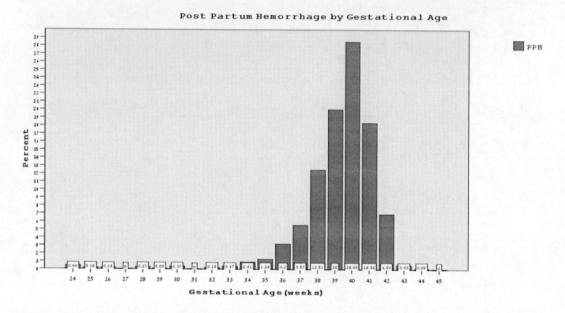

Figure 2. Distribution of all postpartum hemorrhage by gestational age (%); data from Soroka University Medical Center, Beer-Sheva, Israel.

In a Dutch population-based cohort study on PPH, incidence and risk factors were evaluated [14]. Cases were divided into standard and severe PPH; all were vaginally delivering nulliparous women. The incidence of standard PPH (≥500 ml) and severe PPH (≥1000 ml) were 19 and 4.2%, respectively. A retained placenta occurred in 1.8%. These data show higher values compared to other studies in the literature. The most important risk factors for standard and severe PPH were related to prolonged third stage of labor (≥ 30 min) and retained placenta. High birth weight and perineal damage were also independent and significant risk factors.

Treatment

Treatment once PPH is diagnosed should be as an emergency that requires the coordinated functioning of multidisciplinary practitioners—midwife, obstetrician, anesthesiologist, hematologist, and laboratory team including blood bank services. The treatment is built up in steps, from basic actions to treat and simultaneously identify the cause of bleeding, treatment, prevent deterioration, and onto life support and invasive procedures as necessary.

1) Call for assistance! Advise blood bank of possible demand for blood and blood products further on.
2) Uterine massage using bimanual uterine compression technique.
3) IV line, crystalloids, and blood products if needed.
4) Administer uterotonics—oxytocin, ergometrine, prostaglandins (PG)-PGF2α, PGE2, and PGE1.
5) Foley catheter to monitor urinary output.
6) Determine the cause of excessive bleeding. Uterine atony vs. lacerations of the birth canal, or-both.
7) Angiographic embolization or uterine or internal iliac artery ligation to reduce pulse pressure in the distal arteries and by this reduce hemorrhage.
8) Uterine compression sutures, uterine packing.
9) In the face of intractable bleeding, hysterectomy as a life saving procedure.
10) Recombinant activated factor VII.

Before treatment, however, is the prevention of a disease state. Today, the active management of labor and routine prophylactic administration of uterotonic drugs to reduce the risk of PPH has become an integral part of the management of labor and delivery [15]. Active management of labor includes, especially in this context, the active management of the third stage of labor, which is the period of time starting after the delivery of the baby and ending after delivery of the placenta. At this phase the most important mechanism to reduce blood loss from the placental site and to avoid uterine atony is vasoconstriction of blood vessels produced by the firm and steady contraction of the uterine myometrium. Drugs used in this stage act to stimulate uterine contractions and enhance vasoconstriction, and if given immediately after delivery of the baby will also enhance detachment of the placenta. These drugs, which are considered first line, are termed "uterotonic" and include oxytocin, ergometrine, or a regimen of both. Other options are oxytocin agonists and misoprostol, discussed later. The timing of administration of the drug is variable in different institutions, where some prefer administering them immediately after the birth of the fetal shoulders and some only after the placenta is delivered. Other measures of active management of the third stage of labor are clamping of the umbilical cord, controlled cord traction, and guidance of the parturient to bear down.

The next step once this has become evidence-based and a standard of care is the implementation of these strategies. A recent publication describes an intervention to improve obstetrical care, demonstrating the difficulties of these interventions and their reward [16]. Nineteen hospitals in Argentina and Uruguay were randomized to receive an intervention aimed at developing guidelines for the management of the third stage of labor and carrying them out, or to receive no intervention. Primary outcomes were the rates of prophylactic use of oxytocin during the third stage of labor. The main secondary outcome was the rate of PPH. The results speak for themselves: use of prophylactic oxytocin increased from 2.1% at baseline to 83.6% after the end of the intervention at hospitals that received the intervention, compared to a rise from 2.6% to 12.3% at control hospitals (P = 0.01 for the difference in changes). There was also an associated reduction in the rate of PPH of 500 ml or more (relative rate reduction, 45%; 95% CI, 9 to 71) and of 1000 ml or more (relative rate reduction, 70%; 95% CI, 16 to 78).

Medical Treatment

In a thorough review done for the Cochrane Library (2007), including all randomized controlled trials of treatment of primary PPH, only three trials were identified as meeting all requirements [17]. These three trials examined the place of misoprostol in the management of primary PPH. Altogether there were 462 patients. In one trial examining misoprostol versus oxytocin/ergometrine, the use of misoprostol was noted to be superior to oxytocin/ergometrine in subjective cessation of hemorrhage within 20 minutes and significant reduction in the number of women who required additional uterotonics. The two other trials had a different design; they examined misoprostol versus placebo after failure of first line treatment with oxytocin/ergometrine. Misoprostol use was associated with a significant reduction in blood loss of 500 ml or more; however, the additional use of uterotonics, blood transfusion, and evacuation of retained products did not differ between the two groups. Yet, the number of included women is too small to evaluate the effect on maternal mortality and therefore at present there are insufficient data to draw any conclusions about the effectiveness and safety for either first- or second-line therapy with misoprostol in the setting of primary PPH.

The importance of misoprostol is now beyond clinical trials. Having shown that it does work to control excessive bleeding after delivery, its impact is enormous and could save thousands of lives in areas in the world where there is no option to administer injectable uterotonics because they are not available. Misoprostol tablets are administered either by mouth or rectally and are stable in extreme climates. A Cochrane review included 46 trials involving 42,621 women after delivery; of these, 37 trials evaluated misoprostol use [18]. Most trials were conducted in hospital settings where deliveries are performed by skilled caregivers, but still the results are encouraging to implement strategies towards using misoprostol as a modality to prevent PPH in remote areas where out-of-hospital deliveries are the rule. Trials comparing misoprostol with other uterotonics are actually trials designed to evaluate whether misoprostol is as effective as the gold standard drugs given its advantage of oral or rectal route of administration.

A recent advance in the treatment of bleeding disorders is the introduction of recombinant activated factor VIIa (rFVIIa). rFVIIa was initially approved in 1998 for surgery prophylaxis or to treat bleeding in patients with hemophilia who have acquired antibodies to factors VIII or IX, in Glanzmann thrombasthenia, and patients with factor VII deficiency. The drug's 'off-label' use was first reported in trauma and surgical life threatening hemorrhage and the rationale was that no matter what the cause of bleeding is, the clotting system should be maintained and kept from compromise. Recombinant activated factor VII initiates coagulation when tissue factor (TF) has been exposed at the site of injury. They compose a complex that activates factor X and subsequently converts prothrombin into thrombin. This restriction to the local site of damage makes the use of the drug specific. At this stage there are mainly publications of case descriptions of the use of rFVIIa for PPH and guidelines based on specialist opinions and local experience [19]. There are currently no randomized controlled trials. The drug was reported in some case series to save lives and also save fertility, as the last resort before hysterectomy. The major concerns with its use are life-threatening thromboembolism in obstetrical patients known to be already in a hypercoagulable state and its cost [20]. Thus, improvements in conventional and surgical management are necessary before introduction of routine use of rFVIIa.

Conclusions

Postpartum hemorrhage is one of the treatable emergency situations in obstetrics. In many parts of the world, it accounts for up to 55% of the total maternal deaths, which obviously presents a major health problem. Clinicians use different definitions and the estimation of the amount of bleeding is imprecise or missing, making the variations of PPH incidence enormous. Maternal death might occur within a short period of time due to irreversible shock.

Active management of labor, especially the third stage of labor, and routine prophylactic administration of uterotonic drugs to reduce the risk of PPH have become an integral part of the management of labor and delivery. Treatment once PPH is diagnosed as an emergency requires coordinated functioning of multidisciplinary practitioners—midwife, obstetrician, anesthesiologist, hematologist, and laboratory team including blood bank services. The treatment is built up in steps, from basic actions to treat and simultaneously identify the cause of bleeding, to prevent deterioration, and to provide life support and invasive procedures as necessary. The importance of misoprostol is today beyond clinical trials. As a simple administered drug that has been shown to control excessive bleeding after delivery, it could save thousands of lives in areas where there is no option for advanced treatments. Implementation of these strategies is part of the United Nations' Millennium Development Goals to reduce the maternal mortality rate by 75% by 2015.

References

[1] Carroli G, Cuesta C, Abalos E, Gulmezoglu AM. Epidemiology of postpartum haemorrhage: a systematic review. *Best Pract Res Clin Obstet Gynaecol*. 2008;22(6):999-1012. [Epub 2008 Sep. 25]

[2] Sheiner E, Ohel I, Hadar A. Out of hospital deliveries and post partum hemorrhage. In: B-Lynch C, Keith L, Lalonde A, Karoshi M, eds. *A textbook of Post-partum Hemorrhage*. Dumfries, Scotland: Sapiens Publishing, 2006:Chapter 46.

[3] Khan KS, Wojdyla D, Say L, Gülmezoglu AM, Van Look PF. WHO analysis of causes of maternal death: a systematic review. *Lancet*. 2006;9516:1066-1074.

[4] World Health Organization. Health and the Millennium Development Goals. *Geneva: World Health Organization*; 2005.

[5] Hill K. Making deaths count. Editorial. *Bull World Health Organ*. 2006;84:162.

[6] Onakewhor JU, Gharoro EP. Changing trends in maternal mortality in a developing country. *Niger J Clin Pract*. 2008;11:111-120.

[7] Lema VM, Changole J, Kanyighe C, Malunga EV. Maternal mortality at the Queen Elizabeth Central Teaching Hospital, Blantyre, Malawi. *East Afr Med J*. 2005;82:3-9.

[8] Drife J. Maternal mortality in well-resourced countries: is there still a need for confidential enquiries? *Best Pract Res Clin Obstet Gynaecol*. 2008;22:501-515.

[9] Lewis G, ed. *Why Mothers Die 2000–2002: The Sixth Report of the Confidential Enquiries into Maternal Deaths in the United Kingdom*. London: RCOG Press; 2004.

[10] Ford JB, Roberts CL, Simpson JM, Vaughan J, Cameron CA. Increased postpartum hemorrhage rates in Australia. I*nt J Gynaecol Obstet*. 2007;98:237-243.

[11] Joseph KS, Rouleau J, Kramer MS, Young DC, Liston RM, Baskett TF; Maternal Health Study Group of the Canadian Perinatal Surveillance System. Investigation of an increase in postpartum haemorrhage in Canada. *BJOG*. 2007;114:751-759.

[12] Ford JB, Roberts CL, Bell JC, Algert CS, Morris JM. Postpartum haemorrhage occurrence and recurrence: a population-based study. *Med J Aust*. 2007;187:391-393.

[13] Sheiner E, Sarid L, Levy A, Seidman DS, Hallak M. Obstetric risk factors and outcome of pregnancies complicated with early postpartum hemorrhage: A population-based study. *J Matern Fetal Neonatal Med*. 2005;18:149-154.

[14] Bais JM, Eskes M, Pel M, Bonsel GJ, Bleker OP. Postpartum haemorrhage in nulliparous women: incidence and risk factors in low and high risk women. A Dutch population-based cohort study on standard (> or = 500 ml) and severe (> or = 1000 ml) postpartum haemorrhage. *Eur J Obstet Gynecol Reprod Biol*. 2004;2:166-172.

[15] Prendiville W. Active versus expectant management of third stage of labour. *Lancet*. 1998;351:1659.

[16] Althabe F, Buekens P, Bergel E, Belizán JM, Campbell MK, Moss N, Hartwell T, Wright LL; Guidelines Trial Group. A behavioral intervention to improve obstetrical care. *N Engl J Med*. 2008;358:1929-1940.

[17] Mousa HA, Alfirevic Z. Treatment for primary postpartum haemorrhage. *Cochrane Database Syst Rev*. 2007;(1):CD003249. Review.

[18] Gülmezoglu AM, Forna F, Villar J, Hofmeyr GJ. Prostaglandins for preventing postpartum haemorrhage (Review). *Cochrane Database Syst Rev*. 2007;(3):CD000494. Review.

[19] Alfirevic Z, Elbourne D, Pavord S, Bolte A, Van Geifn H, Mercier F, Ahonen J, Bremme K, Bødker B, Magnúsdóttir EM, Salvesen K, Prendiville W, Truesdale A, Clemens F, Piercy D, Gyte G. Use of recombinant activated factor VII in primary postpartum hemorrhage: the Northern European registry 2000-2004. *Obstet Gynecol*. 2007;110:1270-1278.

[20] Welsh A, McLintock C, Gatt S, Somerset D, Popham P, Ogle R. Guidelines for the use of recombinant activated factor VII in massive obstetric haemorrhage. *Aust N Z J Obstet Gynaecol*. 2008;48:12-16.

Maternal and Perinatal Mortality

In: Textbook of Perinatal Epidemiology
Editor: Eyal Sheiner, pp. 691-700

ISBN: 978-1-60741-648-7
© 2010 Nova Science Publishers, Inc.

Chapter XXXII

Epidemiology of Maternal Mortality

Naomi Schneid-Kofman and Eyal Sheiner [*]

From the Department of Obstetrics and Gynecology, Faculty of Health Sciences, Soroka University Medical Center, Ben Gurion University of the Negev, Beer-Sheva, Israel.

Definitions

- Maternal mortality ratio: Number (no) of maternal deaths/100,000 live births.
- Annual mortality rate: Total no. of deaths from all causes in one year X100,000/No. of persons in the population at mid year.
- Case fatality rate: No. of individuals dying during a specific period of time after disease onset or diagnosis X100 / No. of individuals with the specific disease.
- Proportionate mortality (not a rate): No. of deaths from a specific cause X100/ No. of total deaths of all causes

Introduction

Maternal mortality ratio (more commonly cited as maternal mortality rate) is the number of maternal deaths that result from the reproductive process per 100,000 live births[1]. In general, mortality rates serve as measures of disease severity, and can help us determine whether the treatment for a disease has become more effective over time, the denominator for mortality rates is the population at risk and not a subpopulation (live births). This is why maternal mortality is a ratio and not a rate. Maternal mortality ratio represents a range of conditions affecting a specific subgroup. The risk of dying from the reproductive process is

[*] For Correspondence: Eyal Sheiner, M.D, PhD., Department of Obstetrics and Gynecology, Soroka University Medical Center, P.O Box 151, Beer-Sheva, 84101, Israel., Tel 972-8-6400774 Fax 972-8-6275338, E-mail: sheiner@bgu.ac.il

globally perceived as intolerable hence maternal mortality ratio has been extensively explored.

Expressing mortality in quantitative terms denotes differences in the risk of dying from a disease between people in different geographic regions and/or different subgroups in a population. Yet an increase in mortality rates, or lack of expected decrease, may be attributed to a growing awareness to the condition and higher report rates rater than increased severity of the condition. Of note, a mortality rate can be determined only if the size of the population at risk is known, in the case of mortality ratio the number of live births in the studied population.

Quantitative Terms and Definitions

Different quantitative terms are used to describe mortality rates. One example is annual mortality rate. The annual mortality rate for all causes (per 100,000 population) is calculated as the total number of deaths from all causes in one year divided by the number of persons in the population at mid year (x100,000). Since the population changes over time, mid year population is used as an approximation.

Specific mortality rates, such as in a specific age group or a specific geographic region must be calculated as the number of cases in the restricted population, with the denominator expressing the same restricted population.

Mortality from a specific condition can be expressed as case fatality rate: The number of individuals dying during a specific period of time after disease onset or diagnosis divided by the number of individuals with the specific disease (presented as percent, if multiplied by 100). This rate is limited to the risk for a specific sub population who encountered the specific disease. Thus, case fatality rate is a measure of severity of the disease. As therapy improves, case fatality rate would be expected to decline. An obvious limitation in calculating case fatality rate evolves from including death of individuals with the disease that are from other causes. Ideally, only deaths caused by the disease should be included.

As a result of these limitations, unfortunately, it is estimated that more than half of maternal deaths are not recorded in calculated maternal mortality ratios, and accordingly specific case fatality rates are nearly impossible to obtain[2].

Proportionate mortality is a measure of mortality from a specific cause of all mortality causes. It is not a rate. The number of deaths from a specific cause, divided by the number of total deaths of all causes (X100) is the proportionate mortality of that cause. An elevated proportional mortality from a single cause does not mean an increased risk of mortality from that cause in a certain population. This depends upon the overall mortality risk in that population. As an example, a total mortality rate of 30:100,000 in one population, with a proportional mortality from a disease of 10%, results in a mortality rate of 3/100,000. It is equal to the specific mortality rate from the same disease in a different population with an overall mortality rate of 15:100,000, and a proportional mortality of 20%. Hence, proportionate mortality rate represents the major causes of mortality in a certain population but does not convey the risk of dying from a specific cause. For calculation of the risk of dying, mortality rate must be calculated.

Worldwide Data of Maternal Mortality

Worldwide data of maternal mortality is probably based upon pregnancy associated or related deaths only. Persistent efforts are made to assess true mortality rates, though these are considered at most educated guesses. Indirect maternal deaths (estimated 20 percent of all maternal deaths) are likely unreported, as are maternal deaths occurring outside of medical institutions.

Table 1 presents maternal mortality ratios by continent according to the WHO report in 1990[3].

Table 1. Estimated maternal mortality ratio by continent (from WHO report 1990).

Continent	Estimated maternal mortality ratio (per 100,000 live births)
Africa	640
Asia	420
Latin America	270
All developed countries	30
United Kingdoms	12
Northern and Middle Europe	10

Maternal mortality is largely an avoidable cause of death. Lowering maternal mortality ratio has been a target for Millennium Development Goal (MDG) number. However, data weaknesses have made monitoring progress extremely problematic[4].

The worldwide reported data are mainly hospital based. A discrepancy between whole region data and hospital data was noted in several reports. This may indicate inconclusive community based data[5].

Causes of Maternal Mortality

Important causes of maternal death past mid pregnancy are thromboembolism, Amniotic fluid embolism, hemorrhage, hypertension and infection (figure 1). Death during early pregnancy, miscarriage, induced abortion or ectopic pregnancy is prominently from hemorrhage and infection[6]. Other important causes are anesthetic complications and non obstetric infections. Indirect maternal deaths result from preexisting conditions that are exacerbated by the process of pregnancy, abortion or delivery. Table 2 presents a list of direct and indirect mortality causes. Special attention should be given to prevalent risk factors such as high parity which is associated with maternal mortality. Illegal status of abortion in some countries remains an important contributory factor to the abortion related deaths[7].

The proportion of preventable deaths is a main interest of investigation reported as high as 58% of recorded maternal deaths within hospitals[8].

A significant divergence is noted in published data. Increased mortality rate is observed among minority and indigent populations, black race and age are important risk factors[9]. Different regions report death of diverse reasons, sepsis and HIV/AIDS were reported as leading causes of maternal mortality in Africa while toxemia the leading cause of maternal death in the Netherlands[10].

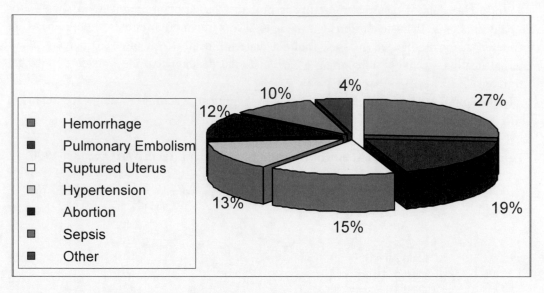

Figure 1. Causes of maternal deaths – WHO and Unicef report 1996

Table 2. Direct and indirect causes of maternal mortality.

Direct causes of maternal mortality (80%)	Indirect causes of maternal mortality (20%)
	Infection
	HIV
	Malaria
Thromboembolism	**Anemia**
Infection	**Sickle cell disease**
Hemorrhage	**Thalassemia**
Hypertension	**Heart disease**
Eclampsia	**Valvular disease**
Uterine rupture	**Cardiomyopathy**
Obstructed labor	**Liver cirrhosis**
Unsafe abortion	**Encephalopathy**
	Collagen vascular disease

Comparison of Mortality Rates between Populations

Comparison of mortality rates between populations must take into account a different age structure of the populations. Other parameters might bias the comparison though age has the most influence upon mortality rates. For example, mortality rates in a low socioeconomic population may be surprisingly lower than in a high socioeconomic population if the oldest age group is smaller in the low socioeconomic population. Specifically, in maternal mortality rate calculations this bias is of less importance, since the population at risk is of a specific age group, and the biologic age of fertility does not differ greatly between different geographic regions.

If a large divergence is noted between compared populations, the population structure should be further evaluated to avoid bias (for example, a very young maternal reproductive age in indigent populations compared with late first pregnancy in advanced age in other populations), an age specific risk for both known population is calculated for a "standard" population, represented as an *age adjusted risk*. These risks can then be compares between the populations.

Applying the methods for comparison of maternal mortality ratio between world sub populations and subsequent to the previously discussed limits, a strong divergence is noted in maternal mortality ratio between populations. Among other tools, multiple regression analyses were used to investigate the variability in reports from different parts of the world. Three country specific variables were noted with the strongest relationship to maternal mortality ratio: proportion of deliveries assisted by a skilled birth attendant, infant mortality rate and health expenditure per capita. Ninety percent of the variability was explained by these models[11].

Safe Motherhood Initiative

Awareness to the geographic gap in maternal mortality ratios led to the Safe Motherhood Initiative launched in 1987. The goal of this project was set at a fifty percent reduction in maternal mortality. A higher goal was further declared in 2000 at a 75% reduction of mortality ratio by the Millennium Development Goal, which was adopted by the UN and heads of state[12]. Since these declarations a reduction was achieved in certain geographic areas such as Latin America and northern Africa yet the gap between developing countries and the rest of the world has widened. Ninety-nine percent of dying mothers are in the developing world, most in sub-Saharan Africa and Asia [13, 14]. An estimated slight reduction of 2.5% per year over fifteen years (1990-2005) is noted in most countries with published data, yet no significant reduction is noted in sub-Saharan Africa during the same period. For example, this region contributed 270,500 maternal deaths in 2005, a mere fifty percent[4].

Evaluation and planning intervention strategies followed world interest in investigating the diversity between nations in maternal mortality ratios. It was concluded that safe motherhood begins with a healthy environment. Women's status, political commitment, and socioeconomic development have crucial effect upon this environment. Obviously, the healthy environment is influenced by women's health and nutritional status, reproductive and health behavior, and access to family planning and maternal care services[15].

Accordingly, a suggested strategy to reduce maternal mortality included adequate primary health care and universally available family planning, adequate prenatal care, including nutrition, with early detection of anemia and other complications, the assistance of a trained personal at births; and appropriate referral of high-risk pregnancies to medical facilities[16].

Many contributing issues have been addressed, for example, lack of trained personal attending deliveries[17], lack of access to emergency care when indicated and funding issues including collaborating with other health organizations (children's health, HIV, family planning). Some authors have questioned the international selected goals and scheduled approach, suggesting that local autonomy over funds for health promotion rather than philanthropic interventions may provide a more gradual improvement however long lasting of a variety of health issues[14].

The Lancet issue published October 13, 2007 is one to review in a few years time. In this issue, some of the influencing figures in the field of global health promotion have declared that joining forces and collaboration are the main means to further reduce maternal mortality rates [12-4, 18-21]. They have all expressed their frustration from not achieving the expected reduction in maternal mortality. Indeed, after two decades of the Safe Motherhood Initiative, meaningful reductions in maternal mortality and disability during pregnancy and childbirth in developing countries have not been realized [22]. Tita et al suggested that among essential elements to achieve safe motherhood, recommended public health strategies should be supported by good quality evidence of effectiveness, through randomized trials when feasible, before their widespread implementation [23].

Local Data

In Israel, maternal mortality has declined since the declaration of the global Safe Motherhood Initiative in 1987, to a low of 1.37 per 100,000 live births in 2004. Setting an example for the divergence between subpopulations in a shared geographic region, a closer examination of the 2004 maternal mortality ratio in Israel is illustrated. Of the 145,207 deliveries in 2004, 12,649(8.7%) were in a single medical center (Soroka medical center), 55.7 percent of deliveries were by women originating from the Bedouin tribal population [24]. 2004 was an exceptional year in the higher rate of mortality in the southern district (figure 2). This may be explicated by the small number of cases that modify the ratio greatly (Table 3).

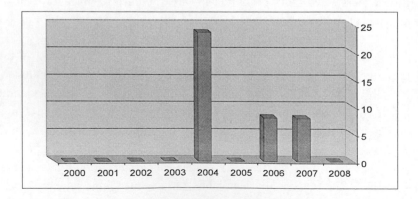

Figure 2. Maternal mortality ratio by year, Soroka University Medical Center.

Table 3: Maternal mortality in Soroka University Medical Center, by year and maternal origin.

Year	Bedouin births	Mortality (no. of cases)	Bedouin Mortality ratio	Jewish births	Mortality (no. of cases)	Jewish Mortality ratio	Total births	Mortality (no. of cases)	Total Mortality ratio
2000	6618	0	0	5700	0	0	12318	0	0
2001	6743	0	0	5990	0	0	12342	0	0
2002	70C3	0	0	5460	0	0	12462	0	0
2003	7340	0	0	5943	0	0	13283	0	0
2004	7042	3	42.6	5607	0	0	12649	3	23.7
2005	6872	0	0	5372	0	0	12244	0	0
2006	6850	0	0	5577	1	17.9	12427	1	8
2007	7089	1	14.1	5522	0	0	12611	1	7.9
2008	7216	1	13.8	5841	1	17.1	13057	2	15.3
2009	7313	0	0	5900	1	16.9	13213	1	7.5
Total	70056	5	7.1	56912	3	5.3	126606	8	6.3

This southern population is distinct, since it can serve as a model for a developing population provided with advanced western world health care systems [25]. Some of the Bedouin tribes have adopted modernization, living in urbanized communities (yet low income and over populated households), preserving tribal costumes as culture heritage rather than way of life, while others conduct third world daily living, residing in unlisted villages throughout the region. Maternal mortality rate for this population during 2003-2006 was 14.2 for every 100,000 live births.

Another interesting aspect of maternal morality ratio in Israel is that prenatal care is subsidized by the government and basic health insurance is provided by law to all citizens. A delivery grant is provided to women who are admitted into a hospital prior or post delivery. These means reflect in a high rate of prenatal care and near 100% of peri-partum hospital admission [26-27], and may contribute to the lower rates of maternal deaths. The Israeli rate of maternal mortality of 3.1/100,000 live births in 2000, must be viewed in light of the Unicef estimated rate of 900/100,000 live births (range of estimation 300-1600) for the Middle east.

In Conclusion

Maternal mortality ratio is the number of maternal deaths that result from the reproductive process per 100,000 live births, representing a range of conditions affecting a specific subgroup. Since dying from the reproductive process is globally perceived as intolerable and frequently avoidable, world initiative was set to reduce mortality by launching global recognition and intervention programs largely based upon epidemiology reports. These reports are strongly limited. Data are inconclusive as they are hospital and not population based, report direct causes omitting indirect important causes of death and inconsistencies are noted between reports. Divergence of death causes and risk factors among populations in different regions of the world (age distribution, parity, infectious disease prevalence) requires a population adjusted approach for reduction of mortality rather than a world wide strategy. Recognizing the limits of data assists in planning appropriate and population targeted means of intervention.

Reassessment of global resources and means of intervention will hopefully result in narrowing the gap between nations, and perhaps further reducing global maternal mortality subsequently creating a safer world for mothers.

References

[1]   Gordis L. Epidemiology. Measuring the occurrence of disease: *Mortality; Chapter 4:59-84.4th Edition*, 2009, Sounders Elsevier, Philadelphia, PA.
[2]   Koonin LM, MacKay AP, Berg CJ. Pregnancy related mortality surveillance – United States, 1987-1990. *MMWR*, 1997; 46:127.
[3]   Pitkin J, Peattie AB, Magowan BA. Obstetrics and Gynecology: An illustrated color text. *Vital statistics page 78-79*; 2003, Churchill Livingstone, London England.

[4]   Hill K, Thomas K, AbouZahr C, Walker N, Say L, Inoue M, Suzuki E; Maternal Mortality working group. Estimates of maternal mortality worldwide between 1990 and 2005: an assessment of available data. *Lancet*, 2007; 370(9595):1311-9.

[5]   Price TG. Preliminary report on maternal deaths in the Southern Highlands of Tanzania in 1983. *J Obstet Gynaecol East Cent Africa*. 1984;3(3):103-10.

[6]   Anachebe JF, Sutton MY. Racial disparities in reproductive health outcomes. *Am J Obstet Gynecol*, 2003; 188:S37.

[7]   Alves SV. Maternal mortality in Pernamuco, Brazil: what has changed in ten years? *Reprod Health Matters*. 2007; 15(30)134-44.

[8]   Varner MW, Daly KD, Goplerud CP, Keettel WC. Maternal mortality in major referral hospital 1926 to1980. *Am J Obstet Gynecol*. 1982;143(3):325-39.

[9]   Chang J, Elam-Evans LD, Berg CJ. Pregnancy related mortality surveillance – United States, 1991-1999. *MMWR*, 2003; 52(SS-2):4.

[10]   Van Dillen J, Stekelenburg J, Schutte J, Walraven G, Van Roosmalen J. The use of audit to identify maternal mortality in different settings Is it just a difference between the rich and the poor? *World Health Popul*. 2007;9(1):5-13.

[11]   Betran AP, Wojdyla D,Posner SF, Gulmezoglu AM. National estimates for maternal mortality: an analysis based on the WHO systematic review of maternal mortality and morbidity. *BMC Public Health*. 2005 ;5:131.

[12]   Freeman LP, Graham WJ, Brazier E, Smith JM, Ensor T, Fauveau V, Themmen E, Currie S, Agrarwl K. Practical lessons from global safe motherhood initiatives: time for a new focus on implementation; *Lancet*, 2007; 307:1383-91.

[13]   Starrs AM, Delivering for women; *Lancet*, 2007; 307:1285-7.

[14]   Hill K, Thomas K, AbouZahr C, Walker N, Say L, Inoue M, Suzuki E; Maternal Mortality Working Group.. Estimates of maternal mortality worldwide between 1990 and 2005: an assessment of available data; *Lancet*, 2007; 307:1311-9.

[15]   Koblinsky MA, Tinker A, Daly P. Programming for safe motherhood: a guide to action. Health Policy Plan. 1994; 9(3):252-66.

[16]   Mahler H. The safe motherhood initiative: a call to action. *Lancet*. 1987; 1(8534):668-70.

[17]   Obaid TA. No women should die giving life; *Lancet*, 2007; 307:1287-8.

[18]   Garrido IG. Women's health and political will; *Lancet*, 2007; 307:1288-91.

[19]   Yazbeck AS. Challenges in measuring maternal mortality; *Lancet*, 2007; 307:1291-2.

[20]   Mushataque A., Chowdhury R. Rethinking interventions for women's health; *Lancet*, 2007; 307:1292-3.

[21]   Kerber KJ, de Graft- Johnson JE, Bhutta ZA, Okong P, Starrs A, Lewn JE. Continuum of care for maternal, newborn, and child health: from slogan to service delivery; *Lancet*, 2007; 307:1358-69.

[22]   Maine D. Detours and shortcuts on the road to maternal mortality reduction; *Lancet*, 2007; 307:1380-2.

[23]   Tita AT, Stringer JS, Goldenberg RL, Rouse DJ. Two decades of the safe motherhood initiative: time for another wooden spoon award? *Obstet Gynecol*. 2007; 110(5):972-6.

[24]   Sheiner E, Levy A, Yerushalmi R, Katz M. Beta-thalassemia minor during pregnancy. *Obstet Gynecol*. 2004; 103(6):1273-7.

[25] Schneid-Kofman N, Sheiner E. Frustration from not achieving the expected reduction in maternal mortality. *Arch Gynecol Obstet*. 2008 ;277:283-4.

[26] Sheiner E, Shoham-Vardi I, Hadar A, Hershkovitz R, Sheiner EK, Mazor M. Accidental out-of-hospital delivery as an independent risk factor for perinatal mortality.*J Reprod Med*. 2002; 47(8):625-30.

[27] Sheiner E, Hershkovitz R, Shoham-Vardi I, Erez O, Hadar A, Mazor M. A retrospective study of unplanned out-of-hospital deliveries. *Arch Gynecol Obstet*. 2004; 269(2):85-8. Epub 2002 Oct 29.

In: Textbook of Perinatal Epidemiology
Editor: Eyal Sheiner, pp. 701-713

ISBN: 978-1-60741-648-7
© 2010 Nova Science Publishers, Inc.

Chapter XXXIII

Epidemiology of Perinatal Mortality

*Rintaro Mori**

Introduction

Perinatal mortality rate is regarded as one of the major health indicators that reflect a community's achievement in health. Perinatal mortality is a sum of early neonatal mortalities (deaths) and late fetal deaths; the denominator for perinatal mortality rate is the number of live births or live births plus fetal deaths, although there is no single widely-accepted international standard regarding the range of gestational age to include in the definition [1-3].

This chapter describes definitions of perinatal mortality rates and the reasons behind the wide variety of its definitions, causes of perinatal mortalities and distribution of perinatal mortalities in the world, as well as some examples of its use.

Definitions of "Perinatal Mortality" and "Perinatal Mortality Rate"

Perinatal Mortality

The definition of the perinatal period in the Tenth Revision of International Classification of Diseases is a period between 22 gestational weeks of age and 7 days after birth [1,4]. The Ninth and Tenth Revisions of International Classification of Diseases recommended that national perinatal statistics should include all fetuses and infants delivered weighing at least 500g (or, when birth weight is unavailable, the corresponding gestational

* For Correspondence: Rintaro Mori MD PhD MSc FRCPCH, Associate Professor, Department of Global Health Policy, Graduate School of Medicine, the University of Tokyo, Japan. E-mail: rintaromori@gmail.com

age [22 weeks] or body length [25cm crown–heel]), whether alive or dead. They also recommended that less mature fetuses and infants should be excluded from perinatal statistics unless there are legal or other valid reasons to the contrary.

However, inclusion of very immature births such as extremely low birth weight infants (weighing up to 1000g) can disrupt international comparisons due to differences in register criteria by countries. Therefore, they also recommended that countries should present, solely for international comparisons, "standard perinatal statistics" in which both the numerator and denominator of all rates are restricted to fetuses and infants weighing 1000g or more (or, where birth weight is unavailable, the corresponding gestational age [28 weeks] or body length [25 cm crown–heel]).

Perinatal Mortality Rate

The definition by the World Health Organization (WHO) is the rate of the number of fetal deaths (28 weeks of gestation or more) plus neonatal deaths (within one week of age), out of the number of 1000 *live births in a year* [1,5]. In many high-income countries, perinatal mortality rate is defined as the rate of the number of fetal deaths (28 weeks of gestation or more) plus neonatal deaths (within one week of age), out of the number of 1000 *fetal deaths* (28 weeks of gestation or more) *plus all live births*. On the other hand, the WHO Expert Committee on the Prevention of Perinatal Mortality and Morbidity recommended a more precise formulation of "late fetal and early neonatal deaths weighing over 1000 g at birth expressed as a ratio per 1000 live births weighing over 1000 g at birth", and this is used in routine statistics in other agencies including the OECD [1].

Definitions by Countries/Agencies

Definitions used in some countries are shown in Table 1.

Table 1. Definitions of perinatal mortality (rates) in selected national governmental agencies and the WHO.

Countries	Fetal numerator	Neonatal numerator	Denominator	Note
WHO definition for international comparison	Fetal deaths (28 weeks of gestation or more)	Neonatal deaths (within 7 days of age)	1000 live births	This is the most widely-used definition where resources are relatively limited
WHO expert group recommendation of precise formulae	Fetal deaths (28 weeks of gestation or more)	Neonatal deaths (within 7 days of age)	1000 live births weighing over 1000 g at birth	
Australia	Fetal deaths (body weight of 400 grams and/or 20 weeks gestation or	Neonatal deaths (babies of at least 400 grams (or at least 20 weeks if	1000 live births and fetal deaths combined (where birth weight is at	

		birth weight is unavailable) up to 28 days)	least 400 grams)	
Austria	Fetal deaths (28 weeks of gestation or more)	Neonatal deaths (within 7 days of age)	1000 live births	
Canada	Fetal deaths (28 weeks of gestation or more)	Neonatal deaths (within 7 days of age)	1000 total births (live births and stillbirths)	Unknown gestational ages are excluded
France	Fetal deaths (body weight of 500 grams and/or 22 weeks gestation or more)	Neonatal deaths (within 7 days of age)	1000 total births (live births and stillbirths)	
Germany	Fetal deaths (28 weeks of gestation or more)	Neonatal deaths (within 7 days of age)	1000 total births (live births and stillbirths)	
Ireland	Fetal deaths (body weight of 500 grams and/or 24 weeks gestation or more)	Neonatal deaths (within 7 days of age)	1000 total births (live births and stillbirths)	
Japan	Fetal deaths (22 weeks of gestation or more)	Neonatal deaths (within 7 days of age)	1000 (all live births + fetal deaths at 22 weeks of gestation or more)	
Netherlands	Fetal deaths (24 weeks of gestation or more)	Neonatal deaths (within 7 days of age)	1000 total births (live births and stillbirths)	
Switzerland	Fetal deaths (body height of 30 cm and/or 28 weeks gestation or more)	Neonatal deaths (within 7 days of age)	1000 total births (live births and stillbirths)	
UK	Fetal deaths (24 weeks of gestation or more)	Neonatal deaths (within 7 days of age)	1000 total births (live births and stillbirths)	Definition of stillbirths was altered on 1 October 1992 from a baby born dead after 28 completed weeks gestation or more
US	Fetal deaths (24 weeks of gestation or more)	Neonatal deaths (within 7 days of age)	1000 total births (live births and stillbirths)	Perinatal Definition I
	Fetal deaths (20 weeks of gestation or more)	Neonatal deaths (within 28 days of age)	1000 total births (live births and stillbirths)	Perinatal Definition II

Effect by difference definitions was evaluated in a previous study. After October 1992, perinatal mortality statistics should include fetal deaths between 24 and 27 weeks of gestation in England and Wales, and Cartlidge et al. showed significant impact by including these fetal deaths [6].

Categories and Causes of Perinatal Mortality

Perinatal mortality is affected by many obstetric and neonatal factors, and therefore it is important to explore its cause. It is often difficult to classify into a single cause of death, though a standardised category of causes of perinatal death allows comparisons of different populations. There have been a number of attempts to explore and categorise causes of perinatal mortality [7-15]. However, again there is no single agreed classification of perinatal mortality in the world, as the classification will be depending upon its purpose. There are three major classifications: (1) the Nordic-Baltic Perinatal Death Classification, (2) the obstetric (Aberdeen) classification, and (3) Wigglesworth classification [14].

The Nordic-Baltic Perinatal Death Classification has its advantages in its simplicity, and this has been used in northern European countries as well as in developing countries. It has been amended and there are several updated versions. Table 2 shows the common Nordic-Baltic Perinatal Death Classification [9,10,16].

Table 2. The Nordic-Baltic Perinatal Death Classification.

There are 13 mutually exclusive groups	
I	Fetal Malformation
II	Antenatal death. Single growth-restricted fetus of 28 weeks of gestation or more
III	Antenatal death. Single fetus of 28 weeks of gestation or more
IV	Antenatal death. Before 28 weeks of gestation
V	Antenatal death. Multiple pregnancy
VI	Intra-partum death. After admission. 28 weeks of gestation or more
VII	Intra-partum death. After admission. Before 28 weeks of gestation
VIII	Neonatal death. 28-33 weeks of gestation. Apgar score higher than 6 after 5 min
IX	Neonatal death. 28-33 weeks of gestation. Apgar score less than 7 after 5 min
X	Neonatal death. After 33 weeks of gestation. Apgar score higher than 6 after 5 min
XI	Neonatal death. After 33 weeks of gestation. Apgar score less than 7 after 5 min
XII	Neonatal death. Before 28 weeks of gestation
XII	Unclassified

Table 3. Obstetric (Aberdeen) Classification.

1	Congenital anomaly	Neural tube defects	Congenital anomaly: any structural or genetic defect at arising at conception or during embryogenesis incompatible with life or potentially treatable but causing death.
2		Other anomalies	
3	Isoimmunisation	Due to Rhesus (D) antigen	Isoimmunisation: death ascribable to blood group incompatibility, rhesus (3) or non-rhesus (4).
4		Due to other antigens	
5	Pre-eclampsia	Without APH	
6		Complicated by APH	
7	Antepartum Haemorrhage	With placenta praevia	Antepartum Haemorrhage: after 20 weeks gestation (140 days) whether revealed or not excluding antepartum haemorrhage secondary to pre-eclampsia (which is classified under pre-eclampsia). Minor degrees of haemorrhage at the start of labour (a
8		With placenta abruption	
9		APH of uncertain origin	

			show), and haemorrhage due to a cervical erosion or polyp should be ignored, bur significant or recurrent bleeding of uncertain origin that is fairly closely followed by preterm labour should not be ignored.
10	Mechanical	Cord prolapsed or compression with vertex or face presentation	Mechanical: any death from uterine rupture and those deaths from birth trauma or intrapartum asphyxia that are associated with problems in labour such as disproportion, malpresentation, cord prolapse, cord compression, or breech delivery in babies of 1000g or more. If there is no evidence of difficulty in labour, deaths from asphyxia or trauma should be classified as unexplained. Antepartum deaths associated with cord entanglement in the absence of strong circumstantial evidence that cord compression caused death (e.g., fetal death soon after external version) should also be classified as unexplained.
11		Other vertex or face presentation	
12		Breech presentation	
13		Oblique or compound presentation, uterine rupture etc.	
14	Maternal disorder	Maternal hypertensive disease	Maternal disorder: include maternal trauma (such as a road traffic accident), diabetes, appendicitis, and cardiac disease etc, if severe enough to jeopardise the baby. Include significant renal disease or essential hypertension known to be present before pregnancy. Also include symptomatic and asymptomatic maternal infection when this resulted in the death of the baby.
15		Other maternal disease	
16		Maternal infection	
17	Miscellaneous	Neonatal infection	Miscellaneous: specific fetal and neonatal conditions only. Do not include conditions directly ascribable to prematurity or anoxia before birth, because these deaths are attributable to the relevant underlying obstetric disorder or are unexplained (see below). Include, however, specific fetal conditions (e.g., twin-to-twin transfusion) or neonatal conditions (e.g., inhalation of milk) where these are not directly ascribable to intrapartum anoxia or preterm delivery. Include, also postnatally acquired infection, except in babies of less than 1000g; here is the reason for the ventilator dependency or low birthweight is the codeable factor
18		Other neonatal diseases	
19		Specific fetal conditions	
20	Unexplained	Equal or greater than 2.5 kg	Unexplained: deaths with no obstetric explanation, including unexplained antepartum stillbirths, deaths resulting from unexplained preterm delivery (including hyaline membrane disease, intraventricular haemorrhage, etc.) an cases of intrapartum anoxia or trauma if the baby weighed less than 1000g at birth or delivery without any obvious associated mechanical problem. Cases should be subclassified into those babies weighing 2500g or more (20) and those of less than 2500g (21) at birth. Unclassifiable: cases where little or nothing is known about pregnancy or delivery and that cannot be fitted into any of the above categories. Use this category as sparingly as possible.
21		Less than 2.5 kg	
22		Unclassifiable	

The Obstetric (Aberdeen) Classification has its focus on obstetric care shown in Table 3 [11,14].

The Wigglesworth Classification has been modified and therefore it has several versions, too. This classification is focused upon pathophysiology. The original classification has 5 major categories including (1) normally formed macerated stillbirths, (2) lethal congenital malformations, (3) conditions associated with immaturity, (4) asphyxia conditions, and (5) other specific conditions. However, an extended Wigglesworth Classification shown in Table 4 is more widely used [7,14].

Table 4. Extended Wigglesworth Classification.

Category 1	Congenital defect/malformation (lethal or severe): Only lethal or potentially lethal congenital malformation should be included here. Serious biochemical abnormalities such as Tay Sach's disease and any known single gene defects known to have a high risk of death should be included.
Category 2	Unexplained antepartum fetal death: Most late fetal losses should be coded here. Where a live-born baby dies due to problems during the antepartum period, code this as 'other specific causes' (category 6).
Category 3	Death from intrapartum 'asphyxia', 'anoxia' or 'trauma': This category covers any baby who would have survived but for some catastrophe occurring during labour. These babies will tend to be normally formed, stillborn or with poor Apgar scores, possible meconium aspiration or evidence of acidosis. Very premature infants (those less than 24 weeks gestation) may be asphyxiated at birth, but should not be entered in this category as a rule.
Category 4	Immaturity: This applies to live births only, who subsequently die from structural pulmonary immaturity, surfactant deficiency, intra ventricular haemorrhage, or their late consequences – including chronic lung damage.
Category 5	Infection: This applies where there is clear microbiological evidence of infection that could have caused death, e.g. maternal infection with Group B streptococci, rubella, parvovirus, syphilis etc; or in the case of a baby dying with overwhelming sepsis.
Category 6	Other specific causes: Use this if there is a specific recognisable fetal, neonatal or paediatric condition not covered under the earlier categories. Examples include: *fetal* conditions; twin-to-twin transfusion and hydrops fetalis; *neonatal* conditions; pulmonary haemorrhage, pulmonary hypoplasia due to prolonged loss of liquor (primary hypoplasia being classed as a malformation), persistent transitional circulation (in the absence of infection, aspiration or surfactant deficiency), blood loss unassociated with trauma (e.g., vasa praevia); *paediatric* conditions; malignancy and acute abdominal catastrophe (such as volvulus without antecedent congenital malrotation).
Category 7	Accident or non-intrapartum trauma: Confirmed non-accidental injury should be coded here. If only suspected, code as a sudden infant death cause unknown (category 8).
Category 8	Sudden infant death, cause unknown: This will include all infants in whom the cause is unknown or unsuspected at the time of death. Modification due to post-mortem information should be notified later.
Category 9	Unclassifiable: To be used as a last resort. Details must be given if this option is ticked.

There are a number of attempts made to develop simpler, more precise and more useful categorisation of perinatal mortality, though no single categorisation has achieved this. The choice of categorisation should be depending upon the purpose of it, knowing the pros and cons of each category.

Distribution of Perinatal Mortality

Perinatal Mortality Rate in Less Developed Countries

The exact number of perinatal mortality is not available in many countries, particularly where resource is limited [5,17]. There is good evidence that availability of these data is associated with better basic health indicators. For the purpose of international comparisons to explore country specific strategies to improve perinatal healthcare and other services, estimation is required to obtain perinatal mortality rates. The below data show that components of perinatal mortality, namely still birth rate and early neonatal rate are unavailable in many countries [5].

This means the current health policy is provided, depending upon no solid information, and this raises real concerns. A model is used to provide the estimates. Early neonatal mortality rate is estimated from regression analysis with neonatal mortality survey data where available or from regression analysis with estimated neonatal mortality extrapolated from under-five mortality rate. Stillbirth rate is less available. Stillbirth rate is estimated with the assumption that ratio of stillbirths and early neonatal mortality is similar for countries for the same mortality sub-region. Figure 1 shows the estimated perinatal mortality rate for each country.

The report shows that 3 million babies die in the early neonatal period worldwide, where 3.3 million babies are stillborn every year. One-third of these fetal deaths occurred during delivery, which could largely be prevented; 98% of the deaths occur in the developing world.

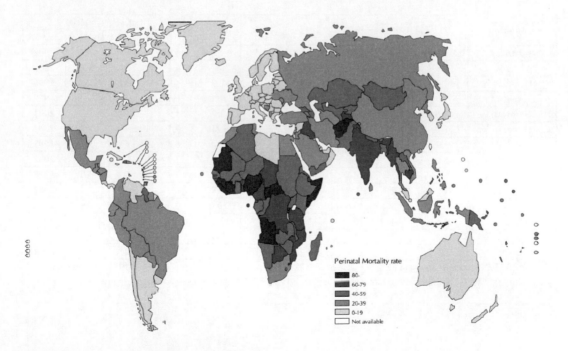

Figure 1. Distribution of estimated perinatal mortality rates in the world by the World Health Organization (WHO, with permission).

**Table 5. Mortality data in the estimation dataset for 192 countries/areas with a
population of 300,000 or more.**

	Stillbirth rate	Early neonatal mortality rate	Neonatal mortality rate	Infant mortality rate	Child mortality rate
Countries with available data in the estimation dataset	102	141	159	159	152
% of countries with data	53%	73%	83%	83%	79%
% of births	40%	76%	95%	95%	91%

Adopted from WHO (2006)

Perinatal Mortality Rate in the More Developed Countries

Perinatal mortality rate is a component of routine national statistics in most of developed countries, regardless of their definitions. Table 6 shows the trend in perinatal mortality rate in selected countries, most of which are high-income countries [18].

Table 6. Trend of perinatal mortality rate in selected countries, 1952–2002.

Countries	1952	1955	1970	1975	1980	1985	Latest available			
							PMR	FMR	NMR	Year
Australia	31.8	28.9	21.5	19.2	13.5	9.5	6.5	2.8	3.7	2002
Canada	35.8	31.5	22.0	14.9	10.9	8.7	6.4	3.3	3.1	2001
Denmark	34.6	33.9	18.0	13.4	9.0	7.9	8.0	4.8	3.2	1996
France	31.0	29.6	20.7	18.3	13.0	10.8	6.6	4.6	2.0	1999
Germany	48.8	44.1	26.7	19.4	11.6	7.9	5.9	3.9	2.0	2001
Hungary	41.0	38.7	34.5	31.6	23.1	19.0	9.1	5.4	3.7	2002
Italy	51.3	46.2	31.7	24.1	17.4	13.5	6.8	3.6	3.1	1997
Japan	45.6	43.9	21.7	16.0	11.7	8.0	3.7	2.0	1.7	2002
Netherlands	31.5	29.3	18.8	14.0	11.1	9.9	7.9	4.9	3.0	1998
New Zealand	31.2	28.2	19.8	16.5	11.8	8.8	6.0	3.1	2.9	2002
Portugal	...	48.3	40.6	31.8	24.2	20.0	6.0	3.4	2.6	2002
Sweden	31.5	28.4	16.5	11.1	8.7	7.3	5.3	3.7	1.7	2002
UK	38.8	28.3	23.8	19.9	13.4	9.9	6.8	3.8	3.0	1997
USA	32.0	30.4	27.8	20.7	14.2	11.2	5.6	3.2	2.4	2001

PMR: Perinatal mortality rate FMR: Fetal deaths at 28 weeks or over per 1000 live births NMR: Early neonatal mortality rate WHO definition for international comparison was used. Data in West Germany were presented for PMR before 1985 for Germany.

Modified from MCHWA (2006)

Perinatal Mortality in Context

Health Service and Perinatal Mortality

Mori et al. examined the effect of national income on association between skilled birth attendant coverage and major perinatal health indicators including neonatal mortality rate, perinatal mortality rate and maternal mortality ratio in an ecological study (Figure 2) by using the data available from the World Health Organization [19,20].

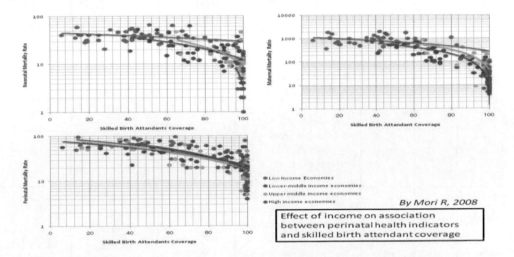

Figure 2. Effect of national income on association between skilled birth attendant coverage and major perinatal health indicators including neonatal mortality rate, perinatal mortality rate and maternal mortality ratio—an ecological study.

The analysis suggests that the association between neonatal mortality rate and skilled birth attendant coverage was most affected by national income, while that between perinatal mortality rate and the coverage is least affected by national income. This means that the choice of appropriate indicator for the purpose of the study is critical even within the major perinatal health indicators.

Perinatal Mortality as an Outcome Measure of Perinatal Clinical Studies

Risks and benefits of each place of delivery were systematically reviewed in a national clinical practice guideline for England and Wales [21,22]. Intrapartum-related perinatal mortality was used to assess the risk of planning home birth compared with planning hospital birth. As suggested in the above analysis of national income, choosing an appropriate indicator is a key, and an outcome indicator for intrapartum care including skilled birth attendance and place of birth should be focused on events directly related to intrapartum care. Intrapartum-related perinatal mortality is **defined as deaths from intrapartum 'asphyxia', 'anoxia' or 'trauma', derived from the extended Wigglesworth classification 3 above.**

Table 7. Intrapartum, perinatal mortality and intrapartum-related perinatal mortality (IPPM) rates for planned home birth compared with planned hospital birth or overall birth.

Authors	Year	Country	Notes on study design	Planned home birth	Planned hospital birth or overall births	Summary statistics
NCC-WCH	1999 – 2003	UK	Booked place of birth A population-based study in the UK. Internal validity was improved by using IPPM rates to control background risk, but the number of planned home births was drawn from transfer rates in previous studies. Sensitivity analyses were conducted to examine the uncertainty in the transfer rates.	IPPM rate 1.37/1000 Upper 1.58, Lower 0.82	IPPM rate Overall: 0.68/1000	IPPM rate RR 2.01 Upper 2.32, Lower 1.21
	1994 – 1998	UK		IPPM rate 1.18/1000 Upper 1.36, Lower 0.71	IPPM rate Overall: 0.90/1000	IPPM rate RR 1.31 Upper 1.51, Lower 0.79
NRPMSCS	1981 – 1994	UK	Booked place of birth A population-based study in the Northern Region on a planned home birth population. Internal validity was improved by using IPPM rates to control background risk.	IPPM rate 1.86/1000 (5/2689)	IPPM rate Overall: 1.23/1000 (642/520 280)	IPPM rate RR 1.51 [95% CI 0.63 to 3.63]
Bastian	1985 – 1990	Australia	Intended place of birth at the onset of labour A population-based study conducted in Australia on an intended home birth population. Internal validity was improved by using IPPM rates to control background risk. However, the intended home birth group included a small number of high-risk women, which may have contributed to the excess. It could also be assumed that there was a higher proportion of high-risk women in the overall birth group.	Intrapartum perinatal mortality rate 2.7/1000 [95% CI 1.5 to 3.9 /1000]	Intrapartum perinatal mortality rate Overall: 0.9/1000 [95% CI 0.85 to 0.95 /1000]	Intrapartum perinatal mortality rate RR 3.02 [95% CI 1.92 to 4.74]

Modified from NCC-WCH (2007

Table 7 shows the results of a systematic review on intrapartum-related mortality or similar indicators of planning home birth compared with planning hospital birth or proxies of it.

**Table 8. Meta-analysis of birth centre and perinatal mortality
Modified from (NCC-WCH 2007).**

	All trials			Trials of separate staff and greater continuity of carer in alongside unit			Trials of same staff and degree of continuity of care between alongside and obstetric units		
	Number of trials	Pooled RR	95% CI	Number of trials	Pooled RR	95% CI	Number of trials	Pooled RR	95% CI
Perinatal Mortality	5	1.83	0.99 to 3.38	2	1.52	0.77 to 3.00	3	2.38	1.05 to 5.41

Table 8 shows the results of a meta-analysis of perinatal mortality by birth centres compared with obstetric maternity units in the same systematic review. It emphasizes the importance of subgroup analysis.

Interventions to Reduce Perinatal Mortality in Areas Where Resources are Limited

A systematic review is conducted of any intervention to reduce perinatal and/or neonatal mortality in areas where resources are limited [23]. There are a number of interventions that have shown evidence of reducing perinatal and/or neonatal mortalities. One of the key messages from the literature is the impact of continuity of care of women before pregnancy through childbirth on the growth and development of their children. The framework of continuity of care is shown in Figure 3 [24].

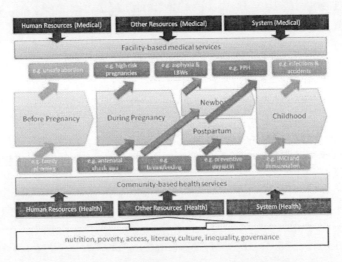

Figure 3. Framework of continuity of care. Modified from Mori (2008, unpublished)

Conclusion

Perinatal mortality rate is widely used as a basic indicator to reflect the health status of a community or country, as well as an outcome measure of perinatal clinical studies. However, differences in definitions and categorisations make any comparison difficult [25]. Although the choice of definitions and categorisations should depend upon the purpose of their use, a standardised measurement is needed not only for vital statistics but also for interventional studies.

References

[1]   Last JM. *A dictionary of epidemiology*. Oxford Press. 2001
[2]   Dunn PM. The search for perinatal definitions and standards. *Acta Paediatr Scand Suppl*. 1985;319:7-16
[3]   Kramer MS, Liu S, Luo Z, Yuan H, Platt RW, Joseph KS; Fetal and Infant Health Study Group of the Canadian Perinatal Surveillance System.Analysis of Perinatal Mortality and Its Components: Time for a Change? *American Journal of Epidemiology*. 2002; 156(6): 493
[4]   World Health Organization. International Classification of Diseases (2008) http://www. who.int/classifications/icd/en/
[5]   World Health Organization Neonatal and Perinatal Mortality. Country, Regional and Global Estimates. (2006) http://whqlibdoc.who.int/publications/2006/9241563206_ eng.pdf
[6]   Cartlidge PHT, Stewart JH. Effect of changing the stillbirth definition on evaluation of perinatal mortality rates. *Lancet*. 1995;346(8973):486-8.
[7]   Amar HSS, Maimunah AH, Wong AL. Use of Wiggleworth pathophysiological classification for perinatal mortality in Malaysia. *Arch Dis Child* 1996;74:F56
[8]   Elamin S, Langhoff-Ross J, Boedker B, Ibrahim SA, Ashmeig AL, and Lindmark G. Classification of perinatal death in a developing country. *Int J Gynaecol Obstet* 2003; 80:327
[9]   Lindmark G, Langhoff-Roos J. Regional quality assessment in perinatal care. *Seminar in Neonatology*. 2004; 9:145
[10]   Borch-Chistensen H, Larsen S, Langhoff-Roos J, Lindberg B, Wennergren M. Potentially avoidable perinatal deaths in Denmark and Sweden 1991. *Acta Obstetricia et Gynecologica Scandinavica* 1996;75:820
[11]   Cole SK, Hey EN, Thomson AM. Classifying perinatal death: an obstetric approach. *BJOG*. 2005; 93: 1204
[12]   Lau SP, Davies DP, Fung KP, Fok TF. Perinatal and neonatal Mortality in Hong Kong: An Appraisal. *Journal of the Hong Kong Medical Association*, 1985; 37(3): 117
[13]   Whitfield CR, Smith NC, Cockburn F, Gibson AA. Perinatally related wastage - a proposed classification of primary obstetric factors. *Br J Obstet Gynaecol*. 1986; 93: 694-703

[14] Confidential Enquiries into Maternal and Child Health (2008). http://www.cemach.org.uk/

[15] Dickson N, Bhula P, Wilson PD. Use of classification of primary obstetric factors in perinatally related mortality surveillance. *N Z Med J.* 1988 May 11;101(845):228-31

[16] Kindato HL, Massave SN, Lindmark G. Analysis of Perinatal mortality at a teaching hospital in Dar es Salaam, Tanzania, 1999-2003. *Afr J Repro Health* 2006;10:72

[17] Zupan J. Perinatal Mortality in Developing Countries. *N Engl J Med* 2005;352:2047

[18] Mothers' and Children's Health and Welfare Association. Maternal and Child Health Statistics of Japan. Mothers' and Children's Health and Welfare Association. 2006

[19] Mori R, Dougherty M, and Whittle M. An estimation of intrapartum-related perinatal mortality rates for booked home births in England and Wales between 1994 and 2003. *BJOG.* 2008;115(5):554-559

[20] Mori R. *Maternal and Child Health in Japan.* 2008 unpublished

[21] Kenyon S, Ullman R, Mori R, and Whittle M. Care of healthy women and their babies during childbirth: summary of NICE Guidance. *BMJ* 2007;335;667-668.

[22] National Collaborating Centre for Women's and Children's Health. *Intrapartum care: management and delivery of care to women in labour.* RCOG Press. September 2007

[23] Bhutta ZA et al. Community-Based Interventions for Improving Perinatal and Neonatal Health Outcomes in Developing Countries: A Review of the Evidence. *Pediatrics* 2005;115;519-617

[24] Mori R. Current Issues in Global Maternal and Child Health. *The Journal of the Japan Pediatric Society.* 2008;112(3)

[25] Berko P. A proposed new interpretation and revised definition of perinatal mortality. *Orv Hetil.* 2006 Feb 12;147(6):269-74

Section III: Ethics

In: Textbook of Perinatal Epidemiology   ISBN: 978-1-60741-648-7
Editor: Eyal Sheiner, pp. 717-729   © 2010 Nova Science Publishers, Inc.

Chapter XXXIV

Ethics of Research on Perinatal Medicine

Frank A. Chervenak[*] *and Laurence B. McCullough*[2]

Center for Medical Ethics and Health Policy, Baylor College of Medicine, Houston,
Texas, USA[2]

Introduction

Less than optimal treatment of pregnant and fetal patients can have serious clinical sequelae. These include ill effects on the pregnant woman's health. A fetal patient's and future child's health-related interests may also be injured by inadequate treatment or non-treatment. These clinical concerns lend urgency to the need to conduct well designed clinical investigations of interventions with pregnant women and fetuses to improve the outcomes of perinatal medicine.

Ethics is an essential component of research in perinatal medicine.[1] This is because investigators in perinatal research must address and responsibly manage ethical challenges related to the protection of both the pregnant patient's and fetal patient's health-related interests. The purposes of this chapter are to identify the international consensus that has formed on research ethics and to the ethics of perinatal research, focusing on research of fetal interventions and obstetric ultrasound. First, we provide key definitions. We then explicate the ethical concept of the fetus as a patient. Third, we identify three components of research ethics. Fourth, we consider the examples of fetal research and of innovation and research in obstetric ultrasound.

[*]For Correspondence: Frank A. Chervenak, M.D., Weill Cornell Medical Center, 525 East 68th Street - J130, New York, N.Y. 10065, Telephone: (212) 746-3045, FAX: (212) 746-8727, fac2001@med.cornell.edu

Key Definitions

The international consensus on research ethics presumes familiarity with a limited number of key definitions and concepts. We provide definitions of medical ethical and the two major ethical principles of beneficence and respect for autonomy.

Medical Ethics

Ethics is the disciplined study of morality. Medical ethics is the disciplined study of morality in medicine and concerns the obligations of physicians and health care organizations to patients as well as the obligations of patients.[2] It is important not to confuse medical ethics with the many sources of morality in a pluralistic society. These include, but are not limited to, law, our political heritage as a free people, the world's religions (most of which now exist in our country), ethnic and cultural traditions, families, the traditions and practices of medicine (including medical education and training), and personal experience. Medical ethics since the eighteenth century European and American Enlightenments has been secular.[3] It makes no reference to God or revealed tradition, but to what rational discourse requires and produces. At the same time, secular medical ethics is not intrinsically hostile to religious beliefs. Therefore, ethical principles and virtues should be understood to apply to all physicians, regardless of their personal religious and spiritual beliefs.[1]

The traditions and practices of medicine constitute an obvious source of morality for physicians. They provide an important reference point for medical ethics because they are based on the obligation to protect and promote the health-related interests of the patient. This obligation tells physicians what morality in medicine ought to be, but in very general, abstract terms. Providing a more concrete, clinically applicable account of that obligation is the central task of medical ethics, using ethical principles.[1,2]

The Principle of Beneficence

The principle of beneficence in its general meaning and application requires one to act in a way that is expected reliably to produce the greater balance of benefits over harms in the lives of others.[2] To put this principle into clinical practice requires a reliable account of the benefits and harms relevant to the care of the patient, and of how those goods and harms should be reasonably balanced against each other when not all of them can be achieved in a particular clinical situation, such as a request for an elective cesarean delivery.[4] In medicine, the principle of beneficence requires the physician to act in a way that is reliably expected to produce the greater balance of clinical benefits clinical over harms for the patient.[1]

Beneficence-based clinical judgment has an ancient pedigree, with its first expression found in the Hippocratic Oath and accompanying texts.[5] It makes an important claim: to interpret reliably the health related interests of the patient from medicine's perspective. This perspective is provided by accumulated scientific research, clinical experience, and reasoned responses to uncertainty. As rigorously evidence-based, beneficence-based judgment is thus not the function of the individual clinical perspective of any particular physician and therefore should not be based merely on the clinical impression or intuition of an individual physician. On the basis of this rigorous clinical perspective, focused on the best available evidence, beneficence-based clinical judgment identifies the benefits that can be achieved for the patient in clinical practice based on the competencies of medicine. The benefits that medicine is competent to seek for patients are the prevention and management of disease, injury, disability, and unnecessary pain and suffering, and the prevention of premature or unnecessary death. Pain and suffering become unnecessary when they do not result in achieving the other goods of medical care, e.g., allowing a woman to labor without effective analgesia.[6]

Nonmaleficence means that the physician should prevent causing harm and is best understood as expressing the limits of beneficence. This is also known as *"Primum non nocere"* or "first do no harm." This commonly invoked dogma is really a Latinized misinterpretation of the Hippocratic texts, which emphasized beneficence while avoiding harm when approaching the limits of medicine.[1,2] Non-maleficence should be incorporated into beneficence-based clinical judgment: when the physician approaches the limits of beneficence-based clinical judgment, i.e., when the evidence for expected benefit diminishes and the risks of clinical harm increase, then the physician should proceed with great caution. The physician should be especially concerned to prevent serious, far-reaching, and irreversible clinical harm to the patient. It is important to note that there is an inherent risk of paternalism in beneficence-based clinical judgment. By this we mean that beneficencebased clinical judgment, if it is *mistakenly* considered to be the sole source of moral responsibility and therefore moral authority in medical care, invites the unwary physician to conclude that beneficence-based judgments can be imposed on the patient in violation of her autonomy. Paternalism is a dehumanizing response to the patient and, therefore, should be avoided in the practice of obstetrics and gynecology.

In clinical practice the preventive ethics response to this inherent paternalism is for the physician to explain the diagnostic, therapeutic, and prognostic reasoning that leads to his or her clinical judgment about what is in the interest of the patient so that the patient can assess that judgment for herself. This general rule can be put into clinical practice in the following way: The physician should disclose and explain to the patient the major factors of this reasoning process, including matters of uncertainty. In neither medical law nor medical ethics does this require that the patient be provided with a complete medical education.[7] The physician should then explain how and why other clinicians might reasonably differ from his or her clinical judgment. The physician should then present a well-reasoned response to this critique. The outcome of this process is that beneficence-based clinical judgments take on a rigor that they sometimes lack, and the process of their formulation includes explaining them to the patient. It should be apparent that beneficence-based clinical judgment will frequently result in the identification of a continuum of clinical strategies that protect and promote the patient's health-related interests, such as the choice of preventing and managing the complications of menopause. Awareness of this feature of beneficence-based clinical judgment provides an important preventive ethics antidote to paternalism by increasing the likelihood that one or more of these medically reasonable, evidence-based alternatives will be acceptable to the patient. This feature of beneficence-based clinical judgment also provides a preventive ethics antidote to "gag" rules that restrict physician's communications with the managed care patient.[8] All beneficence-based alternatives must be identified and explained to all patients, regardless of how the physician is paid, especially those that are well established in evidence-based perinatal medicine.

The Principle of Respect for Autonomy

In contrast to the principle of beneficence, there has been increasing emphasis in the literature of medical ethics on the principle of respect for autonomy.[1,2] This principle requires one always to acknowledge and carry out the value-based preferences of the adult, competent patient, unless there is compelling ethical justification for not doing so, e.g., prescribing antibiotics for viral respiratory infections. The female or pregnant patient increasingly brings to her medical care her own perspective on what is in her interest. The principle of respect for autonomy translates this fact into autonomy-based clinical judgment. Because each patient's perspective on her interests is a function of her values and beliefs, it is impossible to specify the benefits and harms of autonomy-based clinical judgment in advance. Indeed, it would be inappropriate for the physician to do so, because the definition of her benefits and harms and their balancing are the prerogative of the patient. Not surprisingly, autonomy-based clinical judgment is strongly antipaternalistic in nature.[1,2]

To understand the moral demands of this principle in clinical practice, we need an operationalized concept of autonomy to make it relevant to clinical practice. To do this, we identify three sequential autonomy-based behaviors on the part of the patient: 1) absorbing and retaining information about her condition and alternative diagnostic and therapeutic responses to it; 2) understanding that information (i.e., evaluating and rank-ordering those responses and appreciating that she could experience the risks of treatment; and 3) expressing a value-based preference. The physician has a role to play in each of these. They are, respectively, 1) to recognize the capacity of each patient to deal with medical information (and not to underestimate that capacity), provide information (ie, disclose and explain all medically reasonable alternatives, ie, supported in beneficence-based clinical judgment), and recognize the validity of the values and beliefs of the patient; 2) not to interfere with but, when necessary, to assist the patient in her evaluation and ranking of diagnostic and therapeutic alternatives for managing her condition; and 3) to elicit and implement the patient's value-based preference.[1]

The Ethical Concept of the Fetus as a Patient

We now invoke these two principles in explaining the ethical concept of the fetus as a patient, which is a core ethical concept for the ethics of research in perinatal medicine.[1] This is because perinatal investigators have an ethical obligation to protect the health-related interests of both the pregnant woman and the fetus. To say that the fetus has health-related interests invokes the ethical concept of the fetus as a patient.

We have argued that the ethical concept of the fetus as a patient involves dependent moral status.[1] Dependent moral status is conferred on an entity by others freely, not out of an obligation to do so. This contrasts with independent moral status, which others must recognize as a matter of obligation, usually to respect the rights of an entity. The dependent moral status of the fetus as a patient is a function of whether the fetus should be reliably expected later to achieve the moral status of becoming a child (itself a form of dependent moral status) and a person (a form of independent moral status, i.e., a rights-bearer). The previable fetus is a patient when the pregnant woman confers this dependent moral status on it, which she is free to do or not do as she decides. Once she does confer this status, she and her physicians have beneficence-based obligations to protect the fetus' health-related interests. The previable fetus is a patient solely as a function of the pregnant woman's autonomy. The viable fetus is a patient in virtue of both its ability to survive ex utero and access to medical technology that makes this possible, as well as being presented to the physician.

The ethical concept of the fetus as a patient, in sharp contrast to the legal concept of the fetus, does not invoke the divisive discourse of fetal rights. In this discourse some claim that the fetus has moral and therefore legal status as an unborn child. Such claims involve at least two serious, disabling errors. First, such claims, often implicitly and less often explicitly, assert that the fetus, as an unborn child, has the same moral and legal status as a child. This claim ignores the ethical analysis that the moral status of a child involves dependent, not independent, moral status. Thus, the claim that the fetus is an unborn child does not in fact establish that the fetus has independent moral status. Such claims also assert that the fetus has the legal status of a person, which a child surely does. The U.S. Supreme Court, in Roe v. Wade, considered in detail whether the constitutional concept of a person applies to the fetus and showed that it did not. Re-asserting a claim to such legal status without refuting the Court's extensive analysis of the issue is intellectually irresponsible. Second, such claims implicitly assert that the previable fetus has independent moral status, an assertion that requires for its success an indisputable account of why everyone should accept this. In more than 2,000 years of global debate on this subject, no universally agreed-upon method for resolving these deep differences has emerged. Proponents of the claim that the previable fetus is an unborn child ignore this long and contentious history, which is also intellectually irresponsible.

When the fetus is a patient, both the pregnant woman and her physician have beneficence-based obligations to it. As the moral fiduciaries of the fetal patient, the woman and her physician should protect and promote the fetus' health-related interests. The physician's beneficence-based obligations to the fetal patient must in all cases be balanced against the physician's autonomy-based and beneficence-based obligations to the pregnant woman.

The concept of the fetus as a patient has immediate ethical implications for research undertaken for the purpose of meeting the pregnant woman's health needs, because it allows us to identify a central ethical challenge of such research: balancing maternal and fetal interests. Brody is correct to point out that federal regulations in the United States do not require investigators to balance maternal and fetal health-related interests in the design and conduct of such research.[9] Section 36.204 of the U.S. research regulations requires the identification and assessment of risk to the pregnant woman and fetus but does not provide an ethical framework to guide these.[10]

The ethical concept of the fetus as a patient provides the basis for the needed ethical framework. In research designed to determine whether an intervention benefits the fetus, e.g., surgical management of spina bifida, the concept of the fetus as a patient requires a study design in which pregnant subjects take only reasonable risks to their own health.[1,11] In research designed to benefit the pregnant patient, the ethical concept of the fetus as a patient requires a different balancing, namely of her obligation to protect and promote the health-related interests of her fetal patient against her own legitimate interest in participating in research. The physician faces parallel ethical challenges: how to balance these competing beneficence-based obligations in the design and conduct of clinical trials and how to assist the pregnant woman to address her balancing considerations during the informed consent process.

There is an additional ethical consideration pertaining to the investigator's, funder's, and sponsoring organization's legal liability, especially for wrongful injury to a future child. Preventing unnecessary liability of these parties surely counts as legitimate self-interest for all of them. In our judgment, the best way to protect and promote this quite legitimate self-interest is to undertake a thoroughgoing balancing of both maternal and fetal interests, with an emphasis on eliminating major risks to the fetal patient, as required by beneficence-based obligations to the fetal patient. In other words, ethically responsible study design and management can help to manage risks of liability to a minimum. The thorough consent process that we describe below may add additional protection, to the extent that informed consent confers immunity in such cases.

Research Ethics

We next provide a definition of research and describe the three components of research ethics that have emerged from the history of research with human subjects.

Definition of Research

The definition of research in the federal regulations in the United States is the following: "an activity designed to test an hypothesis, permit conclusions to be drawn, and thereby to develop or contribute to generalizable knowledge."[10]

Three Components of Research Ethics

The history of human experimentation appears to be coincident with the history of medicine. Concern about the scientific and ethical quality of research with human subjects begins to emerge in eighteenth-century medical ethics. One of major figures of that period, Dr. John Gregory (1724-1773) of Scotland, wrote the first modern medical ethics in the

English language.[12] He developed a research ethics to address the potential abuse of patients in the Royal Infirmary of Edinburgh by younger physicians anxious to establish their reputations. These physicians would pronounce infirmary patients incurable, not to abandon them (which was the common practice), but to justify introducing experimental medicines into patient care.

Gregory condemned this practice, on two grounds. His first concern was that such experimentation was premature: standard remedies had not yet been attempted and shown to be ineffective in a patient's care. His second concern was that experimentation was often poorly designed. For example, compound drugs would be used without attention to the question of which elements of the compound might cause observed clinical effects. His third concern was that such physicians used the sick poor to advance their own reputational interests, subjecting them to unnecessary risk of clinical harm (a violation of the ethical principle of beneficence) out of personal self-interest. Gregory called this "sporting" with the sick poor; we now call it exploitation.

Gregory's research ethics introduced one of the key components of any adequate research ethics: the protection of research subjects. Such protection was gained by ensuring that there is a clinical justification for research and that the research is scientifically well designed. A second key component of any adequate research ethics, the consent of research subjects, was introduced in the nineteenth century.

Making a reasonable effort to prevent what is known as the *therapeutic misconception* is one of the major responsibilities of clinical investigators in the informed consent process. The therapeutic misconception occurs when potential subjects fail to appreciate that some aspects of what they will experience in a study are not justified by a clinical judgment of what in the patient's health-related interest but by scientific considerations. Subjects, instead, confuse these scientific study design issues with regular medical care.[13] For example, in a randomized study of ultrasound potential subjects would need to understand that whether they would receive an ultrasound examination will be based on a random selection process and not on their physician's clinical judgment.

The need for both scientific and ethical integrity as components of research ethics was reinforced by the scientific and ethical catastrophe of the Nazi medical war crimes. A major result of the trials of the Nazi physicians was the promulgation of the Nuremberg Code. This is regarded as the founding document of contemporary research ethics and insists on sound scientific method and consent, which have become two of the three main components of research ethics globally.[9]

The third and final key component of research ethics was introduced by the Declaration of Helsinki. It requires independent overview of clinical investigation, for both its scientific and its ethical integrity.[9]

As a result of this centuries-long history of medical ethics, there has emerged an international consensus that there are three key components of research ethics:[14]

1) Clinical research with human subjects must be clinically justified and scientifically sound. The clinical need for research should be well established, on the basis of a critical, evidence-based evaluation of current clinical practice. Clinical research should be well designed scientifically, with clearly stated research questions and

testable hypotheses and a method adequate to test the hypotheses and this answer the research questions.

2) Informed consent is required. The Nuremberg Code did not allow any exceptions to this requirement, a position that is no longer part of the international consensus. It has been recognized in recent decades that there are populations of patients for whom we need to improve the quality of medical care but who cannot consent to becoming research subjects. This may be a result of the clinical circumstances of research (e.g., in emergencies for which there is no time for the consent process) or the inability of the potential subject to engage in the informed consent process (e.g., fetuses).

3) Oversight of research is required. Investigators are not obligated to prepare research protocols that establish clinical need, meet standards of scientific integrity, and describe the informed consent process (or justify its waiver) and submit protocols for prospective review by independent committees established for this purpose (known in the United States as Institutional Review Board and in most of the rest of the world as Research Ethics Committees.

Fetal Research

Ethical Criteria for Innovation

Innovation in fetal research begins with the design of an intervention and its implementation in animal models, followed by a single case and then case series. This rigorous approach is required to determine the feasibility, safety, and efficacy of innovations in fetal research. It is a basic tenet of research ethics that potential subjects should be protected from potentially harmful innovation. Three criteria must be satisfied in order to conduct such preliminary investigations in fetal research in an ethically responsible fashion, by taking into account beneficence-based obligations to the fetal patient and beneficence-based obligations to the pregnant woman. The pre-viable fetus is a patient in these cases because, as explained above, the woman has made a decision to continue her pregnancy, in order to have the opportunity to gain the potential benefits of the innovation. She remains free to withdraw that status before viability.

1) The proposed fetal intervention is reliably expected on the basis of previous animal studies either to be life-saving or to prevent serious and irreversible disease, injury, or disability for the fetus;

2) Among possible alternative designs, the intervention is designed in such a way as to involve the least risk of mortality and morbidity to the fetal patient (which is required by beneficence and will satisfy the U.S. research requirement of minimizing risk to the fetus[10]); and

3) On the basis of animal studies and analysis of theoretical risks both for the current and future pregnancies, the mortality risk of the fetal intervention to the pregnant

woman is reliably expected to be low and the risk of disease, injury, or disability to the pregnant woman is reliably expected to be low or manageable. [11]

The first two criteria are based on beneficence-based obligations to the fetal patient. Research on animal models should suggest that there would be therapeutic benefit without disproportionate iatrogenic fetal morbidity or mortality. If animal studies result in high rates of mortality or morbidity for the animal fetal subject, then innovation should not be introduced to human subjects until these rates improve in subsequent animal studies.

The third criterion reflects the fact that fetal intervention in the form of fetal surgery is necessarily also maternal surgery. This criterion reminds investigators that the willingness of a subject, in this case, the pregnant woman, to consent to risk does not by itself establish whether the risk/benefit ratio is favorable. Judgments about an acceptable risk/benefit ratio should not be autonomy-based, but beneficence-based. This is because investigators have an independent beneficence-based obligation to protect human subjects from unreasonably risky research and should use beneficence-based, not autonomy-based, risk-benefit analyses. Phrases such as "maternal-fetal surgery" are useful if they remind investigators of the need for such comprehensive analysis. If they are used systematically to subordinate fetal interests to maternal interest and rights, and therefore to undermine the concept of the fetus as a patient in favor of the concept that the fetus is merely a part of the pregnant woman, such phrases lack ethical utility.

Ethical Criteria in Randomized Trials

Preliminary innovation should end and randomized clinical trials begin when there is clinical equipoise. Clinical equipoise means that there is "a remaining disagreement in the expert clinical community, despite the available evidence, about the merits of the intervention to be tested."[9] Brody notes that one challenge here is identifying how much disagreement can remain for there still to be equipoise.[9] Lilford has suggested that when 2/3 of the expert community, measured reliably, no longer disagrees, equipoise is not satisfied.[15] When the experimental intervention is more harmful than non-intervention, equipoise cannot be achieved.

The satisfaction of the previous three criteria, with slight modifications, should count as equipoise in the expert community.

1) The initial case series indicates that the proposed fetal intervention is reliably expected either to be life saving or to prevent serious and irreversible disease, injury, or disability;

2) Among possible alternative designs, the intervention continues to involve the least risk of morbidity and mortality to the fetus; and

3) The case series indicates that the mortality risk to the pregnant woman is reliably expected to be low and the risk of disease, injury, or disability to the pregnant woman, including for future pregnancies, is reliably expected to be low or manageable. [11]

One useful good test for the satisfaction of the first and third criteria is significant trends in the data from the case series. When equipoise has been achieved on the basis of these three criteria, randomized clinical trials should commence. They must have relevant and clearly defined primary and secondary endpoints and a design and sample size adequate to measure these endpoints.

The above three criteria can be used in a straightforward manner to define stopping rules for such a clinical trial. When the data support a rigorous clinical judgement that the first or third criterion is not satisfied, the trial should be stopped.

Criteria for Defining a Standard of Care

When a clinical trial of a fetal intervention is completed, its outcome can be assessed to determine whether the innovative fetal intervention should be regarded as standard of care. Trial results should meet the following three criteria in order to establish the innovation as a standard of care:

1) The fetal intervention has a significant probability of being life saving or preventing serious or irreversible disease, injury, or disability for the fetus.
2) The fetal intervention involves low mortality and low or manageable risk of serious and irreversible disease, injury, or disability to the fetus, and
3) The mortality risk to the pregnant woman is low and the risk of disease, injury or disability is low or manageable, including for future pregnancies.[11]

Brody has underscored the value of data safety and monitoring boards to prevent investigator bias and to protect subjects.[9] Such boards should be used in fetal research, especially to ensure adherence of the above-mentioned ethical criteria as a basis for monitoring such research.

Research in Obstetric Ultrasound

An important goal of research in obstetric and gynecologic ultrasound is to improve the technique of examination and its interpretation.[16] This process begins with innovation. Innovation or pre-research takes the form of a case report to determine whether an improvement in imaging or interpretation is feasible. This does not involve the production of generalizable knowledge. Reporting feasibility does warrant subsequent investigation of the improvement to determine whether it is promising innovation, i.e., results in trends in findings that support a hypothesis of efficacy. Testing of such hypotheses requires systematic data collection, retrospectively or prospectively, with the explicit purpose of producing generalizable knowledge, i.e., research.

There is no doubt that this last stage in a process of improvement meets the definition of research and should be brought under the legally applicable human subjects protection review process. Innovation is best considered pre-research.

Ultrasound end-users in obstetrics and gynecology should not take this as license to undertake innovation or pre-research without consideration of scientific and ethical rigor. The risk of taking such license is twofold. First, innovation undertaken in a scientifically informal or, worse, haphazard fashion, creates a weak foundation for subsequent research and clinical practice. Moreover, such undisciplined innovation could result in widespread adoption of new "standards" of care in a scientifically premature fashion. Second, innovation can be carried out over a prolonged period of time, to determine whether it is practical and valuable, a form of innovation that can drift into research, e.g., creating a prospective case series without study design or consent and therefore without the transition from innovation to research being managed in a scientifically and ethically responsible fashion.

The key to addressing these two related concerns prospectively is to manage the transition from innovation to research in a scientifically and ethically appropriate fashion. Consider the following recent examples that are in various stages of the progression from innovation, to research, to clinical care. Initially, one might seek to determine, making small modifications of accepted transducer technique, whether a part of fetal anatomy could be measured consistently and thus become a marker for Down syndrome. Another example would be to determine whether aspects of fetal behavior could be assessed in utero. A third example would be to determine whether it is possible to detect coronary artery blood flow in the fetus. Finally, one might attempt to determine whether 4-D ultrasound can improve imaging of fetal anatomy. In none of these examples of innovation would a physician be initially seeking generalizable knowledge, because doing so would be premature. In addition, because there is no departure from accepted practice, there is no increment of harm to the pregnant woman or fetus. These examples did not initially involve research but they did, in our judgment, involve innovation or pre-research to determine the feasibility of an improvement in obstetric ultrasound.

On the basis of innovation, retrospective or prospective case series should be designed and undertaken to obtain results and assess whether they support a hypothesis of efficacy. It is therefore crucial to establish feasibility as the first stage of innovation, so that resources are not wasted on subsequent investigation with little likelihood of generating testable hypotheses and therefore producing generalizable knowledge.

It is very important to encourage innovation, because it is the seedbed of scientific and clinical progress in obstetric and gynecologic ultrasound. If innovation or pre-research with patients were to be treated as human subjects research with its strict requirements, innovation might be discouraged. The central challenge becomes how to manage innovation in a scientifically and ethically disciplined fashion that does not create such a burdensome oversight mechanism that physicians will be discouraged from undertaking improvement in obstetric and gynecologic ultrasound and that protects patients.

The key to managing this challenge is to apply scientific and ethical rigor to innovation or pre-research. Analogous to recent proposals about responsible management of surgical innovation,[11] we propose that academic departments but not institutional review boards or research ethics committees establish oversight mechanisms in which case reports are analyzed for scientific merit and ethical appropriateness before submission for publication. The main scientific concern is whether feasibility has been demonstrated. The goal is to minimize the bias in reaching this judgment by the investigator and in the formulation of hypotheses. The main ethical concern is the level of risk involved in innovation. Ethical review should examine whether the innovation is consistent with accepted principles and practices of obstetric and gynecologic ultrasound, in which case there is no increment of risk. Consent therefore is not required. Of course, if there is any incremental risk, the investigation should immediately come under legally applicable research regulations.

The transition from innovation or pre-research, i.e., case reports, to research, i.e., case series, should always be subject to prospective oversight. This is because initiating a case series to produce results for the purpose of generating or testing hypotheses is always a planned, not serendipitous, decision. As required by human subjects research regulations, oversight should be both scientific and ethical. The scientific review should determine whether the proposed study design for a case series is adequate to generate or test hypotheses. The ethical review centers not just on risk but on the fact the investigator intends now to use patients as subjects, i.e., as sources of generalizable knowledge. Whenever a patient is used prospectively as a scientific subject, consent is required, even when there is no increment of risk. In the technical language of ethics, respect for autonomy is classified as a *deontological* ethical principle, an ethical principle the meaning of which is independent of consequences: patients who will be used prospectively for non-clinical purposes should be respected as persons and autonomous decision makers independently of whether they are at clinical risk.[9] This prospective oversight should be managed at the IRB/IEC level.

Conclusion

Ethics is an essential dimension of research in perinatal medicine. The ethical concept of the fetus as a patient should guide investigators, granting agencies, institutional review board, and clinicians in reaching ethically justified balancing of autonomy-based and beneficence-based obligations to the pregnant patient and beneficence-based obligations to the fetal patient. For research on fetal interventions, ethically justified criteria for the design, conduct, and evaluation of clinical investigation can be identified on the basis of obligations to both the pregnant and fetal patients. For research in obstetric ultrasound ethical criteria for innovation and for the transition from innovation for research can be identified on the basis of obligations to both the pregnant and fetal patients.

References

[1] McCullough LB, Chervenak FA. *Ethics in Obstetrics and Gynecology*. New York: Oxford University Press, 1994.

[2] Beauchamp TL, Childress JF. *Principles of Biomedical Ethics, 6th ed.* New York: Oxford University Press, 2009.

[3] McCullough LB. The discourses of practitioners in eighteenth-century Britain. In Baker RB, McCullough LB, eds. *The Cambridge World History of Medical Ethics*. Cambridge: Cambridge University Press, 2009: 403-413.

[4]   Chervenak FA, McCullough LB. An ethically justified algorithm for offering, recommending, and performing cesarean delivery and its application in managed care practice. *Obstet Gynecol* 1996; 87: 302–305.

[5]   Hippocrates. Oath of Hippocrates.In: Temkin O, Temkin CL, eds. Ancient Medicine: *Selected Papers of Ludwig Edelstein*.Baltimore, Md: Johns Hopkins University Press; 1976: 6.

[6]   Chervenak FA, McCullough LB, Birnbach DJ. Ethics: an essential dimension of clinical obstetric anesthesia. *Anesth Analg* 2003; 96: 1480-1485.

[7]   Faden RR, Beauchamp TL. A History and Theory of Informed Consent.New York, NY: *Oxford University Press*; 1986.

[8]   Brody H, Bonham VL Jr. Gag rules and trade secrets in managed care contracts: ethical and legal concerns. *Arch Intern Med* 1997; 157: 2037-2043.

[9]   Brody BA. *The Ethics of Biomedical Research: An International Perspective*. New York: Oxford University Press, 1998.

[10]   Department of Health and Human Services. Regulations for the Protection of Human Subjects. 45 CFR 46. Available at *http://www.hhs.gov/ohrp/, accessed December 8, 2008.*

[11]   Chervenak FA, McCullough LB: A comprehensive ethical framework for fetal research and its application to fetal surgery for spina bifida. *Am J Obstet Gynecol* 2002; 187: 10-14.

[12]   McCullough LB. *John Gregory and the Invention of Professional Medical Ethics and the Profession of Medicine*. Dordrecht, The Netherlands: Kuwer Academic Publishers, 1998.

[13]   Lidz CW, Appelbaum PS, Grisso T, Renaud M. Therapeutic misconception and the appreciation of risks in clinical trials. *Soc Sci Med* 2004; 58: 1689-1697.

[14]   Brody BA, McCullough LB, Sharp R. Consensus and controversy in research ethics. *JAMA* 2005: 294: 1411-1414.

[15]   Lilford RJ. The substantive ethics of clinical trials. *Clin Obstet Gynecol* 1992; 35: 837-845.

[16]   Chervenak FA, McCullough LB. Scientifically and ethically responsible innovation and research in ultrasound in obstetrics and gynecology. *Ultrasound Obstet Gynecol* 2006; 28: 1-4.

List of Contributors

Jacques S. Abramowicz, MD
Frances T. and Lester B. Knight Professor of Obstetrics and Gynecology
Director, Ob/Gyn Ultrasound
Co-Director, Rush Fetal and Neonatal Medicine Program
Rush University Medical Center, Chicago, IL., USA
E-mail: Jacques_Abramowicz@rush.edu

Robert H. Allen, PhD, PE
Associate Research Professor of Biomedical Engineering and Gynecology/Obstetrics
Johns Hopkins University School of Medicine
Baltimore, Maryland, USA
E-mail: rha@jhu.edu

Cande V. Ananth, PhD, MPH
Professor and Director
Division of Epidemiology and Biostatistics
Department of Obstetrics, Gynecology, and Reproductive Sciences
UMDNJ-Robert Wood Johnson Medical School
125 Paterson Street, New Brunswick NJ 08901, USA
E-mail: cande.ananth@umdnj.edu

Aaron Agopian, MS, CGC
Institute of Biosciences and Technology
2121 W. Holcombe Blvd.
Houston, TX 77030, USA
E-mail: Aaron.Agopian@uth.tmc.edu

Avi Ben-Haroush, MD
Department of Obstetrics and Gynecology,
Helen Schneider Hospital for Women,

Rabin Medical Center, Petah Tiqwa 49100, Israel
E-mail: yudavi@inter.net.il

Frank A. Chervenak, M.D.
Given Foundation Professor and Chairman
Department of Obstetrics and Gynecology
Weill Medical College of Cornell University
New York, New York, USA
E-mail: fac2001@med.cornell.edu

Offer Erez, MD.
Department of Obstetrics and Gynecology,
Soroka University Medical Center, School of Medicine,
Faculty of Health Sciences,
Ben Gurion University of the Negev, Beer Sheva, Israel
E-mail: oerez@med.wayne.edu

Idit Erez-Weiss M.D.
Department of Family Medicine,
School of Medicine, Faculty of Health Sciences,
Ben Gurion University of the Negev, Beer Sheva, Israel

Analee J. Etheredge, MSPH
Institute of Biosciences and Technology
2121 W. Holcombe Blvd.
Houston, TX 77030, USA
E-mail: aetheredge@ibt.tamhsc.edu

J. Brian Fowlkes, PhD
Professor of Radiology and Biomedical Engineering
University of Michigan
Ann Arbor, MI, USA,
E-mail: fowlkes@umich.edu

William D. Fraser MD. FRCSC,
Professor and Chair,
Canada Research Chair in Perinatal Epidemiology,
Department of Obstetrics and Gynecology, Université de Montreal, Canada
E-mail: william.fraser@umontreal.ca

Rafael Gorodischer M.D.
Pediatric Departments, Faculty of Health Sciences,
Ben Gurion University of the Negev, Soroka Medical Center,

BeMORE collaboration (Ben-Gurion Motherisk Obstetric Registry of Exposure collaboration).
E-mail: rgorodischer@gmail.com

Jeffrey B. Gould, MD, MPH
Robert L. Hess Professor of Pediatrics
Department of Pediatrics, Division of Neonatal and Developmental Medicine
Director, Perinatal Epidemiology and Health Outcomes Research Unit
Stanford University School of Medicine
Stanford, CA 94305, USA
E-mail: jbgould@stanford.edu

William A. Grobman, MD, MBA.
Associate Professor, Department of Obstetrics and Gynecology,
Feinberg School of Medicine, 250 East Superior Street, Suite 05-2175
Northwestern University, Chicago, IL, USA.
E-mail: w-grobman@northwestern.edu

Edith Diament Gurewitsch, MD
Associate Professor of Gynecology/Obstetrics and Biomedical Engineering
Johns Hopkins University School of Medicine
Baltimore, Maryland, USA
E-mail: egurewi@jhmi.edu

Xu Hairong, MD, MSc
Department of Obstetrics and Gynecology and Social and Preventive Medicine,
Université de Montréal, Canada.
E-mail: hairongxx@yahoo.ca

Motti Hallak, MD
Professor and Chairman, Department of Obstetrics and Gynecology,
Hillel Yaffe Medical Center, Hadera, Israel.
E-mail: MottiH@hy.health.gov.il

Brady E. Hamilton, Ph.D
Centers for Disease Control & Prevention
National Center for Health Statistics, Division of Vital Statistics
3311 Toledo Road, Rm. 7416
Hyattsville, MD 20782, USA.
E-mail: BHamilton@cdc.gov

Wojciech Hanke PhD, MD
Professor of Epidemiology, Research Director
Unit of Reproductive Environmental Epidemiology
Nofer Institute of Occupational Medicine
91-348 Lodz, Poland
E-mail: wojt@imp.lodz.pl

Avi Harlev, MD.
Department of Obstetrics and Gynecology,
Soroka University Medical Center,
Faculty of Health Sciences, Ben-Gurion University of the Negev,
Be'er-Sheva, Israel.
E-mail: harlev@bgu.ac.il

Julia Harris, BA
School for International Health, Columbia University,
Faculty of Health Sciences, Ben-Gurion University of the Negev,
Be'er-Sheva, Israel.
E-mail: juliaph@gmail.com

Reli Hershkovitz, MD
Associate Professor, Department of Obstetrics and Gynecology,
Soroka University Medical Center, Faculty of Health Sciences,
Ben-Gurion University of the Negev,
Be'er-Sheva, Israel.
E-mail: ralikah@bgu.ac.il

Gershon Holcberg, MD
Professor and Director Maternity C, Department of Obstetrics and Gynecology,
Soroka University Medical Center, Faculty of Health Sciences,
Ben-Gurion University of the Negev, Be'er-Sheva, Israel.
E-mail: holcberg@bgu.ac.il

Joanna Jurewicz PhD
Unit of Reproductive Environmental Epidemiology
Nofer Institute of Occupational Medicine
91-348 Lodz, Poland
E-mail: joannaj@imp.lodz.pl

Mitchell H. Katz, MD
San Francisco Department of Public Health,
San Francisco, CA 94102, USA.
E-mail: mitch.katz@sfdph.org

Vered Kleitman, MD
Department of Obstetrics and Gynecology,
Soroka University Medical Center, Faculty of Health Sciences,
Ben-Gurion University of the Negev,
Be'er-Sheva, Israel.
E-mail: kvered@bgu.ac.il

Gideon Koren MD
The Motherisk Program, Department of Clinical Pharmacology,
Hospital for Sick Children, The University of Toronto, Toronto, Canada,
BeMORE collaboration, (Ben-Gurion Motherisk Obstetric Registry of Exposure collaboration).
E-mail: gkoren@sickkids.ca

Steven J. Korzeniewski Ph.D.-Candidate MA MSc
Director, Statistical Analysis Resource Group,
MPRO- Michigan's Quality Improvement Organization
22670 Haggerty Rd Ste. 100, Farmington Hills, MI 48335, USA
Email: skorzeniewski@mpro.org

Henry Chong Lee, MD, MS
Assistant Clinical Professor of Pediatrics, University of California, San Francisco
Department of Pediatrics, Division of Neonatology
533 Parnassus Avenue, Room U503
San Francisco, CA 94143-0734, USA.
E-mail: LeeHC@peds.ucsf.edu

Amalia Levy PhD
Department of Epidemiology and Health Services Evaluation,
Faculty of Health Sciences, Ben Gurion University of the Negev
Beer-Sheva, Israel,
BeMORE collaboration (Ben-Gurion Motherisk Obstetric Registry of Exposure collaboration).
E-mail: lamalia@bgu.ac.il

Philip J. Lupo, MPH
Institute of Biosciences and Technology
2121 W. Holcombe Blvd.
Houston, TX 77030, USA
E-mail: Philip.J.Lupo@uth.tmc.edu

Ilan Matok
Department of Epidemiology and Health Services Evaluation,
Faculty of Health Sciences,

Ben Gurion University of the Negev, Beer-Sheva, Israel
E-mail: matoki@smile.net.il

Laurence B. McCullough, Ph.D.
Dalton Tomlin Chair in Medical Ethics and Health Policy in
The Center for Medical Ethics and Health Policy,
Baylor College of Medicine
Houston, Texas, USA
E-mail: mccullou@bcm.tmc.edu

Moshe Mazor, MD
Professor and Chairman, Department of Obstetrics and Gynecology B,
Soroka University Medical Center, Faculty of Health Sciences,
Ben-Gurion University of the Negev,
Be'er-Sheva, Israel.
E-mail: mazorm@bgu.ac.il

Ramkumar Menon, Ph.D.
Research Associate Professor,
Department of Epidemiology, Rollins School of Public Health,
Emory University, Atlanta, GA, USA
E-mail: fortunat@edge.net

Laura E. Mitchell, Ph.D.
Associate Professor
Texas A&M University System Health Science Center
Institute of Biosciences and Technology
Center for Environmental and Genetic Medicine
2121 W. Holcombe Blvd.
Houston, Texas 77030, USA
E-mail: Laura.E.Mitchell@uth.tmc.edu

Rintaro Mori MD PhD MSc FRCPCH
Associate Professor, Department of Global Health Policy,
Graduate School of Medicine, the University of Tokyo, Japan
E-mail: rintaromori@gmail.com

Anthony Odibo, MD, MSCE
Associate Professor, Division of Maternal-Fetal Medicine
Washington University in St Louis, USA.
E-mail: odiboa@wudosis.wustl.edu

Iris Ohel, MD
Department of Obstetrics and Gynecology,
Soroka University Medical Center, Faculty of Health Sciences,
Ben-Gurion University of the Negev,
Be'er-Sheva, Israel.
E-mail: ohel@bgu.ac.il

Yinka Oyelese, MD
Associate Professor
Division of Maternal Fetal Medicine, Department of Obstetrics & Gynecology,
Tennessee Institute of Fetal Maternal and Infant Health,
University of Tennessee Health Sciences Center, Memphis, TN, USA
E-mail: yinkamd@aol.com

Nigel Paneth MD MPH
University Distinguished Professor,
Departments of Epidemiology and Pediatrics & Human Development,
College of Human Medicine, Michigan State University, USA
E-mail: paneth@epi.msu.edu

Gali Pariente, MD.
Department of Obstetrics and Gynecology,
Soroka University Medical Center, Faculty of Health Sciences,
Ben-Gurion University of the Negev,
Be'er-Sheva, Israel.
E-mail: galipa@bgu.ac.il

Kinga Polańska PhD
Unit of Reproductive Environmental Epidemiology
Nofer Institute of Occupational Medicine
91-348 Lodz, Poland

Naomi Schneid-Kofman, MD.
Department of Obstetrics and Gynecology, Soroka University Medical Center,
Faculty of Health Sciences, Ben-Gurion University of the Negev,
Be'er-Sheva, Israel.
E-mail: shir2k@zahav.net.il

Eyal Sheiner, MD, PhD.
Associate Professor, Department of Obstetrics and Gynecology,
Soroka University Medical Center,
Faculty of Health Sciences, Ben-Gurion University of the Negev,
Be'er-Sheva, Israel.
E-mail: sheiner@bgu.ac.il

Ilana Shoham-Vardi, PhD
Associate Professor, Department of Epidemiology and Health Services Evaluation,
Faculty of Health Sciences, Ben Gurion University of the Negev,
Beer-Sheva, Israel
E-mail: vilana@bgu.ac.il

Melvin E. Stratmeyer, PhD
Deputy Director, Division of Biology, OSEL
Center for Devices and Radiological Health
Food and Drug Administration
Silver Springs, MD, USA.
E-mail: melvin.stratmeyer@fda.hhs.gov

Digna R. Velez, Ph.D
Miami Institute of Human Genomics and Dr. John T. Macdonald Foundation,
Department of Human Genetics, University of Miami,
Miami, FL, USA

Edi Vaisbuch MD.
Department of Obstetrics and Gynecology,
Kaplan Medical Center, School of Medicine, Hebrew University,
 Jerusalem, Israel

Stephanie J. Ventura, M.A.,
Division of Vital Statistics, National Center for Health Statistics
Hyattsville, MD 20782, USA.

Asnat Walfisch, MD
Department of Obstetrics and Gynecology,
Hillel Yaffe Medical Center,
Hadera, Israel.
E-mail: asnatwalfisch@yahoo.com

Adi Y. Weintraub, MD
Department of Obstetrics and Gynecology,
Soroka University Medical Center, Faculty of Health Sciences,
Ben-Gurion University of the Negev,
Be'er-Sheva, Israel.
E-mail: adiyehud@bgu.ac.il

Arnon Wiznitzer, MD
Professor and Chairman, Department of Obstetrics and Gynecology A,
Soroka University Medical Center, Faculty of Health Sciences,
Ben-Gurion University of the Negev,

Be'er-Sheva, Israel.
E-mail: arnon@clalit.org.il

Yariv Yogev, MD
Department of Obstetrics and Gynecology,
Helen Schneider Hospital for Women,
Rabin Medical Center,
Petah Tiqwa, Israel
E-mail: yarivyogev@hotmail.com

Marvin C. Ziskin, MD
Professor of Radiology and Medical Physics
Director, Center for Biomedical Physics
Temple University Medical School
Philadelphia, PA, 19140, USA.
E-mail: ziskin@temple.edu

Index

B

G

H

I

J

K

L

N

O

T

U

V

W

X

Y

Z